Antitumor and Anti-HIV Agents from Natural Products

Antitumor and Anti-HIV Agents from Natural Products

Editor

Kyoko Nakagawa-Goto

MDPI • Basel • Beijing • Wuhan • Barcelona • Belgrade • Manchester • Tokyo • Cluj • Tianjin

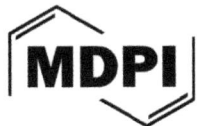

Editor
Kyoko Nakagawa-Goto
Kanazawa University
Japan
The University of North Carolina at Chapel Hill
USA

Editorial Office
MDPI
St. Alban-Anlage 66
4052 Basel, Switzerland

This is a reprint of articles from the Special Issue published online in the open access journal *Molecules* (ISSN 1420-3049) (available at: https://www.mdpi.com/journal/molecules/special_issues/Antitumor_Anti-HIV).

For citation purposes, cite each article independently as indicated on the article page online and as indicated below:

LastName, A.A.; LastName, B.B.; LastName, C.C. Article Title. *Journal Name* **Year**, *Article Number*, Page Range.

ISBN 978-3-03943-008-6 (Hbk)
ISBN 978-3-03943-009-3 (PDF)

© 2020 by the authors. Articles in this book are Open Access and distributed under the Creative Commons Attribution (CC BY) license, which allows users to download, copy and build upon published articles, as long as the author and publisher are properly credited, which ensures maximum dissemination and a wider impact of our publications.

The book as a whole is distributed by MDPI under the terms and conditions of the Creative Commons license CC BY-NC-ND.

Contents

About the Editor vii

Preface to "Antitumor and Anti-HIV Agents from Natural Products" ix

So Ra Kim, Eun Young Lee, Da Jeong Kim, Hye Jung Kim and Hae Ryoun Park
Quercetin Inhibits Cell Survival and Metastatic Ability via the EMT-Mediated Pathway in Oral Squamous Cell Carcinoma
Reprinted from: *Molecules* 2020, 25, 757, doi:10.3390/molecules25030757 1

Elena-Alina Moacă, Ioana Zinuca Pavel, Corina Danciu, Zorin Crăiniceanu, Daliana Minda, Florina Ardelean, Diana Simona Antal, Roxana Ghiulai, Andreea Cioca, Mihnea Derban, Sebastian Simu, Raul Chioibaş, Camelia Szuhanek and Cristina-Adriana Dehelean
Romanian Wormwood (*Artemisia absinthium* L.): Physicochemical and Nutraceutical Screening
Reprinted from: *Molecules* 2019, 24, 3087, doi:10.3390/molecules24173087 17

So Hyun Park, Ji-Young Hong, Hyen Joo Park and Sang Kook Lee
The Antiproliferative Activity of Oxypeucedanin via Induction of G_2/M Phase Cell Cycle Arrest and p53-Dependent MDM2/p21 Expression in Human Hepatoma Cells
Reprinted from: *Molecules* 2020, 25, 501, doi:10.3390/molecules25030501 39

Yu-Ning Teng, Charles C.N. Wang, Wei-Chieh Liao, Yu-Hsuan Lan and Chin-Chuan Hung
Caffeic Acid Attenuates Multi-Drug Resistance in Cancer Cells by Inhibiting Efflux Function of Human P-Glycoprotein
Reprinted from: *Molecules* 2020, 25, 247, doi:10.3390/molecules25020247 55

Hee Jeong Shin, Jang Mi Han, Ye Seul Choi and Hye Jin Jung
Pterostilbene Suppresses both Cancer Cells and Cancer Stem-Like Cells in Cervical Cancer with Superior Bioavailability to Resveratrol
Reprinted from: *Molecules* 2020, 25, 228, doi:10.3390/molecules25010228 73

Simayijiang Aimaiti, Yohei Saito, Shuichi Fukuyoshi, Masuo Goto, Katsunori Miyake, David J. Newman, Barry R. O'Keefe, Kuo-Hsiung Lee and Kyoko Nakagawa-Goto
Isolation, Structure Elucidation, and Antiproliferative Activity of Butanolides and Lignan Glycosides from the Fruit of *Hernandia nymphaeifolia*
Reprinted from: *Molecules* 2019, 24, 4005, doi:10.3390/molecules24214005 89

Zhuo Han, Fang-yuan Liu, Shi-qi Lin, Cai-yun Zhang, Jia-hui Ma, Chao Guo, Fu-juan Jia, Qian Zhang, Wei-dong Xie and Xia Li
Ivalin Induces Mitochondria-Mediated Apoptosis Associated with the NF-κB Activation in Human Hepatocellular Carcinoma SMMC-7721 Cells
Reprinted from: *Molecules* 2019, 24, 3809, doi:10.3390/molecules24203809 105

Chao-Yu Loung, Wasundara Fernando, H.P. Vasantha Rupasinghe and David W. Hoskin
Apple Peel Flavonoid Fraction 4 Suppresses Breast Cancer Cell Growth by Cytostatic and Cytotoxic Mechanisms
Reprinted from: *Molecules* 2019, 24, 3335, doi:10.3390/molecules24183335 115

Krishan Parashar, Siddhartha Sood, Ali Mehaidli, Colin Curran, Caleb Vegh, Christopher Nguyen, Christopher Pignanelli, Jianzhang Wu, Guang Liang, Yi Wang and Siyaram Pandey
Evaluating the Anti-cancer Efficacy of a Synthetic Curcumin Analog on Human Melanoma Cells and Its Interaction with Standard Chemotherapeutics
Reprinted from: *Molecules* 2019, 24, 2483, doi:10.3390/molecules24132483 131

Chih-Ting Chang, Wen-Ni Soo, Yu-Hsin Chen and Lie-Fen Shyur
Essential Oil of *Mentha aquatica var. Kenting Water Mint* Suppresses Two-Stage Skin Carcinogenesis Accelerated by BRAF Inhibitor Vemurafenib
Reprinted from: *Molecules* **2019**, *24*, 2344, doi:10.3390/molecules24122344 149

Michael Kahnt, Sophie Hoenke, Lucie Fischer, Ahmed Al-Harrasi and René Csuk
Synthesis and Cytotoxicity Evaluation of DOTA-Conjugates of Ursolic Acid
Reprinted from: *Molecules* **2019**, *24*, 2254, doi:10.3390/molecules24122254 165

Yu Zhang, Masuo Goto, Akifumi Oda, Pei-Ling Hsu, Ling-Li Guo, Yan-Hui Fu, Susan L. Morris-Natschke, Ernest Hamel, Kuo-Hsiung Lee and Xiao-Jiang Hao
Antiproliferative Aspidosperma-Type Monoterpenoid Indole Alkaloids from *Bousigonia mekongensis* Inhibit Tubulin Polymerization
Reprinted from: *Molecules* **2019**, *24*, 1256, doi:10.3390/molecules24071256 185

Victoria Abzianidze, Petr Beltyukov, Sofya Zakharenkova, Natalia Moiseeva, Jennifer Mejia, Alvin Holder, Yuri Trishin, Alexander Berestetskiy and Victor Kuznetsov
Synthesis and Biological Evaluation of Phaeosphaeride A Derivatives as Antitumor Agents
Reprinted from: *Molecules* **2018**, *23*, 3043, doi:10.3390/molecules23113043 195

Danielly C. Ferraz da Costa, Luciana Pereira Rangel, Mafalda Maria Duarte da Cunha Martins-Dinis, Giulia Diniz da Silva Ferretti, Vitor F. Ferreira and Jerson L. Silva
Anticancer Potential of Resveratrol, β-Lapachone and Their Analogues
Reprinted from: *Molecules* **2020**, *25*, 893, doi:10.3390/molecules25040893 205

Tomhiro Mastuo, Yasuyoshi Miyata, Tsutomu Yuno, Yuta Mukae, Asato Otsubo, Kensuke Mitsunari, Kojiro Ohba and Hideki Sakai
Molecular Mechanisms of the Anti-Cancer Effects of Isothiocyanates from Cruciferous Vegetables in Bladder Cancer
Reprinted from: *Molecules* **2020**, *25*, 575, doi:10.3390/molecules25030575 227

Mohammad Bagher Majnooni, Sajad Fakhri, Antonella Smeriglio, Domenico Trombetta, Courtney R. Croley, Piyali Bhattacharyya, Eduardo Sobarzo-Sánchez, Mohammad Hosein Farzaei and Anupam Bishayee
Antiangiogenic Effects of Coumarins against Cancer: From Chemistry to Medicine
Reprinted from: *Molecules* **2019**, *24*, 4278, doi:10.3390/molecules24234278 249

Karlo Wittine, Lara Saftić, Željka Peršurić and Sandra Kraljević Pavelić
Novel Antiretroviral Structures from Marine Organisms
Reprinted from: *Molecules* **2019**, *24*, 3486, doi:10.3390/molecules24193486 269

Koji Wada and Hiroshi Yamashita
Cytotoxic Effects of Diterpenoid Alkaloids Against Human Cancer Cells
Reprinted from: *Molecules* **2019**, *24*, 2317, doi:10.3390/molecules24122317 305

About the Editor

Kyoko Nakagawa-Goto, Ph.D., is an associate professor in the School of Pharmaceutical Sciences, College of Medical, Pharmaceutical and Health Sciences, Kanazawa University in Japan. She also serves as an adjunct associate professor at Eshelman School of Pharmacy, the University of North Carolina at Chapel Hill. Her research interests include drug discovery and development based on biological natural products. She has published more than 90 research articles in the field of organic, natural products, and medicinal chemistries focused on targeting antitumor and antivirus.

Preface to "Antitumor and Anti-HIV Agents from Natural Products"

Cancers and infectious diseases, including HIV, are major and global health issues to overcome. On the other hand, natural products have contributed to the field of drug discovery for a long time. In this Special Issue, recent notable research works and reviews, regarding the discovery and development of novel anticancer and anti-HIV drug candidates from natural sources, are described.

Kyoko Nakagawa-Goto
Editor

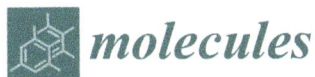

Article

Quercetin Inhibits Cell Survival and Metastatic Ability via the EMT-Mediated Pathway in Oral Squamous Cell Carcinoma

So Ra Kim [1,2], Eun Young Lee [1,2], Da Jeong Kim [1], Hye Jung Kim [2,*] and Hae Ryoun Park [1,2,*]

1. Department of Oral Pathology, and BK21 PLUS Project, School of Dentistry, Pusan National University, Yangsan 50612, Korea; ksr9307@pusan.ac.kr (S.R.K.); eunyeong26@pusan.ac.kr (E.Y.L.); ttakjjung@gmail.com (D.J.K.)
2. Periodontal Disease Signaling Network Research Center (MRC), School of Dentistry, Pusan National University, Yangsan 50612, Korea
* Correspondence: kimhj2850@naver.com (H.J.K.); parkhr@pusan.ac.kr (H.R.P.); Tel.: +82-51-510-8247 (H.J.K.); +82-51-510-8250 (H.R.P.)

Academic Editor: Kyoko Nakagawa-Goto
Received: 31 December 2019; Accepted: 9 February 2020; Published: 10 February 2020

Abstract: This study aimed to investigate whether quercetin exerts anticancer effects on oral squamous cell carcinoma (OSCC) cell lines and to elucidate its mechanism of action. These anticancer effects in OSCC cells were assessed using an MTT assay, flow cytometry (to assess the cell cycle), wound-healing assay, invasion assay, Western blot analysis, gelatin zymography, and immunofluorescence. To investigate whether quercetin also inhibits transforming growth factor β1 (TGF-β1)-induced epithelial–mesenchymal transition (EMT) in human keratinocyte cells, HaCaT cells were treated with TGF-β1. Overall, our results strongly suggest that quercetin suppressed the viability of OSCC cells by inducing cell cycle arrest at the G2/M phase. However, quercetin did not affect cell viability of human keratinocytes such as HaCaT (immortal keratinocyte) and nHOK (primary normal human oral keratinocyte) cells. Additionally, quercetin suppresses cell migration through EMT and matrix metalloproteinase (MMP) in OSCC cells and decreases TGF-β1-induced EMT in HaCaT cells. In conclusion, this study is the first, to our knowledge, to demonstrate that quercetin can inhibit the survival and metastatic ability of OSCC cells via the EMT-mediated pathway, specifically Slug. Quercetin may thus provide a novel pharmacological approach for the treatment of OSCCs.

Keywords: quercetin; oral squamous cell carcinoma cells; metastasis; cell cycle arrest; epithelial-to-mesenchymal transition; matrix metalloproteinase; transforming growth factor-β1

1. Introduction

Oral squamous cell carcinoma (OSCC) is the most common malignancy, accounting for about 90% of head and neck cancers, and develops at the lips, tongue, salivary glands, gums, bottom of the mouth, pharynx, and surfaces within the oral cavity [1–6]. OSCC, an aggressive human cancer with the highest mortality, has a significant impact on the quality of life of patients [6,7]. Early OSCC is treated with a combination of surgery and radiation therapy; however, this strategy does not significantly increase survival in OSCC patients. Thus, many studies have focused on compounds derived from natural products as potential candidate agents for treating or preventing OSCCs. OSCC is known to have multifactorial etiologies, including tobacco, alcohol, and viruses [6,8–10]. Several reviews suggest that periodontal disease (PD) results in a high risk of developing OSCC [8,11]. In "Cancer Facts & Figures 2018" provided by the American Cancer Society, the oral cavity is the most common site of onset of oral cancer, followed by the tongue and pharynx [12]. Therefore, we used oral squamous cell carcinoma HN22 and tongue squamous cell carcinoma such as OSC20 and SAS to confirm the effect of quercetin in oral cancer.

Cancer metastasis involves a complex process that includes primary tumor formation, angiogenesis, invasion, and metastatic colonization [8]. In the initial stages of cancer metastasis, epithelial–to–mesenchymal transition (EMT) causes a loss of adhesion and increases the motility of primary tumor cells [3,13–15]. The matrix metalloproteinase (MMP) is an important extracellular protease that breaks down the extracellular matrix (ECM) and allows cancer cells to migrate into the lymph and blood vessels [16–18]. Some studies have demonstrated that EMT and MMP support the invasion and metastasis of OSCC [19,20]. Therefore, this study investigated whether quercetin exhibits anticancer effects on OSCC cell lines and its mechanism of action.

Quercetin is a plant flavonol of the flavonoid polyphenol group found in many fruits, vegetables, leaves, and grains [21–23]. Although numerous studies have demonstrated that quercetin plays a role in the prevention of various cancers [24–26], it is still an interesting target for OSCCs. Previous studies have reported the antibacterial effects of quercetin against *Actinobacillus actinomycetemcomitans (Aa)* and *Porphyromonas gingivalis (Pg)*, which are the major pathogens in PD [27,28]. Moreover, recently, studies have reported that quercetin inhibits the cell viability, migration, and invasion of OSCC cells [29–32]. However, its potential actions in OSCCs have been poorly explored. Therefore, in this study, we sought to investigate whether quercetin exhibits anticancer effects on OSCC cell lines and to elucidate its mechanism of action.

2. Results

2.1. Quercetin Reduced Cell Viability and Arrested G2 Phase Cell Cycle in OSCC Cells

To determine the effect of quercetin on cell viability, OSCC cell lines (OSC20, SAS, and HN22 cells) were treated with various concentrations (0~160 µM) of quercetin for 24 h, and cell viability was determined using the MTT assay. The results showed that quercetin decreased cell viability in OSCC cell lines (Figure 1A). In particular, cell viability in OSC20 and SAS cells, except HN22 cells, was reduced in a quercetin dose-dependent manner. Treatment with 160 µM quercetin for 24 h reduced cell viability by approximately 50% in all cell lines ($p < 0.01$), whereas treatment with low concentrations (10–40 µM) reduced cell viability slightly (approximately 5–30%) ($p < 0.05$) compared to the control (Figure 1A). To determine the function of quercetin in the regulation of the cell cycle, OSCC cell lines were stimulated with low levels of quercetin (10–40 µM) for 24 h and analyzed the distribution of the cell cycle using flow cytometry. As shown in Figure 1B, the cell populations at the G2/M stage were increased by treatment with quercetin in the OSCC cell lines (OSC20 cell, 7.66% ± 3.92% in the control vs. 36.22% ± 4.10% in quercetin 40 µM, $p < 0.01$; SAS cell, 22.85% ± 3.04% in the control vs. 45.49% ± 1.38% in quercetin 40 µM, $p < 0.005$; and HN22 cell, 23.37% ± 4.13% in control vs. 50.40% ± 5.05% in quercetin 40 µM, $p < 0.05$). However, the cell proportion in the G0/G1 phase decreased (OSC20 cell, 35.99 ± 1.89% in the control vs. 14.06% ± 1.26% in quercetin 40 µM, $p < 0.001$; SAS cell, 33.03% ± 1.12% in the control vs. 8.14% ± 4.39% in quercetin 40 µM, $p < 0.005$; and HN22 cell, 35.05% ± 1.62% in control vs. 6.53% ± 4.34% in quercetin 40 µM, $p < 0.001$). The results indicate that quercetin suppressed the viability of OSCC cells by inducing cell cycle arrest in the G2/M phase.

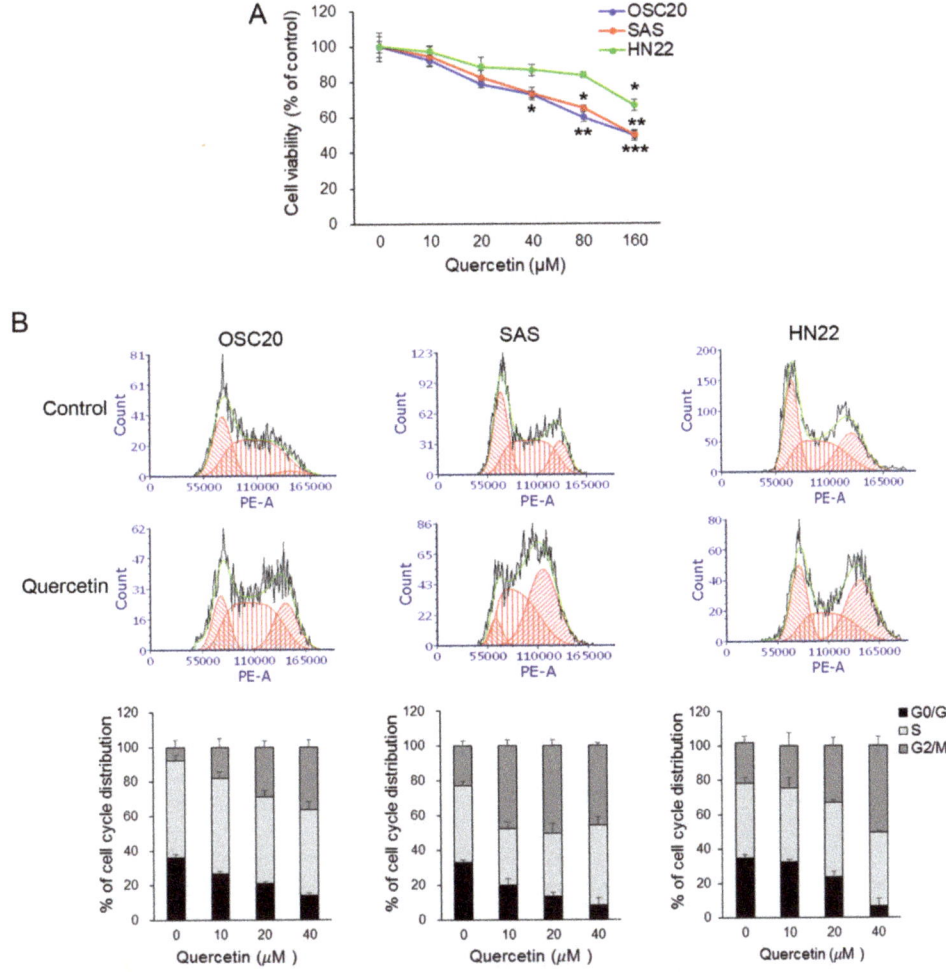

Figure 1. Quercetin reduced cell viability and arrested the G2/M phase cell cycle in oral squamous cell carcinoma (OSCC) cells. (**A**) Cell viability was investigated by an MTT assay. Oral squamous cell carcinoma cell lines (OSC20, SAS, and HN22 cells) were treated with quercetin (10, 20, 40, 80, and 160 μM). (**B**) Quercetin was shown to induce cell cycle arrest in OSC20, SAS, and HN22 cells. Data are the means ± SEM. * $p < 0.05$ and ** $p < 0.01$ vs. corresponding control (quercetin 0 μM).

2.2. Quercetin Suppressed the Migration Potential of OSCC Cells

We performed a wound-healing assay to evaluate the inhibitory effects of quercetin on migration. To observe the effects of quercetin on cell migration, the cell proliferation of OSC20, SAS, and HN22 cells was inhibited by treatment with thymidine (1 mM) for 2 h prior to treatment with quercetin (40 μM). After 24 h, the wound area of the control was almost completely reduced compared to the initial area; however, the quercetin-treated cells did not show any decrease (Figure 2A,B). The migration of quercetin-treated cells was significantly decreased in a dose-dependent manner (not shown). This result suggests that the migratory properties were completely lost upon quercetin treatment for 24 h in the OSCC cell lines.

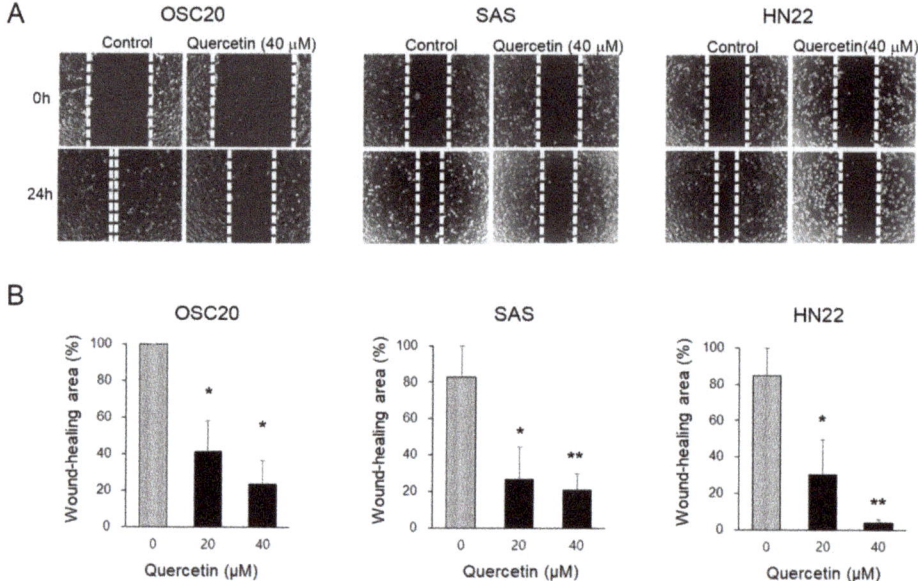

Figure 2. Cell migration ability assessed by a wound-healing assay. (**A**) Changes in the wound area were observed after 24 h. In the quercetin-treated cells, the wound area was less closed. This indicates a decrease in migration capacity. (**B**) The wound area was calculated and presented as a graph. Data are the means ± SEM. * $p < 0.05$ and ** $p < 0.01$ vs. the corresponding control (quercetin 0 µM).

2.3. Quercetin Regulated EMT and MMPs in OSCC Cells

The effects of quercetin treatment on EMT and the activity of ECM-degrading enzymes in OSCC cell lines were analyzed by Western blot or gelatin zymography. OSC20, SAS, and HN22 cells were treated with different concentrations of quercetin (0, 10, 20, and 40 µM) for 24 h. As shown in Figure 3A, quercetin, in a dose-dependent manner, increased the expression of epithelial markers, such as E-cadherin and claudin-1, while decreasing the expression of mesenchymal markers, such as fibronectin, vimentin, and alpha-smooth muscle actin (α-SMA). We observed that 40 µM of quercetin specifically downregulated the expression of the mesenchymal markers in OSCC cells. The activation of MMP-2 and MMP-9 was significantly decreased by quercetin treatment (Figure 3B). These results demonstrate that quercetin suppressed the expression levels of EMT inducers and MMPs in OSCC cells.

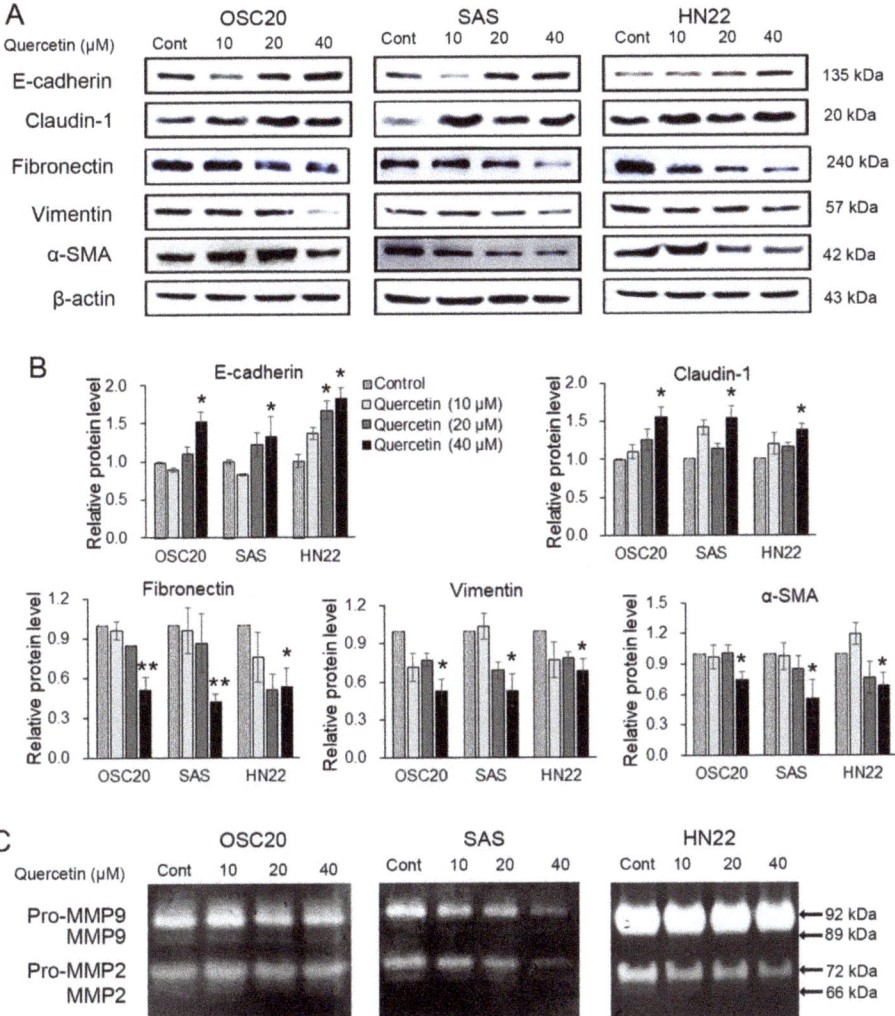

Figure 3. Quercetin is shown to induce regulation of epithelial-mesenchymal transition (EMT) and matrix metalloproteinase (MMP). (**A**) Western blotting was conducted to examine the changes in the EMT inducers. The results showed that the epithelial markers (E-cadherin and claudin-1) were upregulated, and the mesenchymal markers (fibronectin, vimentin, and alpha-smooth muscle actin (α-SMA)) were downregulated upon treatment with quercetin. (**B**) Quantitation of A. The band intensities of each target protein were measured using an image analyzer and presented as relative ratio. (**C**) Gelatin zymography shows the MMP-2 and MMP-9 activities in oral cancer cell lines (OSC20, SAS, and HN22 cells) upon quercetin treatment. Data are the means ± SEM. * $p < 0.05$, and ** $p < 0.01$ vs. the corresponding control (quercetin 0 μM).

2.4. Quercetin Regulated EMT-Activating Transcription Factors in OSCC Cells

EMT-activating transcription factors (EMT-TFs), such as Twist, Slug, and Snail 1, were observed by Western blot and immunofluorescence. Twist and Slug were significantly downregulated in quercetin-treated OSC20 and SAS cells compared to the untreated cells (Figure 4A,B). Slug was significantly downregulated in quercetin-treated HN22 cells compared to untreated cells, but Twist was unchanged (Figure 4A,B). Moreover, upon quercetin treatment, translocation of Twist and Slug expression was observed in the OSC20 and SAS cells by immunofluorescence (Figure 4C,D). The basal level of Twist was observed in the cytosol, and there was no translocation upon quercetin treatment in HN22 cells (Figure 4C). The basal levels of Slug were observed in the nucleus on untreated HN22 cells but were observed in the cytosol upon quercetin treatment (Figure 4D). These data strongly suggest that quercetin inhibits Slug activation by inducing its translocation into the cytoplasm.

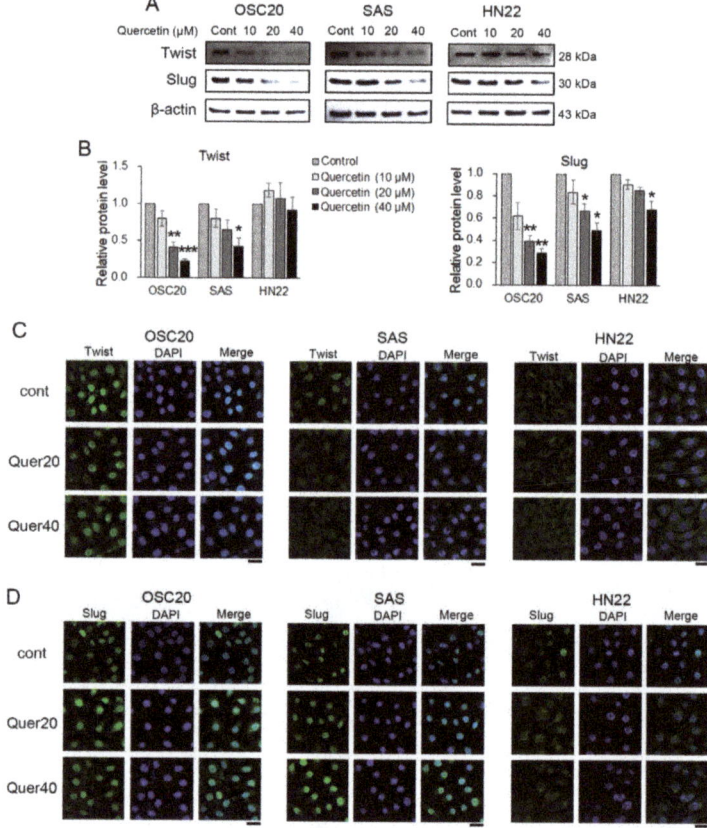

Figure 4. EMT-activating transcription factors were detected using Western blot and immunofluorescence. (**A**) The Western blot showed that quercetin downregulated EMT transcription factors at the protein level. (**B**) Quantitation of A. The band intensities of each target protein were measured using an image analyzer and presented as relative ratio. (**C**) Representative fluorescence microscopy images of Twist in OSCC cell lines. (**D**) Representative fluorescence microscopy images of Slug in OSCC cell lines. Scale bars: 20 µM. Data are the means ± SEM. * $p < 0.05$, ** $p < 0.01$, and *** $p < 0.001$ vs. the corresponding control (quercetin 0 µM).

2.5. Transforming Growth Factor β1 (TGF-β1) Induced EMT in Human Keratinocyte HaCaT Cells

Previous results indicated that quercetin exerts anticancer effects through the regulation of EMT in OSCC cells. To examine the viability effect of quercetin on human keratinocyte cells, HaCaT (immortal keratinocyte) and nHOK (primary normal human oral keratinocyte) cells were treated with various concentrations (0~160 μM) of quercetin for 24 h, and cell viability was determined by an MTT assay. Cell viability of HaCaT cells and nHOK cells was not changed by the low concentration (10–40 μM) of quercetin compared to the control group but was significantly reduced in 160 μM quercetin treatment ($p < 0.05$) (Figure 5A). The results show that quercetin had not much effect on cell viability of HaCaT and nHOK cells in the concentration range of 10–80 μM compared to the OSCC cell lines. To investigate whether quercetin also inhibits TGF-β1-induced EMT in human keratinocyte, HaCaT cells were treated with TGF-β1 (2 ng, 5 ng, and 10 ng) for 24 h. Changes in the expression of EMT inducers upon treatment with TGF-β1 were confirmed by Western blot (Figure 5B). The expression levels of the epithelial markers (E-cadherin and claudin-1) were decreased and those of the mesenchymal markers (fibronectin, vimentin, α-SMA, and Slug) were increased (Figure 5C–H). TGF-β1 (10 ng/mL) was determined to be the optimal concentration for the EMT induction in HaCaT cells. Thus, 10 ng/mL of TGF-β1 was used for the subsequent experiment.

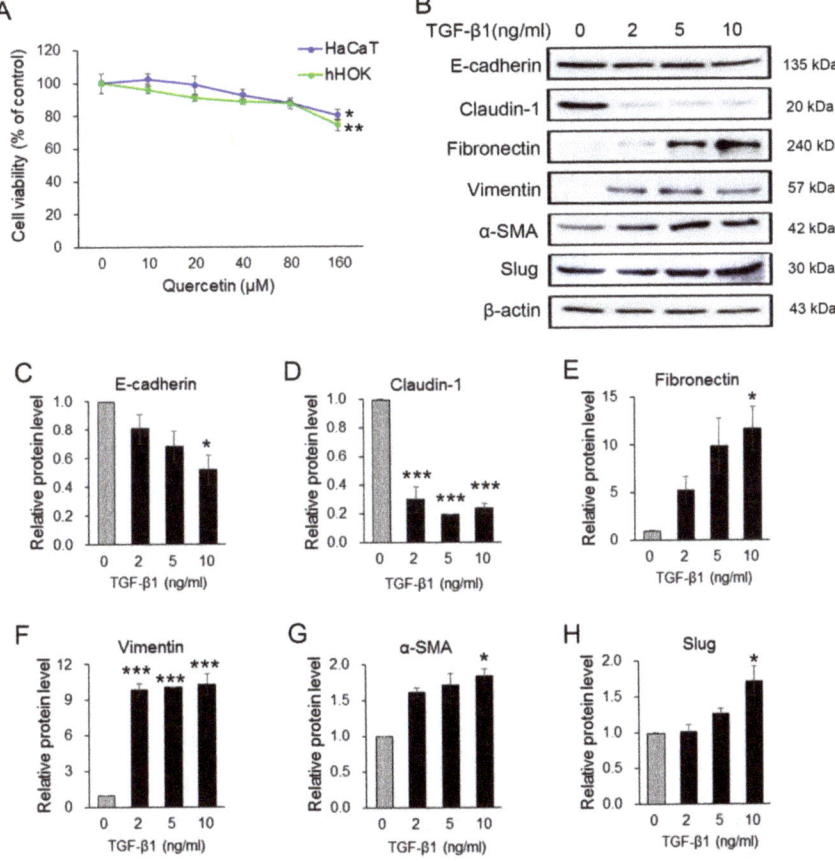

Figure 5. Quercetin was not toxic in normal keratocyte and transforming growth factor β1 (TGF-β1) stimulated EMT in HaCaT cells. (**A**) To examine the effect of quercetin on cell viability, an MTT assay

was conducted on HaCaT and nHOK cells. Data are means ± SEM. * $p < 0.05$ vs. the corresponding control (quercetin 0 µM). (**B**) Expression of EMT-related markers such as in TGF-β1-treated HaCaT cells were analyzed by Western blotting. (**C–H**) Quantitation of B. The band intensities of each target protein were measured using an image analyzer and presented as relative ratio. Data are means ± SEM. * $p < 0.05$ and *** $p < 0.005$ vs. corresponding control (TGF-β1 0 ng/mL).

2.6. Quercetin Attenuated TGF-β1-induced EMT in HaCaT Cells

To investigate whether quercetin also inhibits TGF-β1-induced EMT in normal cells, HaCaT was treated with 10 ng of TGF-β1 for 24 h, followed by various concentrations of quercetin for 24 h without changing the media (Figure 6A). To observe the morphological changes of the treated HaCaT cells, phalloidin staining was conducted. Without treatment, the cells tended to grow together and exhibited a triangle–square shape. However, after treatment with 10 ng of TGF-β1, the HaCaT cells showed morphological changes to their spindle shapes and were spread out (Figure 6B). Additionally, when the cells were treated with TGF-β1 and quercetin together, as explained previously, the morphological changes recovered but the cells did not gather as before (Figure 6B). Western blot data show that quercetin regulated the TGF-β1-induced EMT markers. With regard to the epithelial markers (E-cadherin and claudin-1) of the induced EMT, there were no changes in recovery. In contrast, changes in the mesenchymal markers indicate that treatment with 40 µM quercetin leads to the greatest recovery. Thus, we determined the optimal concentration of quercetin as 40 µM for use in the subsequent experiment (Figure 6C–I). To evaluate the TGF-β1-induced EMT migration ability, a wound-healing assay was performed. The wound area was narrower in the TGF-β1-treated HaCaT cells than in the untreated HaCaT cells (Figure 6J,K). Further, quercetin seemed to inhibit the invasion of EMT-induced HaCaT cells (Figure 6L). The invasion assay also showed that the invasion ability improved upon TGF-β1 treatment. The number of cells that passed the Matrigel and membrane was less in the HaCaT cells treated with quercetin and TGF-β1 than in those treated with only TGF-β1 (Figure 6L). In conclusion, quercetin decreased the TGF-β1-induced EMT in HaCaT cells.

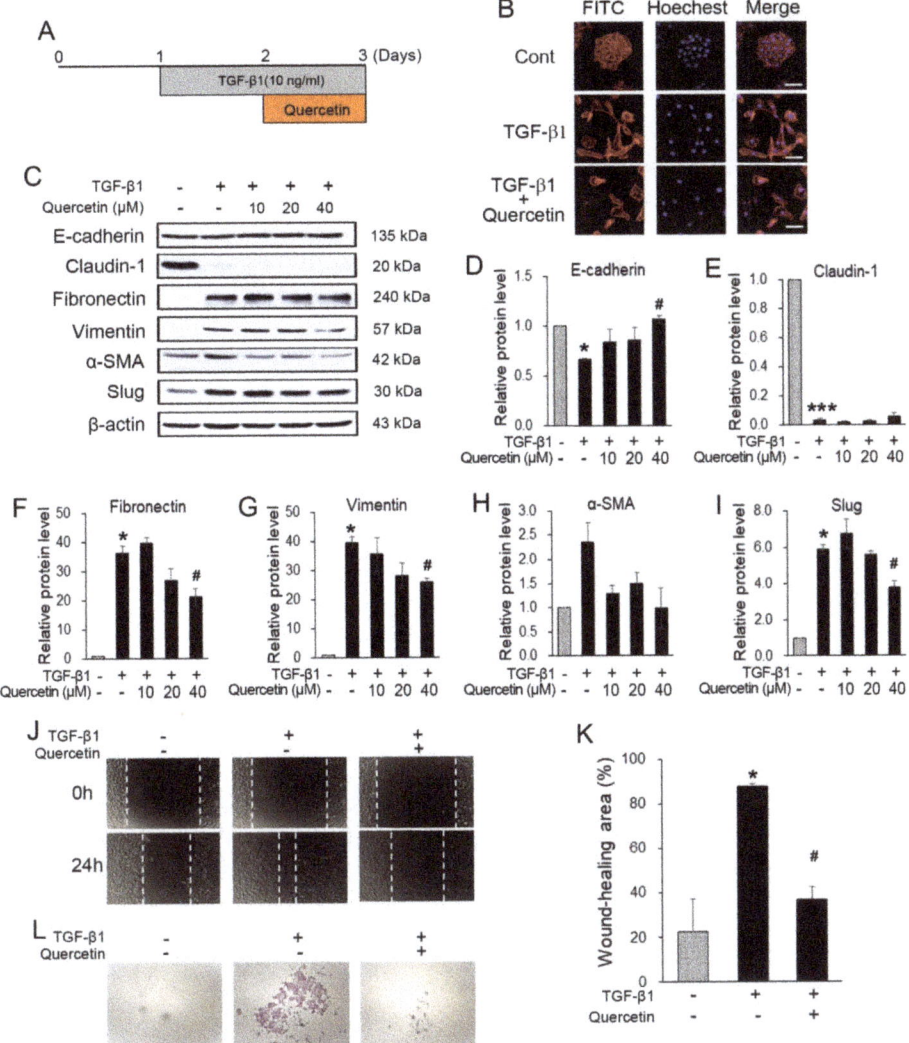

Figure 6. Quercetin inhibited TGF-β1-induced EMT. (**A**) Experimental setup. (**B**) Western blot results showed that quercetin also regulated TGF-β1-induced EMT markers. (**C**) Treatment of TGF-β1 also changed the morphology of HaCaT. Further, quercetin induced morphological recovery. Scale bars: 50 μM. (**D**–**I**) Quantification of hRPTECs viability by MTT assay. (**J**,**K**) A wound-healing assay was conducted to evaluate the TGF-β1-induced EMT migration ability; quercetin attenuated EMT-induced migration in HaCaT cells. (**L**) Quercetin inhibited the invasion capacity of EMT-induced HaCaT cells. Data are the means ± SEM. * $p < 0.05$, and *** $p < 0.001$ vs. the corresponding control (without TGF-β1 and quercetin); # $p < 0.05$ vs. the corresponding control (with TGF-β1 and without quercetin).

3. Discussion

Suppression of cancer metastasis is considered an effective strategy for preventing cancer progression. Many studies have reported that a variety of natural products and compounds exert antitumor effects by inducing apoptosis and cell cycle arrest in cancer cells and reducing their metastatic capacities [33,34]. Thus, the use of dietary biologically active compounds may be a safe and desirable approach for cancer treatment. Quercetin is a potent candidate for cancer treatment, because it is known to have a regulatory effect on apoptosis, migration, and invasion. However, quercetin has limited applications as a therapeutic agent due to problems such as low oral bioavailability (8~16%) and poor water solubility [35]. Numerous studies have used various cancer cell lines to study the anticancer effects of quercetin, and quercetin concentrations vary depending on the cell line and treatment time. Quercetin is used at 10–80 µM concentrations for 24 treatments in cancer cells because of its low bioactivity. Quercetin concentrations 10–80 µM are used under 24-h treatment conditions. Quercetin IC50 values of quercetin are 60–120 µM [36–38]. Especially, quercetin of 25–50 µM had anticancer effects in SAS cells, a typical oral cancer cell [39]. In this study, the anticancer effect of quercetin at 10, 20, 40, 80, and 160 µM was assessed in vitro by MTT assay in the OSCC cell line, such as OSC20, SAS, and HN22 cells. The optimal concentration of quercetin was determined to be 10–40 µM for assessing metastatic capacity in OSCC cells. The 10–40 µM quercetin concentration used in this study is commonly used for cancer cells under 24-h treatment conditions. Quercetin, a flavonoid found in many fruits, vegetables, and grains, has been shown to have an antitumor effect on OSCC cells via the induction of cell cycle arrest [29,40]. Quercetin treatment suppressed cell growth by inducing G2/M arrest and apoptosis in EGFR-overexpressing HSC-3 and TW206 oral cancer cells [30]. Our result show that quercetin inhibits the viability of OSCC cell lines, such as OSC20, SAS, and HN22 cells, in a dose-dependent manner by inducing cell cycle arrest at the G2/M phase (Figure 1A,B).

The EMT process contributes to greater interstitial cell adhesion profiles, as unregulated cellular or cell matrix adhesion and increased migration and invasion are required for the development of metastatic cancer [41]. The ability of cancer cells to migrate and invade is increased by the reduction of the expression of E-cadherin, a cell–cell adhesion molecule, whereas the expression of N-cadherin is decreased, which is inversely proportional to that of E-cadherin [42]. Quercetin regulates the expression of EMT markers, such as E-cadherin, vimentin, and β-catenin, in head and neck cancer-derived sphere cells and breast cancer cells [43,44]. In addition, quercetin prevented the EGF-induced expression of N-cadherin and vimentin and increased the expression of E-cadherin in prostate cells [45]. Based on these reports, it is assumed that quercetin treatment can modulate the expression of EMT-related markers. Additionally, quercetin suppressed cell viability, migration, and invasion by regulating miR-16/HOXA10, which inhibits the expression of MMP-2 and 9 in oral cancer cells [30]. Studies on the mechanism of action of quercetin in the metastasis of OSCCs are still insufficient. In this study, quercetin inhibited EMT by increasing the expression of E-cadherin and claudin-1 and decreasing the expression of fibronectin, vimentin, α-SMA, and Slug in OSCC cell lines (Figures 3 and 4). The activation of MMP-2 and MMP-9 was significantly decreased by quercetin treatment (Figure 3B). Thus, quercetin inhibits cell migration and invasion by regulating the expression of EMT-related genes in OSCC cell lines.

It has been found that transforming growth factor-beta 1 (TGF-β1) induces epithelial mesenchymal transition (EMT) in various cancer cells, promoting motility and invasiveness [46,47]. Additionally, TGF-β1 treatment reduces the enhanced expression of Snail1 and Twist1 and, subsequently, the expression of E-cadherin [47]. We observed whether quercetin reduced EMT-related factors increased by TGF-β1 treatment in human keratinocyte HaCaT cells. TGF-β1 can promote tumor formation by inducing mesenchymal metastasis (via EMT) in the epithelium in various cancer cells. The main TGF-β1-induced effectors in this process are EMT transcription inhibitors, such as Snail 1, Snail 2 (also known as Slug), ZEB1/2, and Twist. HaCaT cells showed morphological changes and induction of EMT-related markers upon TGF-β1 treatment (Figure 6B,C). Quercetin reduced TGF-β1-induced EMT expression in HaCaT cells.

Overall, our results strongly suggest that quercetin suppressed the viability of OSCC cells inducing cell cycle arrest in the G2/M phase (Figure 1). Significantly, our results demonstrate that quercetin suppresses the metastatic ability via EMT and MMP in OSCC cells and decreases the expression level of TGF-β1-induced EMT in human normal HaCaT cells. Thus, quercetin may provide a novel pharmacological approach for the treatment of OSCCs.

4. Materials and Methods

4.1. Reagents and Antibodies

Quercetin was purchased from Sigma-Aldrich (St. Louis, MO) and dissolved in DMSO (DUKSAN, Korea) to prepare stock solutions (100 mM). TGF-β1 was purchased from R&D Systems (Minneapolis, USA) and dissolved in 4 mM HCl containing 0.1% fatty acid-free bovine serum albumin to a concentration of 1.0 mg/mL to prepare stock solutions (20 μg/mL). 3-(4,5-dimethylthiazol-2-yl)-2,5-diphenyltetrazolium bromide (MTT) and thymidine were purchased from Sigma-Aldrich (St. Louis, MO). Antibodies against E-cadherin, vimentin, and Slug were purchased from Cell Signaling Technology (Danvers, MA, USA), whereas fibronectin was purchased from BD Bioscience (San Jose, CA, USA); α-smooth muscle actin was purchased from Abcam (Cambridge, MA, USA), and Twist and beta-actin were purchased from Santa Cruz Biotechnology (Santa Cruz, CA, USA).

4.2. Cell Culture and Treatment

Three OSCC cell lines (OSC20, SAS, and HN22 cells) and human keratinocyte cells such as HaCaT (immortal keratinocyte) and nHOK (primary normal human oral keratinocyte) were used in this study. OSC20 and SAS cells were grown in Dulbecco's modified Eagle's medium F-12, 1:1 mixture (Hyclone, UT, USA); HN22 and HaCaT cells were grown in Dulbecco's modified Eagle's medium with high glucose (DMEM; Hyclone); and nHOK (primary normal human oral keratinocyte) were cultured in KBM^{TM} Gold Keratinocyte growth basal medium (Lonza, MD, USA, #CC-3103) containing KGM^{TM}-2 SingleQuots^{TM} supplements (Lonza, MD, USA, #CC-4152) at 37 °C in 5% CO_2 and 95% O_2 in a humidified environment. Further, both media contained 10% fetal bovine serum (FBS; Hyclone) and 1% penicillin and streptomycin (Thermo Fisher, Waltham, MA, USA). In this study, the three OSCC cell lines were treated with various concentrations of quercetin for 24 h; the HaCaT cells were treated with 10 ng of TGF-β1 for 24 h and then treated with various concentrations of quercetin.

4.3. MTT Assay

An MTT (3-(4,5-dimethylthiazol-2-yl)-2,5-diphenyltetrazolium bromide) assay was conducted to evaluate the cytotoxicity of quercetin on cell viability. Each cell line was seeded at 1×10^4 cells per well in a 96-well plate and incubated with 10% FBS-containing media. However, the exception was that nHOK cells were seeded with 3×10^4 cells per well with serum-free media. After stabilization, the media was replaced with a media containing 10% FBS for 24 h. Then, the cells were treated with various concentrations of quercetin (10, 20, 40, 80, and 160 μM) with media containing 10% FBS. After 24 h, the media were replaced with MTT (500 μg/mL) in a fresh serum-free media, and the cells were incubated for 3 h at 37 °C. Then, the supernatant was removed, and 200 μL of dimethylsulfoxide (DMSO) was added to dissolve the MTT formazan. The absorbance of the plate was read at 570 nm using a Synergy HT micro plate reader (Bio-tek, Winooski, VT, USA).

4.4. Cell Cycle Analysis

A cell cycle analysis was conducted to observe the cell cycle's progression. Cells were seeded at a density of 5×10^5 cells in 60 mm dishes. After cell stabilization, the cells were treated with 40 μM of quercetin for 24 h. Then, the cells were detached using trypsin and washed with phosphate-buffered saline (PBS). The harvested cells were then fixed with 75% ethanol at 4 °C overnight; subsequently, they were centrifuged and incubated with 20 μL RNase A (10 mg/mL) in 1 mL PBS at 4 °C for 30 min. Lastly, cells were stained with 25 μg/mL PI at room temperature for 10 min in the dark. The DNA content was then analyzed using a BD FACSCanto II flow cytometer (BD Bioscience, San Joes, CA, USA).

4.5. Wound-Healing Assay

A wound-healing assay was conducted to evaluate cell migration ability. Cells were seeded in 6-well plates at 5×10^5 per well. At 80% confluence, the cells were treated with 1 mM thymidine for 2 h before reagent treatment. Then, a wound was made in the middle of the well using a sterile 200 µL pipette tip. Further, wells were washed three times with PBS. OSCC cell lines were incubated with media containing 1% FBS and 40 µM of quercetin for 24 h. HaCaT cells were incubated with media containing 1% FBS and 10 ng TGF-β1 for 24 h; then, 40 µM of quercetin was added continuously for 24 h without discarding the existing media. Images were captured using a microscope (Nikon Eclipse TS100, Japan; X100). The rate of reduction of the wound area was calculated as a percentage of the remaining wound area compared to the initial wound area.

4.6. Western Blot Analysis

After treatment, cells were washed three times with cold PBS and lysed with 1X RIPA buffer containing a protease inhibitor cocktail and phosphatase inhibitors. The lysed cells were centrifuged at 12,000 ×g for 24 h. Subsequently, the supernatant was collected. Using the method of Bradford, the protein concentration was quantified as 20 µg. Samples were separated on 10% SDS-polyacrylamide gels. Then, SDS-gels were transferred electrophoretically onto polyvinylidene fluoride membranes (Bio-Rad) using a wet transfer kit. The transferred membranes were blocked with 5% skim milk in Tris-buffered saline containing 0.1% Tween-20 for 1 h at room temperature. The membranes were incubated overnight at 4 °C with the primary antibodies against E-cadherin (cell signaling, #3195, 1:1000); claudin-1 (cell signaling, #4933, 1:1000); fibronectin (BD Bioscience, #610077, 1:1000); vimentin (cell signaling, #5741, 1:1000); α-SMA (Abcam, #ab5694, 1:000); slug (cell signaling, #9585, 1:1000); and Twist (Santa Cruz, #SC-81417, 1:500) and β-actin (Santa Cruz, #SC-47778, 1:4000). Continuously, the membranes were washed three times with 1X TNE buffer, and HRP-conjugated secondary antibodies (ENZO, #ADI-SAB-300-J, and #ADI-SAB-100-J, 1:8000) were applied for 3 h at room temperature. The antigen–antibody complexes were detected using a SuperSignal West–Femto reagent (Thermo Fisher, Waltham, MA, USA).

4.7. Gelatin Zymography

Gelatin zymography was conducted to detect matrix metalloproteinase (MMP) activity using the conditioned media. Each cell line was seeded at 5×10^5 cells per well in a 6-well plate with 10% FBS-containing media. After cell stabilization, the media were transformed into serum-free media and treated with different concentrations of quercetin for 24 h at 37 °C. Subsequently, the supernatant was collected and mixed with a sample buffer (50% 0.5 M Tris-HCl (pH 6.8), 40% glycerol, 8% SDS, and 0.01% bromophenol blue). Further, samples were loaded onto a 7.5% SDS-polyacrylamide gel containing 0.2% gelatin (Sigma). The gels were washed twice with PBS containing 2.5% Triton X-100 for 1 h and incubated with an incubation buffer at 37 °C for 48 h. Then, the gels were stained with Coomassie Blue R-250 (LPS solution, Dae Jeon, Korea) for 1 h. Progressively, the gels were destained with a destaining buffer (8% acetic acid and 4% methanol) until a clear zone was visible.

4.8. Immunofluorescence Staining

Cells were seeded at 2×10^5 cells onto a coverslip in a 6-well plate. In the case of OSCC, the cells were stained for transcription factor expression. The treated cells were fixed in 4% paraformaldehyde at room temperature for 15 min and washed three times with PBS for 10 min. Then, the cells were permeabilized by 0.02% Triton X-100 in PBS at room temperature for 20 min and washed with PBS. Diluted 1:100 primary antibodies (Slug and Twist) were applied to the cells overnight at 4 °C. On the following day, cells were washed three times with PBS, treated with fluorescein isothiocyanate (FITC)-conjugated secondary antibodies for 1 h at 37 °C, and washed three times. Then, 4 µg/mL Hoechst was used to stain the nuclei for 30 min at 37 °C. The treated HaCaT cells were stained to assess changes in their morphology. HaCaT cells were incubated with a phalloidin-conjugate working solution (1:100) and 4 μg/mL Hoechst instead of antibodies. Subsequently, the cells were washed and mounted on a slide glass. An image was then captured via confocal microscopy (LSM780, Carl Zeiss, Jena, Germany).

4.9. Invasion Assay

An 8 μM pore size Transwell (Corning Inc, Corning, NY, USA) was coated with 40 μL of Matrigel (BD Bioscience, San Joes, CA, USA), mixing the serum-free media at a ratio of 1:3 and air drying for 3 h at 37 °C. HaCaT cells were incubated for 24 h with or without 10 ng TGF-β1 and detached using trypsin. The cells were seeded in a Matrigel-coated Transwell culture chamber at 5×10^4 cells with serum-free media containing 10 ng TGF-β1, co-treated with TGF-β1 and quercetin (10 ng TGF-β1 and 40 μM) or without treatment. Then, 600 μL of culture medium containing 10% FBS was placed onto the lower chamber. The cells were next incubated at 37 °C in a 5% CO_2 atmosphere for 44 h. After incubation, the cells on the upper chamber were removed using a cotton swab. The cells passing through the Matrigel and membrane were fixed with cold methanol for 30 min and washed with PBS. The membrane was stained with Mayer's hematoxylin (Muto, Tokyo, Japan) and 1% Eosin Y solution (Muto). Photographs were captured under microscopy (Olympus BX51; 40X).

4.10. Statistical Analyses

Statistical analyses were performed by a one-way analysis of variance (ANOVA) followed by a Bonferroni post-test, whereby three or more experimental groups were compared. *p*-values of < 0.05 were considered statistically significant. All data are the means ± standard error of the mean (SEM).

Author Contributions: Conceptualization and methodology, H.J.K. and H.R.P.; Performing experiments and analyzing data, S.R.K., E.Y.L., and D.J.K.; Validation, H.J.K. and H.R.P.; Writing—Original draft preparation, H.J.K. and S.R.K.; and funding acquisition, H.R.P. All authors have read and agreed to the published version of manuscript.

Funding: This study was supported by and the National Research Foundation of Korea (NRF) Grant funded by the Korea government (MSIT) (No. NRF-2018R1A5A2023879) and the Basic Science Research Program through the National Research Foundation of Korea (NRF) funded by the Ministry of Science and ICT (No. 2017R1A2B4005588).

Conflicts of Interest: The authors declare no conflicts of interest in this manuscript.

References

1. Cooper, J.S.; Porter, K.; Mallin, K.; Hoffman, H.T.; Weber, R.S.; Ang, K.K. National Cancer Database report on cancer of the head and neck: 10-year update. *Head Neck.* **2009**, *31*, 748–758. [CrossRef] [PubMed]
2. Markopoulos, A.K. Current aspects on oral squamous cell carcinoma. *Open Dent. J.* **2012**, *6*, 126–130. [CrossRef] [PubMed]
3. Su, C.W.; Chang, Y.C.; Chien, M.H.; Hsieh, Y.H.; Chen, M.K.; Lin, C.W.; Yang, S.F. Loss of TIMP3 by promoter methylation of Sp1 binding site promotes oral cancer metastasis. *Cell Death Dis.* **2019**, *10*, 793. [CrossRef] [PubMed]
4. Tsantoulis, P.K.; Kastrinakis, N.G.; Tourvas, A.D.; Laskaris, G.; Gorgoulis, V.G. Advances in the biology of oral cancer. *Oral. Oncol.* **2007**, *43*, 523–534. [CrossRef]
5. Gasche, J.A.; Goel, A. Epigenetic mechanisms in oral carcinogenesis. *Future Oncol.* **2012**, *8*, 1407–1425. [CrossRef]
6. Galbiatti, A.L.; Padovani-Junior, J.A.; Maníglia, J.V.; Rodrigues, C.D.; Pavarino, É.C.; Goloni-Bertollo, E.M. Head and neck cancer: Causes, prevention and treatment. *Braz J. Otorhinolaryngol.* **2013**, *79*, 239–247. [CrossRef]
7. Sano, D.; Myers, J.N. Metastasis of squamous cell carcinoma of the oral tongue. *Cancer Metastasis Rev.* **2007**, *26*, 645–662. [CrossRef]
8. Pihlstrom, B.L.; Michalowicz, B.S.; Johnson, N.W. Periodontal diseases. *Lancet* **2005**, *366*, 1809–1820. [CrossRef]

9. Makita, H.; Tanaka, T.; Fujitsuka, H.; Tatematsu, N.; Satoh, K.; Hara, A.; Mori, H. Chemoprevention of 4-nitroquinoline 1-oxide-induced rat oral carcinogenesis by the dietary flavonoids chalcone, 2-hydroxychalcone, and quercetin. *Cancer Res.* **1996**, *56*, 4904–4909.
10. Mehrotra, R.; Yadav, S. Oral squamous cell carcinoma: Etiology, pathogenesis and prognostic value of genomic alterations. *Indian J. Cancer* **2006**, *43*, 60–66. [CrossRef]
11. Javed, F.; Warnakulasuriya, S. Is there a relationship between periodontal disease and oral cancer? A systematic review of currently available evidence. *Crit. Rev. Oncol Hematol.* **2016**, *97*, 197–205. [CrossRef] [PubMed]
12. American Cancer Society. Cancer Facts & Figures: 2018. Available online: https://www.cancer.org/content/dam/cancer-org/research/cancer-facts-and-statistics/annual-cancer-facts-and-figures/2018/cancer-facts-and-figures-2018.pdf (accessed on 26 February 2018).
13. Brabletz, T.; Kalluri, R.; Nieto, M.A.; Weinberg, R.A. EMT in cancer. *Nat. Rev. Cancer.* **2018**, *18*, 128–134. [CrossRef] [PubMed]
14. Bacac, M.; Stamenkovic, I. Metastatic cancer cell. *Annu. Rev. Pathol.* **2008**, *3*, 221–247. [CrossRef]
15. Valastyan, S.; Weinberg, R.A. Tumor metastasis: Molecular insights and evolving paradigms. *Cell* **2011**, *147*, 275–292. [CrossRef] [PubMed]
16. Yoon, S.O.; Park, S.J.; Yun, C.H.; Chung, A.S. Roles of matrix metalloproteinases in tumor metastasis and angiogenesis. *J. Biochem. Mol. Biol.* **2003**, *36*, 128–137. [CrossRef] [PubMed]
17. Kessenbrock, K.; Plaks, V.; Werb, Z. Matrix metalloproteinases: Regulators of the tumor microenvironment. *Cell* **2010**, *141*, 52–67. [CrossRef] [PubMed]
18. Gialeli, C.; Theocharis, A.D.; Karamanos, N.K. Roles of matrix metalloproteinases in cancer progression and their pharmacological targeting. *FEBS J.* **2011**, *278*, 16–27. [CrossRef] [PubMed]
19. Krisanaprakornkit, S.; Iamaroon, A. Epithelial-mesenchymal transition in oral squamous cell carcinoma. *ISRN Oncol.* **2012**, *681469*, 1–10. [CrossRef]
20. Khasigov, P.Z.; Podobed, O.V.; Gracheva, T.S.; Salbiev, K.D.; Grachev, S.V.; Berezov, T.T. Role of matrix metalloproteinases and their inhibitors in tumor invasion and metastasis. *Biochemistry* **2003**, *68*, 711–717.
21. Marunaka, Y.; Marunaka, R.; Sun, H.; Yamamoto, T.; Kanamura, N.; Inui, T.; Taruno, A. Actions of Quercetin, a Polyphenol, on Blood Pressure. *Molecules* **2017**, *22*, 209. [CrossRef]
22. Valentová, K.; Vrba, J.; Bancířová, M.; Ulrichová, J.; Křen, V. Isoquercitrin: Pharmacology, toxicology, and metabolism. *Food Chem Toxicol.* **2014**, *68*, 267–282.
23. Massi, A.; Bortolini, O.; Ragno, D.; Bernardi, T.; Sacchetti, G.; Tacchini, M.; De Risi, C. Research Progress in the Modification of Quercetin Leading to Anticancer Agents. *Molecules* **2017**, *22*, 1270. [CrossRef] [PubMed]
24. Kee, J.Y.; Han, Y.H.; Kim, D.S.; Mun, J.G.; Park, J.; Jeong, M.Y.; Um, J.Y.; Hong, S.H. Inhibitory effect of quercetin on colorectal lung metastasis through inducing apoptosis, and suppression of metastatic ability. *Phytomedicine* **2016**, *23*, 1680–1690. [CrossRef] [PubMed]
25. Rather, R.A.; Bhagat, M. Quercetin as an innovative therapeutic tool for cancer chemoprevention: Molecular mechanisms and implications in human health. *Cancer Med.* **2019**. [CrossRef] [PubMed]
26. Murakami, A.; Ashida, H.; Terao, J. Multitargeted cancer prevention by quercetin. *Cancer Lett.* **2008**, *269*, 315–325. [CrossRef]
27. Geoghegan, F.; Wong, R.W.; Rabie, A.B. Inhibitory effect of quercetin on periodontal pathogens in vitro. *Phytother Res.* **2010**, *24*, 817–820.
28. Palaska, I.; Papathanasiou, E.; Theoharides, T.C. Use of polyphenols in periodontal inflammation. *Eur J. Pharmacol.* **2013**, *720*, 77–83. [CrossRef]
29. Ma, Y.S.; Yao, C.N.; Liu, H.C.; Yu, F.S.; Lin, J.J.; Lu, K.W.; Liao, C.L.; Chueh, F.S.; Chung, J.G. Quercetin induced apoptosis of human oral cancer SAS cells through mitochondria and endoplasmic reticulum mediated signaling pathways. *Oncol. Lett.* **2018**, *15*, 9663–9672. [CrossRef]
30. Zhao, J.; Fang, Z.; Zha, Z.; Sun, Q.; Wang, H.; Sun, M.; Qiao, B. Quercetin inhibits cell viability, migration and invasion by regulating miR-16/HOXA10 axis in oral cancer. *Eur J. Pharmacol.* **2019**, *847*, 11–18. [CrossRef]
31. Li, X.; Guo, S.; Xiong, X.K.; Peng, B.Y.; Huang, J.M.; Chen, M.F.; Wang, F.Y.; Wang, J.N. Combination of quercetin and cisplatin enhances apoptosis in OSCC cells by downregulating xIAP through the NF-κB pathway. *J. Cancer.* **2019**, *10*, 4509–4521. [CrossRef]

32. Huang, C.Y.; Chan, C.Y.; Chou, I.T.; Lien, C.H.; Hung, H.C.; Lee, M.F. Quercetin induces growth arrest through activation of FOXO1 transcription factor in EGFR-overexpressing oral cancer cells. *J. Nutr. Biochem.* **2013**, *24*, 1596–1603. [CrossRef] [PubMed]
33. Surh, Y.J. Cancer chemoprevention with dietary phytochemicals. *Nat. Rev. Cancer.* **2003**, *3*, 768–780. [CrossRef] [PubMed]
34. Kim, H.J.; Kim, S.K.; Kim, B.S.; Lee, S.H.; Park, Y.S.; Park, B.K.; Kim, S.J.; Kim, J.; Choi, C.; Kim, J.S.; et al. Apoptotic effect of quercetin on HT-29 colon cancer cells via the AMPK signaling pathway. *J. Agric Food Chem.* **2010**, *58*, 8643–8650. [CrossRef] [PubMed]
35. Nam, J.S.; Sharma, A.R.; Nguyen, L.T.; Chakraborty, C.; Sharma, G.; Lee, S.S. Application of Bioactive Quercetin in Oncotherapy: From Nutrition to Nanomedicine. *Molecules* **2016**, *21*, 108. [CrossRef]
36. Hashemzaei, M.; Delarami, A.; Yari, A.; Heravi, R.E.; Tabrizian, K.; Taghdisi, S.M.; Sadegh, S.E.; Tsarouhas, K.; Kouretas, D.; Tzanakakis, G.; et al. Anticancer and apoptosis-inducing effects of quercetin in vitro and in vivo. *Oncol. Rep.* **2017**, *38*, 819–828. [CrossRef]
37. Yu, D.; Ye, T.; Xiang, Y.; Shi, Z.; Zhang, J.; Lou, B.; Zhang, F.; Chen, B.; Zhou, M. Quercetin inhibits epithelial-mesenchymal transition, decreases invasiveness and metastasis, and reverses IL-6 induced epithelial-mesenchymal transition, expression of MMP by inhibiting STAT3 signaling in pancreatic cancer cells. *Onco Targets Ther.* **2017**, *10*, 4719–4729. [CrossRef]
38. Cai, W.; Yu, D.; Fan, J.; Liang, X.; Jin, H.; Liu, C.; Zhu, M.; Shen, T.; Zhang, R.; Hu, W.; et al. Quercetin inhibits transforming growth factor β1-induced epithelial-mesenchymal transition in human retinal pigment epithelial cells via the Smad pathway. *Drug Des. Dev. Ther.* **2018**, *12*, 4149–4161. [CrossRef]
39. Lai, W.W.; Hsu, S.C.; Chueh, F.S.; Chen, Y.Y.; Yang, J.S.; Lin, J.P.; Lien, J.C.; Tsai, C.H.; Chung, J.G. Quercetin inhibits migration and invasion of SAS human oral cancer cells through inhibition of NF-κB and matrix metalloproteinase-2/-9 signaling pathways. *Anticancer Res.* **2013**, *33*, 1941–1950.
40. ElAttar, T.M.; Virji, A.S. Modulating effect of resveratrol and quercetin on oral cancer cell growth and proliferation. *Anticancer Drugs* **1999**, *10*, 187–193. [CrossRef]
41. Gupta, G.P.; Massagué, J. Cancer metastasis: Building a framework. *Cell* **2006**, *127*, 679–695. [CrossRef]
42. Thiery, J.P.; Sleeman, J.P. Complex networks orchestrate epithelial-mesenchymal transitions. *Nat. Rev. Mol. Cell. Biol.* **2006**, *7*, 131–142. [CrossRef] [PubMed]
43. Chang, W.W.; Hu, F.W.; Yu, C.C.; Wang, H.H.; Feng, H.P.; Lan, C.; Tsai, L.L.; Chang, Y.C. Quercetin in elimination of tumor initiating stem-like and mesenchymal transformation property in head and neck cancer. *Head Neck.* **2013**, *35*, 413–419. [CrossRef]
44. Srinivasan, A.; Thangavel, C.; Liu, Y.; Shoyele, S.; Den, R.B.; Selvakumar, P.; Lakshmikuttyamma, A. Quercetin regulates β-catenin signaling and reduces the migration of triple negative breast cancer. *Mol. Carcinog.* **2016**, *55*, 743–756. [CrossRef] [PubMed]
45. Bhat, F.A.; Sharmila, G.; Balakrishnan, S.; Arunkumar, R.; Elumalai, P.; Suganya, S.; Raja Singh, P.; Srinivasan, N.; Arunakaran, J. Quercetin reverses EGF-induced epithelial to mesenchymal transition and invasiveness in prostate cancer (PC-3) cell line via EGFR/PI3K/Akt pathway. *J. Nutr. Biochem.* **2014**, *25*, 1132–1139. [CrossRef]
46. Feng, J.; Song, D.; Jiang, S.; Yang, X.; Ding, T.; Zhang, H.; Luo, J.; Liao, J.; Yin, Q. Quercetin restrains TGF-β1-induced epithelial-mesenchymal transition by inhibiting Twist1 and regulating E-cadherin expression. *Biochem. Biophys. Res. Commun.* **2018**, *498*, 132–138. [CrossRef]
47. Zavadil, J.; Bottinger, E.P. TGF-beta and epithelial-to-mesenchymal transitions. *Oncogene* **2005**, *24*, 5764–5774. [CrossRef] [PubMed]

Sample Availability: Samples are available from the corresponding authors.

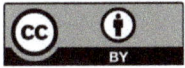 © 2020 by the authors. Licensee MDPI, Basel, Switzerland. This article is an open access article distributed under the terms and conditions of the Creative Commons Attribution (CC BY) license (http://creativecommons.org/licenses/by/4.0/).

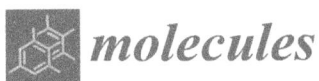

Article

Romanian Wormwood (*Artemisia absinthium* L.): Physicochemical and Nutraceutical Screening

Elena-Alina Moacă [1,†], Ioana Zinuca Pavel [2,†], Corina Danciu [2,*], Zorin Crăiniceanu [3,*], Daliana Minda [2], Florina Ardelean [4], Diana Simona Antal [4], Roxana Ghiulai [5], Andreea Cioca [6], Mihnea Derban [6], Sebastian Simu [7], Raul Chioibaş [8], Camelia Szuhanek [9] and Cristina-Adriana Dehelean [1]

1 Department of Toxicology and Drug Industry, Faculty of Pharmacy, "Victor Babes" University of Medicine and Pharmacy, 2 Eftimie Murgu Square, 300041 Timisoara, Romania
2 Department of Pharmacognosy, Faculty of Pharmacy, "Victor Babes" University of Medicine and Pharmacy, 2 Eftimie Murgu Square, 300041 Timisoara, Romania
3 Department of Plastic and Reconstructive Surgery, Faculty of Medicine, "Victor Babes" University of Medicine and Pharmacy, 2 Eftimie Murgu Square, 300041 Timisoara, Romania
4 Department of Botany, Faculty of Pharmacy, "Victor Babes" University of Medicine and Pharmacy, 2 Eftimie Murgu Square, 300041 Timisoara, Romania
5 Department of Pharmaceutical Chemistry, Faculty of Pharmacy, "Victor Babes" University of Medicine and Pharmacy, 2 Eftimie Murgu Square, 300041 Timisoara, Romania
6 Department of Pathology, CFR Clinical Hospital, 13-15, Tudor Vladimirescu, 300173 Timisoara, Romania
7 Department of Physical Chemistry, Faculty of Pharmacy, "Victor Babes" University of Medicine and Pharmacy, 2 Eftimie Murgu Square, 300041 Timisoara, Romania
8 CBS Medcom Hospital, 12 Popa Sapca Street, 300047 Timisoara, Romania
9 Department of Orthodontics, Faculty of Dentistry, "Victor Babes" University of Medicine and Pharmacy, 2 Eftimie Murgu Square, 300041 Timisoara, Romania
* Correspondence: corina.danciu@umft.ro (C.D.); zcrainiceanu@gmail.com (Z.C.); Tel.: +40-744-648-855 (C.D.); +40-722-356-212 (Z.C.)
† These authors contributed equally to this work.

Received: 15 July 2019; Accepted: 23 August 2019; Published: 25 August 2019

Abstract: *Artemisia* species are used worldwide for their antioxidant, antimicrobial and anti-inflammatory properties. This research was designed to investigate the phytochemical profile of two ethanolic extracts obtained from leaves and stems of *A. absinthium* L. as well as the biological potential (antioxidant activity, cytotoxic, anti-migratory and anti-inflammatory properties). Both plant materials showed quite similar thermogravimetric, FT-IR phenolic profile (high chlorogenic acid) with mild antioxidant capacity [ascorbic acid (0.02–0.1) > leaves (0.1–2.0) > stem (0.1–2.0)]. Alcoholic extracts from these plant materials showed a cytotoxic effect against A375 (melanoma) and MCF7 (breast adenocarcinoma) and affected less the non-malignant HaCaT cells (human keratinocytes) at 72 h post-stimulation and this same trend was observed in the anti-migratory (A375, MCF7 > HaCat) assay. Lastly, extracts ameliorated the pro-inflammatory effect of TPA (12-O-tetradecanoylphorbol-13-acetate) in mice ears, characterized by a diffuse neutrophil distribution with no exocytosis or micro-abscesses.

Keywords: *Artemisia absinthium* L.; antioxidants; total phenolic content; cytotoxicity; melanoma and breast cancer cell line; HaCaT cells; inflammation

1. Introduction

Common wormwood (*Artemisia absinthium* L., Asteraceae) is a woody-based perennial herb which grows widely in dry, sunny regions of Eurasia, Northern Africa, North and South America [1]. It may be recognized by its silver-grey leaves, which have a soft silk texture. The upper parts of the plant have a distinctive aromatic scent when bruised. From a biochemical point of view, wormwood stands out due to the synthesis of bitter-tasting metabolites and essential oils [2]. Bitterness is conferred by sesquiterpenes (0.15–0.4%), including absinthin, artabsin, anabsinthin, and matricin [3]. Essential oils are secreted by numerous glandular hairs and secretory ducts [4], providing a content of 2–6 mL/kg volatiles in the dried herb [5]. Several chemotypes of volatile oils are known from different parts of the world according to the main constituent: α-and β-thujone, *cis*-epoxyocimene, *trans*-sabinyl acetate and chrysanthenyl acetate [6]. Other secondary metabolites in wormwood include flavonoids (myricetin, quercetin, rutin, hesperidin), hydroxybenzoic acids (salicylic acid, gallic acid), hydroxycinnamic acids (caffeic acids, coumaric acids, ferulic acid), resveratrol, and other [7].

Wormwood leaves and stems have traditionally been employed as a bitter tonic in appetite loss. Preparations are also prescribed as a choleretic in dyspeptic disorders, and in liver diseases due to its hepatoprotective effect. The herb is as well known for its anthelmintic, antipyretic, antibacterial and insecticide properties [5]. The importance of the herb is acknowledged by its inclusion in the European Pharmacopoeia and other official compendia, as well as by the monograph of the Committee on Herbal Medicinal Products of the European Medicine Agency (EMA/HMPC/751484/ 2016).

In recent years, wormwood has attracted considerable attention due to its anti-inflammatory effect. Clinical studies could point out favorable effects in Crohn's disease. Patients receiving an herbal blend containing wormwood as an add-up to standard steroids could afford the lowering of steroid doses; the remission of the disease could be pointed out in 65% of the patients after eight weeks of treatment [8]. The favorable evolution was explained by the suppression of tumor necrosis factor alpha (TNF-α) by some metabolites from *A. absinthium* extracts, and the potential of wormwood to treat diseases with an augmented production of pro-inflammatory cytokines was pointed out [9]. Wormwood extracts proved as well efficient in the supportive treatment of early-stage IgA nephropathy [10].

The current research aims to investigate in depth both the chemical composition as well as the biological activity of ethanolic extracts obtained from leaves and stems of wormwood collected from the Southern part of Romania in order to enhance the knowledge about the phytochemistry and bioactivity of this ancient medicinal plant with important medicinal potential. To this end, ethanol extracts of leaves and stems were investigated by liquid chromatography–mass spectrometry (LC-MS), thermal analysis (TG-DSC) and Fourier-transform infrared spectroscopy (FT-IR). The Total Phenolic Content (TPC) was evaluated spectrophotometrically, and radical scavenging effects as well as the cytotoxic and anti-migratory potential on two tumor cell lines–melanoma and breast adenocarcinoma cells and on a non-tumor cell line–HaCaT–keratinocytes was assessed. The anti-inflammatory effects of the extracts were tested in a mouse ear edema model.

2. Results

2.1. Physicochemical Analysis

After lyophilization, both ethanolic extracts, obtained from leaves and stems of wormwood were characterized by thermal analysis (TG-DSC) and Fourier-transform infrared spectroscopy (FT-IR).

2.1.1. Thermal Analysis

TG-DSC curves of dried and lyophilized extracts of *A. absinthium* L. leaves and stems are depicted in Figure 1A,B. Thermal analysis performed for dried and lyophilized wormwood leaves extract revealed a total mass loss of 94.17% in four stages. In the first stage, the wormwood leaves extract loses 66.30% of the total mass and an endothermic process which can be noticed with a maximum at 122.5 °C. The second stage is located between 450 °C and 600 °C; within this interval the sample loses 4.46% of the total mass and shows an exothermic effect with a maximum at 464.5 °C. In the third stage of extract degradation, four exothermic processes occur between 600 °C and 700 °C, and a total mass loss of 20.06% was measured. In the final stage of extract degradation only a slight mass loss (3.35%) without any thermal effect could be determined.

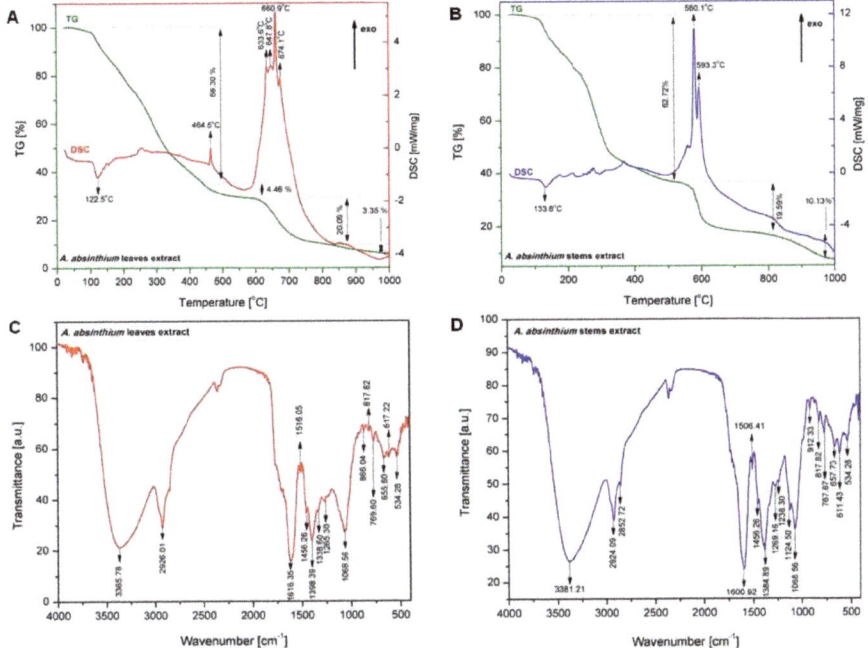

Figure 1. **A**—TG-DSC curves of *A. absinthium* leaves extract, **B**—TG-DSC curves of *A. absinthium* stems extract, **C**—FT-IR spectra of *A. absinthium* leaves extract, **D**—FT-IR spectra of *A. absinthium* stems extract.

Thermal analysis performed for dried and lyophilized wormwood stems extract revealed a total mass loss of 92.44% in three stages. The largest mass loss (about 62.72%) occurs during the first stage; it is accompanied by an endothermic process with a maximum at 133.8 °C. In the second stage (temperature range 500 °C–650 °C) a mass loss of 19.59% was registered, related to two exothermic processes peaking at 580.1 °C and 593.3 °C, respectively. In the final stage of the extract degradation only a mass loss of 10.13% occurred.

2.1.2. FT-IR Investigations

In order to identify the functional groups of the active components which are present in the leaves and stems extracts of *A. absinthium*, the FT-IR analysis was done. The FT-IR analysis is based on the presence of the peak values in the region of IR radiation appeared on different wavenumber. The results of analysis of dried lyophilized leaves and stems extracts based on *A. absinthium* are given in Table 1 and Figure 1C,D. The two lyophilized extracts based on *A. absinthium* exhibited a similar IR profile most probably due to the polar nature of molecules present in both extracts.

Table 1. Peak values and functional groups of *A. absinthium* leaves and stems extracts in the spectrum.

Characteristic Absorptions [cm^{-1}] Leaves Extract/Stems Extract	Functional Group	Bond
3365.78/3381.21	Amines, amide, alcohol	N-H stretching O-H stretch (H-bonded)
2926.01/2924.09; 2852.72	Alkanes	C-H strech
1616.35/1600.92	Amide	N-H bending
1516.05/1506.41	Nitro compounds	N-O asymmetric strech
1456.26	Aromatics	C=C stretch (in ring)
1398.39/1384.89	Alkanes	-C-H bending
1338.60/-	Amines	C-N strech
1265.30/1269.16; 1238.30	Acids	C-O strech
1068.56/1068.56; 1124.50	Alcohols	C-O stretch
866.04/912.33	Alkenes	=C-H bending
817.82/817.82	Alkenes	=C-H bending
769.60/767.67	Alkenes	=C-H bending
655.80/657.73	Alkenes	=C-H bending
617.22/611.43	Alkenes	=C-H bending
534.28/534.28	Alkenes	=C-H bending

2.2. Phenolic Composition

2.2.1. Raw Profiling

The results of our study indicated a higher total phenolic and flavonoid content in the extract obtained from wormwood leaves as compared to the stems extract (Table 2).

Table 2. Total phenolic and flavonoid contents of the ethanolic wormwood extracts.

Extract	Total Phenolic Content (mg GAE/g Extract)	Total Flavonoid Content (mg CE/g Extract)
Leaves extract	54.68 ± 1.93	43.08 ± 2.47
Stems extract	44.15 ± 1.12	34.14 ± 2.16

2.2.2. LC-MS Fingerprint

In Table 3 are presented the polyphenolic content of the *A. absinthium* L. leaves and stems, obtained by LC-MS analysis.

Table 3. Polyphenolic content of extracts analysed by LC-MS.

	Compound Name	Rt (min)	$[M - H^+]^+$ (m/z)	*A. absinthium* Leaves (µg/mg d.w.)	*A. absinthium* Stems (µg/mg d.w.)
1.	Gentisic acid	2.67	153	ND	NQ
2.	Chlorogenic acid	6.45	353	1.94	2.03
3.	Caffeic acid	6.97	179	NQ	NQ
4.	*p*-Coumaric acid	10.56	163	NQ	ND
5.	Isoquercitrin	22.50	463	0.04	0.07
6.	Rutin	23.01	609	0.08	0.55
7.	Quercitrin	26.18	447	0.11	0.05
8.	Luteolin	32.78	285	NQ	ND
9.	Apigenin	36.91	269	NQ	ND

Notes: ND—not detected, below the limit of detection; NQ—not quantified, below the limit of quantification.

2.2.3. Antioxidant Activity

In order to evaluate the antioxidant activity (AOA), both wormwood lyophilized extracts were dissolved in ultra-pure distilled water. The values corresponding to the inhibition percentages of the two extracts of *A. absinthium* (leaves and stems) were evaluated in time, and compared to those of ascorbic acid solution (control) are presented in Figure 2A. As it can be noticed from the graph, both extracts of *A. absinthium* show antioxidant effects during the time frame of the evaluation. Moreover, the AOA values of *A. absinthium* stem extract are slightly higher than the AOA values of *A. absinthium* leaves extract.

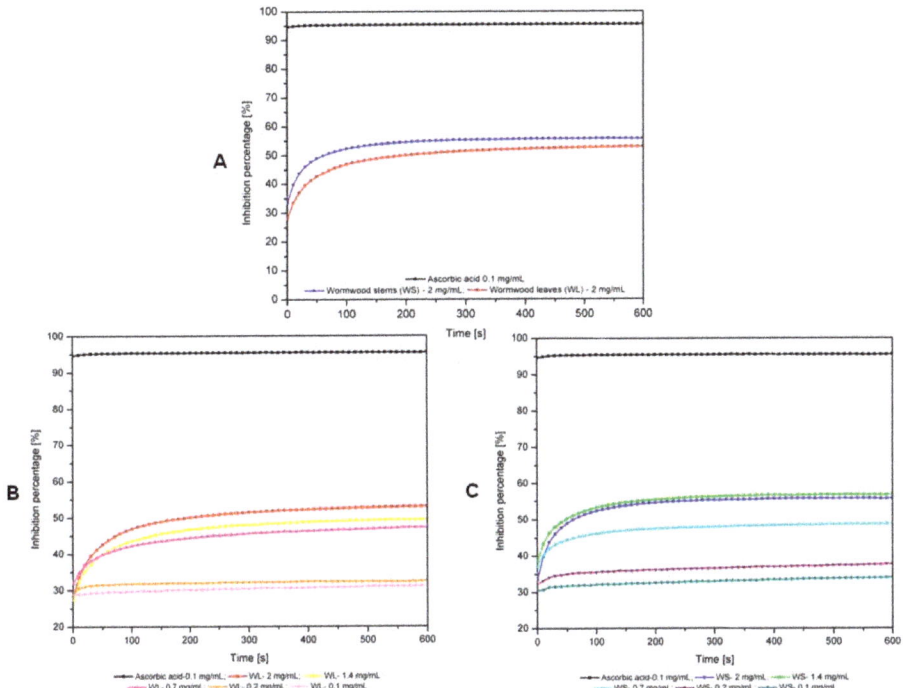

Figure 2. The time dependent inhibition percentage of *A. absinthium* extracts: **A**—*A. absinthium* stock solutions based on leaves and stems vs. ascorbic acid; **B**—extracts of *A. absinthium* leaves vs. ascorbic acid; **C**—extracts of *A. absinthium* stems vs. ascorbic acid.

The reduction rate of DPPH free radical is different for the two extracts. The wormwood stems extract quenches the free radicals after 250 s; subsequently the reaction reaches equilibrium. Wormwood leaves extract quenches the entirety of free radicals after 500 s.

From Figure 2B it can be noted that the antioxidant activity of *A. absinthium* leaves extract is concentration-dependent. In the case of *A. absinthium* stems extracts the values corresponding to inhibition percentages are not directly proportional with their concentration; the maximal inhibition was measured for the sample containing 1.4 mg extract/mL.

Table 4 presents the percent inhibition of leaves and stems extracts. The values were calculated with equation (1) and subsequently used for the determination of IC_{50} values. IC_{50}, characterizing the antioxidant activity as evaluated by the DPPH test, were as follows: for ascorbic acid $IC_{50} = 0.03191 \pm 0.0019$ mg/mL; for wormwood leaves extract $IC_{50} = 0.4993 \pm 0.0201$ mg/mL and for wormwood stems extract $IC_{50} = 0.4865 \pm 0.0182$ mg/mL. The IC_{50} parameter for each sample was determined using GraphPad Prism 8 software. Correlation coefficients were $R^2 = 0.9856$ for wormwood leaves extract and $R^2 = 0.9855$ for wormwood stems extract.

Table 4. The inhibition percentage of *A. absinthium* extracts obtained from leaves and stems, as compared to the inhibition percentage of ascorbic acid [1].

Ascorbic Acid		*A. absinthium* Leaves Extract		*A. absinthium* Stems Extract	
Concentration [mg/mL]	% Inhibition	Concentration [mg/mL]	% Inhibition	Concentration [mg/mL]	% Inhibition
0.1	94.88 ± 0.029	2	53.11 ± 0.014	2	55.77 ± 0.054
0.08	95.47 ± 0.001	1.4	49.47 ± 0.015	1.4	56.84 ± 0.026
0.06	95.06 ± 0.001	0.7	47.32 ± 0.026	0.7	48.79 ± 0.015
0.04	94.85 ± 0.0015	0.2	32.61 ± 0.020	0.2	37.71 ± 0.019
0.02	83.19 ± 0.005	0.1	31.15 ± 0.021	0.1	34.02 ± 0.056

[1] The results are expressed as average ± SD ($n = 3$).

2.3. Bioactivity

2.3.1. Cytotoxicity and Selectivity Index Assessment

The effect of *A. absinthium* ethanolic extracts was evaluated on a non-tumor and two tumor cell lines at different periods of time and compared to the Control group (cells stimulated with ultrapure water). In Supplementary Figure S1 is described the in vitro cytotoxic effect at 24 h and at 48 h post-stimulation. At 24 h post-stimulation, both wormwood leaves and stems extracts showed no cytotoxic effect on the non-tumor cell line, HaCat, regardless of the tested dose. On A375 melanoma cells, *A. absinthium* leaves extract elicited a mild decrease of cell viability at the higher dose tested, 1000 μg/mL (cell viability 86.2 ± 2.2% vs. Control), whereas *A. absinthium* stems extract provoked a slightly more cytotoxic effect at the same dose (cell viability 82.2 ± 4.9% vs. Control). At 24 h, both extracts induced a decrease in MCF7 breast adenocarcinoma cell viability, the most significant results being obtained at the highest tested dose (for *A. absinthium* leaves extract at 1000 μg/mL the cell viability was 84.3 ± 6.1% vs. Control and for the stems extract it was 80.9 ± 3.1% vs. Control).

At 48 h post-stimulation, on HaCaT keratinocytes, wormwood extracts induced a mild decrease in cell viability, the effect being more noticeable in the case of *A. absinthium* leaves extract (at 1000 μg/mL, cells viability was 92.8 ± 4.6% vs. Control). On the tumor cell lines, both wormwood extracts provoked a dose dependent decrease of cells viability, with the best results obtained after stimulation with the stems extract. For A375 cells, at the highest dose, the stems extract decreased the viability to 68.8 ± 4.3% vs. Control, while the same extract induced a viability of 56.9 ± 4.4% in MCF7 cells vs. Control cells. The obtained data shows that the wormwood extracts affect more the cancer cells than the non-tumor cells, especially at higher doses.

Figure 3 presents the effect of wormwood extracts at 72 h post-stimulation. On HaCaT cells, the extracts induced a decrease in cell viability especially at 1000 μg/mL: cell viability was 71.6 ± 7.3% vs. Control in case of *A. absinthium* leaves extract, and 77.6 ± 9.2% vs. Control in case of *A. absinthium* stems extract. These data show that the leaves extract induced a more pronounced decrease in HaCaT cell viability than wormwood stems extract. Regarding the tumor cell lines, *A. absinthium* extracts elicited a significant cytotoxic effect at all the tested doses. Moreover, *A. absinthium* extracts affect rather the tumor cells than the non-tumor cell line, HaCaT. At 1000 μg/mL, on A375 melanoma cells, *A. absinthium* leaves extract decreased cells viability to 38.2 ± 3.8% vs. Control and *A. absinthium* stems extract to 21.06 ± 1.1% vs. Control. On the breast adenocarcinoma cells, at the same dose, *A. absinthium* leaves extract decreased cells viability to 37.6 ± 4.3% vs. Control and the stems extract to 10.8 ± 2.3% vs. Control. For both tumor cell lines, the most potent cytotoxic effect was obtained in the case of the stems extracts and the highest reduction of tumor cells viability was noticed for MCF7 breast cancer cells.

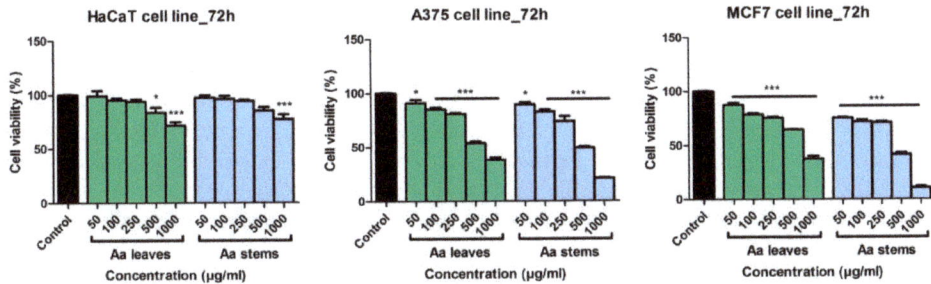

Figure 3. In vitro cytotoxicity assessment of *A. absinthium* leaves and stems ethanolic extracts (50, 100, 250, 500 and 1000 µg/mL) on a non-tumor cell line–HaCaT–human keratinocytes and on two human tumor cell lines A375—melanoma cells and MCF7–breast adenocarcinoma cells at 72 h post-stimulation by the means of Alamar blue assay. The results are expressed as cell viability percentage (%) related to Control (cells stimulated with ultrapure water). The data represent the mean values ± SD of three independent experiments. Comparison among the groups was performed using the One-way ANOVA test followed by Dunnett's post-test. (* $p < 0.05$; *** $p < 0.001$).

The IC$_{50}$ values for the tumor and non-tumor cells following 72 h stimulation with *A. absinthium* extracts are shown in Table 5. The highest IC$_{50}$ value was recorded in the case of HaCaT cells stimulated with *A. absinthium* leaves extract, whereas the lowest values were obtained for the breast cancer cells, MCF7. These data indicate that the tumor cell lines are more affected than the non-cancer cells following stimulation with wormwood extracts.

Table 5. IC$_{50}$ values and selectivity of *A. absinthium* leaves and stems extracts (cancer cells vs. non-malignant HaCaT cells—human keratinocytes) at 72 h post-stimulation.

Extract	HaCaT IC$_{50}$ (µg/mL)	A375 IC$_{50}$ (µg/mL)	MCF7 IC$_{50}$ (µg/mL)	SI *
A. absinthium leaves	397.7 ± 7.2	295.4 ± 7.1	-	1.35
		-	250.6 ± 6.3	1.59
A. absinthium stems	361.8 ± 9.3	312 ± 3.4	-	1.16
		-	246.8 ± 7.2	1.47

* Selectivity index (SI) is calculated as the ratio between the IC$_{50}$ values; IC$_{50}$ [non-malignant HaCaT]/IC$_{50}$ [tumor cell line]. The data represent the mean values ± SD of three independent experiments.

Within this study the Selectivity index (SI) of *A. absinthium* leaves and stems extracts was also determined. The non-malignant HaCaT cells, human keratinocytes, were used as a control in order to evaluate the degree of selectivity of wormwood extracts for the tumor cell lines. The values obtained for the SI range between 1.16 (for A375 cells stimulated 72 h with *A. absinthium* stems extract) and 1.59 (for MCF7 cells stimulated 72 h with *A. absinthium* leaves extract), showing a slightly more active effect of wormwood on the breast adenocarcinoma cells. Following the calculation of SI we can indicate that the extracts did not display a significant selective effect towards the cancer cells.

2.3.2. Scratch Assay Assessment

In order to determine the anti-migratory potential of *A. absinthium* extracts a scratch assay technique was performed. The non-tumor and tumor cell lines were stimulated with different concentrations of wormwood extracts and compared to Control (cells stimulated with ultrapure water).

In Figure 4, the effect of *A. absinthium* leaves and stems extracts on HaCaT, A375 and MCF7 cells is shown. Regarding the effect of *A. absinthium* leaves on HaCaT cells, at low concentrations (50 and 100 µg/mL) stimulation with the extract induced a pro-migratory effect upon the non-tumor cells, the results being similar to those obtained in the Control group. For these concentrations the scratch closure rate after 24 h was 100%. At the concentration of 250 µg/mL, the leaves extract elicited a mild anti-migratory effect, showing a scratch closure rate of 95.4%. On HaCaT cells, at the higher doses tested, *A. absinthium* leaves extract slowed down the migratory effect, showing a scratch closure of 70.8% (500 µg/mL) and 62.7% (1000 µg/mL), respectively. Stimulation with the stems extract elicited a significant pro-migratory effect on the HaCaT cells with scratch closure rate of 100% for concentration ranging from 50 to 500 µg/mL. Only at the highest dose tested, an anti-migratory effect was noticed, having a scratch closure percentage of 85.5%. The data obtained indicate that the stems extract exhibited a superior pro-migratory effect on the non-tumor cells. Furthermore, no changes in the shape and morphology of HaCaT cells were noticed following stimulation with the samples (see Supplementary Figure S2).

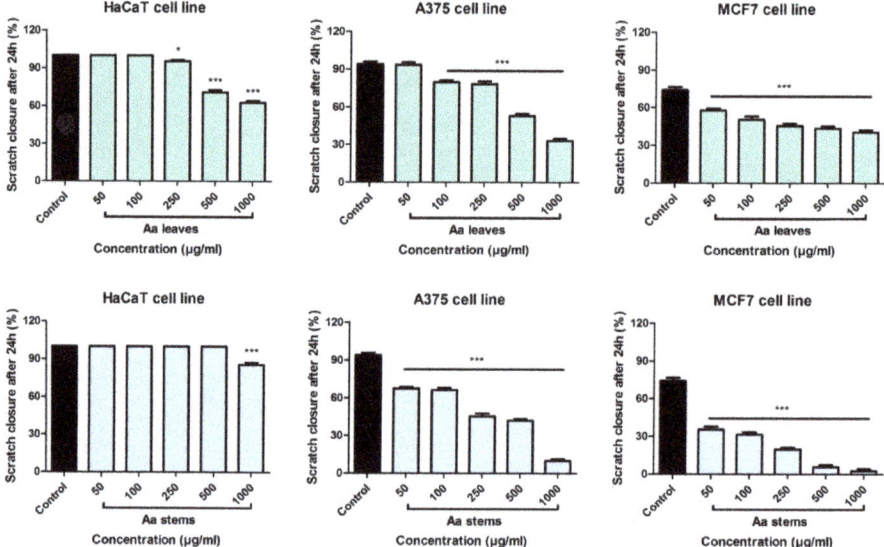

Figure 4. The migratory potential of HaCat, A375 and MCF7 cells following treatment with *A. absinthium* leaves and stems ethanolic extract (50, 100, 250, 500 and 1000 µg/mL). Images were taken by light microscopy at 10× magnification (the scale bars represent 100 µm). The bar graphs are expressed as percentage of scratch closure after 24 h compared to the initial surface. Comparison among the groups was performed using the One-way ANOVA test followed by Dunnett's post-test. (* $p < 0.05$; *** $p < 0.001$ vs. Control-cells stimulated with ultrapure water).

Stimulation of human A375 melanoma cells with *A. absinthium* leaves extract proved to have a dose dependent anti-migratory effect (Figure 4). At the lowest tested dose, 50 µg/mL, the leaves extract provoked a closure of the scratch of 93.3%, similar to the Control group, while at the highest tested dose, 1000 µg/mL, the closure was 32.9%. Moreover, at 24 h post-stimulation, it can be seen in the pictures that at the highest concentration there is a slightly change in the cells shape, some of them displayed round shape, indicating that the leaves extract affects melanoma cells (see Supplementary Figure S2).

A. absinthium stems extract manifested a significant anti-migratory effect on A375 cells at all the tested concentrations. The results show that the stems extract had a stronger inhibitory effect on the migration of melanoma cells. At the highest tested dose, the scratch closure rate was around 9.9%. Furthermore, at this concentration, cells with round shape and detached ones were present, showing the cytotoxic effect of this extract. The results obtained are consistent with the ones from the cell viability assay, proving an anti-migratory and cytotoxic effect of these extracts.

Regarding the anti-migratory effect of *A. absinthium* leaves extract on MCF7 human breast adenocarcinoma cells, at 24 h post-stimulation, all the evaluated concentrations manifested a significant inhibitory effect on cancer cells migration.

The anti-migratory properties on MCF7 cells were more potent after stimulation with *A. absinthium* stems extract compared to the effects obtained in the case of the leaves extract. Application of the stems extract provoked at the concentration of 500 µg/mL a closure percentage of 5.8% and for 1000 µg/mL it was 2.6%. Furthermore, it can be seen in the images from Supplementary Figure S2, that at 500 and 1000 µg/mL, the cells had a modified morphology with round shape and also many cells are detached from the plate (Supplementary Figure S2). These elements suggest that the stems extract had a cytotoxic effect on the breast adenocarcinoma cells.

2.3.3. Anti-Inflammatory Assessment

Skin specimens from the control group had normal histological structures, while the group treated with acetone showed marked edema and congestion of the blood vessels but without inflammation or changes of the epidermal thickness (Figure 5A,B).

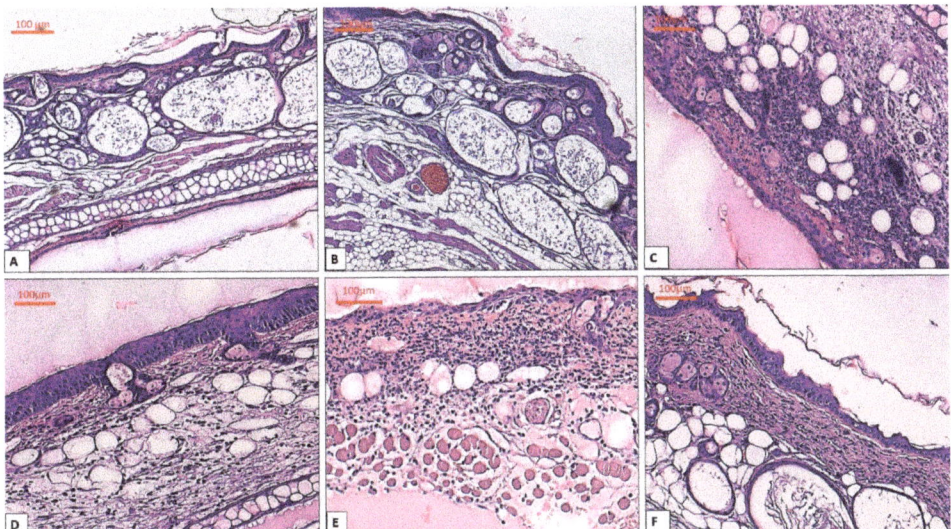

Figure 5. Histological aspects of the skin, H&E stain, **A**: Control group—with no intervention, magnification ×10; **B**: Acetone group showing edema, magnification ×10; **C**: TPA group showing abundant inflammation in the entire dermis with abscess formation, magnification ×20; **D**: TPA + indomethacin group depicting mild inflammation, magnification ×20; **E**: topical application of *A. absinthium* leaves extract indicating moderate inflammation and moderate interstitial edema, magnification ×20; **F**: treatment with *A. absinthium* stems extract having a reduced number of neutrophils and thick collagen fibers in dermis, magnification ×20.

As illustrated in Figure 5C, TPA treatment produced a marked pro-inflammatory action on mice ears. The epidermal thickness was increased and it was accompanied by reactive changes of the cells. We noticed an abundant inflammatory infiltrate composed of neutrophils, disposed in the papillary and reticular dermis and around the dermal appendages. The inflammation showed a diffuse pattern, but it also formed micro-abscesses. In some areas, neutrophils migrated in the epidermal thickness leading to exocytosis. In addition, the blood vessels were congested and some of them displayed leukocytes margination. Intraepidermal and dermal edema was noted in this group.

Topical administration of indomethacin (Figure 5D) provoked a reduction of the inflammatory processes compared to the TPA group. The inflammatory infiltrate was composed of a reduced number of neutrophils that were diffusely disposed in the dermis. Exocytosis and the abcesses were absent in this group and dermal edema was mild.

In the group treated with *A. absinthium* leaves extract (Figure 5E) the epidermis was focally enlarged compared to the untreated group. The inflammation was moderate with a diffuse distribution of the neutrophils in the dermis. No exocytosis or micro-abscesses were observed in this group. Congestion of the blood vessels and interstitial edema were mild and some blood vessels showed leucocytes margination.

In contrast, topical application of the *A. absinthium* stems extract (Figure 5F) showed a clearer anti-inflammatory effect. In this group, the inflammatory infiltrate was mild and diffusely distributed in the dermis and moderate in only few areas. The interstitial edema was mild and focal, while congestion and leucocytes margination of the blood vessels were absent. Moreover, the dermis showed thick collagen fibers organized in compact bundles.

3. Discussion

3.1. Physicochemical Analysis

Thermal analysis is an analytical method used also to characterize the compounds from plant medicine. Figure 1A,B present the TG and DSC signals obtained during thermal decomposition of, lyophilized extracts based on wormwood leaves and stems, in air. In both extracts, there was a substantial mass loss in the first stage of degradation (above 60%). This step was accompanied by an endothermic effect, occurring at: 122.5 °C in the case of wormwood leaves extract and 133.8 °C in the case of wormwood stems extract. We can assume that this endothermic process is in fact an overlap of endothermic effects associated with water elimination and/or partial decomposition of the two extracts. On the TG-DSC curve of wormwood leaves extract, the oxidative degradation occurs with the formation of several exothermic peaks between 464.5 °C and 674.1 °C. The exothermic effect recorded at 464.5 °C, associated with a lower mass loss (4.46%), can be related to the degradation of aromatic amino-acids and/or carbohydrates present in the leaves extract. Continuous exothermic effects can be observed on DSC curve between 633.6 °C and 674.1 °C; these effects could be associated with the oxidative degradation of a wide variety of metabolites, principally phenolics, simple amines and several aromatic compounds. The four exothermic processes recorded on the DSC curve, are accompanied by a mass loss of 20.06% recorded on the TG curve. In the final stage of degradation, only a small mass loss of 3.35% can be seen, which can be assigned to the burning of organic residues (carbon). On the TG-DSC curve of wormwood stems extract, the oxidative degradation occurs with the formation of two exothermic peaks at 580.1 °C and at 593.3 °C, associated with a mass loss of 19.59%. These exothermic effects could be related with the degradation of aromatic compounds, carbohydrates and aromatic amino-acids present in the stems extract.

FT-IR spectroscopy analysis is one of the most widely technique that can be utilized for the qualitative analysis of pharmacologically active compounds from various plant species. The FT-IR spectrum presents unique bands which express the presence of functional groups contained by the molecules in the extracts; it constitutes a chemical fingerprint [11].

Figure 1C,D show that the FT-IR spectra of *A. absinthium* leaves and stems extracts had relevant absorption peaks at 3365.78 cm^{-1} (for leaves) and 3381.21 cm^{-1} (for stems); 2926.01 cm^{-1} (for leaves) and 2924.09 cm^{-1} and 2852.72 cm^{-1} respectively (for stems); 1616.35 cm^{-1} (for leaves) and 1600.92 cm^{-1} (for stems) and at 1068.56 cm^{-1} for both wormwood extracts. The broad bands at 3365.78 (for leaves extract) and 3381.21 cm^{-1} for stems extract correspond both to O-H stretching of hydroxyl groups from alcohols, phenols and carboxylic acids [12] as well as N-H stretching of amines or amides [13]. The peak situated at 2926.01 cm^{-1} for leaves as well as 2924.09 cm^{-1} and 2852.72 cm^{-1} respectively, for stems extract, corresponds to the saturated aliphatic C-H bonds. In the case of stems extract, the two values correspond to C-H stretching which indicate the occurrence of aromatic ring and alkyl group attachment. This may be corresponding to C-C stretching vibration of aromatic amines [14]. Moreover, the band situated at 2926.01 cm^{-1} in case of leaves extract, may correspond to the CH$_3$ vibrations which exist in the functional groups of chlorophyll present in wormwood extract [15]. The peak at 1616.35 cm^{-1} in the case of leaves extract and the peak at 1600.92 cm^{-1} showed in the case of stems extract, confirm the presence of amide functional groups, like N-H bending vibration [16]. The analysis of C-H out-of plane bending can often distinguish substitution patterns which may correspond to N-O asymmetric stretch of nitro functional groups, with bands situated at 1516.05 cm^{-1} in the case of leaves extract and 1506.41 cm^{-1} in the case of stems extract. These two bands confirm the presence of aromatic ring [13]. The bands situated at 1398.39 cm^{-1} (for leaves extract) and 1384.89 cm^{-1} (for stems extract) are attributed to the C-H bending vibration of alkanes, which refer to the binding of the aromatic ring –C-H for the in-plane bending absorption. The band situated at 1265.30 cm^{-1} (for the leaves extract) and the band from 1269.16 cm^{-1} as well as 1238.30 cm^{-1} respectively, in the case of stems extract, corresponds to the aromatic acid ester C-O stretching vibration [17]. The bands located in the range 1068.56 cm^{-1} and 1124.50 cm^{-1} can be attributed to C-O stretch vibration that may come from alcohol functional groups (primary, secondary and tertiary) [17]. The bands in the range 534.28 cm^{-1} and 912.33 cm^{-1} represent the out of plane bending vibration from aromatics alkenes =C-H [18]. The FT-IR spectra reveal only the structural information of some functional groups presents in the plant extract and can be used for authentification of some constituents, but completing information with other techniques for determining the quantitative analysis and confirm the presence of pharmacologically active compounds are required.

3.2. Phenolic Composition

Phenolic compounds are widely distributed in plants and they are associated with the prevention of several diseases where oxidative stress plays an important role [19]. The total phenolic content of the two wormwood extracts was evaluated due to the importance of this class of compounds for the antioxidant activity. The results showed that the leaves extract have a higher phenolic content (54.68 ± 1.93 mg GAE/g extract) compared to the extract from stems (44.15 ± 1.12 mg GAE/g extract).

The total phenolic content of various wormwood extracts was evaluated in several studies. A higher value was observed for the hydroalcoholic extract obtained from the above ground parts of the plant (9.29 ± 0.51 mg GAE/g dry weight) as compared to the hexane and methanol one [20]. Another study estimated a total phenolic content of 123 ± 0.82 mg GAE/g extract for the methanolic extract obtained from aerial parts of the plant [21].

A variation in the total phenolic content depending on the collecting area was observed. Values of the total phenolic content ranging between 49.39 ± 2.20 mg GAE/g dry weight and 99.89 ± 3.30 mg GAE/g dry weight were determined for methanolic extracts obtained from *A. absinthium* aerial parts [22]. In the plant material collected in Romania, a previous study estimated a total phenolic content of 18.14 mg GAE/g dry weight for aerial parts of the plant [23]. The above ground parts of wormwood collected in Turkey presented a total phenolic content of 9.79 µg GAE/mg [24].

Among polyphenols, flavonoids are known for their antioxidant, anti-inflammatory, antibacterial, antiviral and anticancer properties [25]. The total flavonoid content of wormwood extracts was in agreement with the results obtained for total phenolic content, with a lower value for wormwood stems extract (34.14 ± 2.16 mg CE/g extract) compared to leaves extract (43.08 ± 2.47 mg CE/g extract).

Other studies mentioned higher flavonoid content for the ethanolic extract from wormwood aerial parts as compared to chloroform and aqueous extracts [26]. Variations between 3.02 ± 0.05 and 19.28 ± 0.12 mg quercetin equivalents per gram dry weight were observed for different extracts obtained from the above ground plant material [20]. The highest total flavonoid content estimated for plant material collected in different Tunisian areas was 126.4 ± 2.32 mg catechin equivalent per gram dry weight [22].

Both alcoholic extracts were subjected to LC-MS analysis under identical solution and instrumental conditions which enabled the identification and in some cases quantification, consistent with their

Rt and *m/z* values, of 9 polyphenolic acids: gentisic acid, chlorogenic acid, caffeic acid, *p*-coumaric acid, isoquercitrin, rutin, quercitrin, luteolin and apigenin expressed in µg/mg d.w. (Table 3). Obtained results indicated that chlorogenic acid was the most abundant polyphenolic quantified compound. Isoquercitrin, rutin and quercitrin were also detected but in smaller concentrations, accompanied by traces of gentisic acid, caffeic acid, *p*-coumaric acid, luteolin and apigenin which were below the limit of quantification. In terms of their concentration in the two types of extract, it seems that *A. absinthium* stems extract are somehow similar to *A. absinthium* leaves extract, *A. absinthium* stems extracts being slyghtly richer, with one exception (Table 3). Thus, chlorogenic acid, isoquercitrin and rutin have concentrations a bit higher in *A. absinthium* stems while quercitrin is more abundant in *A. absinthium* leaves extract (Table 3).

In a similar approach, Ivanescu and co-workers have conducted a HPLC-DAD-MS study in order to determine the polyphenols from the aerial part of three *Artemisia* species, namely *A. absinthium*, *A. annua*, and *A. vulgaris* before as well as after acid hydrolysis. Results for *A. absinthium* have shown that in case of the un-hydrolyzed extract ferulic acid (0.608 mg/100 g dry herb) and kaempferol (2.456 mg/100 g dry herb) could be identified. On the other hand in case of the hydrolyzed extract *p*-Coumaric acid (12.6 mg/100 g dry herb), ferulic acid (2.432 mg/100 g dry herb), fisetin (0.792 mg/100 g dry herb) and patuletin (0.616 mg/100 g dry herb) could be detected [27]. Also Craciunescu and co-workers, used maceration as a method of extraction but ethanol 70% as solvent. Among the phenolic and flavonoid screened compounds they have detected gallic acid (0.092 ± 0.005 mg/g dry extract), chlorogenic acid (0.077 ± 0.004 mg/g dry extract), caffeic acid (0.181 ± 0.009 mg/g dry extract), coumaric acid (0.112 ± 0.006 mg/g dry extract), ferulic acid (0.100 ± 0.005 mg/g dry extract), rutin (0.089 ± 0.005 mg/g dry extract), luteolin (0.677 ± 0.036 mg/g dry extract), quercetin (2.707 ± 0.135 mg/g dry extract), myricetin (0.201 ± 0.011 mg/g dry extract), apigenin (0.359 ± 0.019 mg/g dry extract) [28]. In a comprehensive study conducted by Aberham and co-workers, sesquiterpene lactones, flavonoids and lignans were detected from an extract of *A. absinthium* obtained by maceration with dichloromethane by HPLC-MS [29]. Sahin and co-workers have tried to increase the amount of bioactive compounds from *A. absinthium* by optimization of ultrasonic-assisted extraction. HPLC-DAD analysis has shown the presence the following polyphenols: protocatechuic acid (0.10 ± 0.01 mg/g dried plant), chlorogenic acid (5.72 ± 0.11 mg/g dried plant), caffeic acid (2.07 ± 0.01 mg/g dried plant), ferulic acid (19.57 ± 0.44 mg/g dried plant), rosmarinic acid (7.82 ± 0.01 mg/g dried plant) [30].

For the prevention of various types of cell damage, antioxidants are widely employed compounds. Antioxidants are natural products with the ability to eliminate reactive oxygen species (ROS) in enzymatic and nonenzymatic processes. Plants contain potent antioxidants which act as radical scavengers and mitigate the damaging effects of ROS to the human body [31].

Regarding the antioxidant activity presented in this study, it was demonstrated that the wormwood extract obtained from stems showed a slightly increased antioxidant effect compared to the leaves extract. Looking at the wormwood extracts obtained from leaves it was showed that with increasing concentration, antioxidant activity increases. Our results are in agreement with those obtained by Kim and co-workers [32]. Lee and co-workers reported an antiradical activity of *A. absinthium* roots (IC_{50} = 271.34 µg/mL). They also found for *A. annua* high IC_{50} values of antiradical activities (IC_{50} = 190.54 µg/mL for leaves extract and IC_{50} = 22.90 µg/mL for stems extracts). Comparable to our results are the values obtained by the same group of authors for *A. capillaries* leaves extract (IC_{50} = 448.15 µg/mL) and *A. selengensis* stems extract (IC_{50} = 411.85 µg/mL) [33].

Slightly higher values regarding the radical-scavenging activities of wormwood extract were reported by Mahmoudi et al. [34]. These authors found IC_{50} values of 612 µg/mL for the DPPH radical-scavenging activity, in case of an *A. absinthium* extract obtained from aerial parts collected during flowering stage.

3.3. Bioactivity

The in vitro studies performed in this paper demonstrate that *A. absinthium* leaves and stems extracts exhibited a dose dependent anti-migratory and cytotoxic effect on the two tumor cell lines, melanoma and breast adenocarcinoma cells. An important aspect is represented by the data obtained for non-tumor cells (human keratinocytes), where *A. absinthium* extracts had no significant cytotoxic effect at 24 and 48 h post-stimulation; at 72 h after stimulation the cytotoxic effect was lower compared to the effect obtained on cancer cells. The differences between the cytotoxic activity on tumor and non-tumor cells suggest that *A. absinthium* extracts affect more the cancer cells.

Our results regarding the fact that wormwood has a more potent effect on cancer cells, are in accordance with the data found in the literature, where Koyuncu [35] evaluated the anticancer activity of *A. absinthium* methanolic extract on DLD-1 colon cancer cells, ECC-1 endometrium cancer cells and HEK-293 embryonic kidney cells and indicated that it had a cytotoxic effect on the cancer cells while showing low cytotoxicity on the kidney cells. Gordanian et al. [36] tested the effect of five *Artemisia* species (*A. absinthium*, *A. vulgaris*, *A. incana*, *A. fragrans* and *A. spicigera*) harvested from Iran against MCF7 breast adenocarcinoma and HEK-293 embryonic kidney cells. *A. absinthium* L. methanolic extract displayed a stronger cytotoxic effect against MCF7 cells than on HEK-293 cells [36]. The same authors evaluated the anti-cancer effect of various *A. absinthium* L. extracts obtained from different parts of the species—flower, leaf, stem or root and demonstrated that the most potent decrease in MCF7 cells viability was obtained after stimulation with the methanolic extract obtained from flowers, followed by the leaf, stem and finally the root methanolic extract [36]. The present study demonstrated strong cytotoxic and anti-migratory activities against both A375 and MCF7 cancer cells after stimulation with *A. absinthium* stems ethanolic extract.

Another aim of the present study was to determine the degree of selectivity of *A. absinthium* leaves and stems extracts. Even though the results obtained in the cytotoxicity assay evidenced that *A. absinthium* extracts affect more the melanoma and breast adenocarcinoma cells rather than the human keratinocytes, the tested samples did not show a selective effect on the cancer cells after the determination of SI; the values obtained were lower than 2. It is considered that the higher the SI is, the more potent and differential a sample is [37]. According to Peña-Morán et al. [38] for a compound to be considered selective the SI value must be higher than 10. The same authors stated that compounds that have the SI between 1 and 10 are considered non-selective [38].

Shafi and co-workers [39] proved that *A. absinthium* methanolic extract obtained from the aerial parts inhibits cell proliferation and triggers apoptosis in two breast cancer cells, namely MDA-MB-231 and MCF7 cells. In a recent study it was shown that *A. absinthium* ethanolic extract inhibited BEL-7404 human hepatoma and H22 mouse hepatoma cells growth and induced apoptosis without affecting the normal hepatic cells [40].

The TPA model of ear inflammation is a very useful tool for assessing anti-inflammatory compounds. When applied to mice ear skin, TPA provokes an influx of mast cells that release mediators responsible for an increased vascular permeability and for neutrophils infiltration [41]. This is consistent with our results, where topical application of TPA led to a massive pro-inflammatory response in mouse ear such as interstitial edema, diffuse inflammation, exocytosis and micro-abscesses.

The group treated with *A. absinthium* leaves extract showed a mild anti-inflammatory effect. By contrast, topical application of *A. absinthium* stems extract elicited a noticeable anti-inflammatory effect in TPA-induced ear inflammation in mice. Histological evaluation showed that *A. absinthium* stems extract inhibited infiltration of neutrophils into the site of inflammation as there was a mild infiltrate with neutrophils at the dermis level, without micro-abscesses, exocytosis or leucocytes margination.

4. Materials and Methods

4.1. Chemicals and Reagents

Ethanol 80% (v/v) and distilled water, purchased from Chemical Company SA (Iasi, Romania) were used to obtain the wormwood extracts (leaves and stems). In order to investigate the antioxidant effect, 2,2-diphenyl-1-picrylhydrazyl (DPPH, Batch No: # STBF5255V, purchased from Sigma Aldrich, Steinheim, Germany) was used The ascorbic acid used as etalon for determination of antioxidant effect, was acquired from Lach-Ner Company (Prague, Czech Republic). For the determination of total phenolic content, were used gallic acid 98% and Na_2CO_3 99%, acquired from Roth (Dautphetal, Germany) and Folin-Ciocalteu reagent, purchased from Merck (Darmstadt, Germany). For the determination of total flavonoid content, were used $NaNO_2$ purchased from Merck; $AlCl_3$ 98% acquired from Roth and NaOH pellets, acquired from ChimReactiv SRL (Bucharest, Romania). (+)-Cathechin hydrate 98% used as standard for the determination of flavonoid content was acquired from Sigma-Aldrich.

The chemicals used for LC-MS analysis were as follows: methanol (99.9% purity) and acetic acid (99.9% purity), purchased from Merck. Standard polyphenolic compounds were: gentisic acid, chlorogenic acid, caffeic acid, p-coumaric acid, isoquercitrin, rutin, quercitrin, luteolin, and apigenin were purchased from Sigma-Aldrich. Ultrapure deionized water was provided by a MiliQ system Milli-Q® Integral Water Purification System (Merck Millipore, Darmstadt, Germany).

The chemicals used for cell culture were purchased from Sigma-Aldrich (Taufkirchen, Germany) and Thermo Fisher Scientific (Boston, MA, USA). TPA (12-O-tetradecanoylphorbol-13-acetate) was acquired from Sigma-Aldrich. For the experimental protocol the substance was dissolved in acetone at a concentration of 8×10^{-4} M. Acetone (analytical purity of 99.92%) was purchased from ChimReactiv SRL.

4.2. Cell Lines

A375-human melanoma cell line (ATCC® CRL-1619 ™) and MCF7—human breast adenocarcinoma cell line (ATCC® HTB-22™) were purchased from the American Type Culture Collection (ATCC, Manassas, VA, USA); HaCaT—human keratinocytes were kindly provided by the University of Debrecen (Debrecen, Hungary). A375 and HaCaT cells were cultured in high glucose Dulbecco's Modified Eagle's Medium (DMEM; Sigma-Aldrich); MCF7 cells were cultured in Eagle's Minimum Essential Medium (EMEM; ATCC). Each cell line was supplemented with 10% fetal bovine serum (FBS; Gibco, Thermo Fisher Scientific) and 1% antibiotic mixture (Penicillin/Streptomycin—Pen/Strep, 10,000 IU/mL; Sigma-Aldrich). The cells were kept under standard conditions (37 °C and humidified atmosphere containing 5% CO_2).

4.3. Plant Material

A. absinthium leaves and stems were collected in June 2018 from Vâlcea county (Romania; coordinates: 44°59′17.46′′ N, 23°52′5.59′′ E) and identified by Professor DS Antal from the Department of Pharmaceutical Botany. A voucher specimen (no. MA_AA1) was deposited at the Herbarium of the Faculty of Pharmacy, Timisoara. After collection, the samples were dried in a plant dryer at room temperature and conserved in a desiccator at 20 °C in darkness until further uses.

4.4. Preparation of A. absinthium L. Ethanolic Extracts

Ethanolic extracts from *A. absinthium* leaves and stems were obtained according to the method of Mau et al., slightly modified [42]. Procedures were as follows: 1 g of dried and ground sample (leaves/stem) was mixed with 60 mL ethanol 80% and sonicated for 1 h at room temperature (amplitude A = 50% and cycle C = 0.5) with an UP200S Ultrasonic Homogenizer from Hielscher (Wanaque, NJ, USA).

After sonication, both samples were filtered through a Whatman no. 4 filter paper and concentrated under reduced pressure at 35 °C using a rotary evaporator. Each dried crude extract was subsequently lyophilized and stored at −4 °C. Lyophilized extracts were further employed for the preparation of aqueous stock solutions (concentration 10 mg/mL). Dispersion in ultrapure water was enhanced by sonication (50% amplitude) for 10 min; finally the obtained stock solutions were filtered. The schematic protocol is depicted in Figure 6.

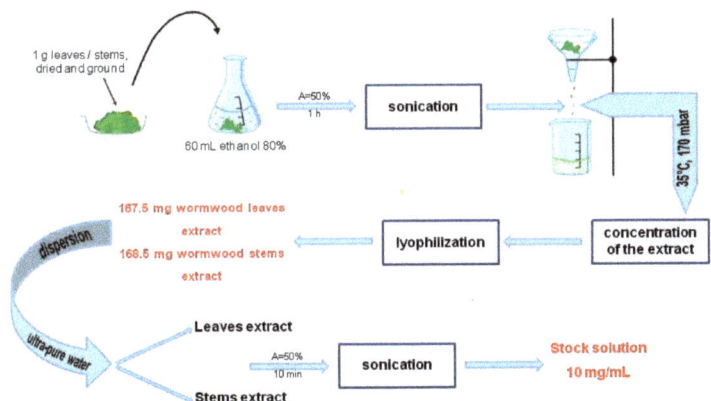

Figure 6. Schematic protocol of *A. absinthium* L. ethanolic extracts preparation.

4.5. Physico-Chemical Characterization

Thermal behavior of the two dried lyophilized extracts was studied using a STA 449C instrument (Netzsch, Selb, Germany) in air atmosphere at a flow rate of 20 mL·min^{-1}. The TG/DSC curves were recorded in the range 25–1000 °C with a heating rate of 10 K·min^{-1}, using alumina crucibles.

The FT-IR spectra of the dried lyophilized of *A. absinthium* leaves and stems extracts were obtained using a Prestige-21 spectrometer (Shimadzu, Duisburg, Germany) at room temperature conditions. The spectral region ranged from 4000–400 cm^{-1} using KBr pellets and a resolution of 4 cm^{-1}.

LC-MS experiments were conducted on an 6120 LC-MS analytical system from Agilent (Santa Clara, CA, USA) consisting of 1260 Infinity HPLC equipped with G1322A degasser, G1311B cuaternary pump, G1316A column thermostat, G1365C MWD detector and G7129A autosampler coupled with a Quadrupolar (Q) mass spectrometer and electrospray ionization source (ESI). LC-MS is connected to a PC computer running the OpenLAB CDS ChemStation Workstation software.

The samples preparation for LC-MS analysis were homogenized with a WisdVM-10vortex mixer (Witeg Labortechnik, Wertheim, Baden-Württemberg, Germany) and centrifuged for 2 min at 10,000 rpm in a ThermoMicro CL17microcentrifuge (Thermo Fisher Scientific). The supernatant was collected and submitted to LC-MS analysis. Polyphenolic compounds were separated on a reverse phase Zorbax Eclipse Plus C18 column (3.0 mm × 100 mm × 3.5 μm). Gradient elution with a mixture of 0.1% acetic acid and methanol as mobile phase consists was performed: the first 5 min 5% methanol, until 38 min in gradient elution up to 42% methanol, proportion kept until 41 min and ending with 5% methanol for 1 more minute as described before [43]. The injection volume was 10 μL, the flow rate was 1 mL/min and the column temperature 40 °C. UV detection was conducted at 330 and 370 nm. MS detection was achieved by electrospray ionization (ESI) in the single ion monitoring mode (SIM) simultaneous for all screened compounds. All mass spectra were recorded in the negative ion mode. Capillary voltage was set at 3500 V, the dry gas flow was 12 L/min at 350 °C, the nebulizer pressure was kept at 55 psi and the fragmentor was set at 70. For the quantification of polyphenolic compounds calibration curves were conducted by the external standard method in the 0.05–2 μg/mL range for a six-point plot for each compound. The *m/z* scale of the mass spectrum was calibrated by use of an external calibration standard ESI Tuning Mix from Agilent.

4.6. Antioxidant Activity Assay

The antioxidant activity of *A. absinthium* extracts was determined by DPPH (2,2-diphenyl-1-picrylhydrazyl) free-radical scavenging assay. The electron donation ability of wormwood leaves and stems extracts was measured spectrophotometrically, leading to the yellow coloration of the initially purple-colored DPPH solution, according to the method of Manzoco et al. [44]. To 0.5 mL ethanolic extract of *A. absinthium* leaves/stems extracts (10–0.5 mg/mL), 2 mL solvent (ultrapure water) and 0.5 mL of 1 mM DPPH ethanolic solution were added. During the incubation period, the extracts were kept within the UV/VIS Spectrophotometer (T 70 type, from PG Instruments Ltd., Leicestershire, United Kingdom) where the absorbance of the samples was read continuously (for 10 min) against a blank at 516 nm. The results were expressed in comparison to an ethanol solution of ascorbic acid 0.1 mg/mL. The inhibition percentage of free radical DPPH, expressed as (IP%), was calculated with the formula below:

$$IP\% = \left[\frac{A_{DPPH} - A_{sample}}{A_{DPPH}}\right] * 100 \qquad (1)$$

where: A_{DPPH} is the absorbance of free radical DPPH (blank), measured at 516 without sample and A_{sample} is the absorbance of each sample in the presence of DPPH radical.

The half maximal inhibitory concentration (IC_{50}) was calculated by linear regression analysis curve plotting between inhibition percentage (IP%) and concentration of the ethanolic wormwood extracts.

4.7. Determination of Total Phenolic Content and Total Flavonoid Content of A. Absinthium

The total phenolic content of the ethanolic extracts from wormwood leaves and stems was evaluated using the Folin-Ciocalteu method, slightly modified [45]. The method was briefly the following: 0.5 mL of extract solutions (1 mg/mL) were mixed with 2.5 mL Folin-Ciocalteu reagent diluted 1:10. Then 2 mL of 7.5% sodium carbonate solution were added. Samples were kept in the dark for 90 min, then the absorbance was read versus blank at 750 nm using a UviLine 9400 Spectrophotometer from SI Analytics (Deutschland, Germany). The total phenolic content was determined using a gallic acid calibration curve (R^2 = 0.996). To this end, a gallic acid calibration curve was obtained, using gallic acid solutions of different concentrations (0.0025–0.1 mg/mL). The total phenolic content of the two extracts was calculated as milligrams of gallic acid equivalents (GAE) per gram extract.

The total flavonoid content of the two ethanolic extracts was evaluated using the following method [22]: an aliquot of 1 mg/mL extract solution (250 µL) was mixed with 5% $NaNO_2$ (75 µL). After 6 min, 10% $AlCl_3$ (150 µL) and 1M NaOH (500 µL) were added. The volume was adjusted to 2.5 mL with distilled water. The absorbance was read at 510 nm versus blank using a UviLine 9400 Spectrophotometer from SI Analytics. The total flavonoid content was calculated using a (+)-Catechin hydrate calibration curve (R^2 = 0.999) in the range 0.005–0.4 mg/mL. The results were expressed as milligrams catechin equivalents per gram extract (mg CE/g extract).

4.8. Alamar Blue Assay–Cell Viability Assessment

The viability was determined using the Alamar blue assay, a technique meant to evaluate the cytotoxic effect caused by different agents. The cells (1×10^4/well) were cultured in 96-well plates, allowed to adhere overnight and then stimulated with different concentrations of the extractive solutions (50, 100, 250, 500 and 1000 µg/mL) for 24, 48 and 72 h. After the stimulation periods, 20 µL of Alamar blue (10% of the volume of cell culture medium—200 µL/well) was added. The cells were incubated for 3h at 37 °C and then the absorbance was measured at two different wavelengths (570 and 600 nm) with an xMark™ Microplate spectrophotometer (BioRad, xMarkTMMicroplate, Serial No. 10578, Tokyo, Japan). The principle of this technique consists of the natural ability of metabolically active cells (viable cells) to reduce resazurin (dark blue compound) to the fluorescent form, resorufin (pink compound with intense fluorescence).

4.9. Selectivity-Index

In order to determine the selectivity of *A. absinthium* leaves and stems extracts, the selectivity index was calculated according to the following formula [38,46]:

$$\text{Selectivity index (SI)} = \frac{IC_{50\,[non-malignant\,HaCaT]}}{IC_{50\,[tumor\,cell\,line]}} \quad (2)$$

4.10. Scratch Assay–Assessment of the Anti-Migratory Potential

This method is an in vitro technique used to determine a possible inhibitory effect of *A absinthium* extractive solutions on the migration and invasion capacity of the tumor cell lines (A375 and MCF7 cells) and of the non-tumor cells (HaCaT). The protocol was applied as previously described in the literature [47]. Briefly, 2×10^5 cells/well were cultured in 12-well plates until 90% confluence was reached. Using a sterile pipette tip scratches were drawn on well-defined zones of the cells monolayer. The detached cells resulted from the procedure were removed by washing with phosphate-buffered saline (PBS) prior to stimulation. The cells were stimulated with different concentrations of the extractive solutions (50, 100, 250, 500 and 1000 µg/mL). Images of the cells in culture were taken at 0 h and 24 h and compared with the control cells (no stimulation). Pictures were taken with Olympus IX73 inverted microscope provided with DP74 camera (Olympus, Tokyo, Japan) and the analysis of the cell growth was performed with cell Sense Dimension software. The migration percentage was calculated according to the formula previously described by Felice et al. [48]:

$$\text{Scratch closure rate} = \left[\frac{A_{t_0} - A_t}{A_{t_0}}\right] * 100 \quad (3)$$

where: A_{t_0} is the scratch area at time 0; A_t is the scratch area at 24 h.

4.11. In Vivo TPA-Induced Ear Inflammation Protocol

In order to evaluate the effect of *A. absinthium* leaves and stems extracts on ear inflammation were performed *in vivo* experiment using SKH1 female mice (n = 3), 6 months old (weigh = 29.70–32.80 g); purchased from Charles River Laboratory (Budapest, Hungary). The mice were kept in standard conditions: a 20–24 °C temperature, humidity between 45–65%, a 12-h light/dark cycle, food *ad libitum* with free access to water, as recommended by the European Directive 2010/63/EU and the national law 43/2014. The protocol used for the euthanasia of the animals followed the Guidelines described by the American Veterinary Medical Association (AVMA) for the Euthanasia of Animals (2013 Edition). The Bioethical Committee of "Victor Babes" University of Medicine and Pharmacy Timisoara, Romania, approved the performed experiment.

The experimental model of TPA-induced ear inflammation was performed according to the following protocol: female mice were anesthetized with Isoflurane and the TPA solution was topically applied (20 µL/mouse ear) and they were assigned to the subsequent groups (Table 6).

Table 6. In vivo experimental design for the local acute inflammation model.

Group No.	Group Name	Description
1	Control	With no intervention
2	Control + Acetone	Acetone (solvent for TPA)—20 µL/mouse ear
3	TPA	TPA solution (20 µL/mouse ear)
4	TPA + Indomethacin	Indomethacine cream (4%) was topically applied after the TPA solution
5	TPA + *A. absinthium* L. leaves extract	*A. absinthium* leaves extract (~2%) was topically applied after the TPA solution
6	TPA + *A. absinthium* L. stems extract	*A. absinthium* stems extract (~2%) was topically applied after the TPA solution

An electronic caliper was used to measure the diameter and length of mice ears (the results were presented in millimeters) before the TPA application and at the end of the experiment. After 24 h the mice were weighted and after that were anesthetized and sacrificed, the ears were measured and collected for histopathological evaluation.

4.12. Histopathological Assessment of Mice Ears

For histopathological analysis, the mice ears were fixed in 10% buffered formalin for 48 h and then they were embedded in paraffin followed the routine automated flow of this procedure. Four μm-thick sections were cut using a Leica Rotary Microtome (Leica Biosystems Nussloch GmbH, Nussloch, Germany) and mounted on glass slides, deparaffinized in xylene and rehydrated. Finally, the samples were stained with the conventional Hematoxylin & Eosin. The slides were examined by two pathologists in a blinded way. Image acquisition and analysis were performed using a Nikon Eclipse E 600 microscope (Nikon Microscopes/Instruments Division, Vienna, Austria) and Lucia G software (Laboratory Imaging, Prague, Czech Republic) for microscopic image analysis.

4.13. Statistical Analysis

The statistical program used in the present study was GraphPad Prism 5 (GraphPad Software, San Diego, CA, USA). The data obtained were expressed as mean ± SD. Regarding the in vitro results, comparison among the groups was performed using the one-way ANOVA followed by Dunnett's multiple comparison test (* $p < 0.05$; ** $p < 0.01$; *** $p < 0.001$).

5. Conclusions

Results of this study showed that the ethanolic extracts from *A. absinthium* leaves and stems collected from Southern Romania contain chlorogenic acid, quercitrin, isoquercitrin and rutin. The IR profiles of extracts from leaves and stems of *A. absinthium* revealed the presence of active components with various functional groups (acid, alcohol, alkane, amine, amide, aromatic radicals). Leaves displayed a higher content of total phenolics and flavonoids than stems. Regarding the activity against cancer cells, at the check point of 72 h a significant cytotoxic activity against both MCF7 and A375 cell lines was detected. Wormwood stems extract were slightly more active than leaves extract. In the experimental conditions of our study, both leaves and stems extracts showed dose-dependent anti-migratory potential, MCF7 being the most sensitive cell line. Moreover, stems extract elicited a stronger anti-migratory activity. In an *in vivo* model of inflammation, the topical application of stems extract led to a noticeable anti-inflammatory effect, while the activity of the leaves extract was milder. Overall, *A. absinthium* from Southern Romania was proved to possess biological activities that can be exploited in further studies.

Supplementary Materials: The supplementary materials are available online.

Author Contributions: Conceptualization, E.-A.M., F.A. and I.Z.P.; methodology, E.-A.M., F.A., D.M., S.S., R.G. and A.C.; software, I.Z.P., F.A. and R.G.; validation, D.S.A., C.D. and C.-A.D.; formal analysis, D.A., C.D. and E.-A.M; investigation, A.C., M.D., S.S., R.G., I.Z.P., D.M., F.A. and E.-A.M.; resources, C.-A.D., Z.C., C.S. and R.C.; data curation, D.S.A., C.D. and C.-A.D.; writing—original draft preparation, E.-A.M., F.A. and I.Z.P.; writing—review and editing, D.S.A., C.-A.D., C.D., Z.C., R.C. and M.D.; visualization, E.-A.M., F.A. and D.S.A.; supervision, D.S.A., C.-A.D., C.S. and C.D.; project administration, C.-A.D.; funding acquisition, Z.C., R.C. and C.-A.D.

Funding: This research was funded by the project CNFIS-FDI-2019, grant number 0393, Project Manager Cristina Adriana Dehelean.

Conflicts of Interest: The authors declare no conflict of interest.

Abbreviations

LC-MS	Liquid chromatography–mass spectrometry
TG-DSC	Thermogravimetry-differential scanning calorimeter analysis
FT-IR	Fourier-transform infrared spectroscopy
Rt	Retention time
DPPH	2,2-Diphenyl-1-picrylhydrazyl
AOA	Antioxidant activity
IC_{50}	Maximal inhibitory concentration
IP	Inhibition percentage
HaCaT	Human keratinocytes
MCF7	Human breast adenocarcinoma cell line
PBS	Phosphate-buffered saline
A375	Human melanoma cell line
ATCC	American Type Culture Collection
DMEM	Dulbecco's Modified Eagle's Medium
EMEM	Eagle's Minimum Essential Medium
FBS	Fetal bovine serum
SD	Standard deviation
TPA	12-O-Tetradecanoylphorbol-13-acetate
ROS	Reactive oxygen species
MS	Mass spectroscopy
ESI	Electrospray ionization
SIM	Single ion monitoring mode
SI	Selectivity index
mg GAE	Milligrams of gallic equivalents
mg CE	Milligrams cathechin equivalents

References

1. Deans, S.G.; Kennedy, A.I. *Artemisia absinthium*. In *Artemisia*, 1st ed.; Wright, C.W., Ed.; CRC Press: London, UK, 2001; pp. 79–90.
2. Bora, K.S.; Sharma, A. The Genus Artemisia: A Comprehensive Review. *Pharm. Biol.* **2011**, *49*, 101–109. [CrossRef] [PubMed]
3. European Medicines Agency. Assessment Report on *Artemisia absinthium L.*, herba. Available online: https://docplayer.net/90203895-Assessment-report-on-artemisia-absinthium-l-herba.html (accessed on 24 August 2019).
4. Ivanescu, B.; Miron, A.; Lungu, C. Histo-anatomy of vegetative organs of some Artemisia species. *Med. Surg. J.* **2015**, *119*, 917–924.
5. Bruneton, J. *Pharmacognosie. Phytochimie. Plantes Médicinales*, 5th ed.; Lavoisier: Paris, France, 2016; pp. 767–769.
6. Hänsel, R.; Sticher, O. *Pharmakognosie–Phytopharmazie*, 8th ed.; Springer: Heidelberg, Germany, 2007; pp. 443–445.
7. Lee, Y.J.; Thiruvengadam, M.; Chung, I.M.; Nagella, P. Polyphenol composition and antioxidant activity from the vegetable plant *Artemisia absinthium* L. *AJCS* **2013**, *7*, 1921–1926.
8. Omer, B.; Krebs, S.; Omer, H.; Noor, T.O. Steroid-sparing effect of wormwood (*Artemisia absinthium*) in Crohn's disease: A double-blind placebo-controlled study. *Phytomedicine* **2007**, *14*, 87–95. [CrossRef] [PubMed]
9. Krebs, S.; Omer, T.N.; Omer, B. Wormwood (*Artemisia absinthium*) suppresses tumour necrosis factor alpha and accelerates healing in patients with Crohn's disease—A controlled clinical trial. *Phytomedicine* **2010**, *17*, 305–309. [CrossRef] [PubMed]
10. Krebs, S.; Omer, B.; Omer, T.N.; Fliser, D. Wormwood (*Artemisia absinthium*) for poorly responsive early-stage IgA nephropathy: A pilot uncontrolled trial. *Am. J. Kidney Dis.* **2010**, *56*, 1095–1099. [CrossRef] [PubMed]

11. Easmin, S.; Sarker, M.Z.I.; Ghafoor, K.; Ferdosh, S.; Jaffri, J.; Ali, M.E.; Mirhosseini, H.; Al-Juhaimi, F.Y.; Perumal, V.; Khatib, A. Rapid investigation of α-glucosidase inhibitory activity of Phaleria macrocarpa extracts using FTIR-ATR based fingerprinting. *J. Food Drug Anal.* **2017**, *25*, 306–315. [CrossRef] [PubMed]
12. Szymczycha-Madeja, A.; Welna, M.; Zyrnicki, W. Multi-element analysis, bioavailability and fractionation of herbal tea products. *J. Braz. Chem. Soc.* **2013**, *24*, 777–787. [CrossRef]
13. Mohani, N.; Ahmad, M.; Mehjabeen; Jahan, N. Evaluation of phytoconstituents of three plants Acorus calamus linn. *Artemisia absinthium* Linn and Bergenia himalaica boriss by FTIR spectroscopic analysis. *Pak. J. Pharm. Sci.* **2014**, *27*, 2251–2255. [PubMed]
14. Malaikozhundan, B.; Vaseeharan, B.; Vijayakumar, S.; Sudhakaran, R.; Gobi, N.; Shanthini, G. Antibacterial and antibiofilm assessment of Momordica charantia fruit extract coated silver nanoparticles. *Biocatal. Agric. Biotechnol.* **2016**, *8*, 189–196. [CrossRef]
15. Chang, H.; Kao, M.J.; Chen, T.L.; Chen, C.H.; Cho, K.C.; Lai1, X.R. Characterization of Natural Dye Extracted from Wormwood and Purple Cabbage for Dye-Sensitized Solar Cells. *Int. J. Photoenergy* **2013**, 1–8. [CrossRef]
16. Kumar, P.; SenthamilSelvi, S.; LakshmiPraba, A.; PremKumar, K.; Ganeshkumar, R.S.; Govindaraju, M. Synthesis of silver nanoparticles from Sargassum tenerrimum and screening phytochemcials for its anti-bacterial activity. *Nano Biomed. Eng.* **2012**, *4*, 12–16. [CrossRef]
17. Li, Y.Q.; Kong, D.X.; Wu, H. Analysis and evaluation of essential oil components of cinnamon barks using GC–MS and FTIR spectroscopy. *Ind. Crops Prod.* **2013**, *41*, 269–278. [CrossRef]
18. Heredia-Guerrero, J.A.; Benítez, J.J.; Domínguez, E.; Bayer, I.S.; Cingolani, R.; Athanassiou, A.; Heredia, A. Infrared and Raman spectroscopic features of plant cuticles: A review. *Front. Plant Sci.* **2014**, *5*, 305. [CrossRef] [PubMed]
19. Dai, J.; Mumper, R.J. Plant phenolics: Extraction, analysis and their antioxidant and anticancer properties. *Molecules* **2010**, *15*, 7313–7352. [CrossRef] [PubMed]
20. Bhat, M.Y.; Gul, M.Z.; Lohamror, L.R.; Qureshi, I.A.; Ghazi, I.A. An in vitro Study of the Antioxidant and Antiproliferative Properties of *Artemisia absinthium*—A Potent Medicinal Plant. *Free Radic. Antioxid.* **2018**, *8*, 18–25.
21. Bora, K.S.; Sharma, A. Evaluation of antioxidant and free-radical scavenging potential of *Artemisia absinthium*. *Pharm. Biol.* **2011**, *49*, 1216–1223. [CrossRef] [PubMed]
22. Msaada, K.; Salem, N.; Bachrouch, O.; Bousselmi, S.; Tammar, S.; Alfaify, A.; Al Sane, K.; Ben Ammar, W.; Azeiz, S.; Haj Brahim, A.; et al. Chemical composition and antioxidant and antimicrobial activities of wormwood (*Artemisia absinthium* L.) essential oils and phenolics. *J. Chem.* **2015**, *804658*, 1–12. [CrossRef]
23. Ivanescu, B.; Vlase, L.; Lungu, C.; Corciova, A. HPLC analysis of phenolic compounds from *Artemisia species*. *Eur. Chem. Bull.* **2016**, *5*, 119–123.
24. Sengul, M.; Ercisli, S.; Yildiz, H.; Gungor, N.; Kavaz, A.; Çetin, B. Antioxidant, antimicrobial activity and total phenolic content within the aerial parts of *Artemisia absinthum*, *Artemisia santonicum* and *Saponaria officinalis*. *Iran. J. Pharm. Res.* **2011**, *10*, 49–56.
25. Kumar, S.; Pandey, A.K. Chemistry and biological activities of flavonoids: An overview. *Sci. World J.* **2013**, 1–16. [CrossRef]
26. Singh, R.; Verma, P.K.; Singh, G. Total phenolic, flavonoids and tannin contents in different extracts of *Artemisia absinthium*. *J. Intercult. Ethnopharmacol.* **2012**, *1*, 101–104. [CrossRef]
27. Ivanescu, B.; Vlase, L.; Corciova, A.; Lazar, M.I. HPLC-DAD-MS study of polyphenols from *Artemisia absinthium*, *A. annua*, and *A. vulgaris*. *Chem. Nat. Compd.* **2010**, *46*, 468–470. [CrossRef]
28. Craciunescu, O.; Constantin, D.; Gaspar, A.; Toma, L.; Utoiu, E.; Moldovan, L. Evaluation of antioxidant and cytoprotective activities of Arnica montana L. and *Artemisia absinthium* L. ethanolic extracts. *Chem. Cent. J.* **2012**, *6*, 97. [CrossRef] [PubMed]
29. Aberham, A.; Cicek, S.S.; Schneider, P.; Stuppner, H. Analysis of Sesquiterpene Lactones, Lignans, and Flavonoids in Wormwood (*Artemisia absinthium* L.) Using High-Performance Liquid Chromatography (HPLC)–Mass Spectrometry, Reversed Phase HPLC, and HPLC–Solid Phase Extraction–Nuclear Magnetic Resonance. *J. Agric. Food Chem.* **2010**, *58*, 10817–10823. [CrossRef]
30. Sahin, S.; Aybastıer, Ö.; Işık, E. Optimisation of ultrasonic-assisted extraction of antioxidant compounds from *Artemisia absinthium* using response surface methodology. *Food Chem.* **2013**, *141*, 1361–1368. [CrossRef]
31. Huang, D. Dietary Antioxidants and Health Promotion. *Antioxidants* **2018**, *7*, 9. [CrossRef]

32. Kim, W.S.; Choi, W.J.; Lee, S.; Kim, W.J.; Lee, D.C.; Sohn, U.D.; Shin, H.S.; Kim, W. Anti-inflammatory, Antioxidant and Antimicrobial Effects of Artemisinin Extracts from *Artemisia annua* L. *Korean J. Physiol. Pharm.* **2015**, *19*, 21–27. [CrossRef]
33. Lee, J.H.; Lee, J.M.; Lee, S.H.; Kim, Y.G.; Lee, S.; Kim, S.M.; Cha, S.W. Comparison of Artemisinin Content and Antioxidant Activity from Various Organs of Artemisia Species. *Hortic. Environ. Biotechnol.* **2015**, *56*, 697–703. [CrossRef]
34. Mahmoudi, M.; Ebrahimzadeh, M.A.; Ansaroudi, F.; Nabavi, S.F.; Nabavi, S.M. Antidepressant and antioxidant activities of Artemisia absinthium L. at flowering stage. *Afr. J. Biotechnol.* **2009**, *8*, 7170–7175.
35. Koyuncu, I. Evaluation of anticancer, antioxidant activity and phenolic compounds of *Artemisia absinthium* L. Extract. *Cell Mol. Biol.* **2018**, *64*, 25–34. [CrossRef]
36. Gordanian, B.; Behbahani, M.; Carapetian, J.; Fazilati, M. In vitro evaluation of cytotoxic activity of flower, leaf, stem and root extracts of five Artemisia species. *Res. Pharm. Sci.* **2014**, *9*, 91–96.
37. Badisa, R.B.; Darling-Reed, S.F.; Joseph, P.; Cooperwood, J.S.; Latinwo, L.M.; Goodman, C.B. Selective cytotoxic activities of two novel synthetic drugs on human breast carcinoma MCF-7 cells. *Anticancer Res.* **2009**, *29*, 2993–2996.
38. Peña-Morán, O.A.; Villarreal, M.L.; Álvarez-Berber, L.; Meneses-Acosta, A.; Rodríguez-López, V. Cytotoxicity, Post-Treatment Recovery, and Selectivity Analysis of Naturally Occurring Podophyllotoxins from Bursera fagaroides var. fagaroides on Breast Cancer Cell Lines. *Molecules* **2016**, *21*, 1013.
39. Shafi, G.; Hasan, T.N.; Syed, N.A.; Al-Hazzani, A.A.; Alshatwi, A.A.; Jyothi, A.; Munshi, A. *Artemisia absinthium* (AA): A novel potential complementary and alternative medicine for breast cancer. *Mol. Biol. Rep.* **2012**, *39*, 7373–7379. [CrossRef]
40. Wei, X.; Xia, L.; Ziyayiding, D.; Chen, Q.; Liu, R.; Xu, X.; Li, J. The Extracts of *Artemisia absinthium* L. Suppress the Growth of Hepatocellular Carcinoma Cells through Induction of Apoptosis via Endoplasmic Reticulum Stress and Mitochondrial-Dependent Pathway. *Molecules* **2019**, *24*, 913. [CrossRef]
41. Bralley, E.E.; Greenspan, P.; Hargrove, J.L.; Wicker, L.; Hartle, D.K. Topical anti-inflammatory activity of Polygonum cuspidatum extract in the TPA model of mouse ear inflammation. *J. Inflamm. (Lond.)* **2008**, *5*, 1. [CrossRef]
42. Mau, J.L.; Chang, C.N.; Huang, S.J.; Chen, C.C. Antioxidant properties of methanolic extracts from Grifola frondosa, Morchella esculenta and Termitomyces albuminosus mycelia. *Food Chem.* **2004**, *87*, 111–118. [CrossRef]
43. Toiu, A.; Mocan, A.; Vlase, L.; Pârvu, A.E.; Vodnar, D.C.; Gheldiu, A.M.; Moldovan, C.; Oniga, I. Comparative Phytochemical Profile, Antioxidant, Antimicrobial and In Vivo Anti-Inflammatory Activity of Different Extracts of Traditionally Used Romanian Ajuga genevensis L. and A. reptans L. (Lamiaceae). *Molecules* **2019**, *24*, 1597. [CrossRef]
44. Manzocco, L.; Anese, M.; Nicoli, M.C. Antioxidant Properties of Tea Extracts as Affected by Processing. *LWT—Food Sci. Technol.* **1998**, *31*, 694–698. [CrossRef]
45. Riahi, L.; Chograni, H.; Elferchichi, M.; Zaouali, Y.; Zoghlami, N.; Mliki, A. Variations in Tunisian wormwood essential oil profiles and phenolic contents between leaves and flowers and their effects on antioxidant activities. *Ind. Crops Prod.* **2013**, *46*, 290–296. [CrossRef]
46. Siewert, B.; Pianowski, E.; Obernauer, A.; Csuk, R. Towards cytotoxic and selective derivatives of maslinic acid. *Bioorg. Med. Chem.* **2014**, *22*, 594–615. [CrossRef]
47. Ghiţu, A.; Schwiebs, A.; Radeke, H.H.; Avram, S.; Zupko, I.; Bor, A.; Pavel, I.Z.; Dehelean, C.A.; Oprean, C.; Bojin, F.; et al. A Comprehensive Assessment of Apigenin as an Antiproliferative, Proapoptotic, Antiangiogenic and Immunomodulatory Phytocompound. *Nutrients* **2019**, *11*, 858. [CrossRef]
48. Felice, F.; Zambito, Y.; Belardinelli, E.; Fabiano, A.; Santoni, T.; Di Stefano, R. Effect of different chitosan derivatives on in vitro scratch wound assay: A comparative study. *Int. J. Biol. Macromol.* **2015**, *76*, 236–241. [CrossRef]

Sample Availability: Not available.

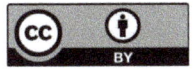

© 2019 by the authors. Licensee MDPI, Basel, Switzerland. This article is an open access article distributed under the terms and conditions of the Creative Commons Attribution (CC BY) license (http://creativecommons.org/licenses/by/4.0/).

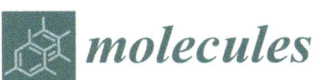

Article

The Antiproliferative Activity of Oxypeucedanin via Induction of G_2/M Phase Cell Cycle Arrest and p53-Dependent MDM2/p21 Expression in Human Hepatoma Cells

So Hyun Park, Ji-Young Hong, Hyen Joo Park and Sang Kook Lee *

College of Pharmacy, Natural Products Research Institute, Seoul National University, Seoul 08826, Korea; hanirela@snu.ac.kr (S.H.P.); jyhong7876@snu.ac.kr (J.-Y.H.); phj00@snu.ac.kr (H.J.P.)
* Correspondence: sklee61@snu.ac.kr; Tel.: +82-2-880-2475

Received: 5 December 2019; Accepted: 21 January 2020; Published: 23 January 2020

Abstract: Oxypeucedanin (OPD), a furocoumarin compound from *Angelica dahurica* (Umbelliferae), exhibits potential antiproliferative activities in human cancer cells. However, the underlying molecular mechanisms of OPD as an anticancer agent in human hepatocellular cancer cells have not been fully elucidated. Therefore, the present study investigated the antiproliferative effect of OPD in SK-Hep-1 human hepatoma cells. OPD effectively inhibited the growth of SK-Hep-1 cells. Flow cytometric analysis revealed that OPD was able to induce G_2/M phase cell cycle arrest in cells. The G_2/M phase cell cycle arrest by OPD was associated with the downregulation of the checkpoint proteins cyclin B1, cyclin E, cdc2, and cdc25c, and the up-regulation of p-chk1 (Ser345) expression. The growth-inhibitory activity of OPD against hepatoma cells was found to be p53-dependent. The p53-expressing cells (SK-Hep-1 and HepG2) were sensitive, but p53-null cells (Hep3B) were insensitive to the antiproliferative activity of OPD. OPD also activated the expression of p53, and thus leading to the induction of MDM2 and p21, which indicates that the antiproliferative activity of OPD is in part correlated with the modulation of p53 in cancer cells. In addition, the combination of OPD with gemcitabine showed synergistic growth-inhibitory activity in SK-Hep-1 cells. These findings suggest that the anti-proliferative activity of OPD may be highly associated with the induction of G_2/M phase cell cycle arrest and upregulation of the p53/MDM2/p21 axis in SK-HEP-1 hepatoma cells.

Keywords: oxypeucedanin; *Angelica dahurica*; antiproliferation; G_2/M phase cell cycle arrest; p53; SK-Hep-1; hepatoma cells

1. Introduction

Hepatocellular carcinoma (HCC) is the sixth most frequently diagnosed cancer and the second most common cause of death from cancer [1]. Approximately 30 to 40% of patients with HCC diagnosed at early stages are potentially effectively treated by surgical therapies such as hepatectomy or liver transplantation [2]. However, the disease diagnosed at an advanced stage or re-progression stage after treatment has poor prognosis due to the fundamental liver disease and lack of other treatment options [2–4]. In accordance, any systemic therapy has not effectively contributed to survival for patients with advanced HCC [5]. Therefore, it is necessary to procure potential chemotherapeutic agents for the treatment of advanced HCC cells.

Angelica dahurica (Umbelliferae) is an indigenous plant mainly distributed in Korea, China, and Russia. The root of *Angelica dahurica* has been used for the control of hysteria, bleeding, menstrual disorder, neuralgia and pain as a traditional medicine in Korea. Previous phytochemical studies revealed that the plant is a rich source of furanocoumarins, including oxypeucedanin [6]. Oxypeucedanin (OPD)

(Figure 1), a coumarin-type major constituent of the root of *Angelica dahurica*, has been reported to have several biological activities, including anti-mutagenic, uterus contraction, blood pressure increase, and cytotoxic and antiproliferative effects against cancer cells [7–9].

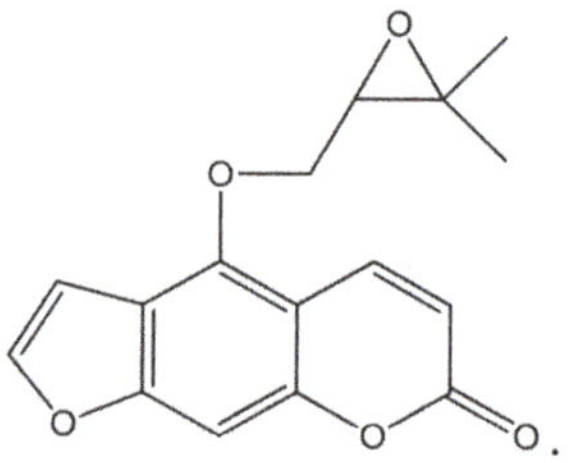

Figure 1. Chemical structure of oxypeucedanin (OPD).

When the DNA damage stimulus comes to the cells, the response of the cellular system is complex and finely controlled. The cellular response involves the functions of gene products that recognize DNA damage signals and activate processes such as the inhibition of proliferation, the stimulation of repair mechanisms, or the induction of apoptosis [10–12]. Generally, the cellular response to DNA damage and the disturbance to replication involve the activation of checkpoints, following signal transduction pathways for regulation of cell cycle progression and cell division [10,11]. Deficiency in these checkpoint responses can induce cell death, genomic instability, or predisposition to cancer [12–14]. In addition, cell cycle progression is finely regulated by cell cycle regulatory proteins and checkpoint proteins depending on the specific cell cycle phase. In particular, the G_2/M phase of the cell cycle is governed by the expression of key G_2/M transition regulatory proteins and the ATR/Chk1 signaling pathways. p53, a tumor suppressor, is also considered to be involved in the transcriptional regulation of a large number of growth-arrest and apoptosis-related genes [15].

Although several biological activities of OPD have been previously reported, the precise molecular mechanism of OPD related to its antiproliferative activity against human liver cancer cells has not been fully elucidated. In the present study, the growth-inhibitory activity and the underlying mechanisms of action of OPD were investigated in SK-Hep-1 human hepatoma cells.

2. Results

2.1. Antiproliferative Effects of Oxypeucedanin (OPD) in SK-Hep-1 Human Hepatoma Cells

To primarily evaluate whether OPD shows potential growth-inhibitory effects on human cancer cells, the anti-proliferative activity of OPD was determined in a panel of human cancer cell lines. As summarized in Table 1, OPD inhibited the growth of human cancer cells. Among the cell lines tested, SK-Hep-1 human hepatoma cells were the most sensitive to OPD. Therefore, further study on the mechanism of action of OPD in the regulation of cell proliferation was conducted in SK-Hep-1 cells. In addition, since OPD was shown to have the anti-proliferative activity against SK-Hep-1 cells, the isolated OPD analogs from the roots of *Angelica dahurica* were also evaluated for their antiproliferative activity in SK-Hep-1 cells. Among the test compounds, OPD was the most active growth inhibitor against SK-Hep-1 cells (Table 2).

Table 1. Anti-proliferative effects of furanocoumarins from *Angelica dahurica* on various human cancer cells.

Compounds	MDA-MB-231 [a]	T47D	SNU638	SK-Hep-1	A549
Isoimperatorin	>100	>100	90.2	>100	>100
Byakangelicol	74.7 [b]	46.0	50.0	72.1	41.1
Oxypeucedanin	50.8	95.5	50.4	32.4	46.3

[a] Cancer cell line: MDA-MB-231 (breast), T47D (breast), SK-Hep-1 (liver), A549 (lung), SNU638 (stomach), [b] IC$_{50}$ value: µM.

Table 2. Anti-proliferative effects of oxypeucedanin analogs on SK-Hep-1 cells.

Compounds	R	IC$_{50}$ (µM)
Oxypeucedanin		32.4
Isooxypeucedanin		91.5
Oxypeucedanin hydrate		81.0
Oxypeucedanin methanolate		77.4

Since the anti-proliferative activity of OPD was found in SK-Hep-1 human hepatoma cells for 72 h, the growth-inhibitory activity of OPD was also investigated for 24 or 48 h in SK-Hep-1 cells. As shown in Figure 2, OPD exhibited growth-inhibitory activity against SK-Hep-1 human hepatoma cells in a concentration- and time-dependent manner.

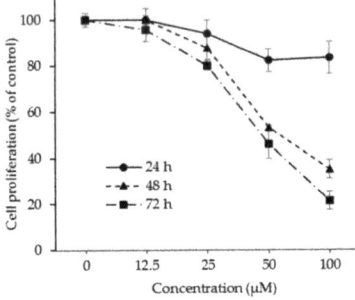
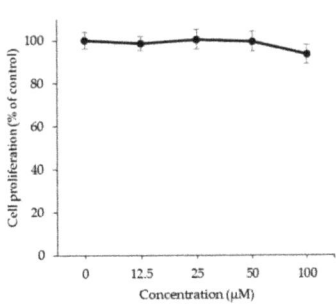

Figure 2. Anti-proliferative effects of OPD in SK-Hep-1 human hepatoma cells (left) and MRC5 human normal cell line (right). SK-Hep-1 cells were cultured in a 96-well plate and treated with the indicated concentrations of OPD for 24–72 h. MRC5 cells were cultured in a 96-well plate and treated with the indicated concentrations of OPD for 72 h. The cell proliferative activity was determined using the SRB assay. The % cell proliferation value was calculated by the mean absorbance of samples/absorbance of the vehicle-treated control as described in the Materials and Methods. Data are presented as the means ± S.E. ($n = 3$).

The IC$_{50}$ value of OPD with a 72 h treatment was 32.4 µM. In addition, the growth-inhibitory activity of OPD was also determined in a normal cell line. OPD was unable to affect the growth rate of MRC5 normal human lung fibroblast cells (IC$_{50}$ >100 µM). These data suggest that OPD may be able to selectively inhibit the proliferation of human hepatoma cancer cells compared to normal cells. Under the same experimental conditions, the IC$_{50}$ value of etoposide, a positive control, was 0.3 µM.

2.2. Effects of OPD on the Cell Cycle Distribution of SK-Hep-1 Cells

To further elucidate the anti-proliferative mechanisms of OPD in SK-Hep-1 cells, the cells were treated with the indicated concentrations of OPD for 24 h, and flow cytometry analysis was performed with PI staining. As shown in Figure 3A, OPD enhanced the accumulation of the G$_2$/M phase peak from 22.66% (control) to 35.90% (75 µM). These data suggest that the antiproliferative activity of OPD in SK-Hep-1 cells is in part associated with the induction of G$_2$/M phase cell cycle arrest. To further investigate whether the G$_2$/M phase cell cycle arrest by OPD is correlated with the regulation of the checkpoint proteins, the expression of the G$_2$/M cell cycle regulatory proteins was determined by western blot analysis. Since OPD did not show significant cytotoxicity at the test concentration up to 100 µM for 24 h (Figure 2), the cells were treated with OPD (50, 75, or 100 µM) for 24 h, and then the checkpoint protein expression related to G$_2$/M phase cell cycle regulation was measured in SK-Hep-1 cells. As shown in Figure 3B, the expression levels of Chk1, p-cdc25c (Ser198), cdc25c, cyclin B1, cdc2, and p-cdc2 (Thr161) were downregulated, but the levels of p-Chk1 (Ser345) were upregulated by OPD treatment. Chk1 (checkpoint kinase 1) is a multifunctional protein kinase that coordinates the response to specific types of DNA damage [16]. Cdc25 is a protein phosphatase responsible for dephosphorylating and activating cdc2, a pivotal step in directing the cells toward mitosis [17]. When DNA damage ocurrs, the Chk1 phosphorylates cdc25c, which then leads to translocation of cdc25c from the cytoplasm to the nucleus, where cdc25c can interact with cdc2/cyclin B during mitosis [18,19]. Moreover, the activity of the cdc2-cyclin B1 complex is dependent on the phosphorylation/dephosphorylation status of cdc2 [11,13,20]. The entry of eukaryotic cells into mitosis is regulated by cdc2 activation, including the binding of cdc2 to cyclin B1 and its phosphorylation at the Thr161 residue. In this study, we found that cdc25c was inactivated by phosphor-Chk1 with OPD treatment, and the activation of the cdc2-cyclin B1 complex was also suppressed by OPD in a concentration-dependent manner, indicating the induction of G$_2$/M phase cell cycle arrest by OPD. These findings suggest that the activation of Chk1 and sequential regulation of signal transduction pathways by OPD may be due to the induction of G$_2$/M phase cell cycle arrest by OPD in SK-Hep-1 cells.

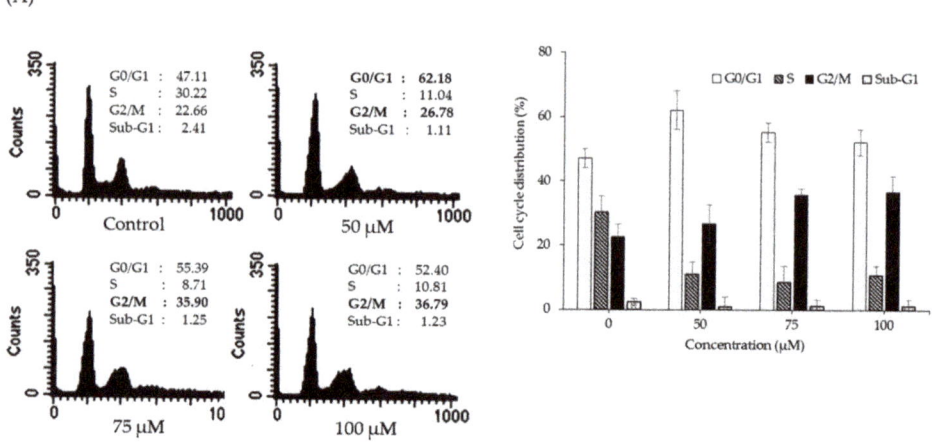

Figure 3. *Cont.*

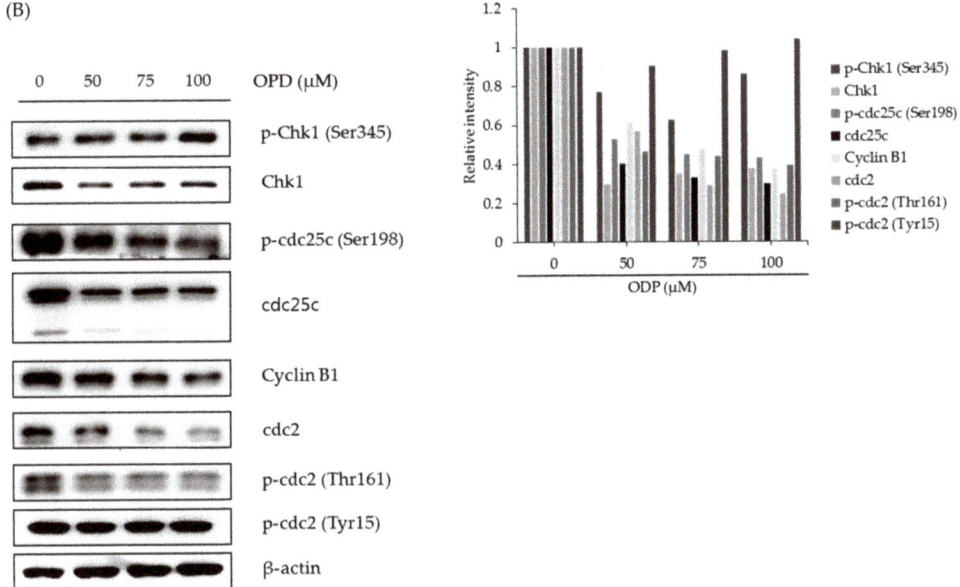

Figure 3. Effects of OPD on the regulation of cell cycle distribution in SK-Hep-1 cells. (**A**) SK-Hep-1 cells were treated with various concentrations of OPD for 24 h. Both adherent and floating cells were collected, fixed with 70% cold ethanol overnight, and then incubated with RNase A and PI for 30 min. The cell cycle distribution was analyzed by flow cytometry. (**B**) The cells were treated with the indicated concentrations of OPD for 24 h, and the expression of cell cycle regulatory proteins was determined by western blot analysis. β-Actin was used as an internal control.

2.3. Effects of OPD on the Regulation of p53-associated Signaling Pathways in SK-Hep-1 Cells

To further validate the association of p53-mediated signaling molecules in the anti-proliferative activity of OPD in SK-Hep-1 cells, the cells was treated with OPD for 24 h, and then the expression of p53-associated molecules were determined by western blot analysis. OPD significantly enhanced the protein expression of p53, p-p53(Ser15), MDM2, p21, and GADD45α in the cells (Figure 4A). Previous studies have reported that the phosphorylation of p53 at Ser15 or Ser20 upregulates p53 stability by disrupting the interaction between p53 and MDM2 [21,22]. Because OPD is able to induce the stability of p53, the accumulation of p53 by OPD may subsequently enhance its downstream target genes, including MDM2, p21, and GADD45α, in the cells. In addition, the expression of p53-associated proteins was also monitored for up to 48 h with treatment with 50 μM OPD and was found to be up-regulated after 4 h of treatment in SK-Hep-1 cells (Figure 4B). Further study was designed to confirm whether the cellular localization of p53 is affected by treatment of cells with OPD. Generally, in the nucleus, MDM2-mediated ubiquitination led to the transportation of p53 into the cytoplasm or its degradation by the 26S proteasome [21,22]. As an important transcriptional factor, the stability and nuclear localization of p53 are considered essential for its tumor suppressor activity [23]. Therefore, we determined the levels of p53 and MDM2 protein expression in both the cytosol and nucleus fraction following treatment with OPD in SK-Hep-1 cells. As shown in Figure 4C, the levels of p53 protein expression were upregulated and localized in the nucleus upon OPD treatment for 24 h in a concentration-dependent manner. The levels of MDM2 protein expression were also shown to be upregulated in the nucleus by OPD treatment in the cells. To further confirm the effects of OPD on the expression of p53-associated proteins, OPD treatment of cells was conducted in the absence or presence of caffeine. Because caffeine is known as an ATR/Chk1 kinase inhibitor [24,25], the effect of caffeine on the enhanced p53-associated protein expression by OPD was investigated in the cells.

As expected, treatment with OPD (50 µM) for 24 h led to a significant upregulation of p53, p21, and MDM2 expression in the absence of caffeine, but the pretreatment with caffeine for 2 h alleviated the enhancement of p53-associated protein expression by OPD in SK-Hep-1 cells (Figure 4D). Although the expression of p53-associated proteins was downregulated by the pretreatment with caffeine, OPD also exhibited a slight upregulation of p53 and p21 expression in the presence of caffeine (Figure 4D). These data suggest that the induction of G_2/M phase cell cycle arrest by OPD seems to be associated with not only the ATR/Chk1 signaling pathway but also the regulation of p53-mediated pathways. Further study examined the maintenance of p53 stability by OPD with the cotreatment of cycloheximide (CHX), a protein synthesis inhibitor [26], in SK-Hep-1 cells. As shown in Figure 4E, OPD significantly suppressed the degradation of p53 in the presence of cycloheximide, suggesting that the half-life of p53 degradation was sustained by OPD treatment compared to vehicle-treated control cells. However, the rate of MDM2 degradation was not greatly affected by the down-regulation of p53 turnover with OPD treatment of cells.

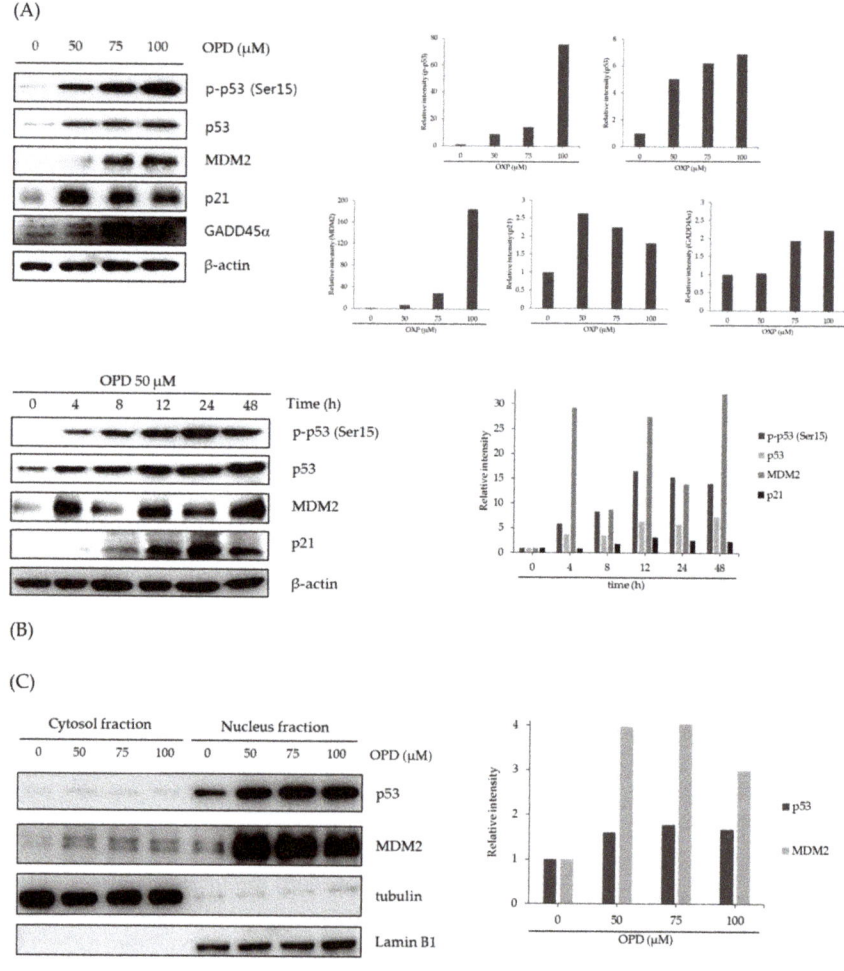

Figure 4. Cont.

(D)

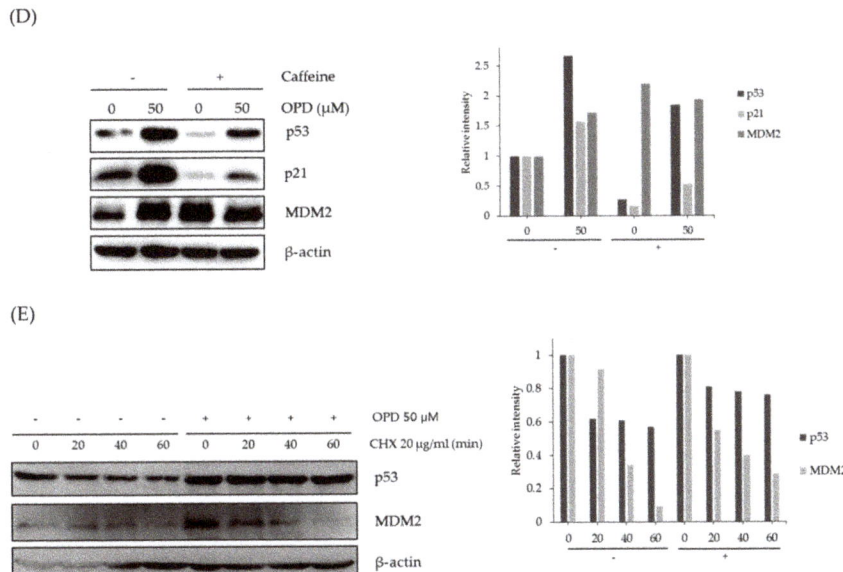

(E)

Figure 4. Effects of OPD on the regulation of p53-associated signaling pathways. (**A**) SK-Hep-1 cells were treated with the indicated concentrations of OPD for 24 h. The expression level of proteins was analyzed by western blot. β-Actin was used as an internal control. (**B**) SK-Hep-1 cells were treated with 50 μM OPD for various time points up to 48 h. The expression level of proteins was analyzed by western blot. β-Actin was used as an internal control. (**C**) SK-Hep-1 cells were treated with various concentrations of OPD for 24 h. After cells were harvested, the proteins were separated into cytosolic and nuclear fractions as described in the Materials and Methods. The protein expression levels were analyzed by western blot. β-Actin was used as an internal control. (**D**) SK-Hep-1 cells were pretreated for 2 h with 1 mM caffeine, and then cultured with 50 μM OPD for an additional 24 h. The expression level of proteins was analyzed by western blot. β-Actin was used as an internal control. (**E**) SK-Hep-1 cells were treated with 50 μM OPD for 24 h and then treated in the absence or presence of 20 μg/mL cycloheximide. The cells were harvested at 0, 20, 40, and 60 min. The expression level of proteins was analyzed by western blot, and the band density was quantified using the NIH ImageJ software (Bethesda, MD).

2.4. Effects of OPD on Cell Proliferation Depending on the p53 Status in Hepatoma Cells

Since p53 seems to be highly associated with the anti-proliferative activity of OPD in SK-Hep-1 cells, the effects of p53 status on the growth-inhibitory activity of OPD were evaluated in human hepatoma cells with different p53 statuses. The cells were treated with various concentrations of OPD for 72 h, and then cell proliferation was determined by the SRB assay. As shown in Figure 5A, wild-type p53 cell lines, such as SK-Hep-1 and HepG2, were more sensitive than the p53-null Hep3B cell line, indicating that p53 plays an important role in the anti-proliferative activity of OPD in human hepatoma cells. To further confirm the involvement of p53 in the antiproliferative activity of OPD, p53 siRNA was transfected into wild-type p53 SK-Hep-1 cells, and the effect of p53 siRNA on the cell proliferation was determined in SK-Hep-1 cells. When the p53 siRNA transfected-SK-Hep-1 cells were treated with OPD (50 μM) for 48 and 72 h, the antiproliferative activity of OPD was decreased compared to that of the control cells (no transfection or scrambled siRNA transfection), suggesting that the anti-proliferative activity of OPD is partly associated with wild-type p53 expression in hepatoma cells (Figure 5B). In addition, the OPD treatment exhibited upregulation of p53 and MDM2 in the control cells. Although p53 expression was not shown in p53 siRNA-treated SK-Hep-1 cells, OPD slightly up-regulated the expression of MDM2 in p53 siRNA-treated SK-Hep-1 cells (Figure 5C).

(A)

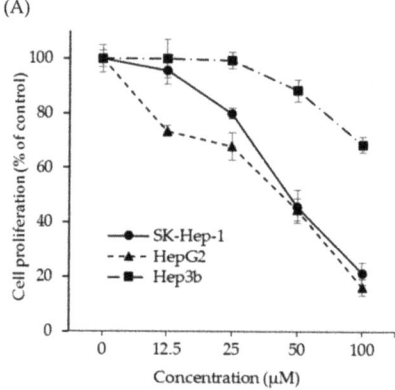

Cell line	IC$_{50}$ (μM)	p53 status
SK-Hep-1	32.4	wild
HepG2	43.8	wild
Hep3B	>100	null

(B)

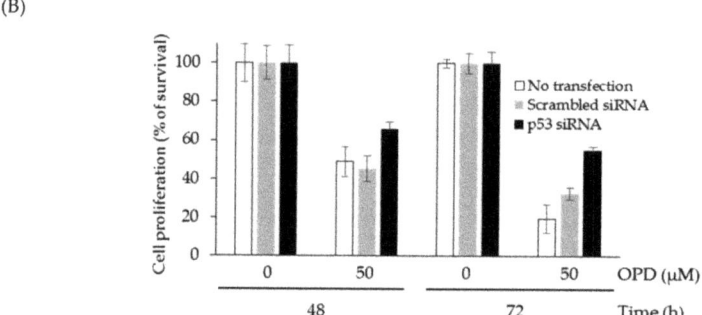

(C)

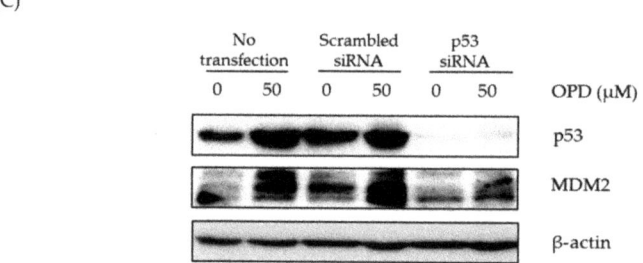

Figure 5. Effects of p53 expression on the cell proliferation of hepatoma cells by OPD. (**A**) SK-Hep-1, HepG2, and Hep3B cells were cultured in a 96-well plate and treated with the indicated concentrations of OPD for 72 h. The cell proliferative effect was determined using the SRB assay. Data are presented as the means ± S.E. (n = 3). (**B**) SK-Hep-1 cells were transfected with 5 nM p53 siRNA or scrambled siRNA for 24 h, and then OPD treatment (50 μM) was given for 48 or 72 h for the measurement of cell proliferation. Data are presented as the means ± S.E. (n = 3). (**C**) The effects of p53 siRNA on the expression level of p53 and MDM2 were analyzed by western blot in control cells and p53 siRNA-transfected SK-Hep-1 cells.

2.5. Effects of OPD in Combination with Gemcitabine on the Cell Proliferation of SK-Hep-1 Cells

To further investigate the effect of the combination of OPD with an anticancer agent on the antiproliferative activity of hepatoma cells, we selected gemcitabine, a pyrimidine-based DNA synthesis inhibitor, as a candidate compound based on the use of patients with liver cancer in the clinic. As shown in Figure 6A, cotreatment with OPD and gemcitabine exhibited a synergistic effect (CI < 1.0) on the antiproliferative activity of SK-Hep-1 cells. The combination of the higher concentrations of OPD and gemcitabine showed a relatively stronger synergistic activity. In accordance, when OPD (20 µM) was treated with various concentrations of gemcitabine (0.1–0.4 µM), the combination with the higher concentration of gemcitabine (0.4 µM) was shown to have a stronger synergistic activity (Figure 6).

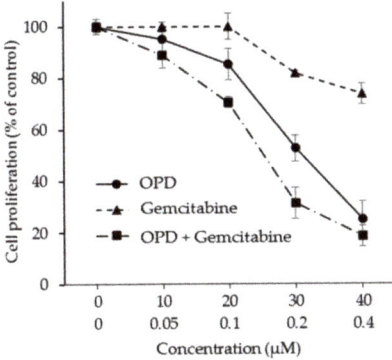

Oxypeucedanin (µM)	Gemcitabine (µM)	Combination index (CI)	Description
20	0.1	1.08	Additive
30	0.2	0.78	Moderate synergism
40	0.4	0.82	Moderate synergism

Figure 6. Combination effect of OPD with gemcitabine on the cell proliferation of SK-Hep-1 cells. (**A**) The cells were treated with the indicated concentrations of OPD and gemcitabine for 72 h, and then cell proliferation was measured by the SRB assay. (**B**) The cells were treated with OPD (20 µM) and various concentrations of gemcitabine (0.1–0.4 µM) for 72 h, and then cell proliferation was measured by the SRB assay. Data are presented as the means ± S.E. ($n = 3$). Based on the cell proliferation data.

Natural products have been used for traditional medicines and also play an important role in drug discovery and development programs. In particular, anticancer drugs are mainly developed based on natural product-originated small molecules. In our continuous efforts to procure small molecules from natural sources in the discovery of antitumor agents, oxypeucedanin (OPD), a furanocoumarin isolated from the root of *Angelica dahurica*, was considered a potential candidate. Previous biological activities of OPD include the effective intervention of sunitinib-induced nephrotoxicity, the hepatoprotective activity of tacrine-induced cytotoxicity in liver cells, and the cytotoxicity against cancer cells such as gastric cancer, prostate cancer, and melanoma cells [27,28]. Although the antiproliferative activities of OPD have been reported in cancer cells, the precise molecular mechanism of OPD in the anticancer activity of human liver cancers remains to be elucidated. This study demonstrates that OPD regulates the induction of G_2/M phase cell cycle arrest and p53-dependent MDM2/p21 signaling pathways in human hepatoma SK-Hep-1 cells.

It is known that the cell cycle is a finely controlled sequence of events in the growth and proliferation of eukaryotic cells. Cell cycle progression occurs in an ordered manner that is monitored by cell cycle checkpoints. Among the checkpoints, the DNA damage-induced G_2/M checkpoint guarantees the fidelity of genomic stability. However, cancer cells have abnormally activated in cell division as a result of diverse factors, including uncontrolled checkpoint protein expression. These defects in the checkpoints lead to genomic instability, cell death, or carcinogenesis. Therefore, the regulation of the G_2/M checkpoint is often applied as a potential therapeutic target to evaluate the efficacy of natural product-derived antitumor agents in cancer cells. In the present study, we found that OPD effectively inhibited the growth of SK-Hep-1 human hepatoma cells. Cell cycle distribution analysis also revealed that the antiproliferative activity of OPD is in part associated with the induction of G_2/M cell cycle arrest in cells. This result was consistent with the previous report of G_2/M phase arrest of OPD in prostate cancer cells [27]. However, a previous study of the antiproliferative activity of OPD on the prostate cancer cells did not investigate in detail the regulatory biomarkers involved in G_2/M phase cell cycle arrest in cancer cells. The present study revealed that the induction of G_2/M phase cell cycle arrest by OPD was correlated with the regulation of Chk1-mediated G_2/M checkpoint proteins, including cdc25c/cdc2 and cdc2/cyclin B1 complex pathways, in hepatoma cells. Chk1 is considered to play an important role in the G_2/M checkpoint via the ATM-RAD3-related (ATR) pathway. Chk1 also regulates the activity of its shared downstream substrate, cell division cycle 25c (cdc25c). OPD effectively modulates the Chk1-cdc25c activation pathway axis, leading to the induction of G_2/M cell cycle arrest in SK-Hep-1 cells. We also found that OPD effectively suppressed the activity of cyclin B1 and its partner cell division cycle 2 (cdc2) expression, which in turn evokes the prevention of entry into the mitosis (M) phase cell cycle transition in hepatoma cells.

Tumor suppressor p53 is mutated, deleted, or rearranged in more than half of all human tumors, and thus, p53 is considered an important target in anticancer drug development [29,30]. p53 is also considered an important factor in the control of the cell cycle at the G_1/S and/or G_2/M transition through diverse mechanisms [31]. In this study, we found that OPD significantly up-regulated the expression of p53 by the accumulation of p53 and increased its stability in SK-Hep-1 cells. The upregulation of p53 levels by OPD led to the activation of downstream target expression such as MDM2, p21 and GADD45α in cells. The association of p53 in G_2/M phase cell cycle signaling was further confirmed by the significant suppression of p53, p21 and MDM2 expression by treatment with caffeine, an ATR/Chk1 inhibitor, in SK-Hep-1 cells. However, OPD did not fully recover the levels of p53 and its downstream target protein expression in the presence of caffeine, indicating that OPD may cause the activation of p53 independently of the ATR/Chk1 pathway. The involvement of p53 in the anti-proliferative activity of OPD in SK-Hep-1 cells was also confirmed using cell types with different p53 statuses and deletion methods. OPD was found to be more effective in p53-wild-type expression cells, and p53 siRNA-transfected cells were less sensitive to the OPD in the antiproliferative activity on liver cancer cells.

The function of p53 is mainly governed by the stability and nuclear localization of p53 in cells. We found that OPD effectively inhibits the degradation of p53 and thus sustains the stability of p53 in cancer cells. In addition, OPD was found to induce the nuclear localization of p53, which may activate the transcriptional activity of its downstream target genes associated with cell cycle regulation in cancer cells.

Gemcitabine (2′,2′-difluorodeoxycytidine), a pyrimidine-based antimetabolite, is currently used to the treatment of pancreatic cancer as well as other cancers [32,33]. Gemcitabine inhibits DNA replication by activating the S-phase checkpoint. A study also showed that gemcitabine activates the ATR/Chk1 pathway [34]. In the present study, we found that OPD in combination with gemcitabine exhibits synergistic anti-proliferative activity in SK-Hep-1 cells. Therefore, OPD might be a promising lead compound in combination with cancer chemotherapeutic agents in advanced liver cancer treatment. In addition, in terms of clinical relevance of furanocoumarins, the bioavailability of oxypeucedanin in plasma samples may be important parameters. In the previous study, Chen et al. [35] reported that the pharmacokinetic parameters of OPD were the Tmax (12 h), T1/2 (2.4 h), and oral bioavailability (F, 10.1%) in rat models by oral administration of OPD. These data suggest that the oral bioavailability of

OPD is a relatively low and thus needed to be further study for improvement of the bioavailability either structural modifications or appropriate formulation of administration of OPD.

3. Materials and Methods

3.1. Chemicals

Dulbecco's modified Eagle's medium (DMEM) and fetal bovine serum (FBS) were purchased from HyClone Laboratories (Logan, UT, USA). Antibiotics-antimycotics solution, Lipofectamine®RNAiMAX, negative control siRNA, and Opti-MEM®Reduced Serum Medium were purchased from Invitrogen (Grand Island, NY, USA). p53-specific siRNA was purchased from Bioneer (Daejeon, Korea). The nuclear extract kit was purchased from Active Motif (Carlsbad, CA, USA). Bovine serum albumin (BSA), dimethyl sulfoxide (DMSO), trichloroacetic acid (TCA), sulforhodamine B (SRB), propidium iodide (PI), ribonuclease A (RNase A), and other agents were purchased from Sigma-Aldrich (St. Louis, MO, CA). Antibodies against p-chk1 (Ser345) (#2348), chk1 (#2360), p-cdc25c (Ser198) (#9529), cdc25c (#4688), p-cdc2 (Tyr15) (#9111), p-cdc2 (Thr161) (#9114), p-p53 (Ser15) (#9284), p21 (#3733), and α/β tubulin (#2148) were purchased from Cell Signaling (Danvers, MA, USA). Antibodies against cyclin B1 (#752), cdc-2 (#54), β-actin, p53 (#126), MDM2 (#965), GADD45α (#797), lamin B1 (#20682) were obtained from Santa Cruz Biotechnology (Dallas, TX, USA)

OPD (Figure 1) and its analogs, isolated from the root of *Angelica dahurica*, were provided by Dr. Jin-Woong Kim (College of Pharmacy, Seoul National University, Seoul, Korea). *Angelica dahurica* (9 kg, dry weight) was purchased from Kyungdong Market Herbal Medicine in Seoul, and ultrasonically extracted three times for 120 min with 100% MeOH. The extract was filtered and concentrated under reduced pressure to obtain MeOH extract (910 g), which was suspended in distilled water to obtain a $CHCl_3$ fraction (229 g). OPD and its analogs were obtained by various column chromatography. Each component was analyzed by ^{1}H-NMR, ^{13}C-NMR, and FABMS, and then identified compared with the literature values of corresponding compounds. OPD and its analogs, dissolved in 100% DMSO.

3.2. Cell Culture

SK-Hep-1, HepG2, and Hep3B cells were purchased from the American Type Culture Collection (Manassas, VA, USA). Cells were cultured in DMEM supplemented with 10% heat-inactivated fetal bovine serum (FBS) and antibiotics-antimycotics (PSF; 100 units/mL penicillin G sodium, 100 μg/mL streptomycin, and 250 ng/mL amphotericin B). Cells were incubated in a humidified atmosphere containing 5% CO_2 at 37 °C.

3.3. Cell Proliferation Assay

Cell proliferation was measured by the sulforhodamine B (SRB) assay [36]. Cells were seeded in 96-well plates (3×10^4 cells/mL), incubated for 24 h, and either fixed (for zero day controls) or treated with various concentrations of test compounds (total volume of 200 μL/well) for 24, 48, and 72 h. After treatment, the cells were fixed with 50% TCA solution and dried at room temperature. Fixed cells were stained in 0.4% SRB in 1% acetic acid, and unbound dye was washed with 1% acetic acid. Stained cells were dried and dissolved in 10 mM Tris (pH 10.0). The absorbance was measured at 515 nm, and cell proliferation was determined as follows: cell proliferation (%) = (average absorbance compound − average absorbance zero day) / (average absorbance control − average absorbance zero day) × 100. IC_{50} values were calculated by non-linear regression analysis using the TableCurve 2D v5.01 software (Systat Software Inc., San Jose, CA, USA).

3.4. Cell Cycle Analysis

SK-Hep-1 cells were plated at a density of 1×10^6 cells per 100-mm culture dish and incubated for 24 h. Fresh media containing various concentrations of test sample were added to the culture dishes. Following a 24 h incubation, the cells were harvested (trypsinization and centrifugation) and fixed with 70% ethanol overnight at 4 °C. Fixed cells were washed with PBS and incubated with a staining solution containing RNase A (50 µg/mL) and propidium iodide (50 µg/mL) in PBS for 30 min at room temperature. The cellular DNA content was analyzed with a FACSCalibur flow cytometer (BD Biosciences, San Jose, CA, USA). At least 20,000 cells were used for each analysis, and the distribution of cells in each phase of the cell cycle was displayed as histograms.

3.5. Western Blot Analysis

SK-Hep-1 human hepatoma cells were exposed to various concentrations of OPD for the indicated times. After incubation, the cells were lysed, and the protein concentrations were determined by the bicinchoninic acid method [37]. Each protein was subjected to 6–15% SDS-PAGE. Proteins were transferred onto PVDF membranes (Millipore, Bedford, MA, USA) by electroblotting, and membranes were blocked for 1 h with blocking buffer [5% bovine serum albumin (BSA) in tris-buffered saline-0.1% Tween 20 (TBST)] at room temperature [38]. Membranes were then incubated with indicated antibodies (mouse anti-β-actin, diluted 1:10,000; other antibodies, diluted 1:500–1:1000 in 5% BSA/TBST) overnight at 4 °C and washed three times for 10 min with TBST. After washing, membranes were incubated with corresponding secondary antibodies diluted 1:2000 in TBST for 2 h at room temperature, washed three times for 10 min with TBST, and visualized with an enhanced chemiluminescence (ECL) detection kit (LabFrontier, Suwon, Korea) using an LAS-4000 Imager (Fuji Film Corp., Tokyo, Japan).

3.6. RNA Interference

RNA interference of p53 was performed using siRNA duplexes purchased from Bioneer (Daejeon, Korea). The coding strand for p53 siRNA was as follows: sense CACUACAACUACA UGUGUA and antisense UACACAUGUAGUUGUAGUG. For transfection, reverse transfection was conducted using Lipofectamine RNAiMAX (Invitrogen) according to the manufacturer's recommendations. Compound treatments occurred 24 h after transfection. Cells were harvested after 24 h and examined by western blotting.

3.7. Combination Assay

Determination of the effect of combination therapy was performed using the SRB assay. On day 1, 3000 cells/well in a volume of 100 µL were plated in 96-well plates. On day 2, gemcitabine (100, 200, or 400 nM) and OPD (20, 30, or 40 µM) were each added in a volume of 50 µL, in all combinations. After 72 h, the cells were fixed with 50% TCA solution for 30 min at 4 °C, rinsed 5 times with water, and air-dried. Fixed cells were colored with 80 µL of 0.4% sulforhodamine B in 0.1% acetic acid) rinsed with 0.1% acetic acid, and air dried. Sulforhodamine was redissolved in 200 µL/well of 10 mM Tris, pH 10, and the absorbance was measured at 515 nm. After calculating the percent of inhibition by OPD and gemcitabine, the combination index (CI) was estimated to evaluate the synergistic effect of OPD and gemcitabine:

$$CI = \frac{(D)_1}{(D_m)_1 [f_a/(1-f_a)]^{\frac{1}{m_1}}} + \frac{(D)_2}{(D_m)_2 [f_a/(1-f_a)]^{\frac{1}{m_2}}}$$

where D = dose; Dm = median-effect dose; m = kinetic order; fa = fraction affected.

The combination index (CI) is a quantitative measure based on the mass-action law of the degree of drug interaction in terms of synergism and antagonism (Table 3) for a given endpoint of the effect measurement.

Table 3. Description and symbols of synergism or antagonism in drug combination studies analyzed with the combination index method.

Range of Combination Index	Description	Symbols
<0.1	Very strong synergism	+++++
0.1–0.3	Strong synergism	++++
0.3–0.7	Synergism	+++
0.7–0.85	Moderative synergism	++
0.85–0.90	Slight synergism	+
0.90–1.10	Nearly addictive	±
1.10–1.20	Slight antagonism	−
1.20–1.45	Moderate antagonism	− −
1.45–3.3	Antagonism	− − −
3.3–10	Strong antagonism	− − − −
>10	Very strong antagonism	− − − − −

3.8. Statistical Analysis

All experiments were repeated at least three times. Data are presented as the means ± standard error (SE) for the indicated number of independently performed experiments and analyzed using Student's *t*-test. Values of $p < 0.05$ were considered statistically significant.

4. Conclusions

In summary, the present study demonstrates the antiproliferative activities of OPD on SK-Hep-1 human hepatoma cells. The inhibition of proliferation of cancer cells was in part associated with cell cycle arrest at the G_2/M phase and the tumor suppressor p53-mediated signaling pahway (Figure 7). These findings suggest that OPD is a promising new chemotherapeutic candidate for the management of human hepatoma cell treatment.

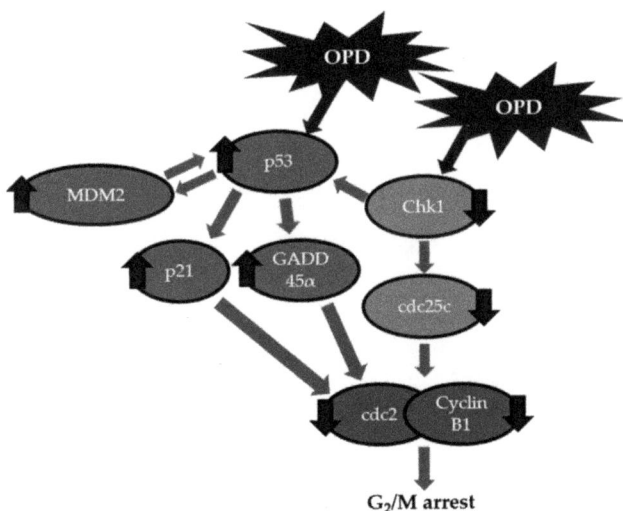

Figure 7. Schematic representation of the mechanisms of action of OPD against SK-Hep-1 human hepatoma cells.

Author Contributions: Conceptualization, S.K.L.; Methodology, S.H.P. and J.-Y.H.; Validation, S.H.P.; Formal Analysis, S.H.P.; Investigation, S.H.P.; Resources, S.K.L.; Data Curation, S.H.P.; Writing-Original Draft Preparation, S.H.P.; Writing-Review & Editing, J.-Y.H., H.J.P. and S.K.L.; Visualization, S.H.P.; Supervision, S.K.L.; Project Administration, S.K.L. All authors have read and agreed to the published version of the manuscript.

Funding: This study was supported by a National Research Foundation of Korea (NRF) Grant funded by the Korean Government (NRF-2016M3A9B6903499) and the Basic Science Research Program through the National Research Foundation of Korea (NRF) funded by the Ministry of Education (2019 R1I1A1A01060558).

Conflicts of Interest: The authors declare no conflict of interest.

References

1. Jemal, A.; Bray, F.; Center, M.M.; Ferlay, J.; Ward, E.; Forman, D. Global cancer statistics. *Ca. Cancer. J. Clin.* **2011**, *61*, 69–90. [CrossRef]
2. Llovet, J.M.; Burroughs, A.; Bruix, J. Hepatocellular carcinoma. *Lancet* **2003**, *362*, 1907–1917. [CrossRef]
3. Bruix, J.; Sherman, M. Management of hepatocellular carcinoma. *Hepatology* **2005**, *42*, 1208–1236. [CrossRef] [PubMed]
4. Bruix, J.; Sherman, M.; Llovet, J.M.; Beaugrand, M.; Lencioni, R.; Burroughs, A.K.; Christensen, E.; Pagliaro, L.; Colombo, M.; Rodes, J. Clinical management of hepatocellular carcinoma. Conclusions of the barcelona-2000 easl conference. European association for the study of the liver. *J. Hepatol.* **2001**, *35*, 421–430. [CrossRef]
5. Llovet, J.M.; Bruix, J. Systematic review of randomized trials for unresectable hepatocellular carcinoma: Chemoembolization improves survival. *Hepatology* **2003**, *37*, 429–442. [CrossRef]
6. Bai, Y.; Li, D.; Zhou, T.; Qin, N.; Li, Z.; Yu, Z.; Hua, H. Coumarins from the roots of angelica dahurica with antioxidant and antiproliferative activities. *J. Funct. Foods* **2016**, *20*, 453–462. [CrossRef]
7. Wall, M.E.; Wani, M.C.; Manikumar, G.; Hughes, T.J.; Taylor, H.; McGivney, R.; Warner, J. Plant antimutagenic agents, 3. Coumarins. *J. Nat. Prod.* **1988**, *51*, 1148–1152. [CrossRef]
8. Cai, Y.; Baer-Dubowska, W.; Ashwood-Smith, M.; DiGiovanni, J. Inhibitory effects of naturally occurring coumarins on the metabolic activation of benzo[a]pyrene and 7,12-dimethylbenz[a]anthracene in cultured mouse keratinocytes. *Carcinogenesis* **1997**, *18*, 215–222. [CrossRef]
9. Oh, H.; Lee, H.S.; Kim, T.; Chai, K.Y.; Chung, H.T.; Kwon, T.O.; Jun, J.Y.; Jeong, O.S.; Kim, Y.C.; Yun, Y.G. Furocoumarins from angelica dahurica with hepatoprotective activity on tacrine-induced cytotoxicity in hep g2 cells. *Planta Med.* **2002**, *68*, 463–464. [CrossRef]
10. Branzei, D.; Foiani, M. Regulation of DNA repair throughout the cell cycle. *Nat. Rev. Mol. Cell Biol.* **2008**, *9*, 297–308. [CrossRef]
11. Goodarzi, A.A.; Block, W.D.; Lees-Miller, S.P. The role of atm and atr in DNA damage-induced cell cycle control. *Prog. Cell Cycle Res.* **2003**, *5*, 393–411. [PubMed]
12. Zhivotovsky, B.; Kroemer, G. Apoptosis and genomic instability. *Nat. Rev. Mol. Cell Biol.* **2004**, *5*, 752–762. [CrossRef] [PubMed]
13. Hartwell, L.H.; Kastan, M.B. Cell cycle control and cancer. *Science* **1994**, *266*, 1821–1828. [CrossRef] [PubMed]
14. Molinari, M. Cell cycle checkpoints and their inactivation in human cancer. *Cell Prolif.* **2000**, *33*, 261–274. [CrossRef]
15. Levine, A.J. P53, the cellular gatekeeper for growth and division. *Cell* **1997**, *88*, 323–331. [CrossRef]
16. Dai, Y.; Grant, S. New insights into checkpoint kinase 1 in the DNA damage response signaling network. *Clin. Cancer Res.* **2010**, *16*, 376–383. [CrossRef]
17. Jessus, C.; Ozon, R. Function and regulation of cdc25 protein phosphate through mitosis and meiosis. *Prog. Cell Cycle Res.* **1995**, *1*, 215–228.
18. Blasina, A.; de Weyer, I.V.; Laus, M.C.; Luyten, W.H.; Parker, A.E.; McGowan, C.H. A human homologue of the checkpoint kinase cds1 directly inhibits cdc25 phosphatase. *Curr. Biol.* **1999**, *9*, 1–10. [CrossRef]
19. Furnari, B.; Blasina, A.; Boddy, M.N.; McGowan, C.H.; Russell, P. Cdc25 inhibited in vivo and in vitro by checkpoint kinases cds1 and chk1. *Mol. Biol. Cell* **1999**, *10*, 833–845. [CrossRef]
20. Porter, L.A.; Donoghue, D.J. Cyclin b1 and cdk1: Nuclear localization and upstream regulators. *Prog. Cell Cycle Res.* **2003**, *5*, 335–347.
21. Chehab, N.H.; Malikzay, A.; Stavridi, E.S.; Halazonetis, T.D. Phosphorylation of ser-20 mediates stabilization of human p53 in response to DNA damage. *Proc. Natl. Acad. Sci. USA* **1999**, *96*, 13777–13782. [CrossRef] [PubMed]
22. Unger, T.; Juven-Gershon, T.; Moallem, E.; Berger, M.; Vogt Sionov, R.; Lozano, G.; Oren, M.; Haupt, Y. Critical role for ser20 of human p53 in the negative regulation of p53 by mdm2. *Embo J.* **1999**, *18*, 1805–1814. [CrossRef] [PubMed]

23. Yuan, J.; Luo, K.; Zhang, L.; Cheville, J.C.; Lou, Z. Usp10 regulates p53 localization and stability by deubiquitinating p53. *Cell* **2010**, *140*, 384–396. [CrossRef] [PubMed]
24. Hall-Jackson, C.A.; Cross, D.A.; Morrice, N.; Smythe, C. Atr is a caffeine-sensitive, DNA-activated protein kinase with a substrate specificity distinct from DNA-pk. *Oncogene* **1999**, *18*, 6707–6713. [CrossRef]
25. Nghiem, P.; Park, P.K.; Kim, Y.; Vaziri, C.; Schreiber, S.L. Atr inhibition selectively sensitizes g1 checkpoint-deficient cells to lethal premature chromatin condensation. *Proc. Natl. Acad. Sci. USA* **2001**, *98*, 9092–9097. [CrossRef]
26. Jin, L.; Li, C.; Xu, Y.; Wang, L.; Liu, J.; Wang, D.; Hong, C.; Jiang, Z.; Ma, Y.; Chen, Q.; et al. Epigallocatechin gallate promotes p53 accumulation and activity via the inhibition of mdm2-mediated p53 ubiquitination in human lung cancer cells. *Oncol. Rep.* **2013**, *29*, 1983–1990. [CrossRef]
27. Kang, T.J.; Lee, S.Y.; Singh, R.P.; Agarwal, R.; Yim, D.S. Anti-tumor activity of oxypeucedanin from ostericum koreanum against human prostate carcinoma du145 cells. *Acta Oncol.* **2009**, *48*, 895–900. [CrossRef]
28. Kimura, Y.; Sumiyoshi, M.; Sakanaka, M.; Taniguchi, M.; Baba, K. In vitro and in vivo antiproliferative effect of a combination of ultraviolet-a and alkoxy furocoumarins isolated from umbelliferae medicinal plants, in melanoma cells. *Photochem. Photobiol.* **2013**, *89*, 1216–1225. [CrossRef]
29. Greenblatt, M.S.; Bennett, W.P.; Hollstein, M.; Harris, C.C. Mutations in the p53 tumor suppressor gene: Clues to cancer etiology and molecular pathogenesis. *Cancer Res.* **1994**, *54*, 4855–4878.
30. Hollstein, M.; Sidransky, D.; Vogelstein, B.; Harris, C.C. P53 mutations in human cancers. *Science* **1991**, *253*, 49–53. [CrossRef]
31. Dai, C.; Gu, W. P53 post-translational modification: Deregulated in tumorigenesis. *Trends Mol. Med.* **2010**, *16*, 528–536. [CrossRef] [PubMed]
32. Carmichael, J. The role of gemcitabine in the treatment of other tumours. *Br. J. Cancer* **1998**, *78* (Suppl. 3), 21–25. [CrossRef]
33. Nabhan, C.; Krett, N.; Gandhi, V.; Rosen, S. Gemcitabine in hematologic malignancies. *Curr. Opin. Oncol.* **2001**, *13*, 514–521. [CrossRef] [PubMed]
34. Arlander, S.J.; Eapen, A.K.; Vroman, B.T.; McDonald, R.J.; Toft, D.O.; Karnitz, L.M. Hsp90 inhibition depletes chk1 and sensitizes tumor cells to replication stress. *J. Biol. Chem.* **2003**, *278*, 52572–52577. [CrossRef] [PubMed]
35. Chen, L.; Jian, Y.; Wei, N.; Yuan, M.; Zhuang, X.; Li, H. Separation and simultaneous quantification of nine furanocoumarins from radix angelicae dahuricae using liquid chromatography with tandem mass spectrometry for bioavailability determination in rats. *J. Sep. Sci.* **2015**, *38*, 4216–4224. [CrossRef] [PubMed]
36. Vichai, V.; Kirtikara, K. Sulforhodamine b colorimetric assay for cytotoxicity screening. *Nat. Protoc.* **2006**, *1*, 1112–1116. [CrossRef] [PubMed]
37. Smith, P.K.; Krohn, R.I.; Hermanson, G.; Mallia, A.; Gartner, F.; Provenzano, M.; Fujimoto, E.; Goeke, N.; Olson, B.; Klenk, D. Measurement of protein using bicinchoninic acid. *Anal. Biochem.* **1985**, *150*, 76–85. [CrossRef]
38. Byun, W.S.; Kim, W.K.; Han, H.J.; Chung, H.-J.; Jang, K.; Kim, H.S.; Kim, S.; Kim, D.; Bae, E.S.; Park, S. Targeting histone methyltransferase dot1l by a novel psammaplin a analog inhibits growth and metastasis of triple-negative breast cancer. *Mol. Ther. -Oncolytics* **2019**, *15*, 140–152. [CrossRef]

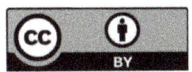

© 2020 by the authors. Licensee MDPI, Basel, Switzerland. This article is an open access article distributed under the terms and conditions of the Creative Commons Attribution (CC BY) license (http://creativecommons.org/licenses/by/4.0/).

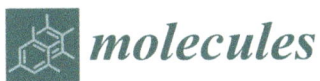

Article

Caffeic Acid Attenuates Multi-Drug Resistance in Cancer Cells by Inhibiting Efflux Function of Human P-Glycoprotein

Yu-Ning Teng [1], Charles C.N. Wang [2], Wei-Chieh Liao [3], Yu-Hsuan Lan [3,*] and Chin-Chuan Hung [3,4,*]

[1] Department of Medicine, College of Medicine, I-Shou University, 8 Yida Road, Kaohsiung 82445, Taiwan; eunicegh520@gmail.com
[2] Department of Bioinformatics and Medical Engineering, Asia University, 500 Lioufeng Rd., Wufeng, Taichung 41354, Taiwan; chaoneng.wang@gmail.com
[3] Department of Pharmacy, College of Pharmacy, China Medical University, 91 Hsueh-Shih Road, Taichung 40402, Taiwan; u102003316@cmu.edu.tw
[4] Department of Pharmacy, China Medical University Hospital, 2 Yude Road, Taichung 40447, Taiwan
* Correspondence: lanyh@mail.cmu.edu.tw (Y.-H.L.); cc0206hung@gmail.com (C.-C.H.); Tel.: +886-4-22053366 (ext. 5138) (Y.-H.L.); +886-4-22053366 (ext. 5155) (C.-C.H.); Fax: +886-4-22078083 (Y.-H.L. & C.-C.H.)

Academic Editor: Kyoko Nakagawa-Goto
Received: 14 November 2019; Accepted: 6 January 2020; Published: 7 January 2020

Abstract: Multidrug resistance (MDR) is a complicated ever-changing problem in cancer treatment, and P-glycoprotein (P-gp), a drug efflux pump, is regarded as the major cause. In the way of developing P-gp inhibitors, natural products such as phenolic acids have gotten a lot of attention recently. The aim of the present study was to investigate the modulating effects and mechanisms of caffeic acid on human P-gp, as well as the attenuating ability on cancer MDR. Calcein-AM, rhodamine123, and doxorubicin were used to analyze the interaction between caffeic acid and P-gp, and the ATPase activity of P-gp was evaluated as well. Resistance reversing effects were revealed by SRB and cell cycle assay. The results indicated that caffeic acid uncompetitively inhibited rhodamine123 efflux and competitively inhibited doxorubicin efflux. In terms of P-gp ATPase activity, caffeic acid exhibited stimulation in both basal and verapamil-stimulated activity. The combination of chemo drugs and caffeic acid resulted in decreased IC_{50} in *ABCB1*/Flp-In^{TM}-293 and KB/VIN, indicating that the resistance was reversed. Results of molecular docking suggested that caffeic acid bound to P-gp through GLU74 and TRY117 residues. The present study demonstrated that caffeic acid is a promising candidate for P-gp inhibition and cancer MDR attenuation.

Keywords: caffeic acid; cancer multidrug resistance; P-glycoprotein; phenolic acid

1. Introduction

As cancer is one of the leading causes of death worldwide, cancer treatment is always on the top of listed hot research topics [1]. With advanced scientific researches and abundant medical resources in recent decades, diverse options have been developed to conquer cancer and related diseases. Nevertheless, the multi-drug resistance (MDR) of cancer treatment is still an ever-changing problem and more in-depth studies have been conducted to unveil the complicated characteristics of cancer treatment. Cancer MDR manifests cross resistance to several structurally and mechanically different chemo-agents and could be contributed to the following reasons [2]. The change in tumor microenvironment [3–5], decreased drug uptake [6], adapted cell apoptotic pathways [7–9], drug inactivation through metabolism [10,11], the influence of epigenetic regulation [12,13], mutation of drug target site [14], and the increased drug efflux [15] have been reported to play important roles in causing cancer MDR. Among the above mechanisms, the increased drug efflux by ATP-binding cassette (ABC) transporters has been regarded as the most influential cause. ABC transporter superfamily consists of several subfamilies, and P-glycoprotein (P-gp) is one of the most comprehensively studied proteins [16]. P-gp is encoded by human *ABCB1* gene and can recognize various clinically used drugs, including antidepressants, HIV protease inhibitors, immunosuppressive agents, and chemotherapeutic drugs [17,18]. The diverse structures recognizing and effluxing the ability of P-gp, result in insufficient chemo-drug concentration inside cancer cells, therefore, causing cancer MDR.

There have been a series of P-gp inhibitor developments along the cancer MDR reversing agents discovering history, and the improvements have been based on previous failure experiences [19]. First generation P-gp inhibitors are potent but toxic as the required dose is high; examples of this are quinidine and verapamil [20]. Second generation inhibitors have exhibited better effects with lower IC_{50}, but the involvement of these inhibitors in CYP450 interaction has impeded their further application [21,22]. Third generation inhibitors, including tariquidar and zosuquidar, have demonstrated prominent MDR reversal effects. However, they have still faced failure in clinical studies [23,24]. Therefore, severe toxicity and interaction of the above chemical reagents have turned the research direction toward natural resources, aiming at discovering low toxic and potent structures from plants, fungi, or marine organisms.

Among various natural resources, phytochemicals such as flavonoids and phenolic acids get much attention due to their multiple pharmacological effects, including antioxidant and antitumor activity [25,26]. Several phytochemicals, such as cyanidin, catechin, quercetin, caffeic acid, and ellagic acid, have been related to the down-regulation of human LDL oxidation [27]. Ellagic acid and ursolic acid have been reported to exhibit preventive and therapeutic effects against breast cancer cells [28]. Caffeic acid (Figure 1), a phenolic acid that widely exists in vegetables, fruits, and tea extracts, is well-known as a natural antioxidant [29]. Besides, caffeic acid has also been identified to have anti-inflammatory, antibacterial, and antiviral effects [30,31]. With regards to cancer treatment, caffeic acid and its derivative, caffeic acid phenethyl ester (CAPE), exhibit some therapeutic effects toward lung cancer and breast cancer cells, as well as breast cancer pre-clinical models [32–34]. CAPE has been well studied in previous researches, including its *MDR1* gene down-regulating effects in MCF-7 and MDA-MB-231 breast cancer cells [34] and P-gp inhibitory effects in HeLa resistant cancer subline and human intestinal LS174T cell line [35,36]. Nevertheless, the P-gp inhibitory and MDR modulating information of the caffeic acid was insufficient and warrants further detailed investigation.

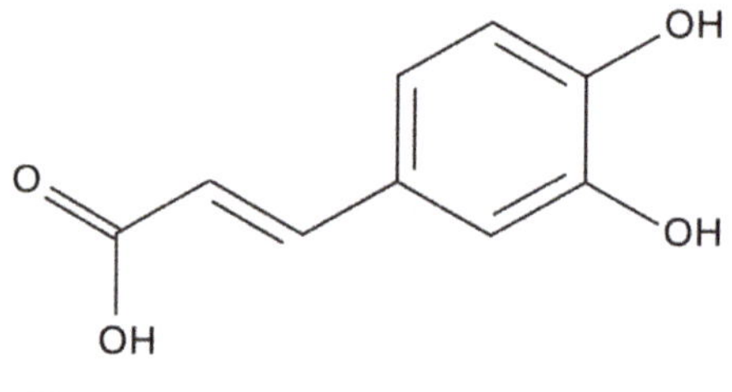

Figure 1. The chemical structure of caffeic acid.

Therefore, in the present study, comprehensive researches of caffeic acid were conducted. The interaction of caffeic acid with human P-gp, as well as the inhibitory effects and mechanisms were assessed in P-gp over-expressing cell line *ABCB1*/Flp-In^{TM}-293. The cancer MDR reversing ability of caffeic acid was then evaluated in both *ABCB1*/Flp-In^{TM}-293 and KB/VIN MDR cancer cell lines. The present study demonstrated that caffeic acid is a promising candidate for P-gp inhibition and cancer MDR attenuation.

2. Results

2.1. Caffeic Acid Is Non-Cytotoxic toward Experimental Cell Lines and Is Not a Substrate of P-gp

Before conducting further experiments, the cytotoxicity of caffeic acid was examined in HeLaS3, KB/VIN, Flp-In^{TM}-293, and *ABCB1*/Flp-In^{TM}-293 cell lines to select a rational concentration range. Caffeic acid exhibited higher than 80% cell viability in all tested cell lines under the treatment of 100 µg/mL for 72 h. Hence, the following assays were conducted with caffeic acid of not more than 100 µg/mL.

The first characteristic of caffeic acid on P-gp was demonstrated through MDR1 shift assay, which revealed whether a compound is a substrate of P-gp. P-gp's substrates activate a conformational change detected by the structure-sensitive UIC2 antibody. As Figure 2 showed, the fluorescent peaks of caffeic acid 20 and 25 µg/mL did not shift to the right as the positive control vinblastine did, indicating that the conformation of P-gp was not influenced by caffeic acid. Therefore, caffeic acid is not P-gp's substrate.

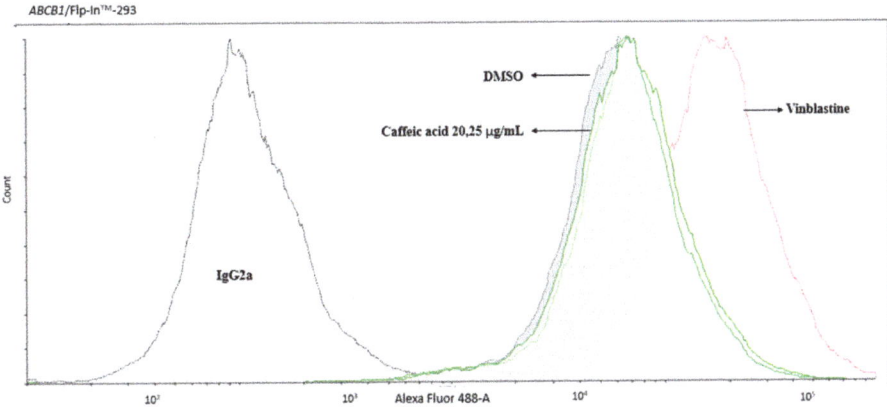

Figure 2. The result of MDR1 shift assay. The conformation of P-gp was not influenced under the treatment of 20 and 25 µg/mL caffeic acid. Vinblastine (a standard substrate of P-gp) was used as a positive control.

2.2. The Inhibitory Effects, Mechanisms and Binding Modes of Caffeic Acid on Human P-gp Function

The inhibitory effect of caffeic acid on P-gp function was screened with calcein-AM accumulation assay. Calcein-AM is a non-florescent substance and P-gp's substrate. It will be transformed to fluorescent calcein (not a P-gp substrate) by cell esterase. Therefore, under the treatment of P-gp's inhibitor, the intracellular calcein fluorescence is higher than the normal condition. The results of caffeic acid are revealed in Figure 3a. When *ABCB1*/Flp-In^{TM}-293 cell line was treated with caffeic acid in amounts of 5, 10, and 20 µg/mL, the intracellular calcein fluorescence was increased in a concentration-dependent manner. Hence, the efflux function of P-gp could be inhibited by caffeic acid.

Caffeic acid's inhibitory effects and mechanisms were further demonstrated via the other two substrates of P-gp, rhodamine123 and doxorubicin. As Figure 3b showed, the efflux of fluorescent substrate rhodamine123 was inhibited by caffeic acid 10 and 20 µg/mL treatment and followed Michaelis-Menten kinetics. The Lineweaver-Burk plot (Figure 3c) indicated that caffeic acid inhibited rhodamine123 efflux in an uncompetitive pattern, both V_{max} and K_m decreased when the *ABCB1*/Flp-In^{TM}-293 cell line was treated with increased caffeic acid concentrations (Table 1). Same as rhodamine123, the efflux of the chemotherapeutic drug doxorubicin was also inhibited by caffeic acid dose-dependently (Figure 3d). However, the inhibitory mechanism of caffeic acid on doxorubicin was competitive inhibition, different from rodamine123 (Figure 3e). When the *ABCB1*/Flp-In^{TM}-293 cell line was treated with an increased concentration of caffeic acid, the K_m (affinity) increased accordingly and the V_{max} remained constant (Table 1).

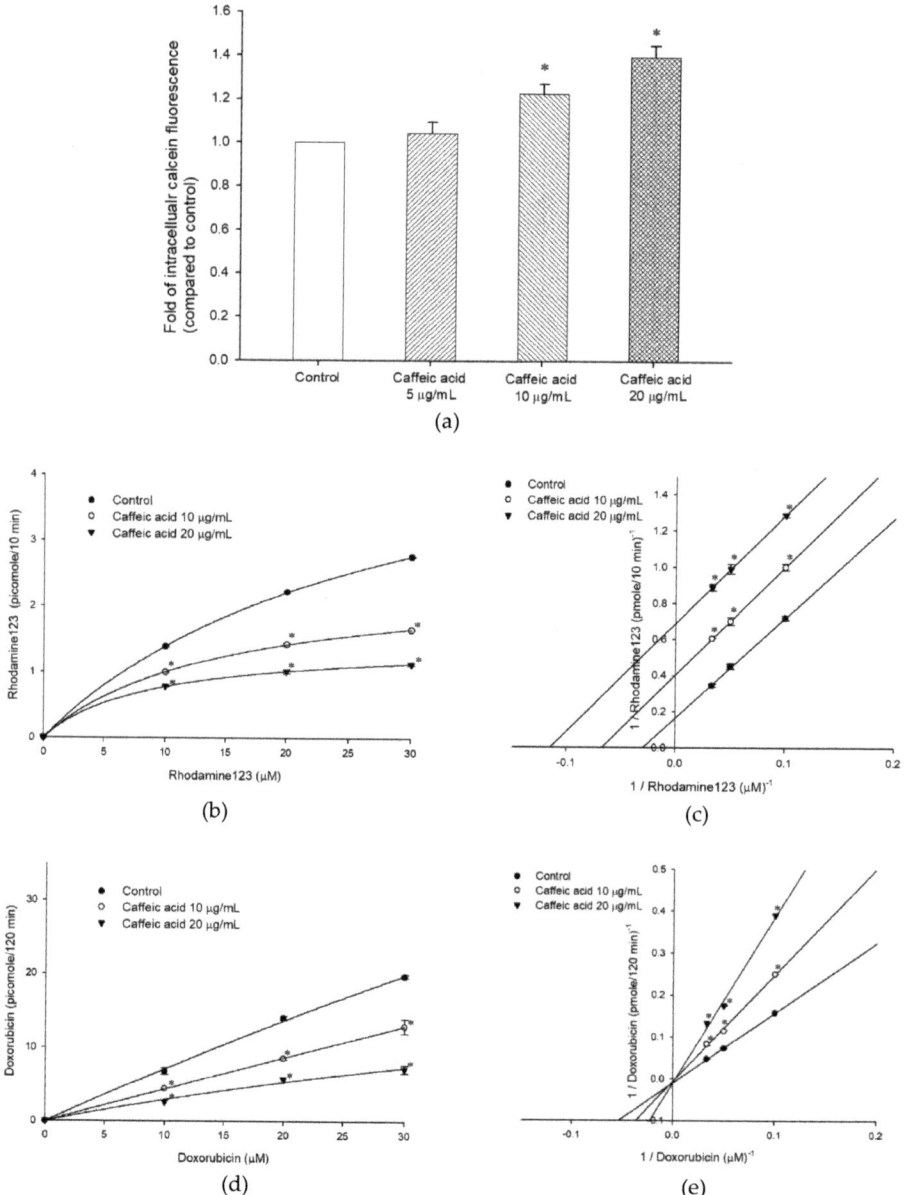

Figure 3. *Cont.*

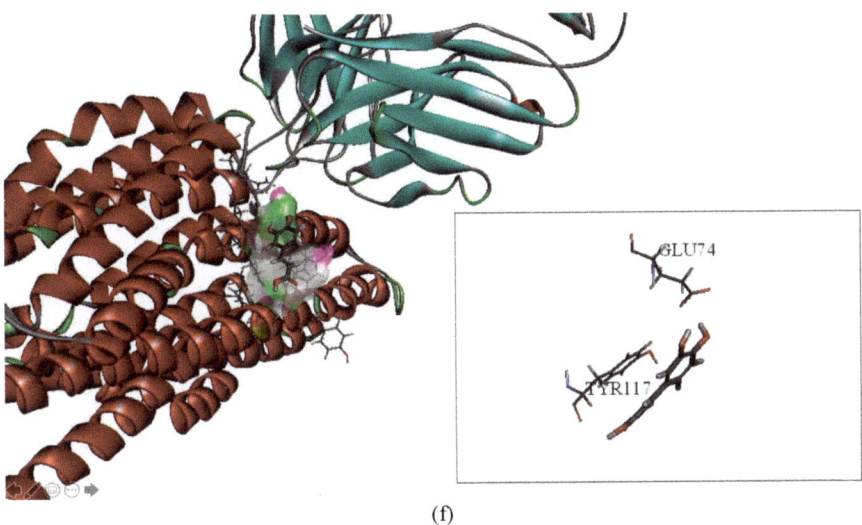

(f)

Figure 3. The effects of caffeic acid on human P-gp efflux function. (**a**) Intracellular calcein fluorescence with or without caffeic acid pretreatment in $ABCB1$/Flp-In^{TM}-293 cell line (over-expressing human P-gp). (**b**) Michaelis-Menten kinetics of rhodamine123 efflux with or without caffeic acid pretreatment in $ABCB1$/Flp-In^{TM}-293. (**c**) Lineweaver-Burk plot analyses of caffeic acid on the transport of rhodamine123 in human P-gp. (**d**) Michaelis-Menten kinetics of doxorubicin efflux with or without caffeic acid pretreatment in $ABCB1$/Flp-In^{TM}-293. (**e**) Lineweaver-Burk plot analyses of caffeic acid on the transport of doxorubicin in human P-gp. * denotes $p < 0.05$ compared with the control group. Data were presented as mean ± SE of at least three experiments, each in triplicate. (**f**) Molecular docking analysis of caffeic acid (PubChem CID: 689043) docked posed of compounds in the P-gp (PDB entry 6QEX) binding pocket of 3D structure.

Table 1. The effects of caffeic acid on the transport of rhodamine123 and doxorubicin by human P-gp.

	Nonlinear Kinetic Parameters		
$ABCB1$/Flp-In^{TM}-293	V_m (pmole/10 min)	K_m (µM)	
Rhodamine123 only	9.04 ± 1.00	56.52 ± 6.97	
+ Caffeic acid, 10 µg/mL	2.47 ± 0.03*	15.93 ± 0.18 *	
+ Caffeic acid, 20 µg/mL	1.57 ± 0.04 *	10.72 ± 0.30 *	
K_i			253.44 ± 2.64
$ABCB1$/Flp-In^{TM}-293	V_m (pmole/120 min)	K_m (µM)	
Doxorubicin only	107.52 ± 0.001	179.81 ± 0.001	
+ Caffeic acid, 10 µg/mL	108.31 ± 0.68	234.76 ± 1.52 *	
+ Caffeic acid, 20 µg/mL	107.52 ± 0.001	426.16 ± 0.00 *	
K_i			14.13 ± 0.005

* $p < 0.05$ as compared to the rhodamine123 or doxorubicin transport without caffeic acid.

In order to investigate the supposed binding pattern and possible interaction between the ligand of caffeic acid and pocket of P-gp, the ligand of caffeic acid was virtually docked to the crystal structures of the ligand-binding domain of P-gp using the docking program CDOCKER. The virtual binding result is shown in Figure 3f. The docking results showed that caffeic acid had the the best binding energies active site of P-gp with a -CDOCKER energy score of 20.1292, and binding energy was 44.4058 Kcal/mol. The binding model clearly indicated that the caffeic acid bound to P-gp with residues GLU74 and TRY117. Our docking results further demonstrated the binding behavior between P-gp and caffeic acid, providing insight into the design of novel P-gp modulators.

The interaction between caffeic acid and ATP binding site of P-gp was carried out with Pgp-Glo™ Assay System. As Figure 4a shows, when the P-gp membrane was treated with caffeic acid with amounts of 1, 10, and 50 µg/mL, the basal P-gp ATPase activity was inhibited. On the other hand, the ATPase activity was stimulated under the treatment of 100 µg/mL caffeic acid. Besides, when combining caffeic acid with 200 µM verapamil, the elevated ATPase activity produced by verapamil was further stimulated and especially high under 100 µg/mL concentration (Figure 4b).

(a)

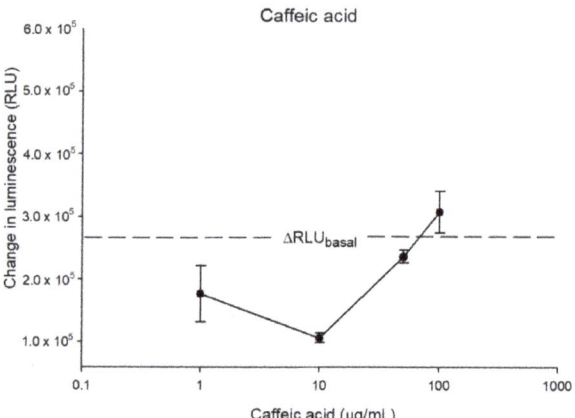

(b)

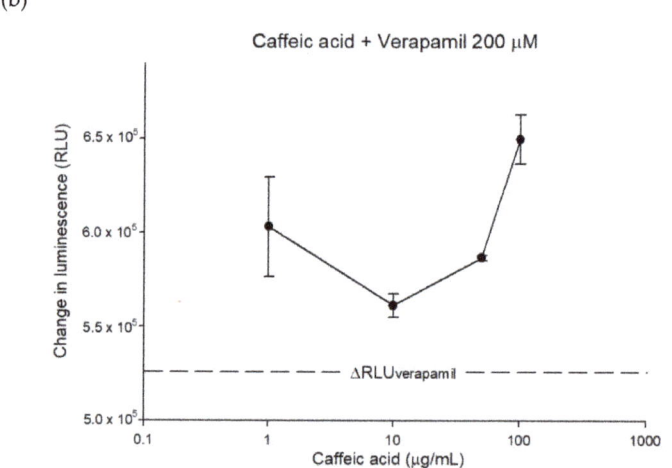

Figure 4. The P-gp ATPase modulating effects of caffeic acid. (**a**) Caffeic acid stimulated ATPase activity dose-dependently (10–100 µg/mL). (**b**) The verapamil-stimulated ATPase activity was further stimulated by caffeic acid. Data were analyzed in terms of the change of luminescence (ΔRLU). Data were presented as mean ± SE of at least three experiments, each in triplicate.

2.3. The Influences of Caffeic Acid on Human P-gp Expression

The modulatory ability of caffeic acid on *ABCB1* gene expression was performed in both *ABCB1*/Flp-In^{TM}-293 and KB/VIN cell lines. In *ABCB1* overexpressing cell line *ABCB1*/Flp-In^{TM}-293, caffeic acid after 72 h treatment slightly down-regulated the expression of P-gp (Figure 5a). Nevertheless, the same treatment for MDR cancer cell line KB/VIN exhibited the opposite phenomenon. Caffeic acid elevated *ABCB1* gene expression under 72 h treatment (Figure 5b).

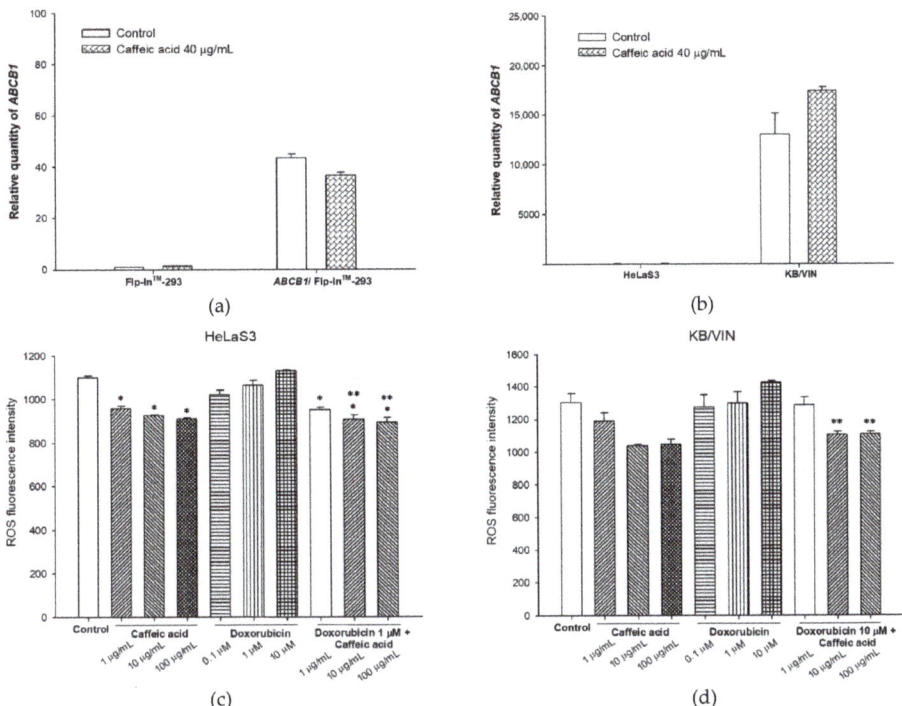

Figure 5. The modulating effects of caffeic acid on human P-gp expression. (**a**) The *ABCB1* expression in *ABCB1*/Flp-In^{TM}-293 was slightly down-regulated after treating the cells with 40 µg/mL caffeic acid for 72 h. (**b**) The *ABCB1* expression in KB/VIN was slightly up-regulated after treating the cells with 40 µg/mL caffeic acid for 72 h. (**c**) The intracellular ROS production under the treatment of caffeic acid with or without doxorubicin in HeLaS3. (**d**) The intracellular ROS production under the treatment of caffeic acid with or without doxorubicin in KB/VIN. Data were presented as mean ± SE of at least three experiments, each in triplicate. * denotes $p < 0.05$ compared with the control group. ** denotes $p < 0.05$ compared with the doxorubicin 1 µM group in Figure 5c and doxorubicin 10 µM group in Figure 5d.

To study whether the regulation of *ABCB1* gene expression was related to the intracellular reactive oxygen species status, the intracellular total ROS activity assay was performed. As Figure 5c,d indicates, caffeic acid significantly decreased ROS production in HeLaS3 cell line and slightly decreased ROS production in KB/VIN cell line. When both cell lines were treated with chemotherapeutic drug doxorubicin and caffeic acid, the ROS production exhibited no difference compared to caffeic acid treatment alone. However, the doxorubicin-induced oxidative challenge was significantly reversed by caffeic acid in amounts of 10 µg/mL and 100 µg/mL in both HeLaS3 and KB/VIN cell lines.

2.4. The Modulating Effects of Caffeic Acid on Cancer Multi-Drug Resistance

The MDR reversal ability of caffeic acid was examined in both P-gp over-expressing cell line ABCB1/Flp-In^{TM}-293 and MDR cancer cell line KB/VIN. As Table 2 shows, 30 µg/mL caffeic acid reversed vincristine, paclitaxel, and doxorubicin resistance by 3.90, 4.96, and 15.11-fold, respectively. The IC$_{50}$ of doxorubicin decreased from 9023.61 nM to 569.90 nM with the treatment of caffeic acid 30 µg/mL in ABCB1/Flp-In^{TM}-293. The MDR reversal phenomenon was further approved and analyzed by cell cycle. Compared to paclitaxel alone treatment, the addition of caffeic acid 20 and 25 µg/mL significantly increased subG1 population (from 11.3% to 24.1% and 33.0%), indicating that the cell underwent obvious apoptosis under combinatorial treatment (Figure 6a and Table 3).

Table 2. The reversal effects of caffeic acid on chemotherapeutic drug resistance in P-gp over-expressing cell line ABCB1/Flp-In^{TM}293.

Cell Line	Flp-In^{TM}293		ABCB1/Flp-In^{TM}293	
Compound	IC$_{50}$ ± S.E. (nM)	RF	IC$_{50}$ ± S.E. (nM)	RF
Vincristine	9.34 ± 0.43	1.00	778.11 ± 14.77	1.00
+ 30 µg/mL Caffeic acid	3.37 ± 4.30	2.77	198.04 ± 6.62	3.90
+ 20 µg/mL Caffeic acid	7.08 ± 0.09	1.31	557.46 ± 8.70	1.40
+ 10 µg/mL Caffeic acid	9.11 ± 0.32	1.02	615.03 ± 3.09	2.26
Paclitaxel	89.99 ± 0.50	1.00	604.09 ± 7.09	1.00
+ 30 µg/mL Caffeic acid	40.9 ± 0.50	2.20	121.55 ± 13.50	4.96 *
+ 20 µg/mL Caffeic acid	79.3 ± 0.67	1.13	313.06 ± 37.71	1.92
+ 10 µg/mL Caffeic acid	86.9 ± 0.12	1.03	597.87 ± 11.25	1.01
Doxorubicin	8.55 ± 0.19	1.00	9023.61 ± 272.90	1.00
+ 30 µg/mL Caffeic acid	4.07 ± 4.49	2.10	596.90 ± 24.18	15.11 *
+ 20 µg/mL Caffeic acid	7.34 ± 4.67	1.20	1299.7 ± 37.18	6.94 *
+ 10 µg/mL Caffeic acid	8.48 ± 2.58	1.00	2628.1 ± 24.49	3.43

* $p < 0.05$ as compared to the chemotherapeutic drug treatment (vincristine, paclitaxel, or doxorubicin) without caffeic acid. The reversal fold (RF) was calculated by dividing the individual IC$_{50}$ of chemotherapeutic drugs by the IC$_{50}$ of chemotherapeutic drugs in the presence of caffeic acid.

Table 3. The percentage of each cell cycle phase under various treatments in ABCB1/Flp-In^{TM}-293 cell line and KB/VIN cell line.

ABCB1/Flp-In^{TM}-293	Percentage of Phase ± SE (%)			
	Sub G1	G0/G1	S	G2/M
Control	0.4 ± 0.17	35.7 ± 1.5	46.2 ± 2.9	17.6 ± 4.3
Paclitaxel 250 nM	11.3 ± 0.2	27.4 ± 0.6	29.3 ± 1.6	31.8 ± 1.3
Caffeic acid 20 µg/mL	3.7 ± 0.6	27.4 ± 0.6	29.3 ± 1.6	31.8 ± 1.3
Caffeic acid 25 µg/mL	1.2 ± 0.1	41.7 ± 0.5	37.7 ± 0.2	19.2 ± 0.6
Paclitaxel 250 nM + Caffeic acid 20 µg/mL	24.1 ± 0.3	36.6 ± 1.4	24.1 ± 1.8	15.0 ± 0.5
Paclitaxel 250 nM + Caffeic acid 25 µg/mL	33.0 ± 9.0	27.5 ± 8.5	29.7 ± 4.8	14.8 ± 0.6
KB/VIN	Percentage of Phase ± SE (%)			
	Sub G1	G0/G1	S	G2/M
Control	0.6 ± 0.07	37.3 ± 4.0	39.2 ± 0.7	22.9 ± 3.3
Paclitaxel 250 nM	12.8 ± 1.5	44.6 ± 1.0	29.2 ± 0.4	13.3 ± 0.1
Caffeic acid 20 µg/mL	1.5 ± 0.04	40.3 ± 0.9	45.5 ± 1.3	12.8 ± 0.5
Caffeic acid 25 µg/mL	1.3 ± 0.1	37.2 ± 0.4	50.1 ± 0.5	11.4 ± 0.3
Paclitaxel 250 nM + Caffeic acid 20 µg/mL	13.2 ± 1.2	44.3 ± 0.5	31.6 ± 1.0	11.0 ± 0.2
Paclitaxel 250 nM + Caffeic acid 25 µg/mL	12.7 ± 1.3	46.9 ± 0.1	23.6 ± 1.5	16.8 ± 0.2

(a)

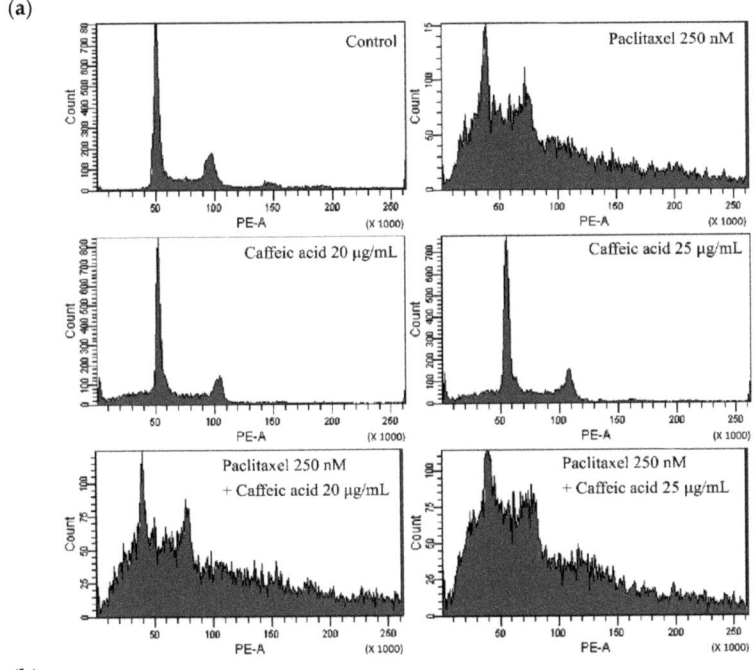

(b)

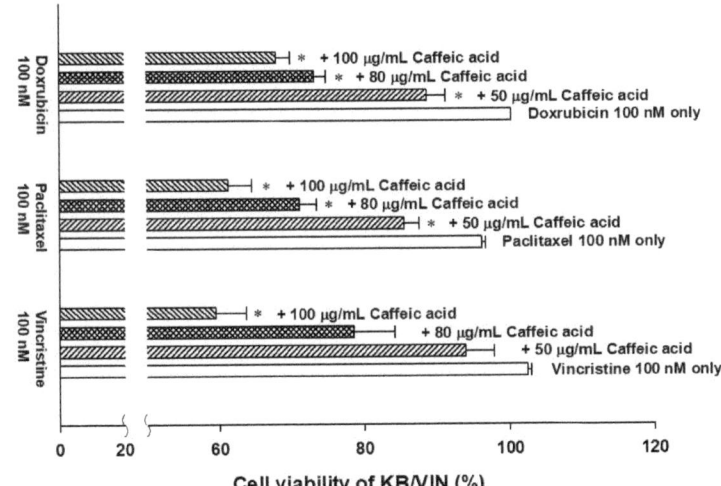

Figure 6. Cont.

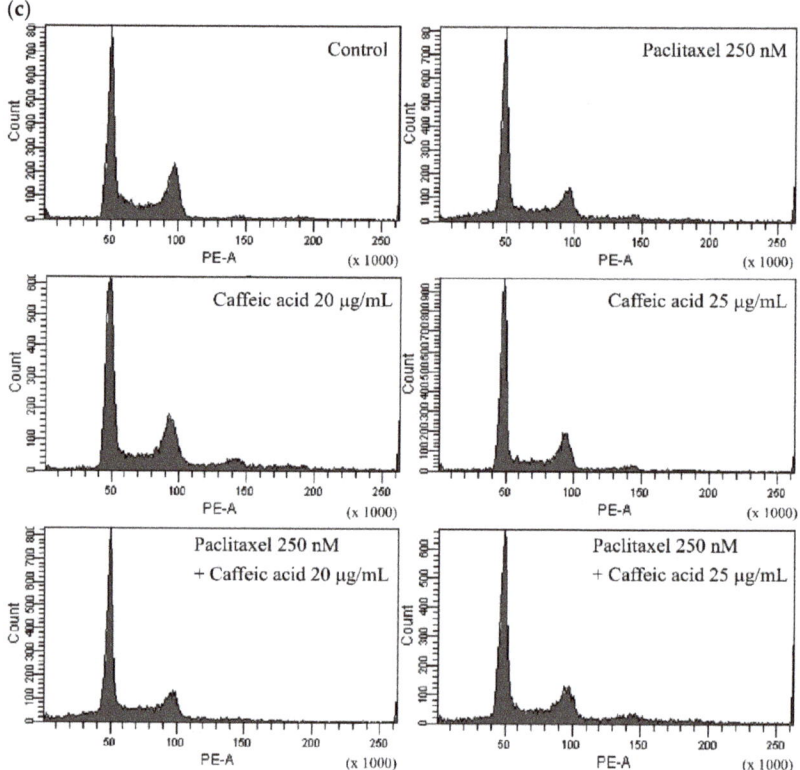

Figure 6. The cytotoxicity-enhancing effects of combinatorial treatment with caffeic acid. (**a**) The cell cycle distribution of 72 h treatment in $ABCB1$/Flp-In^{TM}-293 cell line. (**b**) The cell viability of KB/VIN under the treatment of chemotherapeutic drugs with or without caffeic acid. Data were presented as mean ± SE of at least three experiments, each in triplicate. * $p < 0.05$ as compared to the chemotherapeutic drug treatment (doxorubicin, paclitaxel, or vincristine) without caffeic acid. (**c**) The cell cycle distribution of 72 h treatment in KB/VIN cell line.

In MDR cancer cell line KB/VIN, with 100 μg/mL caffeic acid treatment, the cytotoxicity of 100 nM doxorubicin, paclitaxel, and vincristine significantly increased. The cell viability decreased from nearly 100% to 67.91%, 61.18%, and 59.50% for doxorubicin, paclitaxel, and vincristine, respectively. In addition, the cytotoxic-enhancing ability of caffeic acid on chemotherapeutic drugs was in a dose-dependent manner (Figure 6b). However, the further cell cycle analyses showed that the combination of caffeic acid and paclitaxel did not prominently increase the apoptosis of KB/VIN cells, revealing distinct cell effects among $ABCB1$/Flp-In^{TM}-293 and KB/VIN (Figure 6c and Table 3).

3. Discussion

Caffeic acid, a dietary non-flavonoid phenolic compound, has been a popular candidate among several research fields. The present study has demonstrated its usability in cancer MDR. Caffeic acid can attenuate this severe resistant problem by inhibiting the efflux function of human P-gp. Through diverse modulating mechanisms, caffeic acid helps resistant cancer cells retain chemotherapeutic drugs inside their cells, promoting further apoptosis and cell death.

Through investigating the history of P-gp inhibitor development, the ideal characteristics of potential candidates have been revealed. The inhibitor itself is not a substrate of P-gp, but is one of the favorable properties [19]. Our present research performed an experiment and the results indicated that caffeic acid was not P-gp's substrate. In this way, more caffeic acid could stay inside the cells to help P-gp inhibition, resulting in a higher intracellular chemotherapeutic drugs concentration.

The inhibitory effects of caffeic acid on P-gp efflux function were demonstrated on three P-gp fluorescent substrates, calcein-AM, rhodamine123, and doxorubicin. The different binding modes of each substrate revealed the inhibitory mechanisms of caffeic acid on P-gp drug binding sites. A previous investigation found that doxorubicin was a R-site substrate while rhodamine123 exhibited both M and R sites binding affinity [37–39]. Our efflux assay results indicated that caffeic acid showed uncompetitive inhibition on rhodamine123 transport and competitive inhibition on doxorubicin transport. Therefore, caffeic acid might compete the R drug binding site with doxorubicin, resulting in efflux inhibition. In terms of rhodamine123 inhibition, caffeic acid exhibited an allosteric modulation on M site, indirectly prohibiting the pump out behavior of P-gp.

In addition to drug binding sites, the interaction between caffeic acid and ATP binding sites of P-gp was also studied. According to the tested compound's behavior toward P-gp ATPase regulation, substances could be categorized into three classes: dual regulators, stimulators, and inhibitors [40,41]. Dual regulators stimulate both basal and verapamil-stimulated ATPase activity at a lower dose, but inhibit the activity at a higher dose, such as paclitaxel and vinblastine. Stimulators like valinomycin and bisantrene increase ATPase activity dose-dependently while inhibitors decrease both basal and verapamil-stimulated ATPase activity, such as rapamycin and cyclosporine A. The results of ATPase assay in the present study indicated that caffeic acid exhibited stimulatory activity from 10 μg/mL to 100 μg/mL in a dose-dependent manner. Therefore, caffeic acid was an ATPase stimulator. Besides, the results of verapamil-stimulated ATPase activity further revealed the binding behavior of caffeic acid on ATPase binding sites. Caffeic acid increased verapamil-stimulated ATPase activity regardless of the dose, implying its binding site on ATPase was different from verapamil. This allosteric stimulation advanced the consumption of ATP, indirectly inhibiting P-gp efflux function.

Whether the promising P-gp inhibitory effects of caffeic acid were helpful in reversing cancer MDR was than studied in our following experiments. In $ABCB1$/Flp-In^{TM}-293 P-gp over-expressing cell line, caffeic acid significantly decreased the required doses of chemo-agents, including vincristine, paclitaxel, and doxorubicin. Under the treatment of 30 μg/mL caffeic acid, the IC$_{50}$ of paclitaxel largely decreased from 604.09 nM to 121.55 nM. This advanced cytotoxicity was related to the increased apoptotic effects revealed by cell cycle assay results. With caffeic acid as a combinatory agent, the percentage of subG1 apoptotic population induced by paclitaxel significantly increased in a dose-dependent manner. The above results were consistent with previous researches, which revealed that caffeic acid could sensitize ovarian carcinoma cells and lung cancer cells to cisplatin and paclitaxel, respectively [33,42]. Caffeic acid exhibited chemo-sensitizing effects in the combination group by cell cycle arresting in G2/M (caffeic acid 20 μg/mL with paclitaxel) and G1 (caffeic acid 25 μg/mL with paclitaxel). These effects were not only due to the modulation of P-gp, other cellular targets and multiple mechanistic possibilities may be involved and need further investigation. The MDR reversing ability of caffeic acid was also investigated in MDR cancer cell line KB/VIN. The results exhibited a trend on increasing the cytotoxicity of chemo-agents. With the treatment of 100 μg/mL caffeic acid, the cell viability decreased from nearly 100% to 67.91%, 61.18%, and 59.50% for doxorubicin, paclitaxel, and vincristine, respectively. However, compared to the promising results in $ABCB1$/Flp-In^{TM}-293 cell line, the MDR modulating effects of caffeic acid in KB/VIN seemed to be less potent and did not show increased apoptosis in the cell cycle analyses, exhibiting cell type-dependent effects. This phenomenon could be explained by the regulation of caffeic acid on P-gp expression. As Figure 5a,b shows, caffeic acid slightly decreased $ABCB1$ gene expression in $ABCB1$/Flp-In^{TM}-293 but increased the expression level in KB/VIN cell line. This up-regulating trend in KB/VIN diminished the functional inhibitory potency of caffeic acid, resulting in weaker MDR reversing effects. Previous research has revealed that the oxidative stress might have a role in the regulation of P-gp expression [43]. As caffeic acid exhibited significant ROS-related anti-oxidant effects, the influence of caffeic acid on ROS production in KB/VIN cell line was performed. The results showed that caffeic acid significantly decreased ROS production in HeLaS3 cell line and slightly decreased ROS production in KB/VIN cell line. However, the doxorubicin-induced oxidative challenge was significantly reversed by caffeic acid in amounts of 10 µg/mL and 100 µg/mL in both HeLaS3 and KB/VIN cell lines. Therefore, the relationship between the reactive oxygen species levels and the up-regulation of *ABCB1* gene in KB/VIN might be related to the insufficient ROS regulation of caffeic acid. The above results indicated that the MDR reversal effects of caffeic acid might be cell line-dependent and warrant further detailed investigation.

The present study provided in-depth and comprehensive researches on the relationship between caffeic acid and human P-gp, and demonstrated the ability of caffeic acid on sensitizing MDR cancer cells toward chemotherapeutic drugs treatment. In order for caffeic acid to find a role in clinical application, some attempts could be applied to this phenolic prototype agent, including structural modification and pharmaceutical design.

4. Materials and Methods

4.1. Chemicals and Reagents

Acetic acid, β-Mercaptoethanol (β-ME), caffeic acid, dimethyl sulfoxide (DMSO), ethanol (Absolute; analytical grade), paclitaxel, rhodamine 123, sulforhodamine B (SRB), trichloroacetic acid (TCA), tris base, (±)-verapamil, and vincristine were obtained from Sigma-Aldrich Co. (St Louis, MO, USA). Calcein-AM was from AAT Bioquest (Sunnyvale, CA, USA), and doxorubicin was from US Biological (Woburn, MA, USA). Dulbecco's Modified Eagle Medium, RPMI 1640 medium, fetal bovine serum (FBS), phosphate buffered saline (PBS; pH 7.2), Trypsin-EDTA, and hygromycin B were purchased from Invitrogen (Carlsbad, CA, USA). Zeocin was from InvivoGen (San Diego, CA, USA).

4.2. Cell Lines

Human cervical epithelioid carcinoma HeLaS3 was purchased from Bioresource Collection and Research Center (Hsinchu, Taiwan), and the multi-drug resistant human cervical cancer cell line KB/VIN was kindly provided by Dr. Kuo-Hsiung Lee (University of North Carolina, Chapel Hill, NC, USA) and maintained with vincristine regularly. The human P-gp stable expression cells (*ABCB1*/Flp-In^{TM}-293) and parental cell line Flp-In^{TM}-293 were constructed as previously described [44]. All cells were cultured in DMEM or RPMI-1640 containing 10% FBS at 37 °C in a humidified atmosphere of 5% CO_2.

4.3. Cytotoxicity Determination Assay (SRB Assay)

The method has been described in our previous research [45]. Briefly, after 72 h of treatment of a series of concentrations of chemotherapeutic drugs with or without caffeic acid, 50% trichloroacetic acid (TCA) was added to fix cells for 30 min, and then the cells were washed with water and air-dried. After that, cells were stained with 0.04% sulforhodamine B (SRB) for 30 min, and then the unbound dye was removed by washing cells with 1% acetic acid and air-dried. The bound stain was solubilized in 10 mM Tris Base and the absorbance was measured using a BioTek Synergy HT Multi-Mode Microplate Reader (Winooski, VT, USA) at 515 nm.

4.4. MDR1 Shift Assay

The method has been described in our previous research [46]. The conformation change of P-gp after the addition of caffeic acid was examined by using a MDR1 Shift Assay kit (EMD Millipore Corp., Billerica, MA, USA) according to the manufacturer's protocol. UIC2 shift was shown in the presence of a P-gp substrate such as vinblastine. A total of 5×10^5–1×10^6 cells were prepared per reaction and resuspended with warm UIC2 binding buffer. Cells were incubated at 37 °C for 10 min and then treated with DMSO or vinblastine or test compounds. Cells were incubated at 37 °C for 30 min and then treated with IgG2a (negative control antibody) or UIC2 working solution (P-gp conformational sensitive antibody). Cells were incubated at 37 °C for 15 min and then washed with iced UIC2 binding buffer twice. A secondary antibody, goat anti-mouse IgG ALEXA 488, was added at 4 °C for 15 min, and then iced UIC2 binding buffer was added. The fluorescence was measured by FACS analysis (BD FACSCanto™ II System, South City-I, Haryana, India).

4.5. Intracellular Calcein Accumulation Assay

The method has been described in our previous research [46]. For the screening of an inhibitory effect on human P-gp efflux function, intracellular calcein accumulation assay was performed. Briefly, 1×10^5 cells/well were seeded in 96-well black plates for 24 h. Before the assay, cells were washed and pre-incubated with warm Hanks' balanced salt solution (HBSS) for 30 min and subsequently with caffeic acid for 30 min. After pre-incubation and three times washing with PBS, the calcein-AM was added (substrate of P-gp), and the calcein fluorescence generated within the cells was detected by BioTek Synergy HT Multi-Mode Microplate Reader using an excitation wavelength of 485 nm and emission wavelength of 528 nm at 37 °C temperature every 3 min for 30 min. Each experiment was performed at least three times, each in triplicate on different days.

4.6. Rhodamine123 and Doxorubicin Efflux Assay

The method has been described in our previous research [46]. 1×10^5 cells/well were placed on 96-well plates and incubated overnight. Before the efflux assay, cells were washed and pre-incubated with warm HBSS for 30 min, and subsequently with caffeic acid for 30 min. Then, the cells were treated with rhodamine123 for 30 min or doxorubicin for 3 h at 37 °C. After being washed with warm PBS, cells were allowed to efflux fluorescent rhodamin123 and doxorubicin for 10 min and 2 h, respectively. Supernatant samples (100 μL) were transferred to 96-well black plates. The fluorescence of rhodamine123 and doxorubicin was measured using a BioTek Synergy HT Multi-Mode Microplate Reader (excitation/emission: 485/528 nm for rhodamine123, 485/590 nm for doxorubicin). Each experiment was performed at least three times, each in triplicate on different days. Kinetic parameters were estimated by nonlinear regression using Scientist v2.01 (MicroMath Scientific Software, Salt Lake City, UT, USA) according to the following equation:

$$V = \frac{V_{max} \times C}{K_m + C}$$

where V denoted the efflux rate; V_{max}, the maximal efflux rate; K_m, the Michaelis-Menten constant; and C is the substrate concentration.

4.7. P-gp ATPase Activity Assay

The method has been described in our previous research [46]. For the evaluation of P-gp ATPase activity of caffeic acid, Pgp-Glo™ Assay System from Promega (Madison, WI, USA) was used. In a 96-well untreated white plate, 25 μg of recombinant human P-gp membranes were incubated with Pgp-Glo™ Assay Buffer (untreated control), 200 μM verapamil (positive control for drug induced P-gp ATPase activity), 100 μM sodium orthovanadate (selective inhibitor for P-gp ATPase activity), or a series of concentrations of caffeic acid. The reaction was initiated by adding 5 mM MgATP and incubated for 40 min at 37 °C, followed by stopping the reaction with 50 μL ATPase Detection Reagent for 20 min at room temperature. Luminescence was measured using a BioTek Synergy HT Multi-Mode Microplate Reader, and data were presented as Change in Luminescence (ΔRLU).

4.8. Real-Time Quantitative RT-PCR

The method has been described in our previous research [46]. *ABCB1* mRNA expression levels were quantified by real-time RT-PCR. Total RNA was extracted from HeLaS3, KB/VIN, Flp-In™-293, and *ABCB1*/Flp-In™-293 cells using Qiagen RNeasy kit (Valencia, CA, USA). Taqman Assay-On-Demand™ reagents of primers and probes for *ABCB1* (Hs00184500_m1) and *GAPDH* (Hs02758991_g1) genes were provided by Applied Biosystem (Foster City, CA, USA). The relative *ABCB1* mRNA expression levels were normalized to the amount of *GAPDH* in the same cDNA and evaluated by StepOnePlus™ Real-Time PCR System (Applied Biosystems®).

4.9. Intracellular Total ROS Activity Assay

The influence of caffeic acid on intracellular reactive oxygen species (ROS) was evaluated with Cell Meter™ Fluorimetric Intracellular Total ROS Activity Assay Kit (Catalog number: 22900) purchased from AAT Bioquest (Sunnyvale, CA, USA). Briefly, 4×10^4 cells/well were seeded in 96-well black plates for 24 h. Then the cells were stained with Amplite™ ROS Green working solution for 1 h; after that, caffeic acid with or without chemotherapeutic drugs were added to induce ROS production at room temperature for at least 15 min. The fluorescence was measured using a BioTek Synergy HT Multi-Mode Microplate Reader at 490/525 nm (same as FITC filter).

4.10. Cell Cycle Analysis

The method has been described in our previous research [45]. Cells were plated to 6-well plates with serum-free medium for starvation. Twenty-four hours later, cells were treated with chemotherapeutic drugs with or without caffeic acid for 72 h. After that, cells were harvested and washed in cold phosphate-buffered saline (PBS), followed by fixing in ice-cold 70% ethanol for at least 24 h. Then, cells were incubated with 50 µg/mL PI at 4 °C for 24 h in the dark. Cells were then analyzed by FACS analysis (BD FACSCanto™ II System with excitation laser 488 nm, measuring at emission 575 nm for PI).

4.11. Molecular Docking

Molecular docking helps us in predicting the intermolecular framework formed between a protein and a small molecule and suggests the binding modes responsible for inhibition of the protein. In this study, the existing structure of P-gp (PDB entry 6QEX) was used as a template for docking caffeic acid (PubChem CID: 689043) putative ligands using Discovery Studio 4.5. After removing all crystallized H_2O molecules from the former construction, hydrogen was added into the CDOCKER module. CDOCKER is a powerful CHARMm-based docking method that has been used to generate highly accurate docked poses. In this refinement application, the ligands were conceded to tilt around the rigid receptor [47].

4.12. Statistical Analysis

Statistical differences were evaluated by ANOVA followed by post hoc analysis (Tukey's test) or Student's t-test. The statistical significance was set at p value < 0.05.

Author Contributions: Conceptualization, Y.-N.T. and C.-C.H.; Data curation, Y.-N.T.; Formal analysis, Y.-N.T., C.C.N.W. and W.-C.L.; Funding acquisition, Y.-N.T. and C.-C.H.; Investigation, Y.-N.T., C.C.N.W., W.-C.L. and Y.-H.L.; Methodology, Y.-N.T., C.C.N.W., W.-C.L. and C.-C.H.; Project administration, C.-C.H.; Resources, Y.-H.L. and C.-C.H.; Software, Y.-N.T., C.C.N.W. and W.-C.L.; Supervision, Y.-H.L. and C.-C.H.; Validation, C.-C.H.; Visualization, C.-C.H.; Writing—original draft, Y.-N.T., C.C.N.W. and W.-C.L.; Writing—review & editing, Y.-H.L. and C.-C.H. All authors have read and agreed to the published version of the manuscript.

Funding: This research was funded by China Medical University (CMU108-MF-69), I-Shou University (ISU 108-S-02), and Ministry of Science and Technology (MOST 108-2320-B-039-042 and MOST 108-2320-B-214-009).

Acknowledgments: Flow cytometry analyses were performed at the Medical Research Core Facilities Center, Office of Research & Development at China Medical University, Taichung, Taiwan, R.O.C.

Conflicts of Interest: The authors declare no conflict of interest.

References

1. Silva, R.; Vilas-Boas, V.; Carmo, H.; Dinis-Oliveira, R.J.; Carvalho, F.; de Lourdes Bastos, M.; Remiao, F. Modulation of P-glycoprotein efflux pump: Induction and activation as a therapeutic strategy. *Pharmacol. Ther.* **2015**, *149*, 1–123. [CrossRef] [PubMed]

2. Kumar, A.; Jaitak, V. Natural products as multidrug resistance modulators in cancer. *Eur. J. Med. Chem.* **2019**, *176*, 268–291. [CrossRef] [PubMed]
3. Kathawala, R.J.; Wang, Y.J.; Ashby, C.R., Jr.; Chen, Z.S. Recent advances regarding the role of ABC subfamily C member 10 (ABCC10) in the efflux of antitumor drugs. *Chin. J. Cancer* **2014**, *33*, 223–230. [CrossRef] [PubMed]
4. Shi, R.; Wang, C.; Fu, N.; Liu, L.; Zhu, D.; Wei, Z.; Zhang, H.; Xing, J.; Wang, Y. Downregulation of cytokeratin 18 enhances BCRP-mediated multidrug resistance through induction of epithelial-mesenchymal transition and predicts poor prognosis in breast cancer. *Oncol. Rep.* **2019**, *41*, 3015–3026. [CrossRef]
5. Das, M.; Law, S. Role of tumor microenvironment in cancer stem cell chemoresistance and recurrence. *Int. J. Biochem. Cell Biol.* **2018**, *103*, 115–124. [CrossRef]
6. Giacomini, K.M.; Huang, S.M.; Tweedie, D.J.; Benet, L.Z.; Brouwer, K.L.; Chu, X.; Dahlin, A.; Evers, R.; Fischer, V.; Hillgren, K.M.; et al. Membrane transporters in drug development. *Nat. Rev. Drug Discov.* **2010**, *9*, 215–236.
7. Uddin, M.B.; Roy, K.R.; Hosain, S.B.; Khiste, S.K.; Hill, R.A.; Jois, S.D.; Zhao, Y.; Tackett, A.J.; Liu, Y.Y. An $N(6)$-methyladenosine at the transited codon 273 of p53 pre-mRNA promotes the expression of R273H mutant protein and drug resistance of cancer cells. *Biochem. Pharmacol.* **2019**, *160*, 134–145. [CrossRef]
8. Bedi, A.; Barber, J.P.; Bedi, G.C.; el-Deiry, W.S.; Sidransky, D.; Vala, M.S.; Akhtar, A.J.; Hilton, J.; Jones, R.J. BCR-ABL-mediated inhibition of apoptosis with delay of G2/M transition after DNA damage: A mechanism of resistance to multiple anticancer agents. *Blood* **1995**, *86*, 1148–1158. [CrossRef]
9. Wilson, C.S.; Medeiros, L.J.; Lai, R.; Butch, A.W.; McCourty, A.; Kelly, K.; Brynes, R.K. DNA topoisomerase IIalpha in multiple myeloma: A marker of cell proliferation and not drug resistance. *Mod. Pathol.* **2001**, *14*, 886–891. [CrossRef]
10. Filomeni, G.; Turella, P.; Dupuis, M.L.; Forini, O.; Ciriolo, M.R.; Cianfriglia, M.; Pezzola, S.; Federici, G.; Caccuri, A.M. 6-(7-Nitro-2,1,3-benzoxadiazol-4-ylthio)hexanol, a specific glutathione S-transferase inhibitor, overcomes the multidrug resistance (MDR)-associated protein 1-mediated MDR in small cell lung cancer. *Mol. Cancer Ther.* **2008**, *7*, 371–379. [CrossRef]
11. Rodriguez-Antona, C.; Ingelman-Sundberg, M. Cytochrome P450 pharmacogenetics and cancer. *Oncogene* **2006**, *25*, 1679–1691. [CrossRef] [PubMed]
12. Shoemaker, R.H. Genetic and epigenetic factors in anticancer drug resistance. *J. Natl. Cancer Inst.* **2000**, *92*, 4–5. [CrossRef] [PubMed]
13. Li, H.; Yang, B.B. Friend or foe: The role of microRNA in chemotherapy resistance. *Acta Pharm. Sin* **2013**, *34*, 870–879. [CrossRef] [PubMed]
14. Camidge, D.R.; Pao, W.; Sequist, L.V. Acquired resistance to TKIs in solid tumours: Learning from lung cancer. *Nat. Rev. Clin. Oncol.* **2014**, *11*, 473–481. [CrossRef] [PubMed]
15. Paskeviciute, M.; Petrikaite, V. Overcoming transporter-mediated multidrug resistance in cancer: Failures and achievements of the last decades. *Drug Deliv. Transl. Res.* **2019**, *9*, 379–393. [CrossRef] [PubMed]
16. Yakusheva, E.N.; Titov, D.S. Structure and Function of Multidrug Resistance Protein 1. *Biochem. Biokhimiia* **2018**, *83*, 907–929. [CrossRef]
17. Ling, V.; Thompson, L.H. Reduced permeability in CHO cells as a mechanism of resistance to colchicine. *J. Cell. Physiol.* **1974**, *83*, 103–116. [CrossRef]
18. Mollazadeh, S.; Sahebkar, A.; Hadizadeh, F.; Behravan, J.; Arabzadeh, S. Structural and functional aspects of P-glycoprotein and its inhibitors. *Life Sci.* **2018**, *214*, 118–123. [CrossRef]
19. Leopoldo, M.; Nardulli, P.; Contino, M.; Leonetti, F.; Luurtsema, G.; Colabufo, N.A. An updated patent review on P-glycoprotein inhibitors (2011-2018). *Expert Opin. Ther. Pat.* **2019**, *29*, 455–461. [CrossRef]
20. Joshi, P.; Vishwakarma, R.A.; Bharate, S.B. Natural alkaloids as P-gp inhibitors for multidrug resistance reversal in cancer. *Eur. J. Med. Chem.* **2017**, *138*, 273–292. [CrossRef]
21. O'Brien, M.M.; Lacayo, N.J.; Lum, B.L.; Kshirsagar, S.; Buck, S.; Ravindranath, Y.; Bernstein, M.; Weinstein, H.; Chang, M.N.; Arceci, R.J.; et al. Phase I study of valspodar (PSC-833) with mitoxantrone and etoposide in refractory and relapsed pediatric acute leukemia: A report from the Children's Oncology Group. *Pediatr. Blood Cancer* **2010**, *54*, 694–702. [CrossRef] [PubMed]
22. Li, W.; Zhang, H.; Assaraf, Y.G.; Zhao, K.; Xu, X.; Xie, J.; Yang, D.H.; Chen, Z.S. Overcoming ABC transporter-mediated multidrug resistance: Molecular mechanisms and novel therapeutic drug strategies. *Drug Resist. Updat.* **2016**, *27*, 14–29. [CrossRef] [PubMed]

23. Cripe, L.D.; Uno, H.; Paietta, E.M.; Litzow, M.R.; Ketterling, R.P.; Bennett, J.M.; Rowe, J.M.; Lazarus, H.M.; Luger, S.; Tallman, M.S. Zosuquidar, a novel modulator of P-glycoprotein, does not improve the outcome of older patients with newly diagnosed acute myeloid leukemia: A randomized, placebo-controlled trial of the Eastern Cooperative Oncology Group 3999. *Blood* **2010**, *116*, 4077–4085. [CrossRef] [PubMed]
24. Dash, R.P.; Jayachandra Babu, R.; Srinivas, N.R. Therapeutic Potential and Utility of Elacridar with Respect to P-glycoprotein Inhibition: An Insight from the Published In Vitro, Preclinical and Clinical Studies. *Eur. J. Drug Metab. Pharmacokinet.* **2017**, *42*, 915–933. [CrossRef]
25. Han, R.M.; Zhang, J.P.; Skibsted, L.H. Reaction dynamics of flavonoids and carotenoids as antioxidants. *Molecules* **2012**, *17*, 2140–2160. [CrossRef]
26. Kumar, S.; Pandey, A.K. Chemistry and biological activities of flavonoids: An overview. *Sci. World J.* **2013**, *2013*, 162750. [CrossRef]
27. Meyer, A.S.; Heinonen, M.; Frankel, E.N. Antioxidant interactions of catechin, cyanidin, caffeic acid, quercetin, and ellagic acid on human LDL oxidation. *Food Chem.* **1998**, *61*, 71–75. [CrossRef]
28. Jaman, M.S.; Sayeed, M.A. Ellagic acid, sulforaphane, and ursolic acid in the prevention and therapy of breast cancer: Current evidence and future perspectives. *Breast Cancer (TokyoJpn.)* **2018**, *25*, 517–528. [CrossRef]
29. Xing, Y.; Peng, H.Y.; Zhang, M.X.; Li, X.; Zeng, W.W.; Yang, X.E. Caffeic acid product from the highly copper-tolerant plant Elsholtzia splendens post-phytoremediation: Its extraction, purification, and identification. *J. Zhejiang Univ. Sci. B* **2012**, *13*, 487–493. [CrossRef]
30. Ahmed, N.; Escalona, R.; Leung, D.; Chan, E.; Kannourakis, G. Tumour microenvironment and metabolic plasticity in cancer and cancer stem cells: Perspectives on metabolic and immune regulatory signatures in chemoresistant ovarian cancer stem cells. *Semin. Cancer Biol.* **2018**, *53*, 265–281. [CrossRef]
31. Khan, F.A.; Maalik, A.; Murtaza, G. Inhibitory mechanism against oxidative stress of caffeic acid. *J. Food Drug Anal.* **2016**, *24*, 695–702. [CrossRef] [PubMed]
32. Ahn, C.H.; Choi, W.C.; Kong, J.Y. Chemosensitizing activity of caffeic acid in multidrug-resistant MCF-7/Dox human breast carcinoma cells. *Anticancer Res.* **1997**, *17*, 1913–1917. [PubMed]
33. Lin, C.L.; Chen, R.F.; Chen, J.Y.; Chu, Y.C.; Wang, H.M.; Chou, H.L.; Chang, W.C.; Fong, Y.; Chang, W.T.; Wu, C.Y.; et al. Protective effect of caffeic acid on paclitaxel induced anti-proliferation and apoptosis of lung cancer cells involves NF-kappaB pathway. *Int. J. Mol. Sci.* **2012**, *13*, 6236–6245. [CrossRef] [PubMed]
34. Wu, J.; Omene, C.; Karkoszka, J.; Bosland, M.; Eckard, J.; Klein, C.B.; Frenkel, K. Caffeic acid phenethyl ester (CAPE), derived from a honeybee product propolis, exhibits a diversity of anti-tumor effects in pre-clinical models of human breast cancer. *Cancer Lett.* **2011**, *308*, 43–53. [CrossRef]
35. Nabekura, T.; Kawasaki, T.; Furuta, M.; Kaneko, T.; Uwai, Y. Effects of Natural Polyphenols on the Expression of Drug Efflux Transporter P-Glycoprotein in Human Intestinal Cells. *Acs Omega* **2018**, *3*, 1621–1626. [CrossRef]
36. Takara, K.; Fujita, M.; Matsubara, M.; Minegaki, T.; Kitada, N.; Ohnishi, N.; Yokoyama, T. Effects of propolis extract on sensitivity to chemotherapeutic agents in HeLa and resistant sublines. *Phytother. Res. Ptr.* **2007**, *21*, 841–846. [CrossRef]
37. Montanari, F.; Ecker, G.F. Prediction of drug-ABC-transporter interaction–Recent advances and future challenges. *Adv. Drug Deliv. Rev.* **2015**, *86*, 17–26. [CrossRef]
38. Ferreira, R.J.; Ferreira, M.J.; dos Santos, D.J. Molecular docking characterizes substrate-binding sites and efflux modulation mechanisms within P-glycoprotein. *J. Chem. Inf. Model.* **2013**, *53*, 1747–1760. [CrossRef]
39. Martinez, L.; Arnaud, O.; Henin, E.; Tao, H.; Chaptal, V.; Doshi, R.; Andrieu, T.; Dussurgey, S.; Tod, M.; Di Pietro, A.; et al. Understanding polyspecificity within the substrate-binding cavity of the human multidrug resistance P-glycoprotein. *FEBS J.* **2014**, *281*, 673–682. [CrossRef]
40. Ambudkar, S.V.; Dey, S.; Hrycyna, C.A.; Ramachandra, M.; Pastan, I.; Gottesman, M.M. Biochemical, cellular, and pharmacological aspects of the multidrug transporter. *Ann. Rev. Pharmacol. Toxicol.* **1999**, *39*, 361–398. [CrossRef]
41. Dey, S.; Ramachandra, M.; Pastan, I.; Gottesman, M.M.; Ambudkar, S.V. Evidence for two nonidentical drug-interaction sites in the human P-glycoprotein. *Proc. Natl. Acad. Sci. USA* **1997**, *94*, 10594–10599. [CrossRef] [PubMed]
42. Sirota, R.; Gibson, D.; Kohen, R. The timing of caffeic acid treatment with cisplatin determines sensitization or resistance of ovarian carcinoma cell lines. *Redox Biol.* **2017**, *11*, 170–175. [CrossRef]

43. Huang, C.; Huang, S.; Li, H.; Li, X.; Li, B.; Zhong, L.; Wang, J.; Zou, M.; He, X.; Zheng, H.; et al. The effects of ultrasound exposure on P-glycoprotein-mediated multidrug resistance in vitro and in vivo. *J. Exp. Clin. Cancer Res.* **2018**, *37*, 232. [CrossRef] [PubMed]
44. Sheu, M.J.; Teng, Y.N.; Chen, Y.Y.; Hung, C.C. The functional influences of common ABCB1 genetic variants on the inhibition of P-glycoprotein by Antrodia cinnamomea extracts. *PLoS ONE* **2014**, *9*, e89622. [CrossRef]
45. Teng, Y.-N.; Wang, Y.-H.; Wu, T.-S.; Hung, H.-Y.; Hung, C.-C. Zhankuic Acids A, B and C from Taiwanofungus camphoratus Act as Cytotoxicity Enhancers by Regulating P-Glycoprotein in Multi-Drug Resistant Cancer Cells. *Biomolecules* **2019**, *9*, 759. [CrossRef] [PubMed]
46. Teng, Y.-N.; Hsieh, Y.-W.; Hung, C.-C.; Lin, H.-Y. Demethoxycurcumin Modulates Human P-Glycoprotein Function via Uncompetitive Inhibition of ATPase Hydrolysis Activity. *J. Agric. Food Chem.* **2015**, *63*, 847–855. [CrossRef] [PubMed]
47. Wu, G.; Robertson, D.H.; Brooks, C.L., 3rd; Vieth, M. Detailed analysis of grid-based molecular docking: A case study of CDOCKER-A CHARMm-based MD docking algorithm. *J. Comput. Chem.* **2003**, *24*, 1549–1562. [CrossRef]

Sample Availability: Samples of the compounds are not available from the authors.

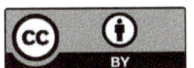

© 2020 by the authors. Licensee MDPI, Basel, Switzerland. This article is an open access article distributed under the terms and conditions of the Creative Commons Attribution (CC BY) license (http://creativecommons.org/licenses/by/4.0/).

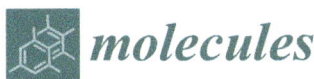

Article

Pterostilbene Suppresses both Cancer Cells and Cancer Stem-Like Cells in Cervical Cancer with Superior Bioavailability to Resveratrol

Hee Jeong Shin [1], Jang Mi Han [1], Ye Seul Choi [1] and Hye Jin Jung [1,2,3,*]

1. Department of Life Science and Biochemical Engineering, Sun Moon University, Asan 31460, Korea; gmlwjd903@naver.com (H.J.S.); gkswkdal200@naver.com (J.M.H.); yesll96@naver.com (Y.S.C.)
2. Genome-based BioIT Convergence Institute, Asan 31460, Korea
3. Department of Pharmaceutical Engineering and Biotechnology, Sun Moon University, Asan 31460, Korea
* Correspondence: poka96@sunmoon.ac.kr; Tel.: +82-41-530-2354

Academic Editor: Kyoko Nakagawa-Goto
Received: 23 November 2019; Accepted: 4 January 2020; Published: 6 January 2020

Abstract: Increasing studies have reported that cancer stem cells (CSCs) play critical roles in therapeutic resistance, recurrence, and metastasis of tumors, including cervical cancer. Pterostilbene, a dimethylated derivative of resveratrol, is a plant polyphenol compound with potential chemopreventive activity. However, the therapeutic effect of pterostilbene against cervical CSCs remains unclear. In this study, we compared the anticancer effects of resveratrol and pterostilbene using both HeLa cervical cancer adherent and stem-like cells. Pterostilbene more effectively inhibited the growth and clonogenic survival, as well as metastatic ability of HeLa adherent cells than those of resveratrol. Moreover, the superior inhibitory effects of pterostilbene compared to resveratrol were associated with the enhanced activation of multiple mechanisms, including cell cycle arrest at S and G2/M phases, induction of ROS-mediated caspase-dependent apoptosis, and inhibition of matrix metalloproteinase (MMP)-2/-9 expression. Notably, pterostilbene exhibited a greater inhibitory effect on the tumorsphere-forming and migration abilities of HeLa cancer stem-like cells compared to resveratrol. This greater effect was achieved through more potent inhibition of the expression levels of stemness markers, such as CD133, Oct4, Sox2, and Nanog, as well as signal transducer and activator of transcription 3 signaling. These results suggest that pterostilbene might be a potential anticancer agent targeting both cancer cells and cancer stem-like cells of cervical cancer via the superior bioavailability to resveratrol.

Keywords: cancer stem cell; cervical cancer; pterostilbene; resveratrol

---

1. Introduction

Cervical cancer is one of the most common types of female malignant tumor, with worldwide incidence of more than 500,000 cases and mortality rate of 9% per year [1]. High-risk human papillomavirus (HPV) types such as HPV-16 and -18 are known to cause cervical cancer through the overexpression of viral oncoproteins E6 and E7 [2]. Although the worldwide death rate from cervical cancer has declined due to the current treatment modalities, including HPV vaccines, surgery, radiation therapy, and chemotherapy, the cancer recurrence, metastasis, and the adverse drug effects remain major problems [3]. Therefore, safer and more effective therapeutic options are needed to improve the treatment of cervical cancer.

Accumulating evidence has demonstrated that cancer stem cells (CSCs), a small subpopulation of tumor cells with self-renewal and multi-lineage differentiation capacities, crucially drive the development, metastasis, relapse, and chemo/radio-resistance of cervical cancer [4,5]. In addition,

HPV oncoprotein E6 has been found to be involved in self-renewal and maintenance of stemness in cervical CSCs by upregulating Hes1, a downstream gene of Notch1 [6]. HPV16 E7 also upregulates the expression of stemness-related genes such as Oct3/4, Sox2, Nanog, and fibroblast growth factor 4 to maintain the self-renewal capacity of cervical CSCs [7]. Accordingly, targeting the cervical CSCs is a promising therapeutic strategy for the high-risk HPV-positive cervical cancer.

Various scientific studies have suggested the potential of natural active compounds isolated from plants or herbs for prevention and treatment of cancer [8,9]. Stilbenes are a class of polyphenolic compounds and naturally found in various dietary sources, such as grapes, blueberries, red wine, peanuts, and some medicinal plants [10]. Recently, stilbenes such as resveratrol (3,4′,5-trihydroxy-trans-stilbene) and its dimethylated analog, pterostilbene (trans-3,5-dimethoxy-4′-hydroxystilbene), have received considerable attention due to their potent antioxidant, anti-inflammatory, antidiabetic, and anticarcinogenic properties (Figure 1) [11,12]. Resveratrol and pterostilbene have been considered as excellent anticancer agents because of their low toxicity and abilities to regulate multiple molecular signaling pathways involved in cancer progression [13,14]. However, resveratrol has a low bioavailability that may lower its biological efficacy, while pterostilbene is more lipophilic, and thus, it exhibits better bioavailability [15]. Pterostilbene shows stronger antiproliferative and apoptotic effects than those shown by resveratrol in the human colon and cervical cancer cells [16,17]. However, the therapeutic effect and anticancer mechanism of pterostilbene against cervical CSCs compared to resveratrol have not been studied.

Here, anticancer effects of resveratrol and pterostilbene were compared using both HeLa cervical cancer adherent and stem-like cells. The abilities of the two compounds to suppress growth, migration, and stemness of HeLa cells were evaluated and the underlying molecular mechanisms were further explored. The results revealed that pterostilbene more effectively inhibited the stem-like properties of HeLa cells than resveratrol through stronger downregulation of specific CSC markers and signal transducer and activator of transcription 3 (STAT3) signaling. This is the first study to demonstrate the potential inhibitory activity of pterostilbene against cervical cancer cell stemness.

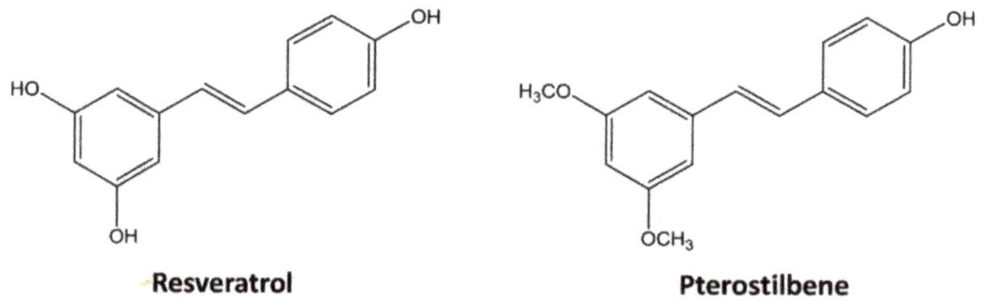

Figure 1. Chemical structures of resveratrol and pterostilbene.

2. Results

2.1. Pterostilbene Inhibited the Growth of Cervical Cancer Cells with Higher Potency Compared to Resveratrol

First, we compared the inhibitory effects of resveratrol and pterostilbene on the growth of HeLa, CaSki, and SiHa cervical cancer adherent cells using the 3-(4,5-dimethylthiazol-2-yl)-2,5-diphenyltetrazolium bromide (MTT) assay at various concentrations (0–200 µM). Resveratrol and pterostilbene suppressed the growth of HeLa, CaSki, and SiHa cells in a concentration-dependent manner (Figure 2A). The results showed that pterostilbene (IC_{50} = 32.67 µM for HeLa; 14.83 µM for CaSki; 34.17 µM for SiHa) exhibited stronger growth inhibitory effect than resveratrol (IC_{50} = 108.7 µM for HeLa; 44.45 µM for CaSki; 91.15 µM for SiHa). Next, we evaluated the effects of pterostilbene and resveratrol on the colony formation of HeLa, CaSki, and SiHa adherent cells. The colony forming ability of the cells was more effectively inhibited by pterostilbene than resveratrol (Figure 2B). These data demonstrate that pterostilbene is more potent in suppressing the growth and clonogenicity of cervical cancer adherent cells compared with resveratrol.

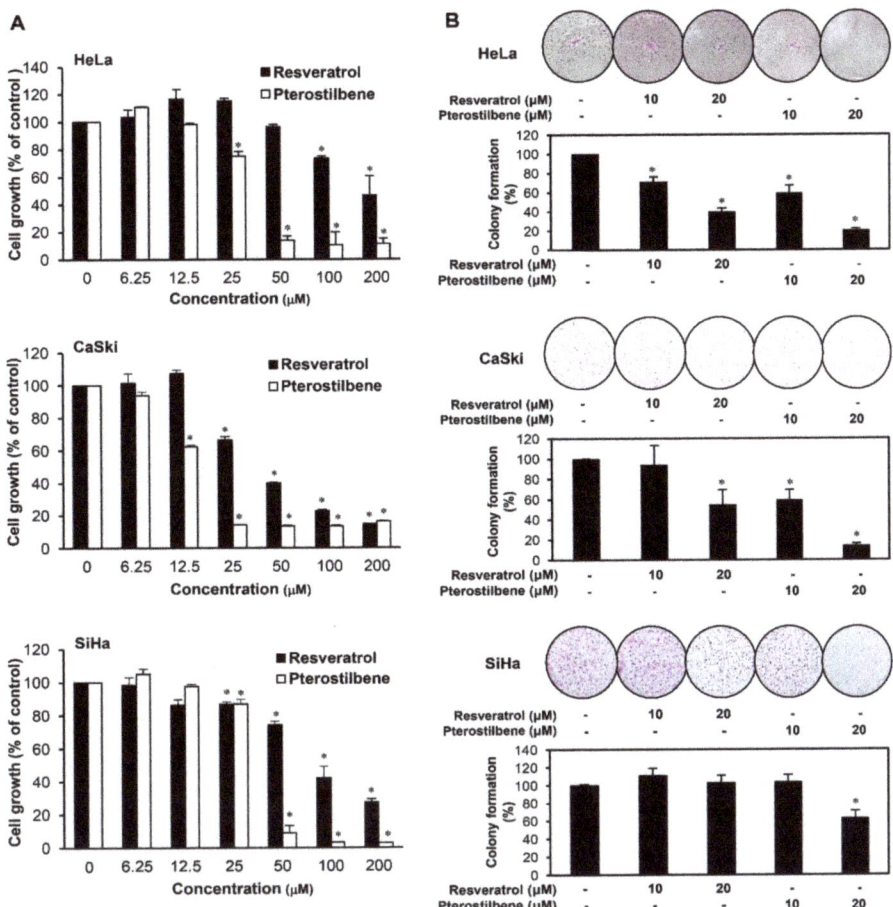

Figure 2. Growth inhibitory effects of resveratrol and pterostilbene on HeLa, CaSki, and SiHa cells. (**A**) The effects of resveratrol and pterostilbene on the growth of HeLa, CaSki, and SiHa adherent cells. The cells were treated with increasing concentrations of the two compounds (0–200 µM) for 72 h, and cell growth was measured by 3-(4,5-dimethylthiazol-2-yl)-2,5-diphenyltetrazolium bromide (MTT) assay. (**B**) The effects of resveratrol and pterostilbene on the colony forming ability of HeLa, CaSki, and SiHa adherent cells. The cells were incubated in the absence or presence of the two compounds (10 and 20 µM) for seven days. The cell colonies were detected by crystal violet staining. * $p < 0.05$ versus the control.

2.2. Pterostilbene Exhibited Stronger Migration Inhibitory Effect than Resveratrol in Cervical Cancer Cells

To compare the effects of resveratrol and pterostilbene on the metastatic ability of cervical cancer cells, we examined whether the two compounds inhibit the migration and invasion of HeLa adherent cells. A monolayer wound healing assay was performed to evaluate their effects on cell migration. Pterostilbene more markedly decreased the migration of HeLa cells at both 24 and 48 h after treatment when compared to resveratrol (Figure 3A). The effects of the two compounds on cell invasion were assessed using a Matrigel-coated Transwell chamber system. Both resveratrol and pterostilbene resulted in a significant reduction in the invasiveness of HeLa cells (Figure 3B). In particular, the invasion inhibitory effect of pterostilbene was more potent than that of resveratrol.

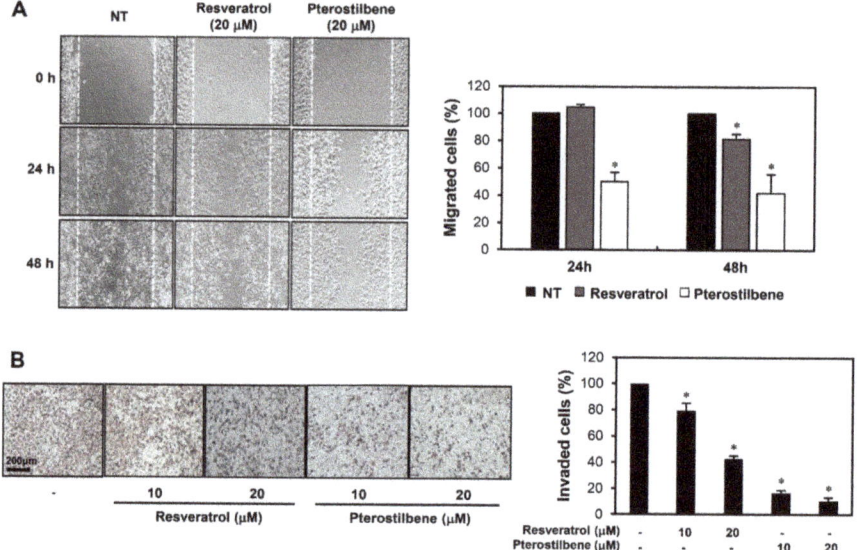

Figure 3. Effects of resveratrol and pterostilbene on the metastatic ability of HeLa cells. (**A**) The effects of resveratrol and pterostilbene on the migration of HeLa adherent cells. The migratory potential of HeLa cells was analyzed using a wound healing assay. The cells were incubated in the absence or presence of the two compounds (20 μM) for 48 h. The cells that migrated into the gap were counted using an optical microscope. Dotted white lines indicate the edge of the gap at 0 h. (**B**) The effects of resveratrol and pterostilbene on the invasion of HeLa adherent cells. The invasiveness of HeLa cells was analyzed using Matrigel-coated polycarbonate filters. The cells were incubated in the absence or presence of the two compounds (10 and 20 μM) for 48 h. The cells penetrating the filters were stained and counted using an optical microscope. * $p < 0.05$ versus the control.

2.3. Comparison of the Cell Cycle Arrest and Apoptosis-Inducing Effects of Resveratrol and Pterostilbene in Cervical Cancer Cells

To determine whether the growth inhibitory effects of resveratrol and pterostilbene on HeLa adherent cells were caused by cell cycle arrest, the effects of the two compounds on the cellular cell cycle distribution were quantified using flow cytometry analysis. Both resveratrol and pterostilbene induced cell cycle arrest at the S and G2/M phases along with a decrease in G0/G1 phase duration when compared with the control cells (Figure 4A). Notably, pterostilbene was more potent than resveratrol in blocking cell cycle progression. The induction of tumor suppressor protein p53 and its downstream target p21 can trigger cell cycle arrest by inhibiting the activity of cyclin-dependent kinase (CDK)–cyclin complexes [18]. Therefore, the effects of resveratrol and pterostilbene on the expression of these cell cycle regulators were assessed. Results revealed that the cell cycle arrest at the S and G2/M phases of HeLa adherent cells by resveratrol and pterostilbene was associated with the promotion of p53 and p21 expression and subsequent downregulation of cyclin E1 and cyclin B1 that are active in the S and G2 phases, respectively (Figure 5B). Furthermore, pterostilbene not only more significantly increased the expression levels of p53 and p21, but also decreased those of cyclin E1 and cyclin B1 compared to resveratrol.

To further elucidate the mechanisms underlying the anticancer effects of the two compounds in cervical cancer cells, cellular apoptosis was quantitatively measured using flow cytometry analysis following annexinV-FITC/propidium iodide (PI) double staining. Annexin V is a marker of early apoptosis and PI is a marker of late apoptosis and necrosis. The total amount of early and late apoptotic cells was markedly increased after resveratrol and pterostilbene treatment in comparison with the control (Figure 4B). Moreover, the apoptosis-inducing effect of pterostilbene was stronger than that of resveratrol in HeLa adherent cells (from 4.67% to 30.58% and 50.46% by resveratrol and pterostilbene, respectively). The elevation of intracellular reactive oxygen species (ROS) plays an important role in mediating apoptotic processes [19]. Thus, to determine whether ROS are involved in the regulation of resveratrol- and pterostilbene-induced apoptosis, the levels of intracellular ROS in HeLa adherent cells were measured using the fluorescent 2′,7′-dichlorofluorescein diacetate (DCFH-DA) product. Pterostilbene more prominently elevated the production of ROS in comparison with resveratrol at the indicated doses (Figure 5A). In addition, the cell apoptosis induced by resveratrol and pterostilbene was involved in the activation of caspase-3 and caspase-9, as well as the downregulation of antiapoptotic proteins such as Bcl-2 and Bcl-XL (Figure 5B) [20]. These data also showed that pterostilbene was more effective in regulating the expression of these apoptosis-related proteins than resveratrol.

Matrix metalloproteinases (MMPs) play a critical role in the degradation of the extracellular matrix (ECM) during cancer metastasis [21]. To further define the mechanism through which resveratrol and pterostilbene reduce cervical cancer cell migration and invasion, the protein expression levels of MMP-2 and MMP-9 in HeLa adherent cells were investigated. Pterostilbene more strongly suppressed the expression of MMP-2 and MMP-9 compared with resveratrol (Figure 5B). These findings suggest that pterostilbene may possess enhanced activity in inhibiting the metastasis of cervical cancer cells than resveratrol, through more effective downregulation of MMP-2 and MMP-9 expression.

Therefore, the superior growth and migration inhibitory effects of pterostilbene compared to resveratrol in HeLa adherent cells were mediated through the enhanced activation of multiple mechanisms, including cell cycle arrest at S and G2/M phases, induction of ROS-mediated caspase-dependent apoptosis, and inhibition of MMP-2/-9 expression.

A

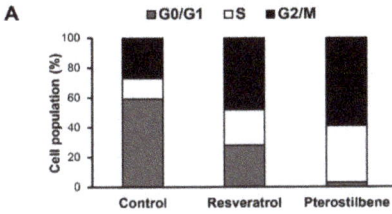

Compound	Cell cycle phase (%)		
	G0/G1	S	G2/M
Control	56.7	13.2	26.1
Resveratrol	25.7	22.1	44.6
Pterostilbene	2.6	34.2	53.5

B

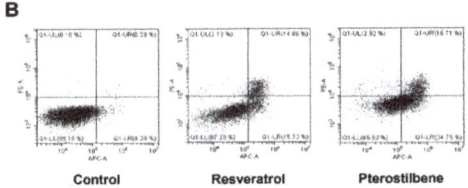

Compound	Annexin V+ /PI − (%)	Annexin V+ /PI + (%)	Apoptotic cells (%)
Control	4.28	0.39	4.67
Resveratrol	15.72	14.86	30.58
Pterostilbene	34.75	15.71	50.46

Figure 4. Effects of resveratrol and pterostilbene on the cell cycle and apoptotic cell death of HeLa cells. (**A**) The cell cycle distribution of HeLa adherent cells was evaluated by flow cytometry after the treatment of the two compounds (40 μM) for 48 h. (**B**) HeLa adherent cells were treated with resveratrol and pterostilbene (40 μM) for 48 h. Apoptotic cells were determined by flow cytometry analysis following annexin V-FITC and propidium iodide (PI) dual labeling.

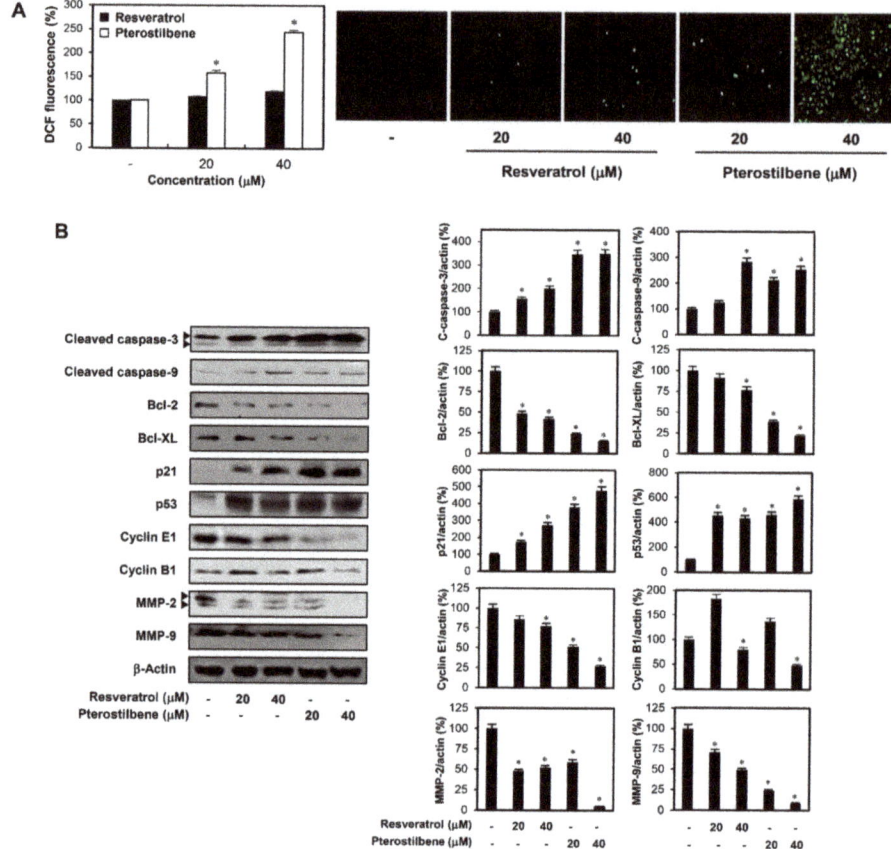

Figure 5. Identification of molecular mechanisms underlying the growth and migration inhibitory effects of resveratrol and pterostilbene in HeLa cells. (**A**) The effects of resveratrol and pterostilbene on reactive oxygen species (ROS) generation in HeLa adherent cells. The cells were treated with resveratrol and pterostilbene (20 and 40 µM) for 48 h. Intracellular ROS levels were detected with 2′,7′-dichlorofluorescein diacetate (DCFH-DA). (**B**) The effects of resveratrol and pterostilbene on the expression of cleaved caspase-3, cleaved caspase-9, Bcl-2, Bcl-XL, p21, p53, cyclin E1, cyclin B1, MMP-2, and MMP-9 in HeLa adherent cells. The cells were treated with the two compounds (20 and 40 µM) for 48 h, and the protein levels were detected by Western blot analysis using specific antibodies. The levels of β-actin were used as an internal control. Arrowheads indicate true bands for the molecular markers. * $p < 0.05$ versus the control.

2.4. Potent Inhibitory Activity of Pterostilbene against the Growth and Migration of Cervical CSCs

CSCs, which play critical roles in therapeutic resistance, recurrence, and metastasis of tumors, have been identified in various solid tumors and hematological cancers including cervical cancer [22,23]. Therefore, anticancer agents with the potential to eliminate cervical CSCs may provide novel therapeutic opportunities for more effective treatment of cervical carcinoma.

To assess the effects of resveratrol and pterostilbene against stem-like properties of cervical cancer cells, the CSC population from HeLa cells was enriched in serum-free suspended spheroid culture condition [24,25]. First, we examined whether the two compounds affect the clonogenic growth as tumorspheres of cancer stem-like cells derived from HeLa cells. The tumorsphere forming ability of HeLa cancer stem-like cells was significantly suppressed by treatment with resveratrol and pterostilbene (Figure 6A). They decreased both the number and size of HeLa cancer stem-like cells. Particularly, pterostilbene was much stronger in inhibiting the tumorsphere formation of HeLa cancer stem-like cells compared with resveratrol.

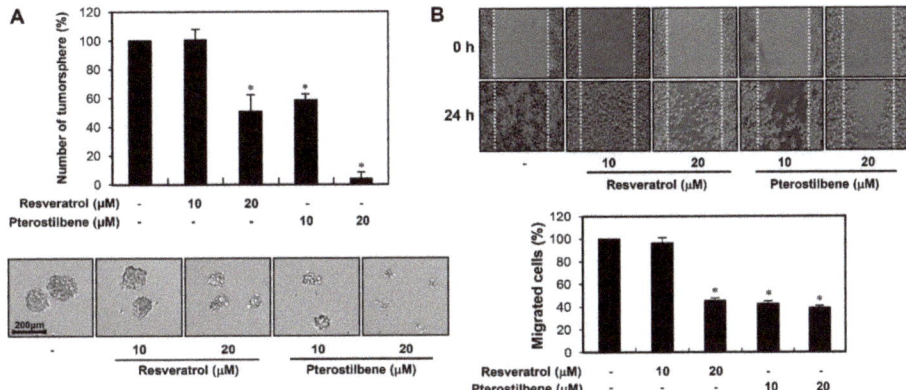

Figure 6. Effects of resveratrol and pterostilbene on the tumorsphere-forming ability and migration of cervical cancer stem cells (CSCs). (**A**) HeLa cancer stem-like cells were treated with the two compounds (10 and 20 µM) and incubated with the CSC culture media for eight days. The number of formed tumorspheres in each well was counted under a microscope. (**B**) HeLa cancer stem-like cells were seeded into laminin-coated culture plate and incubated with the CSC culture media in the absence or presence of resveratrol and pterostilbene (10 and 20 µM) for 24 h. The cells that migrated into the gap were counted under an optical microscope. White lines indicate the edge of the gap at 0 h. * $p < 0.05$ versus the control.

Next, we investigated the effects of resveratrol and pterostilbene on the migration of HeLa cancer stem-like cells. The wound healing assay showed that the two compounds reduced the migration of HeLa cancer stem-like cells when compared to the control conditions (Figure 6B). In addition, the migration inhibition activity of pterostilbene was much more potent than that of resveratrol. These findings underscore the superior therapeutic potential of pterostilbene to eliminate cervical CSCs.

2.5. Pterostilbene Exhibited Better Capacity for Inducing Cell Cycle Arrest and Apoptosis of Cervical CSCs Compared to Resveratrol

To further elucidate the inhibitory effects of resveratrol and pterostilbene on the growth of cervical CSCs, the cell cycle progression and cellular apoptosis of HeLa cancer stem-like cells were measured by flow cytometry analysis. As shown in Figure 7A, both resveratrol and pterostilbene induced S phase arrest (increase in the proportion of arrested cells from 19.87% to 23.83% and 36.93% by treatment with resveratrol and pterostilbene, respectively) when compared with the control cells. Moreover, pterostilbene more strongly induced cell cycle arrest than resveratrol in HeLa cancer stem-like cells. Our data also showed that the number of early and late apoptotic cells was markedly increased after resveratrol and pterostilbene treatment in comparison with the control (Figure 7B). The apoptosis promoting effect of pterostilbene was more potent compared to resveratrol in HeLa cancer stem-like cells (increase in the proportion of total apoptotic cells, from 15.72% to 58.65% and 83.46% by resveratrol and pterostilbene, respectively). These results indicate that pterostilbene has a better capacity for inducing cell cycle arrest and apoptosis of cervical CSCs than resveratrol, thereby causing a stronger inhibition in the tumorsphere-forming ability of cervical CSCs in comparison with resveratrol.

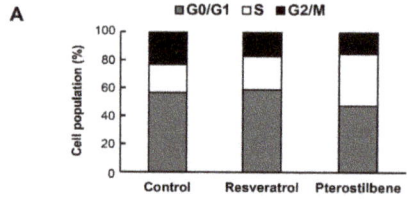

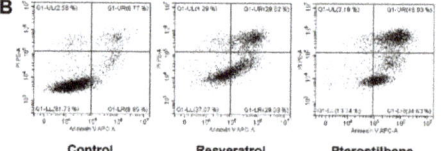

Figure 7. Effects of resveratrol and pterostilbene on the cell cycle and apoptotic cell death of cervical CSCs. (**A**) The cell cycle progression and (**B**) cellular apoptosis of HeLa cancer stem-like cells were measured by flow cytometry analysis after the treatment of resveratrol and pterostilbene (40 μM) for 48 h.

2.6. Effect of Pterostilbene on the Expression of Stemness Markers in Cervical CSCs

To explore the mechanism by which resveratrol and pterostilbene inhibit the growth and migration of cervical CSCs, their effects on the expression of transcription factors, Sox2, Oct4, and Nanog, were investigated. These transcription factors have been reported to induce stem-like properties, in HeLa cancer stem-like cells [26–28]. The two compounds effectively reduced the expression levels of the key stemness-related transcription factors as well as CD133, a cell surface marker for CSCs, suggesting that the inhibitory effects of resveratrol and pterostilbene against cervical CSCs may be associated with the downregulation of these stemness regulators (Figure 8A). Pterostilbene treatment more noticeably decreased the expression levels of stemness markers compared with resveratrol treatment.

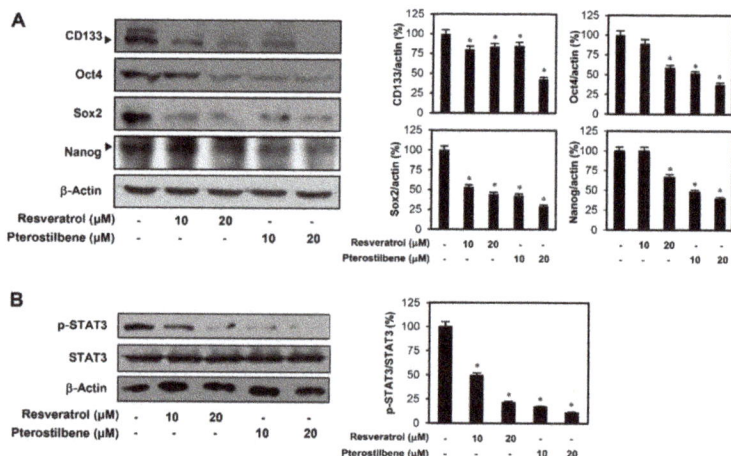

Figure 8. Effects of resveratrol and pterostilbene on stemness markers and signal transducer and activator of transcription 3 (STAT3) signaling in cervical CSCs. (**A**,**B**) HeLa cancer stem-like cells were treated with resveratrol and pterostilbene (10 and 20 μM) for 48 h, and the protein levels were detected by Western blot analysis using specific antibodies. The levels of β-actin were used as an internal control. Arrowheads indicate true bands for the molecular markers. * $p < 0.05$ versus the control.

The STAT3 pathway is involved in the maintenance of cervical CSCs by regulating the expression of stem cell-related transcription factors [29,30]. To further understand the molecular mechanism underlying the anticancer effects of resveratrol and pterostilbene against cervical CSCs, we investigated whether the two compounds affect STAT3 signaling. Our results confirmed that the compounds significantly decreased the expression levels of phosphorylated STAT3, without inhibiting the total protein levels of STAT3 in HeLa cancer stem-like cells (Figure 8B). Furthermore, pterostilbene more profoundly inhibited the phosphorylation of STAT3 than resveratrol. These results demonstrate that pterostilbene is more effective in suppressing the stem-like properties of cervical cancer cells than resveratrol through stronger downregulation of specific CSC markers and STAT3 signaling.

3. Discussion

The health beneficial effects of stilbene, a class of natural polyphenolic compounds, have been extensively studied in the past several decades [10,11]. Resveratrol and pterostilbene, the most widely known stilbenes, have gained increasing attention due to their roles in the potential prevention of major non-infectious chronic diseases such as cancer, cardiovascular disease, diabetes, and neurological degeneration [12–14]. Although both resveratrol and pterostilbene possess the therapeutic activities to inhibit various mechanisms for these human diseases, the bioavailability of pterostilbene with two methoxy groups is higher than resveratrol with two hydroxyl groups [12]. According to several studies, resveratrol and pterostilbene exhibit bioavailability at approximately 20% and 80% in vivo, respectively [31,32]. Such structural differences between the two compounds are expected to make pterostilbene more easily absorbed by oral ingestion through the promotion of lipophilicity and membrane permeability, compared with resveratrol.

The superior anticancer effects of pterostilbene have been reported in various tumors including lung, colon, breast, and cervical cancers [13]. Pterostilbene effectively suppressed cancer progression and metastasis by regulating apoptosis-dependent and apoptosis-independent signaling pathways. Accumulating evidence has shown that the anticancer effects of pterostilbene against cervical cancer are associated with the induction of apoptosis by activating the endoplasmic reticulum (ER)/nuclear factor erythroid 2-related factor 2 (Nrf2) pathway and downregulating the HPV oncoprotein E6 that causes the degradation of tumor suppressor protein p53 [17,33].

In the current study, we thoroughly investigated the cellular mechanisms responsible for the improved anticancer effects of pterostilbene compared to resveratrol in cervical cancer. Our results revealed that the superior growth and migration inhibitory effects of pterostilbene than resveratrol in HeLa cervical cancer cells could be attributed to the following reasons: the enhanced activation of multiple mechanisms, including cell cycle arrest at S and G2/M phases through the reduction of cyclin E1 and cyclin B1 expression following the induction of p53 and its downstream target p21; apoptosis through the activation of caspase-3 and caspase-9 mediated by ROS, as well as the downregulation of antiapoptotic proteins such as Bcl-2 and Bcl-XL; and the inhibition of MMP-2 and MMP-9 expression.

In addition, this is the first study to investigate the suppressive activities of pterostilbene and resveratrol against cervical cancer stemness. The critical role of CSCs in cancer progression and metastasis has already been identified and validated in many studies [4,5,22,23]. Notably, CSCs display resistance to many types of therapies, which results in cancer recurrence. Thus, it is important to suppress the self-renewal, proliferation, and metastasis abilities of CSCs for more reliable cancer treatment. In several cancers, the therapeutic effects of pterostilbene to eradicate CSCs have been confirmed. Pterostilbene inhibits the tumorsphere formation, migration, and stemness-related gene expression of CD133+ CSCs by downregulating multifaceted oncoprotein (MUC1), NF-κB, and Wnt/β-catenin-dependent signaling pathways in lung, breast, brain, and liver tumors [34–38]. However, the inhibitory effect of pterostilbene against cervical CSCs has not been studied previously.

In this study, pterostilbene significantly suppressed both the tumorsphere-forming ability and migration of HeLa cancer stem-like cells. Particularly, the therapeutic potential of pterostilbene to suppress cervical CSCs was markedly stronger than resveratrol. A tumorsphere is a solid, spherical structure developed from the proliferation of the cancer stem/progenitor cells. In these results, pterostilbene showed a better capacity for inducing cell cycle arrest and apoptosis of cervical CSCs in comparison with resveratrol. Therefore, the cell cycle arrest and apoptosis promoting effect of pterostilbene compared to resveratrol led to a stronger inhibition in the tumorsphere formation of HeLa cancer stem-like cells.

The stemness supporting transcription factors, such as Sox2, Klf4, c-Myc, Oct4, and Nanog, are upregulated in various types of CSCs [22,23,26–28]. Our results demonstrated that pterostilbene effectively decreased the expression levels of the major stemness transcription factors, including Sox2, Oct4, and Nanog, as well as a cell surface marker for CSCs, CD133, suggesting that the inhibitory effect of pterostilbene against cervical CSCs may be associated with the downregulation of these stemness regulators. In addition, pterostilbene more markedly suppressed the expression of stemness markers than resveratrol.

STAT3 is a transcription factor that is activated in many cancer types and can regulate pathways involving cell proliferation, cell survival, angiogenesis, and tumorigenesis [39]. Recent studies have revealed that STAT3 is an important regulator for self-renewal and survival of CSCs in various tumors [40]. In cervical carcinoma, STAT3 upregulates the stem-like characteristics of cervical cancer cells by increasing the expression of the stemness supporting markers such as Sox2, Oct4, and Nanog [29,30]. Therefore, targeting STAT3 signaling may be a promising approach to combat the survival of cervical CSCs. In the present study, pterostilbene resulted in a reduction in the expression levels of phosphorylated STAT3, without affecting the total protein levels of STAT3 in HeLa cancer stem-like cells. Furthermore, pterostilbene was more effective in suppressing the phosphorylation of STAT3 than resveratrol.

Our results collectively demonstrate that pterostilbene can suppress the stem-like properties of cervical cancer cells by downregulating specific CSC markers and STAT3 signaling. Thus, pterostilbene might serve as a potential anticancer agent for more effectively eradicating cervical cancer by targeting both cancer cells and CSCs, with superior bioavailability compared to resveratrol. However, the precise mechanism underlying how pterostilbene modulates the phosphorylation of STAT3 remains unclear. It is well known that STAT3 is phosphorylated by various protein kinases, including epidermal growth factor receptor (EGFR), Janus kinases (JAK), and Src family kinases (SFKs) [41]. Accumulating evidence has revealed that pterostilbene and resveratrol can induce cell cycle arrest and apoptosis by inhibiting the upstream kinase activities of STAT3 signaling in several cancers such as breast, pancreatic, prostate, and bone tumors [42–45]. Further studies to understand the mechanism of action of pterostilbene against cervical CSCs will help the discovery of the upstream cellular mediators of STAT3 activity regulated by pterostilbene. Moreover, further in vivo experiments using tumor xenograft animal models will be required to better verify the therapeutic potential of pterostilbene for cervical cancer compared to resveratrol.

4. Materials and Methods

4.1. Materials

Resveratrol and pterostilbene were purchased from Sigma-Aldrich (Saint Louis, MO, USA) and dissolved in dimethyl sulfoxide (DMSO) at a concentration of 100 mM to prepare a stock solution. Matrigel and gelatin were obtained from BD Biosciences (San Jose, CA, USA). Laminin and the Transwell chamber system were obtained from Koma Biotech (Seoul, Korea) and Corning Costar (Acton, MA, USA), respectively. Antibodies against p21, p53, MMP-2, MMP-9, Bcl-2, Bcl-XL, cleaved caspase-3, cleaved caspase-9, cyclin E1, cyclin B1, STAT3, phospho-STAT3, Sox2, Oct4, Nanog, β-actin, rabbit IgG, and mouse IgG were purchased from Cell Signaling Technology (Danvers, MA, USA). Anti-CD133 antibody was obtained from MiltenyiBiotec GmbH (BergischGladbach, Germany).

4.2. Cell Culture

Human cervical cancer HeLa, CaSki, and SiHa cell lines were obtained from the Korean Cell Line Bank (KCLB). The cells were cultured in Dulbecco's modified Eagle medium (DMEM; Gibco, Grand Island, NY, USA) supplemented with 10% fetal bovine serum (FBS; Gibco) and 1% penicillin–streptomycin–amphotericin B (Lonza, Walkersville, MD, USA) and then maintained at 37 °C in a 5% CO_2 humidified incubator.

4.3. Cell Growth Assay

HeLa, CaSki, and SiHa cells (3×10^3 cells/well) were seeded in a 96-well culture plate and then treated with various concentrations of resveratrol and pterostilbene (0–200 µM) for 72 h. Cell growth was measured with the 3-(4,5-dimethylthiazol-2-yl)-2,5-diphenyltetrazolium bromide (MTT) colorimetric assay (Sigma-Aldrich). The absorbance of each well was determined at a wavelength of 540 nm using a microplate reader (Thermo Fisher Scientific, Vantaa, Finland). The IC_{50} values from obtained data were analyzed using the curve-fitting program GraphPad Prism 5 (GraphPad Software, La Jolla, CA, USA).

4.4. Colony Formation Assay

To evaluate the colony forming inhibitory effects of resveratrol and pterostilbene, HeLa, CaSki, and SiHa cells (2.5×10^2 cells/well) were seeded in a six-well culture plate. After 24 h incubation, the cells were treated with resveratrol and pterostilbene (10 and 20 µM) and incubated for 7 days until colonies were formed. Following this, the colonies were fixed with 4% formaldehyde and stained with 0.5% crystal violet solution for 10 min and washed with double-distilled water. The number of colonies on each well was counted and the percentage of compound-treated colonies relative to DMSO-treated control colonies was calculated.

4.5. Wound Healing Assay

HeLa cells (2.5×10^5 cells/well) were seeded in a 24-well culture plate. The confluent monolayer cells were scratched using a tip and each well was washed with PBS to remove non-adherent cells. The cells were treated with resveratrol and pterostilbene (20 µM) and then incubated for up to 48 h. The perimeter of the central cell-free zone was observed under an optical microscope (Olympus, Center Valley, PA, USA).

4.6. Invasion Assay

The invasiveness of cells was examined using Transwell chamber inserts with a pore size of 8.0 µm. The lower surface of the polycarbonate filter was coated with 10 µL of gelatin (1 mg/mL), while the upper surface was coated with 10 µL of Matrigel (3 mg/mL). HeLa cells (5×10^4 cells/well) were seeded in the upper chamber of the filter; resveratrol and pterostilbene (10 and 20 µM) were added to the lower chamber filled with medium. The chamber was incubated at 37 °C for 48 h, and then the cells were fixed with 70% methanol and stained with hematoxylin and eosin (H and E). The total number of cells that invaded the lower chamber of the filter was counted using an optical microscope (Olympus).

4.7. Cell Cycle Analysis

The cell cycle distribution was analyzed using the Muse Cell Cycle Assay Kit (Millipore, Hayward, CA, USA) according to the manufacturer's instructions. To this end, HeLa cells (5×10^5 cells/dish) were seeded in a 60-mm culture dish and treated with resveratrol and pterostilbene for 48 h. The cells were collected by centrifugation and washed using PBS and fixed in ice cold 70% ethanol at −20 °C for more than 3 h. The cells were then incubated with the Muse Cell Cycle reagent for 30 min at room temperature in the dark. The cell cycle analysis was carried out using the Muse Cell Analyzer (Millipore).

4.8. Apoptosis Analysis

The apoptotic cell distribution was determined using the Muse Annexin V and Dead Cell Kit (Millipore) according to the manufacturer's instructions. Briefly, after treatment with resveratrol and pterostilbene, HeLa cells were collected and diluted with PBS containing 1% bovine serum albumin (BSA) as a dilution buffer to a concentration of 5×10^5 cells/mL. The single cell suspension was mixed with the Muse Annexin V/Dead Cell reagent at a 1:1 ratio and incubated in the dark for 20 min at room temperature. The cells were then analyzed using the Muse Cell Analyzer (Millipore).

4.9. Reactive Oxygen Species (ROS) Measurement

Intracellular ROS levels were measured using a ROS-sensitive fluorescence indicator, 2′,7′-dichlorofluorescein diacetate (DCFH-DA; Sigma-Aldrich). HeLa cells (1×10^5 cells/well) were seeded in a 96-black well culture plate and treated with resveratrol and pterostilbene (20 and 40 µM) for 48 h. The cells were then incubated with 10 µM of DCFH-DA for 20 min and washed with PBS. The fluorescence intensity of DCF was detected using a multimode microplate reader (Biotek, Inc., Winooski, VT, USA) at the excitation and emission wavelengths of 495 and 529 nm, respectively. The fluorescent images were also acquired using an Optinity KI-2000F fluorescence microscope (Korea Lab Tech, Seong Nam, Korea).

4.10. Western Blot Analysis

Cells were lysed using RIPA buffer (Sigma-Aldrich) supplemented with a protease inhibitor cocktail (Roche Diagnostics, Mannheim, Germany) on ice. Protein concentrations of the extracts were determined using a BCA Protein Assay kit (Pierce; Thermo Fisher Scientific, Inc., Waltham, MA, USA). Equal amounts of cell lysate were separated by 10% sodium dodecyl sulfate-polyacrylamide gel electrophoresis (SDS-PAGE), and the separated proteins were transferred to polyvinylidene difluoride (PVDF) membranes (EMD Millipore) using standard electroblotting procedures. The blots were blocked in Tris-buffered saline with Tween-20 (TBST) containing 5% skim milk at room temperature for 1 h and immunolabeled with primary antibodies against p21, p53, MMP-2, MMP-9, Bcl-2, Bcl-XL, cleaved caspase-3, cleaved caspase-9, cyclin E1, cyclin B1, STAT3, phospho-STAT3, Sox2, Oct4, Nanog, CD133 (dilution 1:2000), and β-actin (dilution 1:10000) overnight at 4 °C. After washing with TBST three times, the membranes were incubated with horseradish peroxidase-conjugated anti-rabbit or anti-mouse (dilution 1:3000) secondary antibody for 1 h at room temperature. Immunolabeling was detected with an enhanced chemiluminescence (ECL) kit (Bio-Rad Laboratories, Inc., Hercules, CA, USA) according to the manufacturer's instructions. The band density was analyzed using ImageJ software (version 1.5; NIH).

4.11. CSC Culture

CSCs were cultured using a non-adhesive culture method [24,25]. To propagate cervical cancer stem-like cells, HeLa cells grown in the serum-based media were cultured in Dulbecco's modified Eagle medium/nutrient mixture F-12 (DMEM/F12; Gibco) containing 1× B-27 serum-free supplement (Gibco), 5 µg/mL heparin (Sigma-Aldrich), 2 mM L-glutamine (Gibco), 20 ng/mL epidermal growth factor (EGF; Gibco), 20 ng/mL basic fibroblast growth factor (bFGF; Gibco), and 1% penicillin/streptomycin (Gibco). Tumorspheres grown in the serum-free media were subcultured every 7 days by dissociating with Accutase (Millipore) and maintained at 37 °C in a 5% CO_2 humidified incubator.

4.12. CSC Tumorsphere Formation Assay

HeLa cancer stem-like cells were seeded in a 96-well culture plate at a density of 500 cells/well using the serum-free media with EGF and bFGF. After 8 days of resveratrol and pterostilbene treatment (10 and 20 µM), the number of tumorspheres formed in each well was counted under an optical microscope (Olympus).

4.13. CSC Migration Assay

For the CSC migration assay, the ibidi culture inserts (IBIDI GmbH, Martinsried, Germany) were placed in a laminin-coated 24-well culture plate. HeLa cancer stem-like cells were prepared at a density of 5×10^5 cells/mL, of which 70 µL was transferred to each chamber. After cell attachment for 24 h, the culture inserts were removed, and the attached cells were incubated with the serum-free media containing EGF and bFGF, in the absence or presence of resveratrol and pterostilbene (10 and 20 µM) for 24 h. The perimeter of the central cell-free zone was confirmed under an optical microscope (Olympus).

4.14. Statistical Analysis

The data were presented as the mean ± standard error (SE) of three independent experiments. Student's *t*-test was used to determine statistical significance between the control and the test groups. A *p*-value of <0.05 was considered to indicate a statistically significant difference.

5. Conclusions

The present study focused on the therapeutic effect and mechanism underlying the anticancer effects of pterostilbene against both cancer cells and cancer stem-like cells in cervical cancer compared to resveratrol. Our results demonstrated that the superior inhibitory effects of pterostilbene compared to resveratrol were associated with the enhanced activation of multiple mechanisms, including cell cycle arrest at S and G2/M phases through the induction of p53 and p21 and subsequent reduction of cyclin E1 and cyclin B1; apoptosis through the activation of caspase-3 and -9 mediated by ROS and the downregulation of Bcl-2 and Bcl-XL antiapoptotic proteins; and the inhibition of MMP-2 and -9 expression. Notably, pterostilbene exhibited a greater inhibitory effect against HeLa cancer stem-like cells than resveratrol through more potent inhibition of the expression levels of stemness markers, such as CD133, Oct4, Sox2, and Nanog, as well as STAT3 signaling. Based on these findings, we conclude that pterostilbene is a better potential candidate than resveratrol for more effectively treating cervical carcinoma.

Author Contributions: H.J.J. conceived and designed the experiments; H.J.S., J.M.H. and Y.S.C. performed the experiments and analyzed the data; H.J.S. and H.J.J. wrote the paper. All authors have read and agreed to the published version of the manuscript.

Funding: This research was supported by the Basic Science Research Program through the National Research Foundation of Korea (NRF) funded by the Ministry of Education (NRF-2016R1D1A1B03932956) and the NRF grant funded by the Ministry of Science and ICT (No. 2019R1A2C1009033). This work was also supported by the Brain Korea 21 Plus Project, Republic of Korea.

Conflicts of Interest: The authors declare no conflict of interest.

References

1. Torre, L.A.; Bray, F.; Siegel, R.L.; Ferlay, J.; Lortet-Tieulent, J.; Jemal, A. Global cancer statistics, 2012. *CA Cancer J. Clin.* **2015**, *65*, 87–108. [CrossRef]
2. Schiffman, M.; Castle, P.E.; Jeronimo, J.; Rodriguez, A.C.; Wacholder, S. Human papillomavirus and cervical cancer. *Lancet* **2007**, *370*, 890–907. [CrossRef]
3. Liontos, M.; Kyriazoglou, A.; Dimitriadis, I.; Dimopoulos, M.A.; Bamias, A. Systemic therapy in cervical cancer: 30 years in review. *Crit. Rev. Oncol. Hematol.* **2019**, *137*, 9–17. [CrossRef]
4. Ortiz-Sánchez, E.; Santiago-López, L.; Cruz-Domínguez, V.B.; Toledo-Guzmán, M.E.; Hernández-Cueto, D.; Muñiz-Hernández, S.; Garrido, E.; Cantú De León, D.; García-Carrancá, A. Characterization of cervical cancer stem cell-like cells: Phenotyping, stemness, and human papilloma virus co-receptor expression. *Oncotarget* **2016**, *7*, 31943–31954. [CrossRef]
5. Huang, R.; Rofstad, E.K. Cancer stem cells (CSCs), cervical CSCs and targeted therapies. *Oncotarget* **2017**, *8*, 35351–35367. [CrossRef]
6. Tyagi, A.; Vishnoi, K.; Mahata, S.; Verma, G.; Srivastava, Y.; Masaldan, S.; Roy, B.G.; Bharti, A.C.; Das, B.C. Cervical cancer stem cells selectively overexpress HPV oncoprotein E6 that controls stemness and self-renewal through upregulation of HES1. *Clin. Cancer Res.* **2016**, *22*, 4170–4184. [CrossRef] [PubMed]
7. Organista-Nava, J.; Gómez-Gómez, Y.; Ocadiz-Delgado, R.; García-Villa, E.; Bonilla-Delgado, J.; Lagunas-Martínez, A.; Tapia, J.S.; Lambert, P.F.; García-Carrancá, A.; Gariglio, P. The HPV16 E7 oncoprotein increases the expression of Oct3/4 and stemness-related genes and augments cell self-renewal. *Virology* **2016**, *499*, 230–242. [CrossRef]

8. Cragg, G.M.; Newman, D.J. Plants as a source of anti-cancer agents. *J. Ethnopharmacol.* **2005**, *100*, 72–79. [CrossRef] [PubMed]
9. Yin, S.Y.; Wei, W.C.; Jian, F.Y.; Yang, N.S. Therapeutic applications of herbal medicines for cancer patients. *Evid. Based Complement. Alternat. Med.* **2013**, *2013*, 302426. [CrossRef] [PubMed]
10. Chong, J.; Poutaraud, A.; Hugueney, P. Metabolism and roles of stilbenes in plants. *Plant Sci.* **2009**, *177*, 143–155. [CrossRef]
11. Akinwumi, B.C.; Bordun, K.M.; Anderson, H.D. Biological activities of stilbenoids. *Int. J. Mol. Sci.* **2018**, *19*, 792. [CrossRef]
12. Tsai, H.Y.; Ho, C.T.; Chen, Y.K. Biological actions and molecular effects of resveratrol, pterostilbene, and 3′-hydroxypterostilbene. *J. Food Drug Anal.* **2017**, *25*, 134–147. [CrossRef]
13. Chen, R.J.; Kuo, H.C.; Cheng, L.H.; Lee, Y.H.; Chang, W.T.; Wang, B.J.; Wang, Y.J.; Cheng, H.C. Apoptotic and nonapoptotic activities of pterostilbene against cancer. *Int. J. Mol. Sci.* **2018**, *19*, 287. [CrossRef]
14. Xiao, Q.; Zhu, W.; Feng, W.; Lee, S.S.; Leung, A.W.; Shen, J.; Gao, L.; Xu, C. A review of resveratrol as a potent chemoprotective and synergistic agent in cancer chemotherapy. *Front. Pharmacol.* **2019**, *9*, 1534. [CrossRef] [PubMed]
15. Asensi, M.; Medina, I.; Ortega, A.; Carretero, J.; Baño, M.C.; Obrador, E.; Estrela, J.M. Inhibition of cancer growth by resveratrol is related to its low bioavailability. *Free Radic. Biol. Med.* **2002**, *33*, 387–398. [CrossRef]
16. Nutakul, W.; Sobers, H.S.; Qiu, P.; Dong, P.; Decker, E.A.; McClements, D.J.; Xiao, H. Inhibitory effects of resveratrol and pterostilbene on human colon cancer cells: A side-by-side comparison. *J. Agric. Food Chem.* **2011**, *59*, 10964–10970. [CrossRef] [PubMed]
17. Chatterjee, K.; AlSharif, D.; Mazza, C.; Syar, P.; Al Sharif, M.; Fata, J.E. Resveratrol and pterostilbene exhibit anticancer properties involving the downregulation of HPV oncoprotein E6 in cervical cancer cells. *Nutrients* **2018**, *10*, 243. [CrossRef] [PubMed]
18. Libra, M.; Scalisi, A.; Vella, N.; Clementi, S.; Sorio, R.; Stivala, F.; Spandidos, D.A.; Mazzarino, C. Uterine cervical carcinoma: Role of matrix metalloproteinases (review). *Int. J. Oncol.* **2009**, *34*, 897–903. [CrossRef]
19. Wu, G.; Lin, N.; Xu, L.; Liu, B.; Feitelson, M.A. UCN-01 induces S and G2/M cell cycle arrest through the p53/p21(waf1) or CHK2/CDC25C pathways and can suppress invasion in human hepatoma cell lines. *BMC Cancer* **2013**, *13*, 167. [CrossRef]
20. Redza-Dutordoir, M.; Averill-Bates, D.A. Activation of apoptosis signalling pathways by reactive oxygen species. *Biochim. Biophys. Acta* **2016**, *1863*, 2977–2992. [CrossRef]
21. Wu, P.P.; Chung, H.W.; Liu, K.C.; Wu, R.S.; Yang, J.S.; Tang, N.Y.; Lo, C.; Hsia, T.C.; Yu, C.C.; Chueh, F.S.; et al. Diallyl sulfide induces cell cycle arrest and apoptosis in HeLa human cervical cancer cells through the p53, caspase- and mitochondria-dependent pathways. *Int. J. Oncol.* **2011**, *38*, 1605–1613. [PubMed]
22. Reya, T.; Morrison, S.J.; Clarke, M.F.; Weissman, I.L. Stem cells, cancer, and cancer stem cells. *Nature* **2001**, *414*, 105–111. [CrossRef]
23. Jordan, C.T.; Guzman, M.L.; Noble, M. Cancer stem cells. *N. Engl. J. Med.* **2006**, *355*, 1253–1261. [CrossRef]
24. Cao, H.Z.; Liu, X.F.; Yang, W.T.; Chen, Q.; Zheng, P.S. LGR5 promotes cancer stem cell traits and chemoresistance in cervical cancer. *Cell Death Dis.* **2017**, *8*, e3039. [CrossRef]
25. Kim, B.; Jung, N.; Lee, S.; Sohng, J.K.; Jung, H.J. Apigenin inhibits cancer stem cell-like phenotypes in human glioblastoma cells via suppression of c-Met signaling. *Phytother. Res.* **2016**, *30*, 1833–1840. [CrossRef] [PubMed]
26. Yao, T.; Lu, R.; Zhang, Y.; Zhang, Y.; Zhao, C.; Lin, R.; Lin, Z. Cervical cancer stem cells. *Cell Prolif.* **2015**, *48*, 611–625. [CrossRef] [PubMed]
27. Li, Z. CD133: A stem cell biomarker and beyond. *Exp. Hematol. Oncol.* **2013**, *2*, 17. [CrossRef]
28. Bigoni-Ordóñez, G.D.; Ortiz-Sánchez, E.; Rosendo-Chalma, P.; Valencia-González, H.A.; Aceves, C.; García-Carrancá, A. Molecular iodine inhibits the expression of stemness markers on cancer stem-like cells of established cell lines derived from cervical cancer. *BMC Cancer* **2018**, *18*, 928. [CrossRef]
29. Wang, H.; Cai, H.B.; Chen, L.L.; Zhao, W.J.; Li, P.; Wang, Z.Q.; Li, Z. STAT3 correlates with stem cell-related transcription factors in cervical cancer. *J. Huazhong Univ. Sci. Technol.* **2015**, *35*, 891–897. [CrossRef]
30. Wang, H.; Deng, J.; Ren, H.Y.; Jia, P.; Zhang, W.; Li, M.Q.; Li, S.W.; Zhou, Q.H. STAT3 influences the characteristics of stem cells in cervical carcinoma. *Oncol. Lett.* **2017**, *14*, 2131–2136. [CrossRef]
31. Kapetanovic, I.M.; Muzzio, M.; Huang, Z.; Thompson, T.N.; McCormick, D.L. Pharmacokinetics, oral bioavailability, and metabolic profile of resveratrol and its dimethylether analog, pterostilbene, in rats. *Cancer Chemother. Pharmacol.* **2011**, *68*, 593–601. [CrossRef]

32. Francioso, A.; Mastromarino, P.; Masci, A.; d'Erme, M.; Mosca, L. Chemistry, stability and bioavailability of resveratrol. *Med. Chem.* **2014**, *10*, 237–245. [CrossRef] [PubMed]
33. Zhang, B.; Wang, X.Q.; Chen, H.Y.; Liu, B.H. Involvement of the Nrf2 pathway in the regulation of pterostilbene-induced apoptosis in HeLa cells via ER stress. *J. Pharmacol. Sci.* **2014**, *126*, 216–229. [CrossRef]
34. Mak, K.K.; Wu, A.T.; Lee, W.H.; Chang, T.C.; Chiou, J.F.; Wang, L.S.; Wu, C.H.; Huang, C.Y.; Shieh, Y.S.; Chao, T.Y.; et al. Pterostilbene, a bioactive component of blueberries, suppresses the generation of breast cancer stem cells within tumor microenvironment and metastasis via modulating NF-κB/microRNA 448 circuit. *Mol. Nutr. Food Res.* **2013**, *57*, 1123–1134. [CrossRef]
35. Huang, W.C.; Chan, M.L.; Chen, M.J.; Tsai, T.H.; Chen, Y.J. Modulation of macrophage polarization and lung cancer cell stemness by MUC1 and development of a related small-molecule inhibitor pterostilbene. *Oncotarget* **2016**, *7*, 39363–39375. [CrossRef] [PubMed]
36. Huynh, T.T.; Lin, C.M.; Lee, W.H.; Wu, A.T.; Lin, Y.K.; Lin, Y.F.; Yeh, C.T.; Wang, L.S. Pterostilbene suppressed irradiation-resistant glioma stem cells by modulating GRP78/miR-205 axis. *J. Nutr. Biochem.* **2015**, *26*, 466–475. [CrossRef] [PubMed]
37. Lee, C.M.; Su, Y.H.; Huynh, T.T.; Lee, W.H.; Chiou, J.F.; Lin, Y.K.; Hsiao, M.; Wu, C.H.; Lin, Y.F.; Wu, A.T.; et al. Blueberry isolate, pterostilbene, functions as a potential anticancer stem cell agent in suppressing irradiation-mediated enrichment of hepatoma stem cells. *Evid. Based Complement. Alternat. Med.* **2013**, *2013*, 258425. [CrossRef] [PubMed]
38. Paul, S.; DeCastro, A.J.; Lee, H.J.; Smolarek, A.K.; So, J.Y.; Simi, B.; Wang, C.X.; Zhou, R.; Rimando, A.M.; Suh, N. Dietary intake of pterostilbene, a constituent of blueberries, inhibits the beta-catenin/p65 downstream signaling pathway and colon carcinogenesis in rats. *Carcinogenesis* **2010**, *31*, 1272–1278. [CrossRef]
39. Chai, E.Z.; Shanmugam, M.K.; Arfuso, F.; Dharmarajan, A.; Wang, C.; Kumar, A.P.; Samy, R.P.; Lim, L.H.; Wang, L.; Goh, B.C.; et al. Targeting transcription factor STAT3 for cancer prevention and therapy. *Pharmacol. Ther.* **2016**, *162*, 86–97. [CrossRef]
40. Galoczova, M.; Coates, P.; Vojtesek, B. STAT3, stem cells, cancer stem cells and p63. *Cell. Mol. Biol. Lett.* **2018**, *23*, 12. [CrossRef]
41. Bromberg, J., Jr.; Darnell, J.E. The role of STATs in transcriptional control and their impact on cellular function. *Oncogene* **2000**, *19*, 2468–2473. [CrossRef]
42. Kotha, A.; Sekharam, M.; Cilenti, L.; Siddiquee, K.; Khaled, A.; Zervos, A.S.; Carter, B.; Turkson, J.; Jove, R. Resveratrol inhibits Src and Stat3 signaling and induces the apoptosis of malignant cells containing activated Stat3 protein. *Mol. Cancer Ther.* **2006**, *5*, 621–629. [CrossRef] [PubMed]
43. McCormack, D.; Schneider, J.; McDonald, D.; McFadden, D. The antiproliferative effects of pterostilbene on breast cancer in vitro are via inhibition of constitutive and leptin-induced Janus kinase/signal transducer and activator of transcription activation. *Am. J. Surg.* **2011**, *202*, 541–544. [CrossRef]
44. Liu, Y.; Wang, L.; Wu, Y.; Lv, C.; Li, X.; Cao, X.; Yang, M.; Feng, D.; Luo, Z. Pterostilbene exerts antitumor activity against human osteosarcoma cells by inhibiting the JAK2/STAT3 signaling pathway. *Toxicology* **2013**, *304*, 120–131. [CrossRef] [PubMed]
45. Chen, R.J.; Tsai, S.J.; Ho, C.T.; Pan, M.H.; Ho, Y.S.; Wu, C.H.; Wang, Y.J. Chemopreventive effects of pterostilbene on urethane-induced lung carcinogenesis in mice via the inhibition of EGFR-mediated pathways and the induction of apoptosis and autophagy. *J. Agric. Food Chem.* **2012**, *60*, 11533–11541. [CrossRef] [PubMed]

Sample Availability: Samples are available from the first or corresponding author.

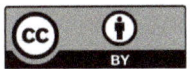

© 2020 by the authors. Licensee MDPI, Basel, Switzerland. This article is an open access article distributed under the terms and conditions of the Creative Commons Attribution (CC BY) license (http://creativecommons.org/licenses/by/4.0/).

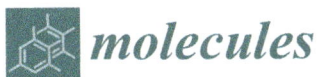

Article

Isolation, Structure Elucidation, and Antiproliferative Activity of Butanolides and Lignan Glycosides from the Fruit of *Hernandia nymphaeifolia*

Simayijiang Aimaiti [1], Yohei Saito [1], Shuichi Fukuyoshi [1], Masuo Goto [2], Katsunori Miyake [3], David J. Newman [4], Barry R. O'Keefe [5,6], Kuo-Hsiung Lee [2,7] and Kyoko Nakagawa-Goto [1,2,*]

1. School of Pharmaceutical Sciences, College of Medical, Pharmaceutical and Health Sciences, Kanazawa University, Kanazawa 920-1192, Japan; ismayil507@stu.kanazawa-u.ac.jp (S.A.); saito-y@staff.kanazawa-u.ac.jp (Y.S.); fukuyosi@p.kanazawa-u.ac.jp (S.F.)
2. Natural Products Research Laboratories, UNC Eshelman School of Pharmacy, University of North Carolina at Chapel Hill, Chapel Hill, NC 27599-7568, USA; goto@med.unc.edu (M.G.); khlee@unc.edu (K.-H.L.)
3. Tokyo University of Pharmacy and Life Sciences, Hachioji, Tokyo 192-0392, Japan; miyake@toyaku.ac.jp
4. NIH Special Volunteer, Wayne, PA 19087, USA; newmand@mail.nih.gov
5. Natural Products Branch, Developmental Therapeutics Program, Division of Cancer Treatment and Diagnosis, National Cancer Institute, NCI at Frederick, Frederick, MD 21702-1201, USA; okeefeba@mail.nih.gov
6. Molecular Targets Program, Center for Cancer Research, National Cancer Institute, NCI at Frederick, Frederick, MD 21702-1201, USA
7. Chinese Medicine Research and Development Center, China Medical University and Hospital, Taichung 40447, Taiwan
* Correspondence: kngoto@p.kanazawa-u.ac.jp; Tel.: +81-762-264-6305

Academic Editor: Maria Carla Marcotullio
Received: 9 October 2019; Accepted: 31 October 2019; Published: 5 November 2019

Abstract: Seven new butanolides, peltanolides A–G (**1–7**), and two lignan glucosides, peltasides A (**8**) and B (**9**), along with eleven known compounds, **10–20**, were isolated from a crude CH_3OH/CH_2Cl_2 (1:1) extract of the fruit of *Hernandia nymphaeifolia* (Hernandiaceae). The structures of **1–9** were characterized by extensive 1D and 2D NMR spectroscopic and HRMS analysis. The absolute configurations of newly isolated compounds **1–9** were determined from data obtained by optical rotation and electronic circular dichroism (ECD) exciton chirality methods. Butanolides and lignan glucosides have not been isolated previously from this genus. Several isolated compounds were evaluated for antiproliferative activity against human tumor cell lines. Lignans **15** and **16** were slightly active against chemosensitive tumor cell lines A549 and MCF-7, respectively. Furthermore, both compounds displayed significant activity (IC_{50} = 5 µM) against a P-glycoprotein overexpressing multidrug-resistant tumor cell line (KB-VIN) but were less active against its parent chemosensitive cell line (KB).

Keywords: *Hernandia nymphaeifolia*; butanolides; lignan glycosides; antiproliferative activity

1. Introduction

Plants in the genus *Hernandia* (Hernandiaceae) are found in subtropical and tropical areas [1]. They contain diverse bioactive secondary metabolites, especially lignans, including podophyllotoxin analogues [2,3], and benzylisoquinolines [4], including aporphines [5–7]. These compounds exhibit various biological activities, including significant cytotoxic [8,9], antiplasmodial [9,10], and antibacterial activities [2]. *H. nymphaeifolia* (C.Presl) Kubitzki (synonym: *H. peltata* Meisn.) is a common coastal tree and grows to 12–20 m in height. This plant has been used for the treatment of abdominal pains, boils, cough, diarrhea, eye problems, and convulsions as a traditional medicine in western Samoa [11]. A CH$_3$OH/CH$_2$Cl$_2$ (1:1) extract of *H. nymphaeifolia* (N053499, originally described as *H. peltata*) provided by the U.S. National Cancer Institute Natural Products Branch (NCI, Frederick, MD, USA) exhibited broad cytotoxicity in the NCI-60 human tumor cell line (HTCL) assay, possibly due to the above or similar cytotoxic constituents. To supplement the reported phytochemical research on *H. nymphaeifolia* [2,4,9,12–14], we conducted a thorough study to identify new chemical compounds as part of our continuing investigation of rainforest plants. Accordingly, the extract of N053499 yielded seven new butanolides, peltanolides A–G (**1–7**), and two new lignan glycosides, peltasides A (**8**) and B (**9**), as well as eleven known compounds **10–20** (Figure 1). Herein, we report the details of isolation, structure elucidation, and cytotoxicity of isolated compounds from *H. nymphaeifolia*.

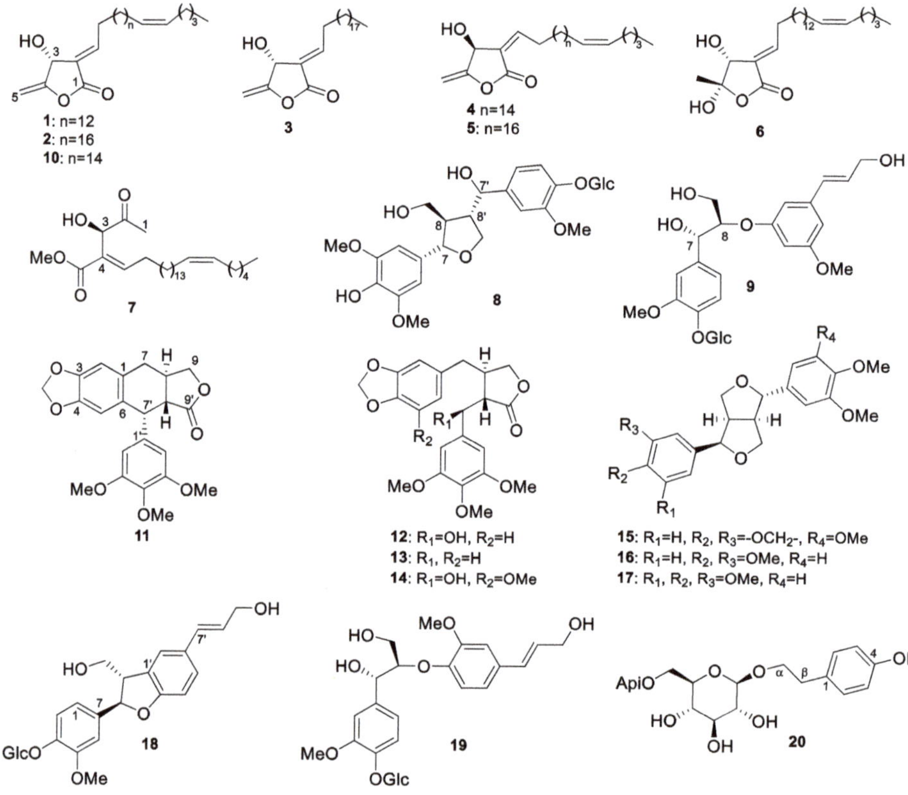

Figure 1. Isolated compounds (**1–20**) from *H. nymphaeifolia*.

2. Results and Discussion

2.1. Structure Elucidation of Isolated Compounds from H. nymphaeifolia

The CH$_3$OH/CH$_2$Cl$_2$ (1:1) extract of *H. nymphaeifolia* (fruit, N053499) was firstly partitioned with water and *n*-hexane. The water fraction was further partitioned with EtOAc and *n*-BuOH. All fractions were subjected to a combination of column chromatography, preparative HPLC, and preparative TLC using silica gel and octadecylsilyl (ODS) to give seven new butanolides, peltanolides A–G (**1–7**), and two new lignan glycosides, peltasides A (**8**) and B (**9**), as well as eleven known compounds, tambouranolide (**10**) [15], deoxypodophyllotoxin (**11**) [16], podorhizol (**12**) [17], bursehernin (**13**) [18], (2*S*,3*S*)-(+)-5′-methoxyyatein (**14**) [19], epiashantin (**15**) [20], epieudesmin (**16**) [21], (1*S*,3a*R*,4*R*,6a*R*)-

1-(3,4-dimethoxyphenyl)-4-(3′,4′,5′-trimethoxyphenyl)tetrahydro-1H,3H-furo-[3–c]furan (**17**) [20], (7R,8S)-dehydrodiconiferyl alcohol-4-O-β-D-glucoside (**18**) [22], alaschanioside A (**19**) [23], and osmanthuside H (**20**) [24]. The structures of all known compounds were identified by comparison of their spectroscopic data with reported values.

Compound **1** was obtained as a yellow amorphous solid: $[\alpha]^{25}_D$ + 27.3 (c 0.075, CHCl$_3$). It gave a [M]$^+$ peak at m/z 390.3137, appropriate for a molecular formula of C$_{25}$H$_{42}$O$_3$. The ^{1}H and ^{13}C NMR spectra (Tables 1 and 2) contained signals attributed to oxymethine [δ_H 5.26 (1H, brs); δ_C 66.5, C-3], methylidene [δ_H 4.96 (1H, dd, J = 2.8, 1.4 Hz), 4.72 (1H, dd, J = 2.8, 1.4 Hz); δ_C 91.4, 157.6, C-4,5], vinyl [δ_H 7.09 (1H, td, J = 7.8, 2.2 Hz); δ_C 127.3, 150.3, C-2,6], and carbonyl (δ_C 166.5, C-1) groups, consistent with a β-hydroxy-γ-methylene-α,β-unsaturated-γ-lactone. The chemical shifts of H-6 (δ_H 7.09) and H-7 (δ_H 2.48) as well as allylic carbon C-3 (δ_C 66.5) and olefinic carbon C-6 (δ_C 150.3) were identical with those of tambouranolide (**10**) [15] and related linderanolides and isolinderanolides [25,26] with an E-configured double bond [$\Delta^{2(6)}$]. This assignment was also supported by a cross-peak between H-3 and H-7 in the NOESY spectrum (Figure 3). The presence of a long aliphatic chain containing a double bond was suggested by NMR resonances for olefinic and multiple methylene carbons. The allylic (δ_C 27.0, 27.2) and olefinic (δ_C 129.8, 129.9) carbon signals in the ^{13}C NMR spectrum of **1** suggested that the internal olefin has the typical Z-configuration, comparable with those of **10** as well as the abovementioned linderanolides and isolinderanolides with Z-double bonds in the side chain. In a related E-isomer, the allylic and olefinic carbons appeared at 32.6 and 25.6 ppm and at 131.9 and 129.3 ppm, respectively [25]. The location of the olefinic bond at Δ^{20} was based on HMBC and COSY correlations (Figure 2). From the NMR and HREIMS data, compounds **10** and **1** differ only in the number of methylene groups (16 in **10**, 14 in **1**) in the long aliphatic chain. The absolute configuration of **1** was determined from its optical rotation, which was the same as that of **10**. Furthermore, the total synthesis of peumusolide A analogues clearly proved that the optical rotation is positive for 3R compounds and negative for 3S [27,28]. Therefore, compound **1** (peltanolide A) was assigned as (2E,3R)-3-hydroxy-4-methylidene-2-[(15Z)-15-icosenylidene]butanolide.

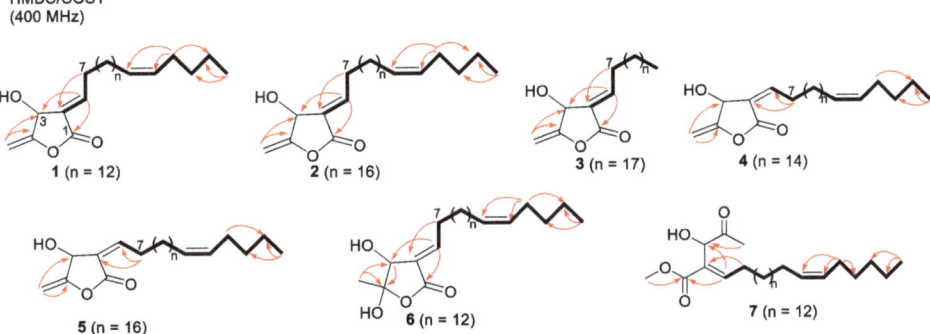

Figure 2. Selected HMBC correlations (arrows in red), COSY connectivities (bold lines) for compounds **1–7**.

Compound **2** was isolated as a yellow solid, $[\alpha]^{25}_D$ +26.1 (c 0.12, CHCl$_3$). The HREIMS data supported a molecular formula of C$_{29}$H$_{51}$O$_3$ from the peak at m/z 446.3743 [M]$^+$. The MS data and NMR spectra indicated four additional methylene units compared with **1**, and the optical rotation suggested the same configuration as that of **1**. Thus, compound **2** (peltanolide B) was defined as (2E,3R)-3-hydroxy-4-methylidene-2-[(19Z)-19-tetracosenylidene]butanolide.

Compound **3** was obtained as a colorless oil: $[\alpha]^{25}_D$ +26.0 (c 0.07, CHCl$_3$). The HREIMS data indicated a molecular formula of C$_{25}$H$_{44}$O$_3$ from the peak at m/z 392.3302 [M]$^+$, which was identical to that of miaolinolide [29]. One dimensional NMR spectra of **3** also displayed the similar signal pattern with one exception: the chemical shift of H-6 is δ_H 7.10 (1H, td, J = 7.8, 2.2 Hz) in **3** and δ_H 6.70 (1H, td, J = 8.0, 2.0 Hz) in miaolinolide. Thus, the $\Delta^{2(6)}$ double bond has an E configuration in **3**, rather than the Z configuration in miaolinolide [29]. This assignment was also proved that the chemical shift of H-6 in **3** was close to that of related butanolides with an E configuration of the $\Delta^{2(6)}$ double bond [15,25,26,30], including compounds **1** and **2**. A NOESY correlation between H-3 and H-7 (Figure 3) supported this conclusion. Based on their optical rotations, compound **3** and miaolinolide have the same absolute configuration. Hence, the structure of **3** (peltanolide C) was established as (2E,3S)-3-hydroxy-4-methylidene-2-icosylidenebutanolide.

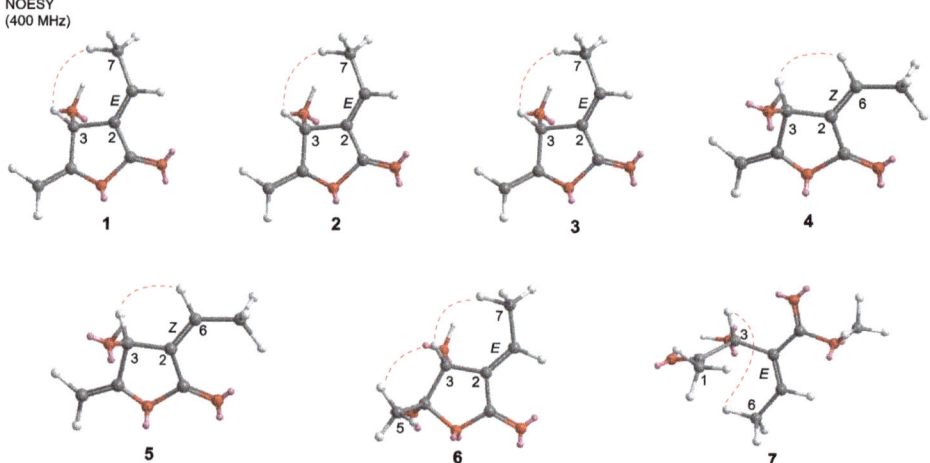

Figure 3. Key NOESY (red dashed lines) correlations for compounds **1–7**.

HRFABMS of compound **4** showed a molecular formula $C_{27}H_{46}O_3$ with a molecular ion at m/z 441.3357 [M + Na]$^+$. The ^{1}H and ^{13}C NMR spectra of **4** (Tables 1 and 2) were comparable to those of **10** but suggested different double bond [$\Delta^{2(6)}$] configurations and C-3 stereochemistries. For **4**, the $\Delta^{2(6)}$ configuration was determined as Z from a NOESY correlation between H-3 and H-6 (Figure 3) and the chemical shift of H-6 at 6.69 ppm rather than ca. 7.10 ppm for the E form. The C-3 stereochemistry was determined as S by comparison of optical rotations, $[\alpha]^{25}_D$ −29.7 (c 0.02, CHCl$_3$) for **4** and $[\alpha]^{25}_D$ + 18.0 (c 0.03, CHCl$_3$) for **10** with 3R. Thus, compound **4** (peltanolide D) was determined as (2Z,3S)-3-hydroxy-4-methylidene-2-[(17Z)-17-docosenylidene]butanolide.

Table 1. ^{1}H NMR Spectroscopic data of compounds 1–7.

Position	1^a (CDCl$_3$) δ_H (J in Hz)	2^b (CDCl$_3$) δ_H (J in Hz)	3^b (CDCl$_3$) δ_H (J in Hz)	4^b (CDCl$_3$) δ_H (J in Hz)	5^b (CDCl$_3$) δ_H (J in Hz)	6^a (CDCl$_3$) δ_H (J in Hz)	7^b (CDCl$_3$) δ_H (J in Hz)
1							2.15 s
3	5.26 brs	5.26 brs	5.26 brd (5.6)	5.11 m	5.10 brd (7.3)	4.82 brs	4.89 d (4.2)
5a	4.72 dd (2.8, 1.4)	4.72 dd (2.8, 1.4)	4.72 dd (2.8, 1.4)	4.67 dd (2.8, 1.4)	4.66 dd (2.8, 1.4)	1.62 s	7.07 t (8.0)
5b	4.96 dd (2.8, 1.4)	4.96 dd (2.8, 1.4)	4.96 dd (2.8, 1.4)	4.89 dd (2.8, 1.4)	4.89 dd (2.8, 1.4)		
6	7.09 td (7.8, 2.2)	7.09 td (7.8, 2.2)	7.10 td (7.8, 2.2)	6.69 td (7.8, 2.2)	6.67 td (7.8, 2.2)	7.04 td (7.8, 2.2)	2.34 td (14.8, 8.0)
7	2.48 m	2.48 m	2.48 m, 2.43 m	2.78 m	2.76 m	2.38 m	1.50 m
8	1.52 m	1.52 m	1.53 m	1.46 m	1.45 m	1.52 m	1.25 m^p
9–18	1.26 m^c	1.26 m^e	1.25 m^g	1.25 m^h	1.25 m^j	1.25 m^m	1.25 m^p
19	2.00 m	1.26 m^e	1.25 m^g	1.25 m^h	1.25 m^j	2.01 m^n	2.00 m^q
20	5.36 m^d	1.26 m^e	1.25 m^g	1.25 m^h	1.25 m^j	5.34 t (4.8)^o	5.34 t (4.8)^r
21	5.36 m^d	1.26 m^e	1.25 m^g	2.02 m	1.25 m^j	5.34 t (4.8)^o	5.34 t (4.8)^r
22	2.02 m	1.26 m^e	1.25 m^g	5.35 m^i	1.25 m^j	2.01 m^n	2.00 m^q
23	1.26 m^c	2.00 m	1.25 m^g	5.35 m^i	2.01 m^k	1.25 m^m	1.25 m^p
24	1.32 m	5.36 m^f		2.02	5.33 m^l	1.31	1.25 m^p
25	0.89 t (6.9)	5.36 m^f	0.89 br t (7.3)	1.25 m^h	5.33 m^l	0.89 t (6.0)	1.31 m
26		2.02 m		1.33 m	2.01 m^k		0.89 t (6.0)
27		1.26 m^e		0.88 t (6.9)	1.25 m^j		
28		1.32 m			1.32 m		
29		0.89 t (7.3)			0.87 t (6.9)		
2-OH		2.26 m					
3-OH							4.00 brs
OCH$_3$							3.72 s

^{a} 600 MHz, ^{b} 400 MHz, $^{c-r}$ Overlapping signals.

Table 2. ^{13}C NMR Spectroscopic data in CDCl$_3$ of compounds 1–7.

Position	1[a] δ_c	2[b] δ_c	3[b] δ_c	4[b] δ_c	5[b] δ_c	6[a] δ_c	7[b] δ_c
1	166.5	166.5	166.3	163.1		166.4	24.8
2	127.3	127.3	127.2	127.4	127.3	125.2	206.3
3	66.5	66.5	66.6	68.9	68.9	70.9	73.4
4	157.6	157.6	157.5	160.1	160.2	100.1	129.8
5	91.4	91.4	91.5	90.3	90.4	26.8	149.0
6	150.3	150.3	150.3	151.4	151.4	151.9	28.7
7	29.8	29.8	29.8	29.8	29.8	30.1	29.3
8	28.4	28.4	28.4–29.6[d]	28.4	28.4	29.5–29.9[g]	29.4–30.0[h]
9–18	29.4–30.0	29.4–30.0[c]	28.4–29.6[d]	29.4–30.0[e]	29.4–30.0[f]	29.5–29.9[g]	29.4–30.0[h]
19	27.0	29.4–30.0[c]	28.4–29.6[d]	29.4–30.0[e]	29.4–30.0[f]	27.0	27.2
20	129.8	29.4–30.0[c]	28.4–29.6[d]	29.4–30.0[e]	29.4–30.0[f]	129.8	129.8
21	129.9	29.4–30.0[c]	28.4–29.6[d]	27.0	29.4–30.0[f]	129.9	129.9
22	27.2	29.4–30.0[c]	28.4–29.6[d]	129.8	27.0	27.7	27.2
23	32.0	27.0	32.0	129.9	129.8	32.1	29.8
24	22.4	129.8	22.8	27.2	129.9	22.5	31.9
25	14.0	129.9	14.1	32.0	27.2	14.1	22.7
26		27.2		22.3	32.0		14.1
27		32.0		14.0	32.0		
28		22.4			22.4		
29		14.0			14.0		
COO							166.5
OCH$_3$							52.0

[a] 150 MHz, [b] 100 MHz, [c–h] Overlapping signals.

Compound **5** was obtained as a yellow solid and displayed a peak at *m/z* 446.3749 [M]$^+$ in the HREIMS spectrum, which agreed with a molecular formula of $C_{29}H_{50}O_3$ and two additional methylene units (C_2H_4) compared with **4**. This finding was also supported by the two NMR spectra. Both compounds also have the same absolute configurations based on their optical rotations, $[\alpha]^{25}_D$ −21.1 (*c* 0.015, CHCl$_3$) for **5** and $[\alpha]^{25}_D$ −29.7 (*c* 0.02, CHCl$_3$) for **4**. Thus, compound **5** (peltanolide E) was defined as (2Z,3S)-3-hydroxy-4-methylidene-2-[(15Z)-15-icosenylidene]butanolid.

Compound **6** was isolated as a colorless oil. The HREIMS data indicated a molecular formula of $C_{25}H_{44}O_4$ from the peak at *m/z* 408.3230 [M]$^+$. Compared with **1**, the ^{1}H and ^{13}C NMR spectra of **6** (Tables 1 and 2) showed the absence of signals for a methylidene group and the presence of signals for a methyl group [δ_H 1.62 (3H, s)/δ_C 26.8] and a doubly oxygenated carbon (δ_C 100.1). The doubly oxygenated carbon was assigned as C-4 with an attached methyl group; these assignments were confirmed by HMBC correlations (Figure 2). A NOESY correlation between H-7 and H-3 as well as the chemical shift of H-6 at 7.04 ppm were consistent with $\Delta^{2(6)}$ being the *E*-isomer. The stereochemistry of C-3 was determined as *R* based on the optical rotation $[\alpha]^{25}_D$ +116.0 (*c* 0.015, CHCl$_3$) by comparison with related 4-hydroxybutanolides [31–33]. The NOESY correlation between H-3 and H-5 supported the 4*S* stereochemistry (Figure 3). TDDFT-ECD calculation was also sorted the (3*R*,4*S*) absolute configuration (Figure 4). Therefore, compound **6** (peltanolide F) was assigned as (2*E*,3*R*,4*S*)-3,4-dihydroxy-5-methyl-2-[(15Z)-15-icosenylidene]butanolide.

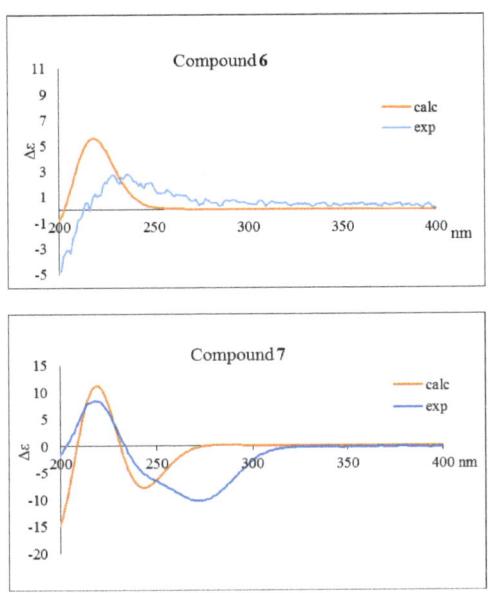

Figure 4. Experimental and calculated ECD spectra of compounds **6** and **7**.

Compound **7** has the molecular formula, $C_{28}H_{50}O_4$, based on the peak at *m/z* 450.3702 [M]$^+$ in the HREIMS. All NMR data and EIMS fragment peaks (Figure 5) of **7** were identical to those of illigerone A [34]. However, the ECD spectrum of **7** exhibited a different Cotton effect from that of illigerone A, and TDDFT-ECD calculation was indicated the 3*R* absolute configuration (Figure 4). In addition, the experimental optical rotation, $[\alpha]^{25}_D$ −78.5 (*c* 0.03, acetonitrile), of **7** had a negative (levorotary) rather than positive (dextrorotary) value, as found with illigerone A [34]. We concluded that compound **7** (peltanolide G) is (3*R*,4*E*,20*Z*)-3-hydroxy-4-(2-methoxy-2-oxo)hexacosa-4,20-dien-2-one, the enantiomer of illigerone A.

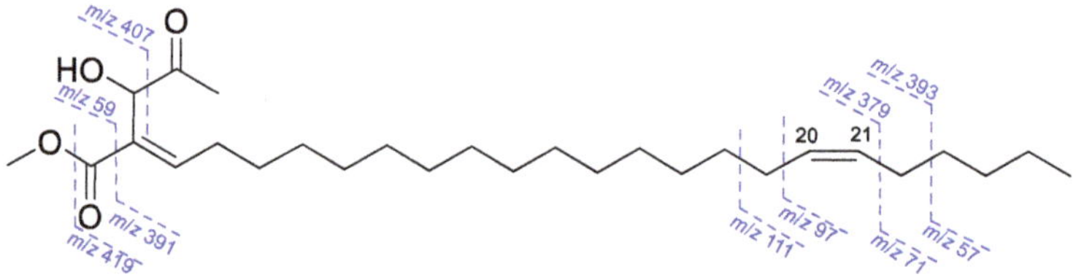

Figure 5. EIMS fragmentation of **7**.

Compound **8** was obtained as a yellow solid, and its molecular formula was determined to be $C_{27}H_{36}O_{13}$ on the HRFABMS ion at *m/z* 591.2022 [M + Na]$^+$. The ^{1}H NMR data displayed five aromatic [δ_H 7.11 (1H, d, *J* = 8.2 Hz), 6.92 (1H, d, *J* = 1.8 Hz), 6.82 (1H, dd, *J* = 8.2, 1.8 Hz), and 6.52 (2H, s, overlap)], two oxymethine [δ_H 4.63 (1H, d, *J* = 7.3 Hz), 4.52 (1H, d, *J* = 8.2 Hz)], four oxymethylene protons [δ_H 4.26 (1H, dd (*J* = 9.0, 4.6 Hz), 3.92 (1H, m), 3.87 (1H, m), and 3.63 (1H, m)], three methoxy groups [δ_H 3.84 (6H, s), and 3.83 (3H, s)], and two methine protons [δ_H 2.53 (1H, m), 1.89 (1H, m)]. In addition, a glucopyranosyl anomeric proton was observed at δ_H 4.84 (1H, m). The ^{13}C NMR spectrum showed 27 carbon signals, six from a glucose unit and three methoxy groups and the remaining 18 carbons from the lignan skeleton. The spectroscopic data of **8** resembled those of the known compound, (7*S*,8*R*,7'*S*,8'*S*)-4,9,7'-trihydroxy-3,3'-dimethoxy-7,9'-epoxylignan-4'-*O*-β-D-glucopyrano-side [35], except for the absence of the H-3 aromatic proton in the ^{1}H NMR spectrum and the presence of an additional methoxy group in **8**. The HMBC (Figure 6) and NOESY (Figure 7) spectra agreed with this structure, and the observed ROESY correlations between H-7/H-9, H-8/H-7′, and H-8′/H-9 (Figure 7) strongly suggested trans configurations of H-7/H-8 and H-8/H-8′. The CD spectrum of **8** showed positive Cotton effects at 237 nm and 274 nm (Figure 8), which were identical with those of the known compound [35]. Thus, the structure of **8** (peltaside A) was determined as (7*S*,8*R*,7'*S*,8'*S*)-4,9,7'-trihydroxy-3,5,3'-trimethoxy-7,9'-epoxylignan-4'-*O*-β-D-glucopyranoside.

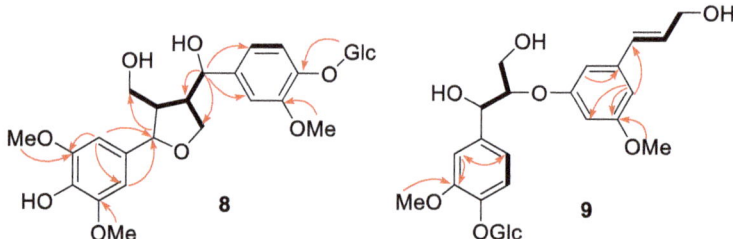

Figure 6. Selected HMBC correlations (arrows in red), COSY connectivities (bold lines) for **8** and **9**.

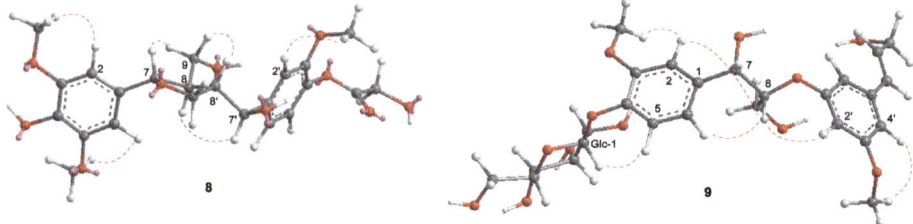

Figure 7. Key NOESY correlations (red lines) and Key ROESY correlations (blue lines) for **8** and **9**.

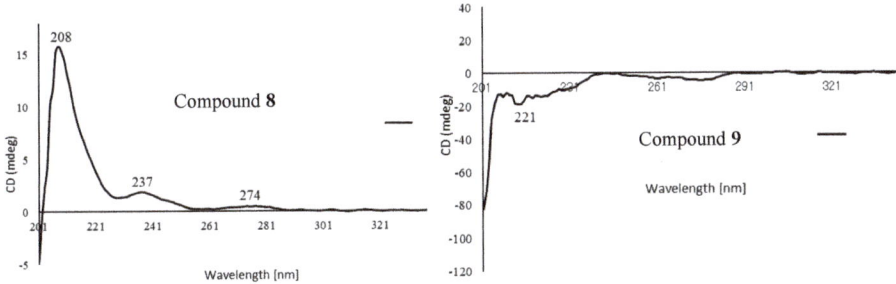

Figure 8. Experimental ECD spectra of compounds 8 and 9.

Compound **9** was obtained as a yellow solid and its HRFABMS (m/z 561.1958 [M + Na]$^+$) indicated the molecular formula $C_{26}H_{34}O_{12}$. The 1H NMR spectrum of **9** displayed the signals for a trans-olefinic, two oxygenated methine, two oxygenated methylene, and six aromatic protons, as well as a β-glucose and two methoxy groups (Table 3). In addition, its ^{13}C-NMR spectrum showed the signals for 26 carbons, including 12 aromatic, two methoxy, two olefinic, and six glucopyranosyl carbons (Table 3). The COSY, HMQC, HMBC, and NOESY spectra suggested that the glucopyranosyl moiety was attached to C-4 (Figures 5 and 6). The relative configuration between C-7 and C-8 was assigned as erythro based on the small coupling constant (J = 4.8 Hz) in ^{1}H NMR (Figure S57). The absolute configuration of **9**, which showed a negative Cotton effect at 221 nm in the CD spectrum (Figure 8), was determined to be 7S,8R via a comparison with that of reported analogues [36–38]. Hence, compound **9** (peltaside B) is (7S,8R,7'E)-7,9,9'-trihydroxy-3,5'-dimethoxy-8-3'-oxyneolign-7'-ene-4-O-β-D-glucopyranoside.

Table 3. ^{1}H and ^{13}C NMR Spectroscopic Data of Compounds 8 and 9.

Position	8 (CD$_3$OD)		9 (CD$_3$OD)	
	$\delta_C{}^a$	δ_H (J in Hz)^b	$\delta_C{}^a$	δ_H (J in Hz)^b
1	134.1		131.5	
2	104.6^c	6.52 s^d	112.3	7.09 brs
3	149.3		147.4	
4	135.9		150.5	
5	149.3		120.6	7.06 d (8.2)
6	104.6^c	6.52 s^d	121.1	6.96 dd (2.2, 8.2)
7	85.1	4.63 d (7.3)	74.9	4.85 overlap
8	53.7	1.89 m	85.9	4.36 m
9	62.3	3.87 m	62.2	3.82 m
		3.63 m		3.47 m
1'	139.5		137.8	
2'	112.2	6.92 d (1.8)	118.7^g	6.86 brs^g
3'	150.7		149.2	
4'	147.5		118.7^g	6.86 brs^g
5'	117.5	7.11 d (8.2)	151.2	
6'	120.9	6.82 dd (8.2, 1.8)	111.3	6.97 d (2.2)
7'	74..8	4.52 d (8.2)	132.9	6.52 d (15.4)
8'	50.7	2.53 m	111.3	6.27 dd (5.7, 15.4)
9'	76.2	4.26 dd (9.0, 4.6)	63.8	4.19 d (5.9)
		3.92 m		
3-OMe	56.9	3.84 s^e	56.7	3.81 s
5-OMe	56.8	3.84 s^e	56.5	3.79 s
3'-OMe	56.7	3.83 s		

Table 3. Cont.

Position	8 (CD$_3$OD)		9 (CD$_3$OD)	
	$\delta_C{}^a$	δ_H (J in Hz)^b	$\delta_C{}^a$	δ_H (J in Hz)^b
Glc-1	102.7	4.84 m	103.1	4.81 d (6.9)
Glc-2	74.9	3.4–3.8 m^f	73.9	3.4–3.8 m^h
Glc-3	78.2	3.4–3.8 m^f	78.2	3.4–3.8 m^h
Glc-4	71.4	3.4–3.8 m^f	71.4	3.4–3.8 m^h
Glc-5	77.9	3.4–3.8 m^f	77.9	3.4–3.8 m^h
Glc-6	62.5	3.4–3.8 m^f	62.5	3.4–3.8 m^h

^{a} 100 Hz, ^{b} 400 Hz, $^{c-h}$ Overlapping signals.

2.2. Antiproliferative Activity of Isolated Compounds from H. nymphaeifolia

Compounds **1**, **2**, **8**, **10**, and **13–18** were evaluated for antiproliferative effects against five human tumor cell lines, A549 (lung carcinoma), MCF-7 (estrogen receptor-positive and HER2-negative breast cancer), MDA-MB-231 (triple negative breast cancer), KB (cervical cancer cell line HeLa derivative), and P-glycoprotein (P-gp)-overexpressing multidrug-resistant (MDR) KB subline, KB-VIN (Table 4). The remaining compounds were not tested due to insufficient quantities. Butanolide **10** slightly inhibited MCF-7 and KB-VIN tumor cell growth with an IC$_{50}$ value of 9 µM. Both lignans **15** and **16** showed antiproliferative activity against chemosensitive A549 and MCF-7 tumor cell lines, while **16** was also active against MDA-MB-231. Interestingly, compounds **15** and **16** also displayed moderate activity against the MDR cell line (KB-VIN) with an IC$_{50}$ value of 5 µM but were less active against its parent chemosensitive cell line (KB). Compounds **1**, **2**, **8**, **14** and **18** exhibited no activity against all tested cell lines. These results demonstrated that the CH$_3$OH/CH$_2$Cl$_2$ (1:1) extract of *H. nymphaeifolia* contained antiproliferative natural products, which showed broad spectrum against HTCLs including MDR cells and could also work synergistically against MDR cells.

Table 4. Antiproliferative Activity of the Isolated Compounds.

Compounds	Cell Lines^a (IC$_{50}$ µM)^b				
	A549	MDA-MB-231	MCF-7	KB	KB-VIN
1	>40	22.5	>40	25.7	31.7
2	21.9	24.6	24.6	22.6	21.4
8	35.1	35.3	35.7	32.7	21.7
10	12.5	10.8	8.8	18.6	8.8
13	32.8	37.7	33.5	>40	8.7
14	23.2	32.9	32.8	23.2	19.9
15	8.1	20.8	6.8	20.3	5.4
16	5.7	8.2	8.1	12.6	5.3
17	37.8	>40	38.0	>40	8.2
18	>40	>40	>40	>40	>40
Paclitaxel (nM)	6.5	8.4	12.1	7.1	2213

^{a} A549 (lung carcinoma), MDA-MB-231 (triple-negative breast cancer), MCF-7 (estrogen receptor-positive & HER2-negative breast cancer), KB (cervical cancer cell line HeLa derivative), KB-VIN (P-gp-overexpressing multidrug-resistant (MDR) subline of KB). ^{b} Antiproliferative activity expressed as IC$_{50}$ values for each cell line cultured with compound for 72 h, the concentration of compound that caused 50% reduction relative to untreated cells determined by the SRB assay. IC$_{50}$ of all compounds were calculated.

3. Materials and Methods

3.1. General Experimental Procedures

Infrared spectra (IR) were obtained with a Thermo Fisher Scientific (Waltham, MA, USA) NICOLET iS5 FT-TR spectrometer from samples in CHCl$_3$ and MeOH. NMR spectra were measured on JEOL

(Akishima, Tokyo, Japan) JNM-ECA600 and JNM-ECS400 spectrometers with tetramethylsilane as an internal standard, and chemical shifts are stated as δ values. HRMS data were recorded on a JEOL JMS-700 Mstation (FAB or EI) mass spectrometer. Analytical and preparative TLC were carried out on precoated silica gel 60F254 and RP-18F254 plates (0.25 or 0.50 mm thickness; Merck, Darmstadt, Germany). MPLC was performed on a Combiflash R_f (Teledyne Isco, Lincoln, NE, USA) with silica gel and C18 cartridges (Biotage, Uppsala Sweden). Preparative HPLC was carried out with a GL Science (Shinjuku, Tokyo, Japan) recycling system (PU714 pump and UV702 UV-Vis detector) using an InertSustain C18 column (5 μM, 20 × 250 mm).

3.2. Plant Material

The crude CH_3OH/CH_2Cl_2 (1:1) extract (#N053499) from fruit of *H. nymphaeifolia* (Presl) Kubitzki (originally identified as *H. peltata*), collected in Java (Indonesia) was provided by NCI/NIH. The plant was collected on May 25, 1992 in a sandy habitat in the Ujung Kulon Reserve by A. McDonald. A voucher specimen for the plant collection was deposited at the Smithsonian Institution (Washington, WA, USA) and voucher extracts were deposited at the NCI (Frederick, MD, USA) and Kanazawa University (Kanazawa, Ishikawa, Japan).

3.3. Extraction and Isolation

The crude extract N053499 (25.0 g) was dissolved in CH_3OH/H_2O (9:1) then partitioned with n-hexane, EtOAc, and *n*-BuOH, yielding *n*-hexane (17.4 g), EtOAc (3.94 g), *n*-BuOH (1.72 g), and H_2O (0.997 g) fractions. The EtOAc-soluble fraction was subjected to silica gel column chromatography (CC) with a gradient system [*n*-hexane/EtOAc 100:0 (500 mL)→90:10 (500 mL)→70:30 (1000 mL)→50:50 (1000 mL)→30:70 (1000 mL)→10:90 (1000 mL)→0:100 (500 mL)→EtOAc/MeOH 50:50 (500 mL)→MeOH (1000 mL)] to yield nine fractions, F1–F9. F3 (123 mg) was subjected to silica gel MPLC (RediSep Rf GOLD High Performance 4 g) eluted with *n*-hexane/EtOAc (9:1 to 0:1) to afford five subfractions 3a–e. Subfraction 3b (21.6 mg) was purified by repeated recycling reversed-phase preparative HPLC with H_2O/MeOH (1:19) to provide compounds **2** (2.2 mg), **3** (1.4 mg), and **10** (1.2 mg). F4 (77.9 mg) was subjected to silica gel CC eluted with CH_2Cl_2 followed by MeOH to yield eight subfractions 4a–h. Subfraction 4d (1.0 mg) was further separated by preparative normal-phase TLC with CH_2Cl_2 to afford compound **5** (0.4 mg). Subfraction 4f (4.6 mg) was purified by repeated recycling preparative HPLC with H_2O/MeOH (1:2) to afford compound **7** (0.6 mg). Subfraction 4h (54.0 mg) was purified by preparative normal-phase TLC with CH_2Cl_2/EtOAc (19:1) to afford compounds 13 (13.2 mg) and 15 (2.1 mg). F6 was subjected to silica gel CC eluted with CH_2Cl_2/EtOAc (19:1 to 0:1) followed by MeOH to obtain six subfractions, 6a–f. Subfraction 6b (37.5 mg) was purified by repeated recycling preparative HPLC with H_2O/MeOH (1:2) to afford compounds **12** (7.1 mg) and **16** (20.3 mg). Subfraction 6c (15.9 mg) was purified by repeated recycling preparative HPLC with H_2O/MeOH (1:2), to provide compound **17** (4.1 mg). The *n*-hexane fraction (12.0 g) was subjected to silica gel MPLC (RediSep R_f GOLD High Performance 120 g) with a gradient system [*n*-hexane/CH_2Cl_2 1:1 (600 mL)→2:3 (1400 mL)→3:7 (1200 mL)→4:1 (1400 mL)→CH_2Cl_2 (1200 mL)→CH_2Cl_2/EtOAc 1:1 (1000 mL)→EtOAc (1000 mL)→MeOH (1400 mL)] to yield 15 fractions, F1–F15. F6 (695 mg) was applied to silica gel MPLC (RediSep Rf GOLD High Performance 24 g) eluted with *n*-hexane/EtOAc (9:1 to 0:1) followed by MeOH to yield ten subfractions 6a–j. Subfraction 6e (197 mg) was subjected to silica gel CC eluted with *n*-hexane/EtOAc (2:3 to 0:1) followed by MeOH to yield 11 subfractions 6e1–11. Subfraction 6e5 (4.9 mg) was purified by preparative normal-phase TLC with *n*-hexane/CH_2Cl_2 (3:1) to afford compound **6** (0.4 mg). F11 (1.12 g) was applied to silica gel MPLC (RediSep Rf GOLD High Performance 24 g) with *n*-hexane/EtOAc (9:1 to 0:1) followed by MeOH to yield seven subfractions 11a–g. Subfraction 11f (535 mg) was purified by MPLC on ODS-25 (YMC-DispoPack AT 12 g) with H_2O/CH_3OH (1:3), followed by recycling preparative HPLC with H_2O/MeOH (1:2) to afford compounds **13** (0.4 mg) and **14** (0.2 mg). F13 (1.35 g) was subjected to silica gel MPLC (RediSep Rf GOLD High Performance 24 g) with *n*-hexane/CH_2Cl_2/EtOAc (1:1:0 to 0:0:1) followed by MeOH to yield ten subfractions 13a–j.

Subfraction 13e (48.2 mg) was purified by ODS preparative TLC eluted three times using MeOH to afford compounds **1** (3.2 mg), **2** (1.1 mg), and **10** (1.0 mg). The *n*-BuOH-soluble fraction (1.72 g) was subjected to silica gel MPLC (RediSep R_f GOLD High Performance 120 g) with a gradient system [CHCl$_3$/MeOH 1:0 (1000 mL)→10:1 (1400 mL)→5:1 (1200 mL)→1:1 (1800 mL)→MeOH (1400 mL)] to yield nine fractions, F1–F9. F1 (147 mg) was subjected to silica gel CC eluted with CH$_2$Cl$_2$/EtOAc (1:0 to 0:1) followed by MeOH to obtain 14 subfractions, 1a–n. Compound **4** (0.3 mg) was obtained from subfraction 1e. Subfraction 1g (3.3 mg) was purified by preparative normal-phase TLC with CH$_2$Cl$_2$/EtOAc (95:5) to afford compound **10** (1.3 mg). Subfraction 1k was purified by recycling preparative HPLC with H$_2$O/MeOH (1:3) to afford compounds **11** (1.8 mg), **14** (0.3 mg), and **17** (0.4 mg). F2 (44.3 mg) was subjected to silica gel CC eluted with CH$_2$Cl$_2$/EtOAc (9:0 to 0:1) followed by MeOH to obtain nine subfractions, 2a–i. Subfraction 2b (1.1 mg) was purified by ODS preparative TLC eluted three times using H$_2$O/MeOH (1:8) to yield compound **13** (0.6 mg). F3 (33.8 mg) was purified by preparative normal-phase TLC with CHCl$_3$/MeOH (9:1) to afford compound **8** (1.0 mg). F5 (149 mg) was subjected to silica gel CC eluted with CH$_2$Cl$_2$/MeOH (10:1 to 1:1) followed by MeOH to obtain seven subfractions, 5a–g. Subfraction 5d (75.6 mg) was purified by MPLC on ODS-25 (YMC-DispoPack AT 12 g) with H$_2$O/MeOH (1:3), followed by recycling preparative HPLC with H$_2$O/MeOH (2:3) to afford compounds **9** (1.3 mg), **18** (2.3 mg), **19** (1.0 mg), and **20** (1.2 mg).

3.3.1. Peltanolide A (**1**)

Yellow amorphous solid; $[\alpha]^{25}_D$ +27.3 (*c* 0.075, CHCl$_3$); IR ν_{max} (CHCl$_3$) cm^{-1} 2923, 2853, 2017, 1733, 1457, 1278, 1219; ^{1}H and ^{13}C NMR, Tables 1 and 2; HREIMS *m/z* 390.3137 [M]$^+$ (calcd for C$_{25}$H$_{42}$O$_3$, 390.3134).

3.3.2. Peltanolide B (**2**)

Yellow amorphous solid; $[\alpha]^{25}_D$ +26.1 (*c* 0.12, CHCl$_3$); IR ν_{max} (CHCl$_3$) cm^{-1} 2923, 2852, 1731, 1464, 1265, 1074; ^{1}H and ^{13}C NMR, Tables 1 and 2; HREIMS *m/z* 446.3743 [M]$^+$ (calcd for C$_{29}$H$_{51}$O$_3$, 446.3760).

3.3.3. Peltanolide C (**3**)

Colorless oil; $[\alpha]^{25}_D$ +26.0 (*c* 0.07, CHCl$_3$); IR ν_{max} (CHCl$_3$) cm^{-1} 2916, 2849, 2016, 1750, 1678, 1470, 1278, 1184; ^{1}H and ^{13}C NMR, Tables 1 and 2; HREIMS *m/z* 392.3302 [M]$^+$ (calcd for C$_{25}$H$_{44}$O$_3$, 392.3290).

3.3.4. Peltanolide D (**4**)

Yellow amorphous solid; $[\alpha]^{25}_D$ −29.7 (*c* 0.02, CHCl$_3$); IR ν_{max} (CHCl$_3$) cm^{-1} 2923, 2852, 1783, 1733, 1465, 1373, 1287; ^{1}H and ^{13}C NMR, Tables 1 and 2; HRFABMS *m/z* 441.3357 [M + Na]$^+$ (calcd for C$_{27}$H$_{46}$O$_3$Na, 441.3345).

3.3.5. Peltanolide E (**5**)

Yellow amorphous solid; $[\alpha]^{25}_D$ −21.1 (*c* 0.015, CHCl$_3$); IR ν_{max} (CHCl$_3$) cm^{-1} 2922, 2852, 2017, 1770, 1731, 1557, 1458, 1375, 1287; ^{1}H and ^{13}C NMR, Tables 1 and 2; HREIMS *m/z* 446.3749 [M]$^+$ (calcd for C$_{29}$H$_{50}$O$_3$, 446.3760).

3.3.6. Peltanolide F (**6**)

Colorless oil; $[\alpha]^{25}_D$ +116.0 (*c* 0.015, CHCl$_3$); IR ν_{max} (CHCl$_3$) cm^{-1} 2923, 2852, 1733, 1558, 1540, 1456, 1287; ^{1}H and ^{13}C NMR, Tables 1 and 2; HREIMS *m/z* 408.3230 [M]$^+$ (calcd for C$_{25}$H$_{44}$O$_4$, 408.3240).

3.3.7. Peltanolide G (7)

Colorless oil; $[\alpha]^{25}_D$ −78.5 (c 0.03, acetonitrile); IR ν_{max} (CHCl$_3$) cm^{-1} 2922, 2852, 2016, 1717, 1669, 1558, 1456, 1436; ^{1}H and ^{13}C NMR, Tables 1 and 2; HREIMS m/z 450.3702 [M]$^+$ (calcd for C$_{28}$H$_{50}$O$_4$, 450.3709).

3.3.8. Peltaside A (8)

Yellow solid; $[\alpha]^{25}_D$ +5.6 (c 0.055, MeOH); IR ν_{max} (CHCl$_3$) cm^{-1} 3330, 2945, 2833, 1645, 1514, 1450, 1112; ^{1}H and ^{13}C NMR, Table 3; HRFABMS m/z 591.2022 [M + Na]$^+$ (calcd for C$_{27}$H$_{36}$O$_{13}$Na, 591.2054).

3.3.9. Peltaside B (9)

Yellow solid; $[\alpha]^{25}_D$ −71.8 (c 0.065, MeOH); IR ν_{max} (CHCl$_3$) cm^{-1} 3386, 3293, 1657, 1511, 1265; ^{1}H and ^{13}C NMR, Table 3; HRFABMS m/z 561.1958 [M + Na]$^+$ (calcd for C$_{26}$H$_{34}$O$_{12}$Na, 561.1948).

3.4. Calculation of ECD Spectra

Preliminary conformational analysis for each compound was carried out by using CONFLEX8 with the MMFF94 force field. The conformers were further optimized in MeCN by density functional theory (DFT) method with the B3LYP functional and 6–31(d) basis set. The ECD spectrum was calculated by the time-dependent DFT (TDDFT) method with the CAM-B3LYP functional and TZVP basis set. The calculation was completed by the use of conformers within 2 kcal/mol predicted in MeCN. The solvent effect was introduced by the conductor-like polarizable continuum model (CPCM). The DFT optimization and TDDFT-ECD calculation were performed using Gaussian09 (Gaussian, Inc., Wallingford, CT, USA). The calculated spectrum was displayed by GaussView 5.0.920 with the peak half-width at half height being 0.333 eV. The Boltzmann-averaged spectrum at 298.15K was calculated using Excel 2016 (Microsoft Co., Redmond, WA, USA). The calculations were re-optimized according to the literature [39].

3.5. Assay for Antiproliferative Activity

Antiproliferative activity of the compounds was determined by the sulforhodamine B (SRB) assay as described previously [40]. Briefly, cell suspensions were seeded on 96-well microtiter plates at a density of 4000–12,000 cells per well and cultured for 72 h with test compound. The cells were fixed in 10% trichloroacetic acid and then stained with 0.04% SRB. The absorbance at 515 nm of 10 mM Tris base-solubilized protein-bound dye was measured using a microplate reader (ELx800, BioTek, Winooski, VT, U.S) operated by Gen5 software (BioTek). IC$_{50}$ data were calculated statistically (MS Excel) from at least three independent experiments performed with duplication (n = 6). All human tumor cell lines, except KB-VIN, were obtained from the Lineberger Comprehensive Cancer Center (UNC-CH, Chapel Hill, NC, USA) or from ATCC (Manassas, VA, USA). KB-VIN was a generous gift from Professor Y.-C. Cheng of Yale University (New Haven, CT, USA).

4. Conclusions

As part of our continuing investigation of rainforest plants, we conducted a thorough study to identify new chemical compounds to supplement the reported phytochemical research on *H. nymphaeifolia*. Consequently, a CH$_3$OH/CH$_2$Cl$_2$ (1:1) extract of *H. nymphaeifolia* (N053499) provided by NCI yielded seven new butanolides, peltanolides A–G (1–7), and two new lignan glycosides, peltasides A (8) and B (9), as well as eleven known compounds 10–20. This is the first report to identify butanolides and lignan glucosides from this genus. The evaluation of antiproliferative activity against human tumor cell lines revealed that lignans 15 and 16 were slightly active against chemosensitive tumor cell lines A549 and MCF-7, respectively. Interestingly, both compounds displayed significant activity with IC$_{50}$ valued of 5 µM against a P-glycoprotein overexpressing MDR tumor cell line (KB-VIN) although they were less active against its parent chemosensitive cell line (KB).

Supplementary Materials: NMR spectra and HRMS of new compounds are available online at http://www.mdpi.com/1420-3049/24/21/4005/s1.

Author Contributions: S.A., Y.S; investigation, performed the chemical experiments and data collection, S.F.; ECD calculation and analysis, M.G.; investigation, performed cytotoxic experiments using SRB assay, M.G., K.M., D.J.N, B.R.O. K.-H.L.; editing and guidance, K.N.-G; writing, conceptualization, and supervision.

Funding: This study was supported by JSPS KAKENHI Grant Number JP25293024, awarded to K.N.G. This work was also supported partially by NIH grant CA177584 from the National Cancer Institute, awarded to K.H.L., as well as the Eshelman Institute for Innovation, Chapel Hill, North Carolina, awarded to M.G. The content of this publication does not necessarily reflect the views or policies of the Department of Health and Human Services, nor does mention of trade names, commercial products, or organizations imply endorsement by the U.S. Government.

Acknowledgments: We appreciate critical comments, suggestions, and editing on the manuscript by Susan L. Morris-Natschke (UNC-CH).

Conflicts of Interest: The authors declare no conflict of interest.

References

1. Lakshmi, V.; Pandey, K.; Mishra, S.K.; Srivastava, S.; Mishra, M.; Agarwa, S.K. An overview of family *Hernandiaceae*. *Rec. Nat. Prod.* **2009**, *3*, 1–22.
2. Pettit, G.R.; Meng, Y.H.; Gearing, R.P.; Herald, D.L.; Pettit, R.K.; Doubek, D.L.; Chapuis, J.C.; Tackett, L.P. Antineoplastic Agents. 522. *Hernandia peltata* (Malaysia) and *Hernandia nymphaeifolia* (Republic of Maldives). *J. Nat. Prod.* **2004**, *67*, 214–220. [CrossRef] [PubMed]
3. Udino, L.; Abaul, J.; Bourgeois, P.; Corrichon, L.; Duran, H.; Zedde, C. Lignans from the seeds of *Hernandia sonora*. *Planta Med.* **1999**, *65*, 279–281. [CrossRef] [PubMed]
4. Chalandre, M.C.; Bruneton, J.; Cabalion, P.; Guinaudeau, H. Hernandiaceae. XII. Aporphine-benzylisoquinoline dimers isolated from *Hernandia peltata*. *Can. J. Chem.* **1986**, *64*, 123–126. [CrossRef]
5. Wei, C.Y.; Wang, S.W.; Ye, J.W.; Hwang, T.L.; Cheng, M.J.; Sung, P.J.; Chang, T.H.; Chen, J.J. New anti-inflammatory aporphine and lignan derivatives from the root wood of *Hernandia nymphaeifolia*. *Molecules* **2018**, *23*, 2286. [CrossRef]
6. Lavault, M.; Cabalion, P.; Bruneton, J. Study on Hernandiaceae. IV. Alkaloids of *Hernandia peltata*. *Planta Med.* **1982**, *46*, 119–121. [CrossRef]
7. Chen, J.J.; Tsai, I.L.; Chen, I.S. New Oxoaporphine Alkaloids from *Hernandia nymphaeifolia*. *J. Nat. Prod.* **1996**, *59*, 156–158. [CrossRef]
8. Chen, J.J.; Ishikawa, T.; Duh, C.Y.; Tsai, I.L.; Chen, I.S. New dimeric aporphine alkaloids and cytotoxic constituents of *Hernandia nymphaefolia*. *Planta Med.* **1996**, *62*, 528–533. [CrossRef]
9. Angerhofer, C.K.; Guinaudeau, H.; Wongpanich, V.; Pezzuto, J.M.; Cordell, G.A. Antiplasmodial and cytotoxic activity of natural bisbenzylisoquinoline alkaloids. *J. Nat. Prod.* **1999**, *62*, 59–66. [CrossRef]
10. Rasoanaivo, R.; Urverg, R.; Rafatro, H.; Ramanitrahasimbola, D.; Palazzino, G.; Galeffi, C.; Nicoletti, M. Alkaloids of *Hernandia voyronii*. Chloroquine-potentiating activity and structure elucidation of herveline D. *Planta Med.* **1998**, *64*, 58–62. [CrossRef]
11. Dittmar, A. The effectiveness of *Hernandia* spp. (Hernandiaceae) in traditional Samoan medicine and according to scientific analyses. *J. Ethnopharmacol.* **1991**, *33*, 243–251. [CrossRef]
12. Bruneton, J.; Shamma, M.; Minard, R.D.; Freyer, A.J.; Guinaudeau, H. Novel biogenetic pathways from (+)-reticuline. Three dimeric alkaloids: (+)-vanuatine, (+)-vateamine, and (+)-malekulatine. *J. Org. Chem.* **1983**, *48*, 3957–3960. [CrossRef]
13. Chen, I.S.; Chen, J.J.; Duh, C.Y.; Tsai, I.L. Cytotoxic lignans from Formosan *Hernandia nymphaeifolia*. *Phytochemistry* **1997**, *45*, 991–996. [CrossRef]
14. Chen, I.J.; Chang, Y.L.; Teng, C.M.; Chen, I.S. Anti-platelet aggregation alkaloids and lignans from *Hernandia nymphaefolia*. *Planta Med.* **2000**, *66*, 251–256. [CrossRef] [PubMed]
15. Yoder, B.J.; Cao, S.; Norris, A.; Miller, J.S.; Ratovoson, F.; Andriantsiferana, R.; Rasamison, V.E.; Kingston, D.G.I. Tambouranolide, a new cytotoxic hydroxybutanolide from a *Tambourissa* sp. (Monimiaceae). *Nat. Prod. Res.* **2007**, *21*, 37–41. [CrossRef] [PubMed]

16. Muto, N.; Tomokuni, T.; Haramoto, M.; Tatemoto, H.; Nakanishi, T.; Inatomi, Y.; Murata, H.; Inada, A. Isolation of apoptosis- and differentiation-inducing substances toward human promyelocytic leukemia HL-60 cells from leaves of *Juniperus taxifolia*. *Biosci. Biotechnol. Biochem.* **2008**, *72*, 477–484. [CrossRef] [PubMed]
17. Trazzi, G.; André, M.F.; Coelho, F.J. Diastereoselective synthesis of β-piperonyl-γ-butyrolactones from Morita-Baylis-Hillman adducts. Highly efficient synthesis of (±)-yatein, (±)-podorhizol and (±)-*epi*-podorhizol. *Braz. Chem. Soc.* **2010**, *21*, 2327–2339. [CrossRef]
18. Okunishi, T.; Umezawa, T.; Shimada, M. Enantiomeric compositions and biosynthesis of *Wikstroemia sikokiana* lignans. *J. Wood Sci.* **2000**, *46*, 234–242. [CrossRef]
19. Li, N.; Wu, J.L.; Sakai, J.I.; Ando, M. Dibenzylbutyrolactone and Dibenzylbutanediol Lignans from *Peperomia duclouxii*. *J. Nat. Prod.* **2003**, *66*, 1421–1426. [CrossRef]
20. Ahmed, A.A.; Mahmoud, A.A.; Ali, E.T.; Tzakou, O.; Couladis, M.; Mabry, T.J.; Gáti, T.; Tóth, G. Two highly oxygenated eudesmanes and ten lignans from *Achillea holosericea*. *Phytochemistry* **2002**, *59*, 851–856. [CrossRef]
21. Iida, T.; Nakano, M.; Ito, K. Hydroperoxysesquiterpene and lignan constituents of *Magnolia kobus*. *Phytochemistry* **1982**, *21*, 673–675. [CrossRef]
22. Asikin, Y.; Takahashi, M.; Mizu, M.; Takara, K.; Okua, H.; Wada, K. DNA damage protection against free radicals of two antioxidant neolignan glucosides from sugarcane molasses. *J. Sci. Food Agric.* **2016**, *96*, 1209–1215. [CrossRef] [PubMed]
23. Calis, I.; Kirmizibekmez, H.; Beutler, J.A.; Donmez, A.A.; Yalc, F.N.; Kilic, I.E.; Ozlap, M.; Ruedi, P.; Tasdemir, D. Secondary metabolites of *Phlomis viscosa* and their biological activities. *Turk. J. Chem.* **2005**, *29*, 71–81.
24. Sugiyama, M.; Kikuchi, M. Phenylethanoid glycosides from *Osmanthus asiaticus*. *Phytochemistry* **1993**, *32*, 1553–1555. [CrossRef]
25. Seki, K.; Sasaki, T.; Wano, S.; Haga, K.; Kaneko, R. Linderanolides and isolinderanolides, ten butanolides from *Lindera glauca*. *Phytochemistry* **1995**, *40*, 1175–1181. [CrossRef]
26. Anderson, J.E.; Ma, W.; Smith, D.L.; Chang, C.J.; Mclaughlin, J.L. Biologically active γ-lactones and methylketoalkenes from *Lindera benzoin*. *J. Nat. Prod.* **1992**, *55*, 71–83. [CrossRef]
27. Tamura, S.; Doke, S.; Murakami, N. Total synthesis of peumusolide A, NES non-antagonistic inhibitor for nuclear export of MEK. *Tetrahedron* **2010**, *66*, 8476–8480. [CrossRef]
28. Tamura, S.; Tonokawa, M.; Murakami, N. Stereo-controlled synthesis of analogs of peumusolide A, NES non-antagonistic inhibitor for nuclear export of MEK. *Tetrahedron Lett.* **2010**, *51*, 3134–3137. [CrossRef]
29. Tsenga, M.; Su, Y.S.; Cheng, M.J.; Liu, T.W.; Chen, I.S.; Wu, M.D.; Chang, H.S.; Yuan, G.F. Chemical constituents from a soil-derived actinomycete, Actinomadura miaoliensis BCRC 16873, and their inhibitory activities on lipopolysaccharide-induced tumor necrosis factor production. *Chem. Biodivers.* **2013**, *10*, 303–312. [CrossRef]
30. Tanaka, H.; Takaya, Y.; Toyoda, J.; Yasuda, T.; Sato, M.; Murata, J.; Murata, H.; Kaburagi, K.; Iida, O.; Sugiyama, K.; et al. Two new butanolides from the roots of *Litsea acuminate*. *Phytochemistry Lett.* **2015**, *11*, 32–36. [CrossRef]
31. Cheng, H.I.; Lin, W.Y.; Duh, C.Y.; Lee, K.H.; Tsai, I.L.; Chen, I.S. New cytotoxic butanolides from *Litsea acutivena*. *J. Nat. Prod.* **2001**, *64*, 1502–1505. [CrossRef] [PubMed]
32. Juan, C.; Martinez, V.; Yoshida, M.; Gottlieb, O.R. The chemistry of Brazilian Lauraceae. Part LXI. ω-Ethyl, ω-ethenyl and ω-ethynyl-α-alkylidene-γ-lactones from *Clinostemon mahuba*. *Phytochemistry* **1981**, *20*, 459–464. [CrossRef]
33. Takeda, K.I.; Sakurawi, K.; Ishi, H. Components of the Lauracea family. I. New lactonic compounds from *Litsea japonica*. *Tetrahedron* **1972**, *28*, 3757–3766. [CrossRef]
34. Li, X.J.; Dong, J.W.; Cai, L.; Wang, J.P.; Yu, N.X.; Ding, Z.T. Illigerones A and B, two new long-chain secobutanolides from *Illigera henryi* W. W. Sm. *Phytochem. Lett.* **2017**, *19*, 181–186. [CrossRef]
35. Yang, Y.N.; Huang, X.Y.; Feng, Z.M.; Jiang, J.S.; Zhang, P.C. Hepatoprotective Activity of Twelve Novel 7′-Hydroxy Lignan Glucosides from Arctii Fructus. *J. Agric. Food Chem.* **2014**, *62*, 9095–9102. [CrossRef] [PubMed]
36. Greca, M.D.; Molinaro, A.; Monaco, P.; Previtera, L. Neolignans from *Arum italicum*. *Phytochemistry* **1994**, *35*, 777–779. [CrossRef]

37. Arnoldi, A.; Merlini, L. Asymmetric synthesis of 3-methyl-2-phenyl-1,4-benzodioxanes. Absolute configuration of the neolignans eusiderin and eusiderin C and D. *J. Chem. Soc. Perkin Trans. 1* **1985**, 2555–2557. [CrossRef]
38. Gan, M.; Zhang, Y.L.; Lin, S.; Liu, M.T.; Song, W.X.; Zi, J.C.; Yang, Y.C.; Fan, X.N.; Shi, J.G.; Hu, J.F.; et al. Glycosides from the root of *Iodes cirrhosa*. *J. Nat. Prod.* **2008**, *71*, 647–654. [CrossRef]
39. Pascitelli, G.; Bruhn, T. Good Computational Practice in the Assignment of Absolute Configurations by TDDFT Calculations of ECD Spectra. *Chirality* **2016**, *28*, 466–474. [CrossRef]
40. Nakagawa-Goto, K.; Oda, A.; Hamel, E.; Ohkoshi, E.; Lee, K.H.; Goto, M. Development of a novel class of tubulin inhibitors from desmosdumotin B with a hydroxylated bicyclic B-ring. *J. Med. Chem.* **2015**, *58*, 2378–2389. [CrossRef]

Sample Availability: Not available.

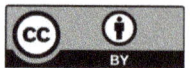

© 2019 by the authors. Licensee MDPI, Basel, Switzerland. This article is an open access article distributed under the terms and conditions of the Creative Commons Attribution (CC BY) license (http://creativecommons.org/licenses/by/4.0/).

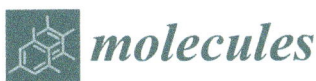

Article

Ivalin Induces Mitochondria-Mediated Apoptosis Associated with the NF-κB Activation in Human Hepatocellular Carcinoma SMMC-7721 Cells

Zhuo Han [1,†], Fang-yuan Liu [1,†], Shi-qi Lin [1,†], Cai-yun Zhang [1], Jia-hui Ma [1], Chao Guo [1], Fu-juan Jia [1], Qian Zhang [1], Wei-dong Xie [1] and Xia Li [1,2,*]

1. Marine college, Shandong University, Weihai 264209, China; hanzhuo1013@gmail.com (Z.H.); fangyuan617@outlook.com (F.L.); lsqsd@outlook.com (S.L.); caiyun617@outlook.com (C.Z.); sdumjh@hotmail.com (J.M.); super70732635@163.com (C.G.); jfj1996@outlook.com (F.J.); zhangqianzq@sdu.edu.cn (Q.Z.); wdxie@sdu.edu.cn (W.X.)
2. School of Pharmaceutical Sciences, Shandong University, Jinan 250012, China
* Correspondence: xiali@sdu.edu.cn; Tel.: +86-631-5688303
† These authors contributed equally to this study.

Academic Editor: Kyoko Nakagawa-Goto
Received: 6 September 2019; Accepted: 22 October 2019; Published: 22 October 2019

Abstract: Ivalin, a natural compound isolated from *Carpesium divaricatum*, showed excellent microtubule depolymerization activities among human hepatocellular carcinoma in our previous work. Here, we investigated its functions on mitochondria-mediated apoptosis in hepatocellular carcinoma SMMC-7721 cells. DAPI (4′,6-diamidino-2-phenylindole) staining, annexin V-fluorexcein isothiocyanate (FITC) apoptosis detection, and western blotting were applied to explore the apoptotic effect of Ivalin. Next, the induction effect of Ivalin on the mitochondrial pathway was also confirmed via a series of phenomena including the damage of mitochondria membrane potential, mitochondria cytochrome c escape, cleaved caspase-3 induction, and the reactive oxygen species generation. In this connection, we understood that Ivalin induced apoptosis through the mitochondrial pathway and the overload of reactive oxygen species. Furthermore, we found that the activation of nuclear factor-κB (NF-κB) and subsequent p53 induction were associated with the apoptotic effect of Ivalin. These data confirmed that Ivalin might be a promising pro-apoptotic compound that can be utilized as a potential drug for clinical treatment.

Keywords: Ivalin; *Carpesium divaricatum*; hepatocellular carcinoma; mitochondria-mediated apoptosis; NF-κB

1. Introduction

Clinical data have shown that hepatocellular carcinoma (HCC) is the most common and dominating primary tumor with a high incidence rate in adults worldwide [1–3]. Since many advanced treatments have been used in recent years, chemotherapy is still widely applied to treat HCC in the research of clinical trials [4]. However, both the occurrence of drug resistance and recurrences are the key hurdles associated with chemotherapy [5]. Therefore, the exploration and evolution of novel therapeutic agents for the treatment of HCC are greatly of need.

Abstracted compounds from plants utilized into an effective anticancer drug is one of the fastest developing therapeutics for chemotherapy [6,7]. The large family Asteraceae contains over 25,000 species (such as *Aster* and *Carpesium*) and many species have shown that it is best utilized as sources of edible oils, vegetables, pesticides, medicines and so on. In addition, it is considered to be an ideal source of effective natural compounds with the structure of sesquiterpenoids, particularly, an eudesmane framework [8]. Eudesmane-type sesquiterpenoids and their biological functions including antifungal, antitumor, and antibacterial have been the fastest growing field of pharmacological and synthetic studies during the last two decades [9]. Telekin and 1-oxoeudesm-11(13)-eno-12,8a-lactone (OEL), examples of compounds with an eudesmane framework, have been reported to strongly restrain cell proliferation via the induction of mitochondria-mediated apoptosis [10,11]. Ivalin (Figure 1), another compound with an eudesmane framework, was abstracted from the traditional herb *Carpesium divaricatum* [12]. Our previous works demonstrated that Ivalin can serve as a novel microtubule inhibitor by depolymerizing microtubules and resulted in cell proliferation inhibition in hepatocellular carcinoma SMMC-7721 cells [13]. Here, we report that Ivalin enforced the procedure of apoptosis in the same cells by triggering reactive oxygen species (ROS) generation and the participation of the mitochondria pathway.

Nuclear factor-κB (NF-κB), a conventional transcription factor, is important for the execution and control of apoptosis [14]. NF-κB, in different given stimulations such as in ROS accumulation and cancer therapeutic agents, complexly regulates the program of apoptosis via its downstream target genes, which include the p53 protein and so on [15,16]. Detecting both the protein and mRNA levels of NF-κB and p53 will help us to further perceive and recognize the influence of pro-apoptosis and underlying theory of Ivalin. The results from these experiments showed that the initiate of NF-κB and subsequent p53 induction were associated with the apoptotic effect of Ivalin in SMMC-7721 cells.

2. Results

2.1. Apoptotic Effect of Ivalin

Our previous studies confirmed that Ivalin (Figure 1) was significantly cytotoxic to SMMC-7721 cells (IC50: 4.34 ± 0.10) with a lower effect toward the normal cell line HL7702 (IC50: 25.86 ± 0.87) [13]. In response to characterizing the cell growth inhibition effect of Ivalin, we monitored morphological changes in SMMC-7721 cells after 24 h of treatment. Compared to the untreated cells, Ivalin treatment increased the apoptotic body formation as well as nuclear condensation, which were the significant morphologic alterations related to apoptosis (Figure 2A).

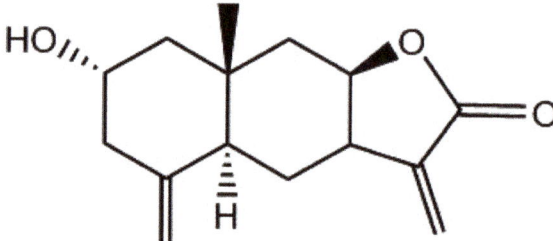

Figure 1. Structure of Ivalin.

When cells were undergoing apoptosis, the phosphatidylserine in the inter surface of the plasma membrane transforms to the outer surface, which can be stained with Annexin V. In this connection, we performed flow cytometry to further quantify the apoptotic effect of Ivalin via dual stained cells with Annexin V-fluorexcein isothiocyanate and propidium iodide. The results shown in Figure 2B revealed that the proportion of Annexin V-stained cells increased with the percentages increased from 4.57%, 9.28%, 16.6%, to 47.32% after treating with 0 to 8 μmol/L Ivalin, respectively. Therefore, we believe that Ivalin may strongly increase the ratio of apoptotic cells in SMMC-7721 cells.

The Bcl-2 family consists of members with a pro-apoptotic or the opposite effect and the balance between them may regulate the fate of cells [17,18]. Bcl-2 and Bax, the most common proteins with vital roles in the Bcl-2 family, were analyzed by western blot after Ivalin treatment. Results revealed that Ivalin-treatmen triggered the altered expression of Bcl-2 and Bax in SMMC-7721 cells (Figure 2C).

The increase in the Bax protein and decrease in the Bcl-2 protein expression levels further confirmed the pro-apoptotic effect of Ivalin as suggested above.

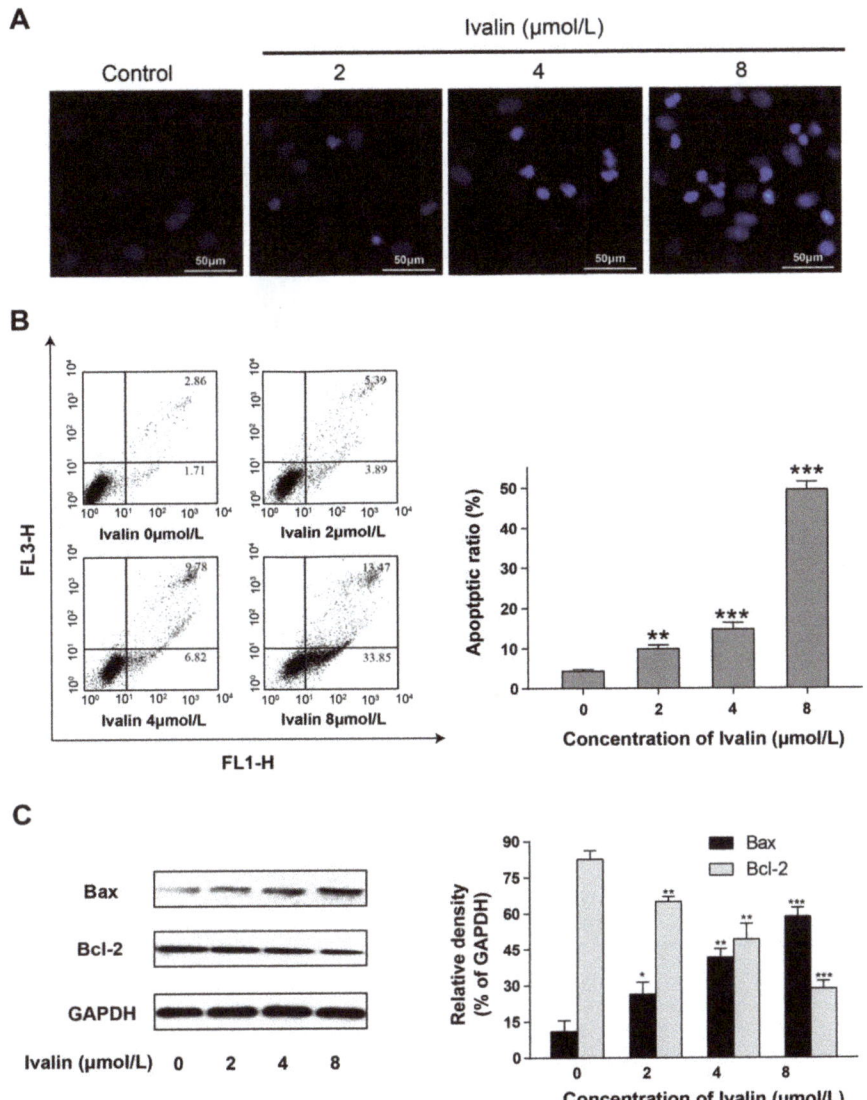

Figure 2. SMMC-7721 cells treated with Ivalin causing apoptosis. (A) Fluorescence micrographs of untreated and Ivalin treated SMMC-7721 cells with 4′,6-diamidino-2-phenylindole (DAPI). Magnification: 100×. (B) Results from the flow cytometry analysis, the quantification of the apoptotic cells after indicate treatment. (C) Western blot showed that Ivalin induced apoptosis by enhancing the Bax and declining the Bcl-2 expression. * $p < 0.05$; ** $p < 0.01$, *** $p < 0.001$ vs. the control group.

2.2. Ivalin Triggered the Loss of Mitochondrial Membrane Potential (MMP) in SMMC-7721 Cells

We next stained the cells with JC-1 to measure the cellular MMP in response to Ivalin treatment. Cells treated with Ivalin led to the loss of MMP in a concentration-dependent manner (Figure 3).

Meanwhile, the increased mitochondrial membrane permeability in treated cells may result in the translocation of mitochondria cytochrome c to cytosol. Figure 4A illustrates an apparent release of cytochrome c from the mitochondria to cytosol in the experimental groups. Furthermore, the treatment with Ivalin concentration-dependent increased the level of cleaved caspase-3 in the experimental groups (Figure 4B). The above findings indicate that the mitochondria-mediated pathway was associated with Ivalin-induced apoptosis.

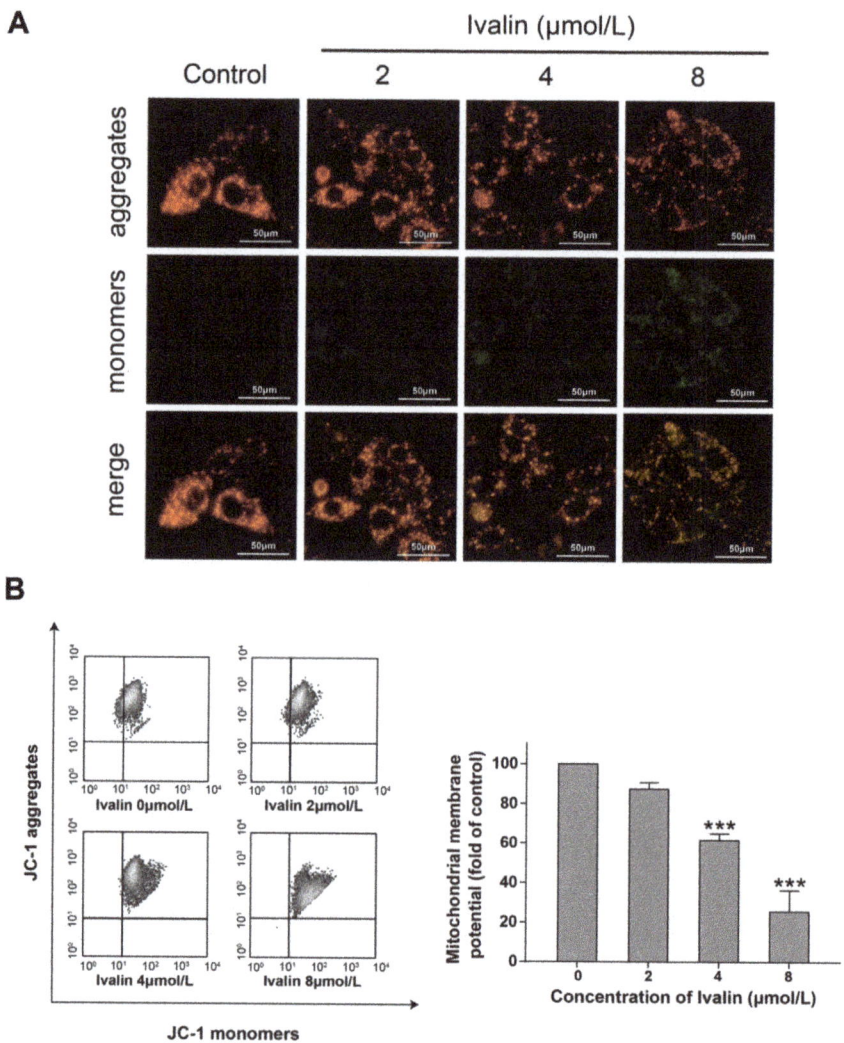

Figure 3. Effects of MMP generation in Ivalin-treated cells. (**A,B**) After Ivalin treatment for 24 h, flow cytometry and fluorescence microscope were used to detect cellular mitochondrial membrane potential. (**A**) Ivalin treatment decreased the red fluorescence intensity (aggregates) and increased green fluorescence intensity (monomers) in SMMC-7721 cells, indicating that Ivalin reduced the mitochondrial membrane potential, thereby leading to mitochondrial dysfunction. (**B**) Ivalin induced the loss of mitochondrial membrane potential as shown by flow cytometry. *** $p < 0.01$ vs. the control group.

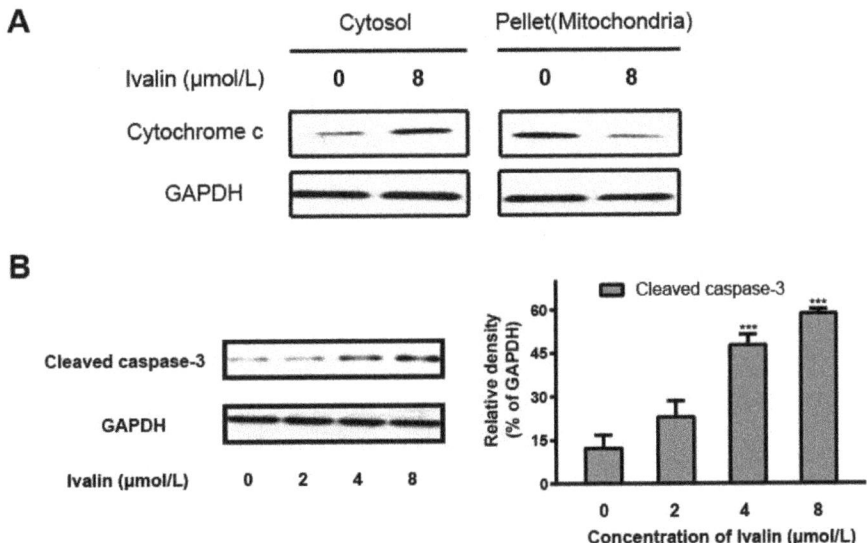

Figure 4. Ivalin trigged apoptosis by means of the mitochondria activation. (**A**) The cytochrome c in mitochondria with the stimulation of Ivalin inflowed into the cytosol. (**B**) Cleaved caspase-3 was increased with the treatment of Ivalin. *** $p < 0.001$ vs. the control group.

2.3. The Generation of ROS Appeared in Ivalin-Treated Cells

Intracellular ROS generation always appears during the process of mitochondrial obstruction. Therefore, we detected the fluorescence produced by dichlorofluorescein (DCF) by evaluating the possession of ROS by the flow cytometric assay to determine whether Ivalin can induce the accumulation of ROS. The group of treated and untreated cells were incubated with DCF-DA for 30 min and analyzed via flow cytometry. The results are shown in Figure 5 with a greater generation of ROS in the experimental groups in contrast to the untreated group.

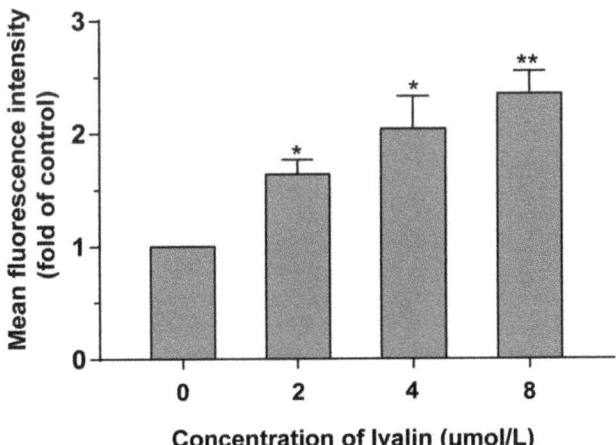

Figure 5. Ivalin induced the generation of intracellular ROS. Graph shows the fluorescence intensities of DCF in the SMMC-7721 cells exposed to Ivalin in contrast to control. The fluorescence intensity of control group was set as 1. * $p < 0.05$; ** $p < 0.01$ vs. the control group.

2.4. Ivalin Modulated the Protein and mRNA Levels of NF-κB, IκB, and p53

Currently, a large member of anticancer compounds take effect in coping with hazardous substances by targeting transcription activators like nuclear factor-κB (NF-κB) and p53 regulating ROS [19–21]. In order to further perceive and recognize the role of Ivalin in apoptotic induction, we experimented with the expression of NF-κB, IκB, and p53 through western blot analysis. Ivalin-treatment enhanced the expressions of NF-κB and p53, but decreased that of IκB protein (Figure 6A).

We also performed real-time PCR to evaluate if there had been any alteration in the NF-κB, p53, and Bax mRNA levels in the presence of Ivalin treatment. The data revealed that Ivalin time-dependently induced the gene expressions of NF-κB, p53, and Bax (Figure 6B). NF-κB was activated before p53, and the activation of NF-κB mRNA reached the highest levels early, about 4 h. Therefore, the effective activation of NF-κB was associated with the apoptotic effect of Ivalin.

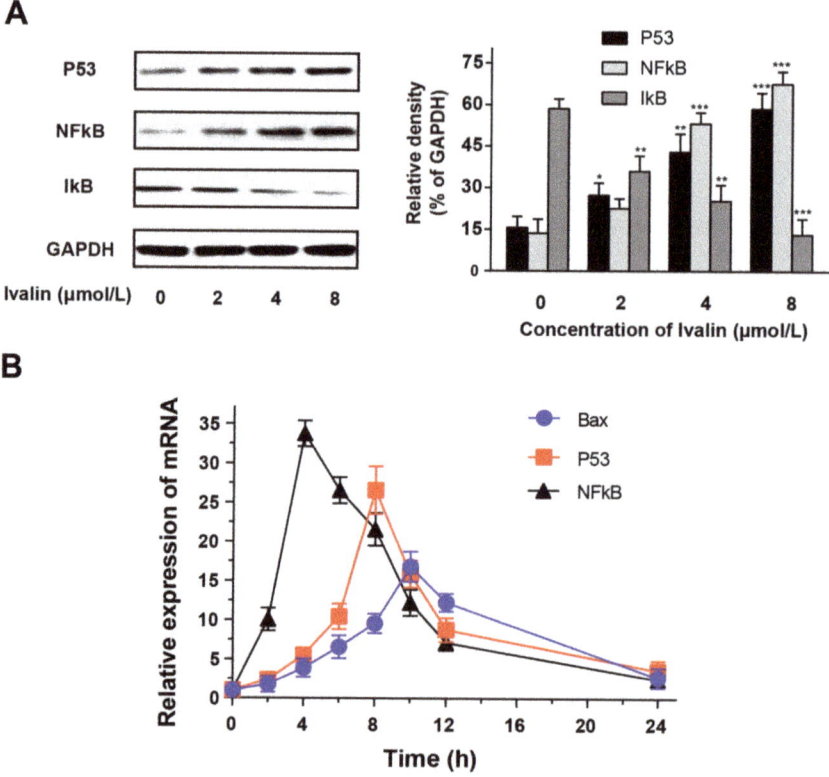

Figure 6. Trends of Ivalin on the p53, NF-κB and IκB expression. (**A**) The expressions of relative proteins were measured by western blotting. * $p < 0.05$; ** $p < 0.01$, *** $p < 0.001$ vs. the control group. (**B**) Relative mRNA expression values were calculated by real-time PCR. The quantity of each mRNA was relative to the glyceraldehyde-3-phosphate dehydrogenase (GAPDH) mRNA levels.

3. Discussion

In our previous work, we reported the ideal microtubule depolymerization activities of Ivalin in SMMC-7721 cells [13]. In this study, we found that Ivalin treatment may lead to obviously apoptotic features including apoptotic body formation and nuclear condensation in the same cells. Furthermore, in the presence of an indicated concentration of Ivalin, a significant increase in the proportion of apoptotic cells was observed through double staining by annexin V-FITC and PI. In this connection, we presumed the apoptotic effect of Ivalin in SMMC-7721 cells.

Apoptosis can be induced by the extrinsic (death receptor pathway) and intrinsic pathways (mitochondria-mediated pathway). During the mitochondria-mediated pathway, the increase in mitochondria membrane permeability led to the subsequent release of mitochondria cytochrome c to cytosol, activated the caspase-9 and its downstream effector caspases including caspase-3, and finally induced apoptosis [22]. The Bcl-2 family proteins such as Bax and Bcl-2 mediate the intrinsic pathway by changing the mitochondria outer membrane permeabilization [23]. In particular, a common gateway for the mitochondria-mediated apoptotic pathway is the required level of Bax protein [24]. Ivalin treatment resulted in inducing the expression of Bax and attenuating that of Bcl-2 protein in SMMC-7721 cells. Additionally, treatment with Ivalin also caused the increase in the mitochondria membrane permeability, which was confirmed by the loss of MMP and an obvious release of cytochrome c from mitochondria into cytosol. Furthermore, the induction of cleaved caspase-3 expression in Ivalin-treated cells was also observed in the experiment. All of these results confirmed the effective mitochondria-mediated apoptotic effect of Ivalin among SMMC-7721 cells.

NF-κB, a transcription factor first identified in 1986, provides an effective goal for the progress of inflammation and apoptosis [25]. Nowadays, more and more evidence suggests the positive role of NF-κB in apoptosis, while the negative role of it in the apoptosis process has been discussed for many years [26]. In fact, the function of NF-κB in mediating apoptosis strongly relies on the type of cancer, the stimulation, and the related subunit [27–30]. When under non-stimulated status, NF-κB is in a complex formed with IκB in the cytoplasm without activation. Extracellular stimuli bring about rapid phosphorylation of IκB, which will be further degraded by ubiquitinase or protease [31]. When the degradation of IκB is finished, NF-κB activates rapidly and subsequently translocates into the nucleus to react with the downstream targets [32–34]. A key example was a report that confirmed the important role of NF-κB in the induction of wild type p53 expression to initiate pro-apoptotic signaling in response to ROS accumulation [21].

Here, Ivalin treatment led to a greater generation of ROS in SMMC-7721 cells. In this connection, further investigation was performed to confirm whether NF-κB was involved in the mitochondria-mediated apoptotic effect of Ivalin. Western blot analysis revealed that Ivalin increased the expression of NF-κB and p53, but decreased the expression of IκB. Moreover, rt-PCR revealed that the mRNA levels of NF-κB, p53, and Bax increased after Ivalin treatment in a time-dependent manner. NF-κB was activated first, followed by the activation of p53 and Bax, and the expression of NF-κB mRNA reached the highest levels as early as about 4 h. This finding indicates that the NF-κB signaling pathway is involved in Ivalin-induced mitochondria-mediated apoptosis in SMMC-7721 cells.

To sum up, this study is the first to report that Ivalin induced mitochondria-mediated apoptosis associated with the NF-κB activation in SMMC-7721 cells. Ivalin treatment resulted in a significant generation of ROS in SMMC-7721 cells. In response to this, NF-κB was activated and served as a transcription factor to induce p53 activation, which subsequently induced Bax while decreasing Bcl-2 protein expression, which eventually led to mitochondria-mediated apoptosis in SMMC-7721 cells. However, the detail mechanisms responsible for the pro-apoptotic activity of Ivalin need to be explored further. Hence, Ivalin deserves further research to develop it into a promising chem-therapeutic agent or leading compound for anti-cancer agent searching.

4. Materials and Methods

4.1. Chemicals and Reagents

Ivalin (>98%), provided by Dr. Xie (Shandong University, Weihai, China) [12], was dissolved and its concentration adjusted by dimethylsulfoxide (DMSO) when required. DAPI (4′,6-diamidino-2-phenylindole) was acquired from Sigma-Aldrich Corp. (St. Louis, MO, USA). An Annexin V-fluorexcein isothiocyanate (FITC) Apoptosis Detection Kit was purchased from BD Biosciences (San Jose, CA, USA).

Caspase-3, cytochrome c, p53, and NF-κB antibodies were obtained from Cell Signaling Technology (CST, Inc, Beverly, MA, USA). Bcl-2, Bax, and GAPDH antibodies were obtained from Abcam Inc. (Cambridge, MA, USA). Beyotime Institute of Biotechnology (Shanghai, China) supplied the cell mitochondria/cytosol isolation kit, JC-1 and DCFH-DA, to us.

4.2. Human Hepatocellular Carcinoma and Cell Culture

Shanghai Institute for Biological Sciences (SIBS) of Chinese Academy of Sciences (Shanghai, China) supplied the SMMC-7721 cell line (human hepatocellular carcinoma cell line) and we cultured the cells according to the supplier's instructions.

4.3. DAPI Staining

DAPI staining assay, as previously described [35], was used to observe the change in the nucleus after Ivalin treatment.

4.4. Mitochondrial Membrane Potential

We performed JC-1 staining to measure the changes in mitochondrial membrane potential ($\Delta\Psi m$) in SMMC-7721 cells after Ivalin treatment. Cells were treated with Ivalin (0 μM to 8 μM) for 24 h and dealt with JC-1 in the light of the instructions from the manufacturer. Stained cells were collected for flow cytometric analysis or fluorescence microscope observation. The results contained three independent experiments.

4.5. Apoptosis Detection

The apoptosis rate of SMMC-7721 cells after Ivalin 24 h treatment was evaluated by Annexin V-FITC and Propidium Iodide (PI) double staining, according to our previously described study [13].

4.6. Measurement of Intracellular ROS Levels

Cells were treated with Ivalin, as described above, for 24 h. The working principle of the kit was that with an increase in ROS, DCFH-DA can transform into DCFH, which reacts with ROS, presenting the fluorescence property. We took advantage of this to measure the change of intracellular ROS content via flow cytometry as previously described [35].

4.7. Western Blot Analysis

Western blot analysis, performed as previously described [36], was used to detect the expression levels of indicated protein. In the assay for cytochrome c measurement, we used a mitochondria/cytosol isolation kit to separate the mitochondrial proteins from cytosol proteins.

4.8. Real-Time PCR Analysis

Real-time PCR assay, as described in our previous work [36], was used to detect the mRNA levels of the NF-κB, p53, and Bax genes. We designed all needed primers using primer premier 5 and synthesis by Sangon Biotech Co Ltd. (Shanghai, China) for the NF-κB gene (sense primer: 5'-TAGAAACAGACCGAGGAG-3' and anti-sense primer: 5'-ACTGGCTAATAAAGTGAATG-3'), p53 gene (sense primer: 5'-GTTTCCGTCTGGGCTTCT-3' and anti-sense primer: 5'-CCTCAGGCGGCTCATAG-3'), and Bax gene (sense primer: 5'-TCAACTGGGGCCGGGTTGTC-3' and anti-sense primer: 5'-CCTGGTCTTGGATCCAGCC-3').

4.9. Statistical Analysis

All data are presented as mean ± SD (standard deviation) if appropriate. A comparison between two groups was performed with the Student's t-test. * $p < 0.05$; ** $p < 0.01$, *** $p < 0.001$ vs. the control group.

Author Contributions: Conceptualization, X.L.; Formal analysis, Z.H. and F.L.; Funding acquisition, X.L.; Investigation, Z.H., F.L., S.L., C.Z., J.M., C.G., F.J. and Q.Z.; Resources, W.X. and X.L.; Paper writing, S.L.; Paper review and editing, X.L.

Funding: This work was supported by Natural Science Foundation of Shandong Provincial under Grant (No. ZR2019MH001), the Fundamental Research Funds for the Central Universities under Grant (No. 2019ZRJC004), and the National Natural Science Foundation of China under Grant (No. 81273532).

Conflicts of Interest: The authors declare no conflicts of interest.

References

1. Siegel, R.L.; Miller, K.D.; Jemal, A. Cancer statistics, 2019. *Ca-A. Cancer J. Clin.* **2019**, *69*, 7–34. [CrossRef] [PubMed]
2. Abdalla, E.K.; Vauthey, J.N. Focus on treatment of large hepatocellular carcinoma. *Ann. Surg. Oncol.* **2004**, *11*, 1035–1036. [CrossRef] [PubMed]
3. Yan, M.-D.; Yao, C.-J.; Chow, J.-M.; Chang, C.-L.; Hwang, P.-A.; Chuang, S.-E.; Whang-Peng, J.; Lai, G.-M. Fucoidan Elevates MicroRNA-29b to Regulate DNMT3B-MTSS1 Axis and Inhibit EMT in Human Hepatocellular Carcinoma Cells. *Mar. Drugs* **2015**, *13*, 6099–6116. [CrossRef] [PubMed]
4. Mor, E.; Kaspa, R.T.; Sheiner, P.; Schwartz, M. Treatment of hepatocellular carcinoma associated with cirrhosis in the era of liver transplantation. *Ann. Intern. Med.* **1998**, *129*, 643–653. [CrossRef]
5. Li, X.; Zhao, Y.; Wu, W.K.K.; Liu, S.; Cui, M.; Lou, H. Solamargine induces apoptosis associated with p53 transcription-dependent and transcription-independent pathways in human osteosarcoma U2OS cells. *Life Sci.* **2011**, *88*, 314–321. [CrossRef]
6. Wiseman, L.R.; Markham, A. Irinotecan—A review of its pharmacological properties and clinical efficacy in the management of advanced colorectal cancer. *Drugs* **1996**, *52*, 606–623. [CrossRef]
7. Perez, E.A. Microtubule inhibitors: Differentiating tubulin-inhibiting agents based on mechanisms of action, clinical activity, and resistance. *Mol. Cancer Ther.* **2009**, *8*, 2086–2095. [CrossRef]
8. Wu, Q.-X.; Shi, Y.-P.; Jia, Z.-J. Eudesmane sesquiterpenoids from the Asteraceae family. *Nat. Prod. Rep.* **2006**, *23*, 699–734. [CrossRef]
9. Da Costa, F.B.; Terfloth, L.; Gasteiger, J. Sesquiterpene lactone-based classification of three Asteraceae tribes: A study based on self-organizing neural networks applied to chemo systematics. *Phytochemistry* **2005**, *66*, 345–353. [CrossRef]
10. Zheng, B.; Wu, L.; Ma, L.; Liu, S.; Li, L.; Xie, W.; Li, X. Telekin Induces Apoptosis Associated with the Mitochondria-Mediated Pathway in Human Hepatocellular Carcinoma Cells. *Biol. Pharm. Bull.* **2013**, *36*, 1118–1125. [CrossRef]
11. Cui, M.; Zhang, Y.; Liu, S.; Xie, W.; Ji, M.; Lou, H.; Li, X. 1-Oxoeudesnn-11(13)-ene-12,8 alpha-lactone-induced Apoptosis via ROS Generation and Mitochondria Activation in MCF-7 Cells. *Arch. Pharmacal Res.* **2011**, *34*, 1323–1329. [CrossRef] [PubMed]
12. Xie, W.-D.; Wang, X.-R.; Ma, L.-S.; Li, X.; Row, K.-H. Sesquiterpenoids from Carpesium divaricatum and their cytotoxic activity. *Fitoterapia* **2012**, *83*, 1351–1355. [CrossRef] [PubMed]
13. Liu, F.; Lin, S.; Zhang, C.; Ma, J.; Han, Z.; Jia, F.; Xie, W.; Li, X. The Novel Nature Microtubule Inhibitor Ivalin Induces G2/M Arrest and Apoptosis in Human Hepatocellular Carcinoma SMMC-7721 Cells In Vitro. *Medicina* **2019**, *55*, 470. [CrossRef] [PubMed]
14. Bonvin, C.; Guillon, A.; Van Bemmelen, M.X.; Gerwins, P.; Johnson, G.L.; Widmann, C. Role of the amino-terminal domains of MEKKs in the activation of NF kappa B and MAPK pathways and in the regulation of cell proliferation and apoptosis. *Cell. Signal.* **2002**, *14*, 123–131. [CrossRef]
15. Zhang, Y.; Wu, Y.; Wu, D.; Tashiro, S.-i.; Onodera, S.; Ikejima, T. NF-kappa b facilitates oridonin-induced apoptosis and autophagy in HT1080 cells through a p53-mediated pathway. *Arch. Biochem. Biophys.* **2009**, *489*, 25–33. [CrossRef] [PubMed]
16. Liao, G.; Gao, B.; Gao, Y.; Yang, X.; Cheng, X.; Ou, Y. Phycocyanin Inhibits Tumorigenic Potential of Pancreatic Cancer Cells: Role of Apoptosis and Autophagy. *Sci. Rep.* **2016**, *6*, 34564. [CrossRef] [PubMed]
17. Nascimento, P.D.S.; Ornellas, A.A.; Campos, M.R.M.; Scheiner, M.A.M.; Fiedler, W.; Alves, G. Bax and Bcl-2 imbalance and HPB infection in penile tumors and adjacent tissues. *Prog. En Urol.* **2004**, *14*, 353–359.

18. Cheng, E. Molecular Control of Mitochondrial Apoptosis by the BCL-2 Family. *Blood* **2009**, *114*, 1577–1578. [CrossRef]
19. Ye, J.; Ma, J.; Liu, C.; Huang, J.; Wang, L.; Zhong, X. A novel iron(II) phenanthroline complex exhibits anticancer activity against TFR1-overexpressing esophageal squamous cell carcinoma cells through ROS accumulation and DNA damage. *Biochem. Pharmacol.* **2019**, *166*, 93–107. [CrossRef]
20. Galadari, S.; Rahman, A.; Pallichankandy, S.; Thayyullathil, F. Reactive oxygen species and cancer paradox: To promote or to suppress? *Free Radic. Biol. Med.* **2017**, *104*, 144–164. [CrossRef]
21. Fujioka, S.; Schmidt, C.; Sclabas, G.M.; Li, Z.K.; Pelicano, H.; Peng, B.; Yao, A.; Niu, J.G.; Zhang, W.; Evans, D.B.; et al. Stabilization of p53 is a novel mechanism for proapoptotic function of NF-kappa B. *J. Biol. Chem.* **2004**, *279*, 27549–27559. [CrossRef] [PubMed]
22. Kroemer, G.; Galluzzi, L.; Brenner, C. Mitochondrial membrane permeabilization in cell death. *Physiol. Rev.* **2007**, *87*, 99–163. [CrossRef] [PubMed]
23. Czabotar, P.E.; Lessene, G.; Strasser, A.; Adams, J.M. Control of apoptosis by the BCL-2 protein family: Implications for physiology and therapy. *Nat. Rev. Mol. Cell Biol.* **2014**, *15*, 49–63. [CrossRef] [PubMed]
24. Wei, M.C.; Zong, W.X.; Cheng, E.H.Y.; Lindsten, T.; Panoutsakopoulou, V.; Ross, A.J.; Roth, K.A.; MacGregor, G.R.; Thompson, C.B.; Korsmeyer, S.J. Proapoptotic BAX and BAK: A requisite gateway to mitochondrial dysfunction and death. *Science* **2001**, *292*, 727–730. [CrossRef] [PubMed]
25. Sen, R.; Baltimore, D. Inducibility of kappa immunoglobulin enhancer-binding protein Nf-kappa B by a posttranslational mechanism. *Cell* **1986**, *47*, 921–928. [CrossRef]
26. Lee, C.H.; Jeon, Y.-T.; Kim, S.-H.; Song, Y.-S. NF-kappa B as a potential molecular target for cancer therapy. *Biofactors* **2007**, *29*, 19–35. [CrossRef] [PubMed]
27. Bernard, D.; Monte, D.; Vandenbunder, B.; Abbadie, C. The c-Rel transcription factor can both induce and inhibit apoptosis in the same cells via the upregulation of MnSOD. *Oncogene* **2002**, *21*, 4392–4402. [CrossRef]
28. Kaltschmidt, B.; Kaltschmidt, C.; Hofmann, T.G.; Hehner, S.P.; Droge, W.; Schmitz, M.L. The pro- or anti-apoptotic function of NF-kappa B is determined by the nature of the apoptotic stimulus. *Eur. J. Biochem.* **2000**, *267*, 3828–3835. [CrossRef]
29. Sheehy, A.M.; Schlissel, M.S. Overexpression of RelA causes G1 arrest and apoptosis in a pro-B cell line. *J. Biol. Chem.* **1999**, *274*, 8708–8716. [CrossRef]
30. Tarabin, V.; Schwaninger, M. The role of NF-kappa B in 6-hydroxydopamine- and TNF alpha-induced apoptosis of PC12 cells. *Naunyn-Schmiedebergs Arch. Pharmacol.* **2004**, *369*, 563–569. [CrossRef]
31. Yeh, P.Y.; Chuang, S.E.; Yeh, K.H.; Song, Y.C.; Ea, C.K.; Cheng, A.L. Increase of the resistance of human cervical carcinoma cells to cisplatin by inhibition of the MEK to ERK signaling pathway partly via enhancement of anticancer drug-induced NF kappa B activation. *Biochem. Pharmacol.* **2002**, *63*, 1423–1430. [CrossRef]
32. Liu, S.; Wu, D.; Li, L.; Sun, X.; Xie, W.; Li, X. NF-kappa B activation was involved in reactive oxygen species-mediated apoptosis and autophagy in 1-oxoeudesm-11(13)-eno-12,8 alpha-lactone-treated human lung cancer cells. *Arch. Pharmacal Res.* **2014**, *37*, 1039–1052. [CrossRef] [PubMed]
33. Liang, Y.; Zhou, Y.; Shen, P. NF-kappa B and Its Regulation on the Immune System. *Cell. Mol. Immunol.* **2004**, *1*, 343–350. [PubMed]
34. Perkins, N.D. Integrating cell-signalling pathways with NF-kappa B and IKK function. *Nat. Rev. Mol. Cell Biol.* **2007**, *8*, 49–62. [CrossRef] [PubMed]
35. Wang, Q.-L.; Guo, C.; Qi, J.; Ma, J.-H.; Liu, F.-Y.; Lin, S.-Q.; Zhang, C.-Y.; Xie, W.-D.; Zhuang, J.-J.; Li, X. Protective effects of 3-angeloyloxy-8, 10-dihydroxyeremophila-7(11)-en-12, 8-lactone on paraquat-induced oxidative injury in SH-SY5Y cells. *J. Asian Nat. Prod. Res.* **2019**, *21*, 364–376. [CrossRef] [PubMed]
36. Lin, S.; Zhang, C.; Liu, F.; Ma, J.; Jia, F.; Han, Z.; Xie, W.; Li, X. Actinomycin V Inhibits Migration and Invasion via Suppressing Snail/Slug-Mediated Epithelial-Mesenchymal Transition Progression in Human Breast Cancer MDA-MB-231 Cells In Vitro. *Mar. Drugs* **2019**, *17*, 305. [CrossRef]

Sample Availability: Samples of the compounds are available from the authors.

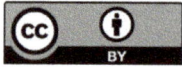 © 2019 by the authors. Licensee MDPI, Basel, Switzerland. This article is an open access article distributed under the terms and conditions of the Creative Commons Attribution (CC BY) license (http://creativecommons.org/licenses/by/4.0/).

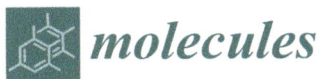

Article

Apple Peel Flavonoid Fraction 4 Suppresses Breast Cancer Cell Growth by Cytostatic and Cytotoxic Mechanisms

Chao-Yu Loung [1,†], Wasundara Fernando [1,†], H.P. Vasantha Rupasinghe [1,2] and David W. Hoskin [3,*]

[1] Department of Pathology, Faculty of Medicine, Dalhousie University, Halifax, NS B3H 4R2, Canada; joe.loung@dal.ca (C.-Y.L.); wasufer@dal.ca (W.F.); vrupasinghe@dal.ca (H.P.V.R.)
[2] Department of Plant, Food, and Environmental Sciences, Faculty of Agriculture, Dalhousie University, Truro, NS B2N 5E3, Canada
[3] Department of Pathology, Department of Microbiology and Immunology, Department of Surgery, Faculty of Medicine, Dalhousie University, Halifax, NS B3H 4R2, Canada
* Correspondence: d.w.hoskin@dal.ca
† These authors contribute equally to this work.

Received: 7 June 2019; Accepted: 11 September 2019; Published: 13 September 2019

Abstract: Many dietary flavonoids possess anti-cancer activities. Here, the effect of apple peel flavonoid fraction 4 (AF4) on the growth of triple-negative (MDA-MB-231, MDA-MB-468), estrogen receptor-positive (MCF-7), and HER2-positive (SKBR3) breast cancer cells was determined and compared with the effect of AF4 on normal mammary epithelial cells and dermal fibroblasts. AF4 inhibited breast cancer cell growth in monolayer cultures, as well as the growth of MCF-7 spheroids, without substantially affecting the viability of non-malignant cells. A sub-cytotoxic concentration of AF4 suppressed the proliferation of MDA-MB-231 cells by inhibiting passage through the G_0/G_1 phase of the cell cycle. AF4-treated MDA-MB-231 cells also exhibited reduced in vitro migration and invasion, and decreased Akt (protein kinase B) signaling. Higher concentrations of AF4 were selectively cytotoxic for MDA-MB-231 cells. AF4 cytotoxicity was associated with the intracellular accumulation of reactive oxygen species. Importantly, intratumoral administration of AF4 suppressed the growth of MDA-MB-231 xenografts in non-obese diabetic severe combined immunodeficient (NOD-SCID) female mice. The selective cytotoxicity of AF4 for breast cancer cells, combined with the capacity of sub-cytotoxic AF4 to inhibit breast cancer cell proliferation, migration, and invasion suggests that flavonoid-rich AF4 (and its constituents) has potential as a natural therapeutic agent for breast cancer treatment.

Keywords: apoptosis; breast cancer; cell cycle; flavonoids; reactive oxygen species; tumor suppression

1. Introduction

The regular consumption of fruits and vegetables that are rich in flavonoids and other bioactive molecules is associated with a reduced risk of developing various types of cancers [1–5]. It is unlikely that any single natural source-derived compound is responsible for this beneficial effect since multiple bioactive molecules in flavonoid-rich foods are likely to act in a synergistic fashion. Numerous studies on phytochemicals as potential anti-cancer agents have found that these natural compounds affect many different signaling pathways involved in cancer development and progression [6,7]. It is hoped that further research on the anti-cancer properties of phytochemicals will lead to the development of plant-based therapeutics for the prevention or treatment of cancer.

Apples, which are a common source of dietary flavonoids, have been widely investigated for their disease-fighting properties [8–11]. Apple peel flavonoid fraction 4 (AF4) is a flavonoid-rich ethanolic extract of the Northern Spy apple cultivar [12]. AF4 contains a number of polyphenolic compounds, including flavonols, anthocyanins, dihydrochalcones, phenolic acids, and flavan-3-ols. Quercetin glycosides (quercetin-3-*O*-galactoside, quercetin-3-*O*-rutinoside, quercetin-3-*O*-glucoside and quercetin-3-*O*-rhamnoside) comprise approximately 70% of the phenolic content of AF4. Previous studies have established the neuroprotective and anti-inflammatory properties of AF4 in different mouse models [12,13]. AF4 also inhibits the growth of hepatocellular carcinoma (HepG2) cells by causing cell cycle arrest and apoptosis, as well as acting as a topoisomerase toxicant [14].

Breast cancer is the most common cancer among North American women and the second highest cause of cancer-related deaths [15]. The poor prognosis of metastatic breast cancer mandates the development of novel treatment strategies. The impact of AF4 treatment on breast cancer cells has not yet been determined. In the current study we used in vitro and in vivo approaches to elucidate the selective cytotoxic, anti-proliferative, anti-migratory and tumor suppressor effects of AF4 on breast cancer cells.

2. Results

2.1. Apple Peel Flavonoid Fraction 4 (AF4) Selectively Inhibits the Growth of Breast Cancer Cells

Exposure to AF4 reduced the number of viable triple-negative (MDA-MB-231, MDA-MB-468), estrogen receptor-positive (MCF-7), and HER2 receptor-positive (SKBR3) breast cancer cells in monolayer cultures in a dose- and time-dependent manner, as indicated by reduced cellular metabolic activity measured by 3-(4,5-dimethythiazol-2-yl)-2,5-diphenyltetrazolium bromide (MTT) assays (Figure 1A). Sensitivity to AF4 (100 µg/mL) at 72 h was as follows: MDA-MB-231 (39% ± 3% viable) and MDA-MB-468 (38% ± 3% viable) > SKBR3 (48% ± 2% viable) > MCF-7 (56% ± 2% viable). AF4 was selective for breast cancer cells since a concentration of AF4 (100 µg/mL) that was cytotoxic for breast cancer cells had little effect on the viability of nonmalignant human mammary epithelial cells (HMEC) and MCF-10A mammary epithelial cells (Figure 1B). In comparison to quercetin, AF4 was a less potent inhibitor of breast cancer cell growth but had greater selectivity (Figure S1). MCF-7 spheroids that were grown in the presence of AF4 (100 µg/mL) were smaller than vehicle-treated control spheroids (Figure 1C). In addition, numerous floating cells with morphology characteristic of dead or dying cells were present in AF4-treated cultures, and there was a significant decrease in the number of viable MCF-7 cells, as indicated by reduced phosphatase activity, within spheroids treated with AF4 (100 µg/mL) relative to vehicle-treated controls. Therefore, AF4 inhibited breast cancer cell growth in both 2-dimensional and 3-dimensional culture systems. Subsequent experiments focused on the effect of AF4 on MDA-MB-231 cells as this breast cancer cell line was most sensitive to AF4 and readily forms tumors in immune-deficient mice.

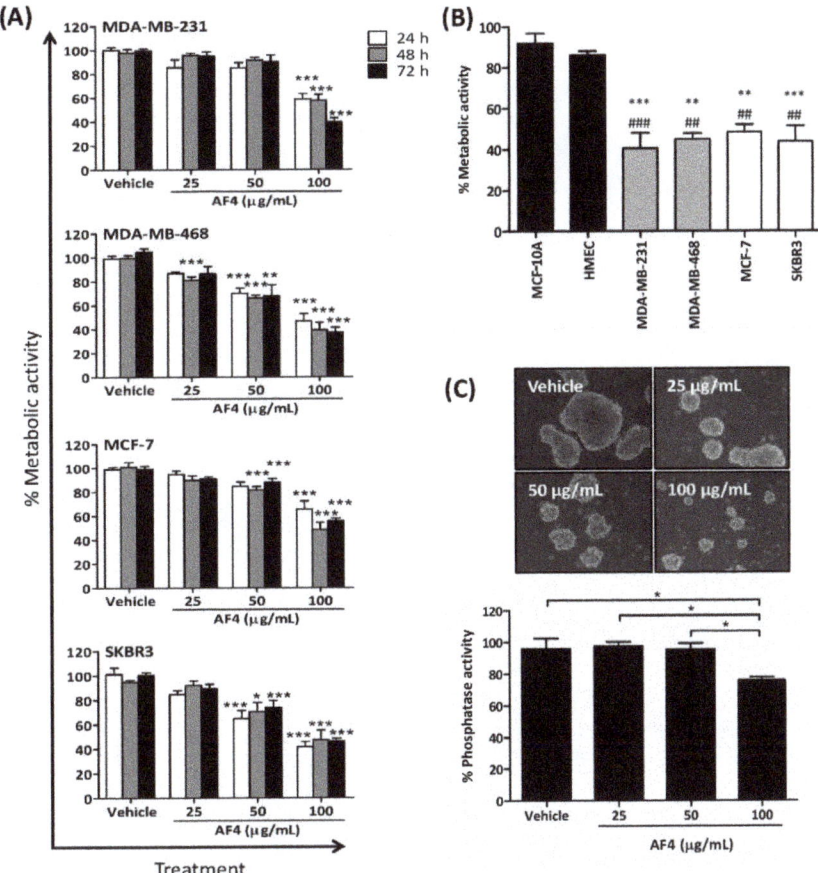

Figure 1. Apple peel flavonoid fraction 4 (AF4) is selectively cytotoxic to breast cancer cells. (**A**) MDA-MB-231, MDA-MB-468, MCF-7 and SKBR3 cells were cultured in the absence or presence of the indicated concentrations of AF4 for the indicated times. The % metabolic activity of AF4-treated cells was determined using an MTT (3-(4,5-dimethythiazol-2-yl)-2,5-diphenyltetrazolium bromide) assay. Data are expressed as mean ± standard error of the mean (SEM). (**B**) The % metabolic activity of AF4-treated (100 μg/mL) breast cancer cells was compared to MCF-10A cells (#) and HMECs (*) cells. Data from MTT assays are expressed as mean ± SEM. (**C**) MCF-7 spheroids were cultured for 72 h in the absence or presence of the indicated concentrations of AF4. Relative cell number of viable cells was determined by acid phosphatase assay. Data are shown as mean ± SEM. (A–C) Statistical analysis of 3 independent experiments was performed using analysis of variance (ANOVA) and Tukey's multiple comparisons test; * $p < 0.05$, ** and ## $p < 0.01$, *** and ### $p < 0.001$.

2.2. AF4 Suppresses the Proliferation of MDA-MB-231 Cells

Next, we determined whether a non-cytotoxic concentration of AF4 could impact breast cancer cell growth. As shown in Figure 2, flow cytometric analysis of Oregon Green 488-stained MDA-MB-231 cells that were treated with a sub-cytotoxic dose of AF4 (40 μg/mL) revealed a significant reduction in the number of cell divisions (Figure 2A). In addition, cell cycle analysis showed that AF4-treated MDA-MB-231 cells accumulated in the G_0/G_1 phase of the cell cycle, with a corresponding reduction in the number of MDA-MB-231 cells in the S phase of the cell cycle (Figure 2B). The same effect was observed in AF4-treated MDA-MB-468 cells (Figure S2). Consistent with an AF4-induced partial block at G_0/G_1, there was reduced expression of CDK4 and cyclin D3 in AF4-treated MDA-MB-231 cells (Figure 2C).

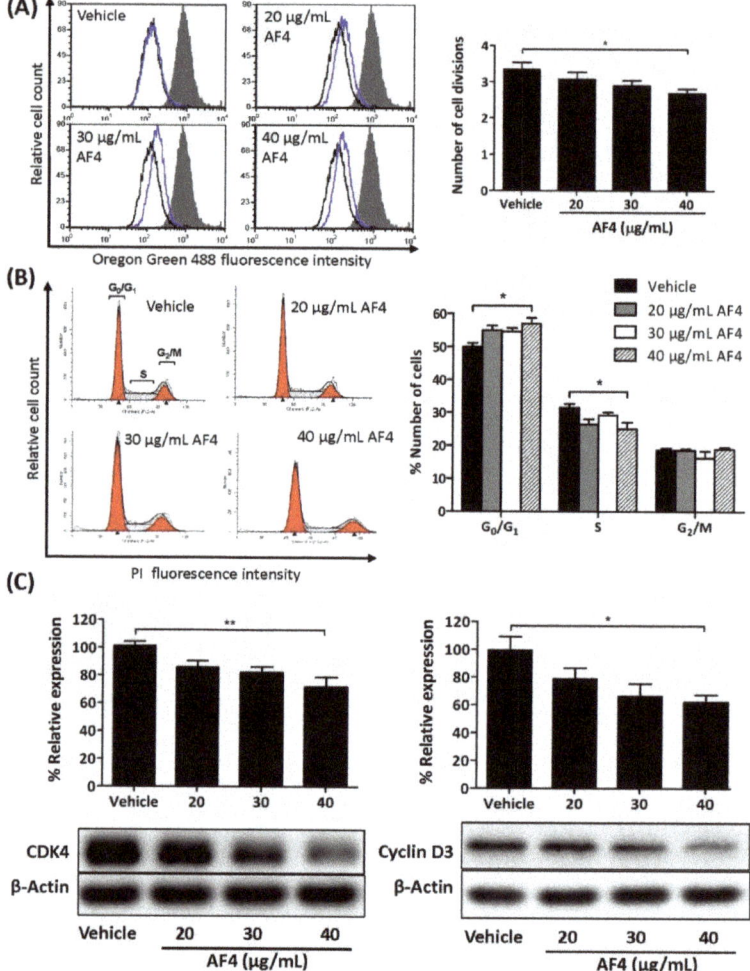

Figure 2. AF4 inhibits breast cancer cell proliferation. (**A**) MDA-MB-231 cells were stained with Oregon Green 488 dye and then cultured for 72 h in the absence or presence of the indicated concentrations of AF4. Fluorescence was measured by flow cytometry. Data are shown as representative histograms (filled peak, non-proliferating cells; black peak, vehicle; blue peak, AF4) and mean number of cell divisions ± SEM. (**B**) MDA-MB-231 cells were cultured for 72 h in the absence or presence of the indicated concentrations of AF4. Cells were stained with propidium iodide (PI) and cell cycle analysis was performed by flow cytometry. Data are shown as representative histograms and mean % number of cells ± SEM in each phase of the cell cycle. (**C**) MDA-MB-231 cells were cultured for 24 h in the absence or presence of the indicated concentrations of AF4. The relative expression of CDK4 and cyclin D3 was determined using Western blot analysis. Equal protein loading was confirmed by probing for β-actin. Data shown are representative blots and mean % relative expression ± SEM. (**A**–**C**) Statistical analysis of 3 independent experiments was performed using ANOVA and Tukey's multiple comparisons test; * $p < 0.05$, ** $p < 0.01$.

2.3. AF4 Inhibits the Migration and Invasion of MDA-MB-231 Cells

Gap closure and trans-well migration assays were used to determine the effect of sub-cytotoxic AF4 on the migration and invasion capacity of MDA-MB-231 cells. These experiments used AF4 at a final concentration of 20 μg/mL in order to ensure that there would be no AF4-associated cytotoxic activity. As shown in Figure 3, a sub-cytotoxic concentration of AF4 (20 μg/mL) inhibited the migration of MDA-MB-231 cells by 65% in gap closure assays and by 87% in trans-well migration assays (Figure 3A and B, respectively). In addition, the invasion of MDA-MB-231 cells through a fibronectin-coated porous membrane was reduced by 80% in the presence of sub-cytotoxic AF4 (Figure 3C). Expression of invasion-promoting matrix metalloproteinase 2 (MMP2) was also significantly reduced when MDA-MB-231 cells were cultured in the presence of sub-cytotoxic AF4 (Figure 3D).

2.4. AF4-Induced Apoptosis Is Associated with Oxidative Stress

To determine the mechanism by which AF4 killed breast cancer cells, MDA-MB-231 cells were stained with Annexin V-488 and propidium iodide (PI) prior to culture for 24 h in the presence of a cytotoxic concentration of AF4 (100 μg/mL). As shown in Figure 4A, flow cytometric analysis revealed that a high concentration of AF4 caused MDA-MB-231 cells to die by apoptosis (Figure 4A). In contrast, neither MCF-10A epithelial cells nor dermal fibroblasts were sensitive to AF4, suggesting a selective cytotoxic effect on neoplastic cells. As shown in Figure 4B,C, treatment of MDA-MB-231 cells with an apoptosis-inducing concentration of AF4 resulted in the generation of reactive oxygen species (ROS), as indicated by Amplex Red assays and flow cytometric analysis of cells stained with the ROS-sensitive dye 5-(and-6)-chloromethyl-2′,7′-dichlorodihydrofluorescein diacetate, acetyl ester (CM-H_2DCFDA). MCF-10A cells that were cultured in the presence of AF4 (100 μg/mL) also exhibited increased levels of intracellular ROS (Figure S3). Oxidative stress was at least in part responsible for the cytotoxic action of AF4 since apoptosis of AF4-treated MDA-MB-231 cells was reduced in the presence of the antioxidant N-acetyl cysteine (NAC). In comparison to MDA-MB-231 cells, non-malignant MCF-10A epithelial cells were relatively resistant to oxidative stress (Figure S4).

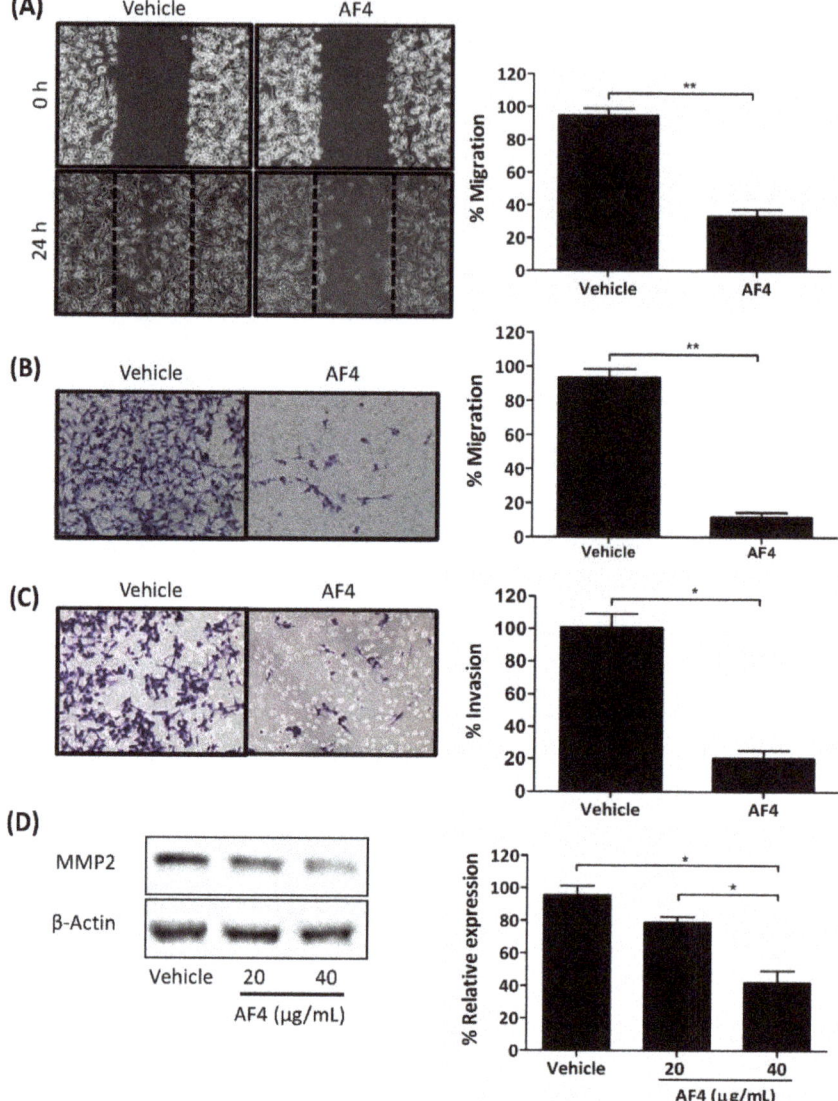

Figure 3. AF4 inhibits breast cancer cell motility and invasion. (**A**) Mitomycin C-treated MDA-MB-231 cells were cultured in wells containing cell culture inserts, which were removed at 0 h. After 24 h culture in the absence or presence of 20 µg/mL AF4 cultures were photographed. Representative images and mean % migration ± SEM of 3 independent experiments are shown. (**B**) Serum-starved MDA-MB-231 cells were treated with 20 µg/mL AF4 for 24 h. Mean % migration ± SEM through an 8 µm porous membrane and (**C**) mean % invasion ± SEM through a fibronectin-coated 8 µm porous membrane were determined as described in the Methods. (**D**) MDA-MB-231 cells were cultured for 24 h in the absence or presence of the indicated concentrations of AF4. Relative expression of MMP2 was determined using Western blot analysis. Equal protein loading was confirmed by probing for β-actin expression. Data shown are representative blots and mean % relative expression ± SEM. Statistical analysis of 3 independent experiments was performed using (A–C) Student's t-test or (D) ANOVA and Tukey's multiple comparisons test; * $p < 0.01$, ** $p < 0.001$.

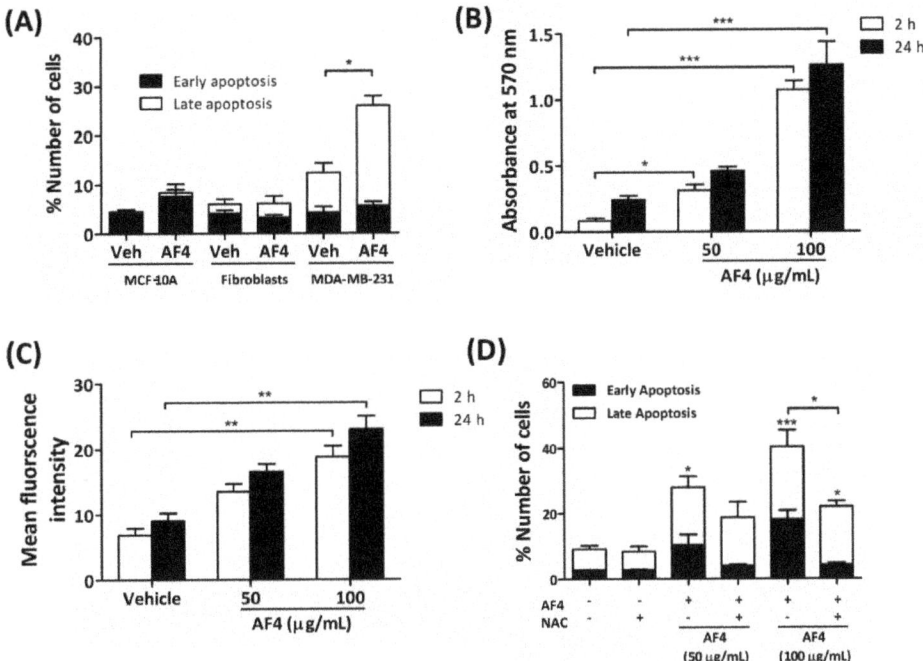

Figure 4. AF4-induced apoptosis of breast cancer cells is reactive oxygen species (ROS)-dependent. (**A**) MCF-10A cells, fibroblasts and MDA-MB-231 cells were cultured for 24 h in the absence or presence of 100 µg/mL AF4, and then stained with Annexin-V-488 and propidium iodide (PI) for flow cytometric analysis. Data are shown as mean % cell number ± SEM of 3 independent experiments. (**B**) MDA-MB-231 cells were cultured in the absence or presence of the indicated concentrations of AF4 for 2 h or 24 h and relative ROS in cultures was determined by Amplex Red assay. Data are shown as mean absorbance at 570 nm ± SEM of 3 independent experiments. (**C**) CM-H$_2$DCFDA-stained MDA-MB-231 cells were cultured in the absence or presence of the indicated concentrations of AF4 for 2 h or 24 h and the relative amount of intracellular ROS was determined by fluorescence at 529 nm. Data are shown as mean fluorescence intensity ± SEM of 3 independent experiments. (**D**) MDA-MB-231 cells were cultured for 24 h in the absence or presence of 100 µg/mL AF4 without or with 5 mM N-acetyl cysteine (NAC), and then stained with Annexin-V-488 and PI for flow cytometric analysis. Data are shown as mean % cell number ± SEM of 3 independent experiments. (**A–D**) Statistical analysis was performed using ANOVA and Tukey's multiple comparisons test; * $p < 0.05$, ** $p < 0.01$, *** $p < 0.001$.

2.5. AF4 Inhibits Akt Signaling

To determine a possible mechanism to account for the growth inhibitory effect of AF4, we examined the impact of AF4 on Akt (protein kinase B) signaling in MDA-MB-231 cells. A sub-cytotoxic concentration of AF4 (40 µg/mL) was used in these experiments in order to obtain sufficient protein for western blot analysis. Figure 5 shows that AF4 inhibited the phosphorylation-induced activation of Akt at Thr308. AF4 also suppressed Ser380 phosphorylation of phosphatase and tensin homolog (PTEN), which is the upstream inhibitor of Akt. Both PTEN and Akt phosphorylation were restored when AF4-treated MDA-MB-231 cells were cultured in the presence of the antioxidant NAC. The importance of the Akt signaling pathway for the growth and survival of MDA-MB-231 cells was confirmed using 2 different Akt inhibitors (MK2206 and SC66). Figure S5 shows that the percentage of apoptotic MDA-MB-231 cells increased significantly when Akt activation was inhibited.

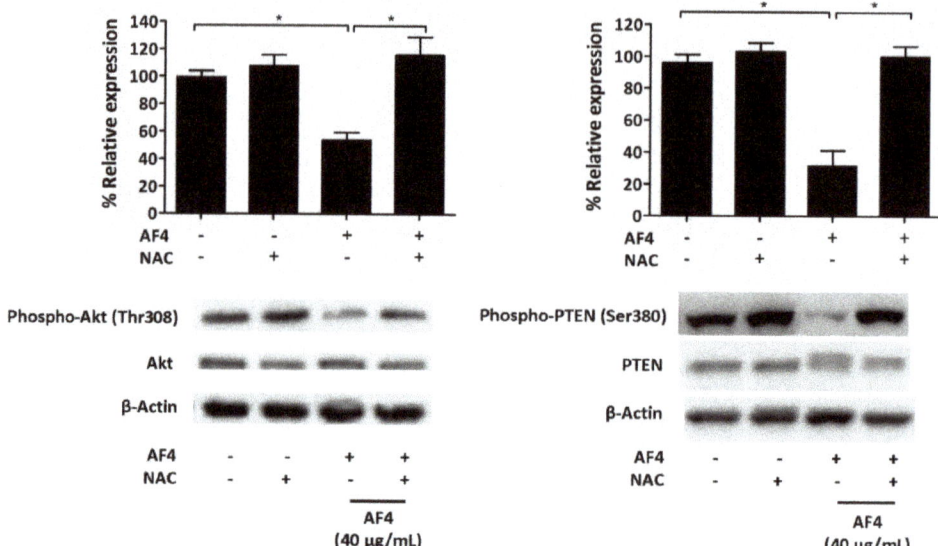

Figure 5. AF4 inhibits Akt and phosphatase and tensin homolog (PTEN) phosphorylation in breast cancer cells. MDA-MB-231 cells were cultured for 24 h in the absence or presence of 40 μg/mL AF4 without or with 5 mM NAC. Relative expression of phospho-Akt (Thr308), total Akt, phospho-PTEN (Ser380), and total PTEN was determined using Western blot analysis. Equal protein loading was confirmed by probing for β-actin expression. Data are shown as representative blots and mean % relative expression ± SEM of 3 independent experiments. Statistical analysis was performed using ANOVA and Tukey's multiple comparisons test; * $p < 0.05$.

2.6. AF4 Suppresses Growth of MDA-MB-231 Xenografts

The effect of AF4 on in vivo tumor growth was determined by intratumoral administration of AF4 (0.5 mg/kg) to MDA-MB-231 xenografts grown in female non-obese diabetic severe combined immunodeficient (NOD-SCID) mice. Dosage that was predicted to suppress MDA-MB-231 tumor growth was based on the total concentration of quercetin, quercetin glycosides, catechin, epicatechin, cyanidin-3-O-galactoside, phloridzin, chlorogenic acid and cafeic acid within AF4. Consistent with our in vitro findings regarding the anti-proliferative and cytotoxic activities of AF4, Figure 6A shows that treatment with AF4 significantly slowed the growth of MDA-MB-231 xenografts. Examination of tumor sections stained with hematoxylin and eosin revealed larger areas of necrosis in AF4-treated tumors (Figure 6B). Moreover, in comparison to saline-treated tumors, expression of the endothelial cell marker CD31 was reduced in the interior and periphery of AF4-treated tumors. No adverse effects were noted in AF4-treated mice, including no significant difference in average body weight between the treatment groups at day 15 (saline-treated group, 24.5 ± 0.6 g; AF4-treated group, 26.3 ± 0.5 g; $p > 0.05$ by Student's t-test).

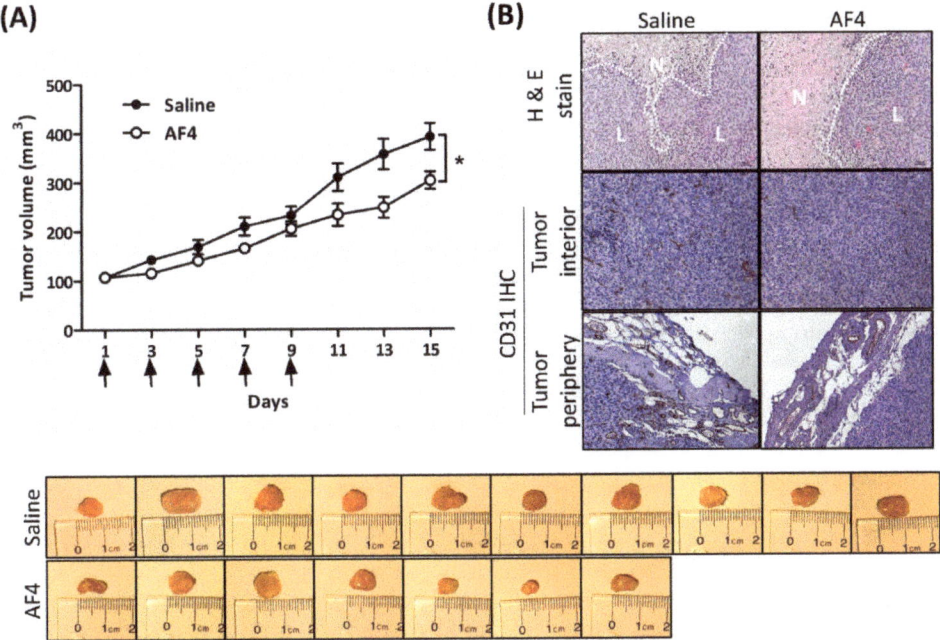

Figure 6. AF4 suppresses MDA-MB-231 xenograft growth. MDA-MB-231 cells were xenografted into the left flank of non-obese diabetic severe combined immunodeficient (NOD-SCID) female mice and AF4 (0.5 mg/kg) or saline was injected directly into the resulting tumors every second day (day 1, 3, 5, 7 and 9, indicated by arrows) for 9 days. The control group consisted of 10 animals and the AF4 treatment group was 7 animals. (**A**) Mean tumor volume ± SEM was determined every second day. Statistical analysis was determined by Student's *t*-test; * $p < 0.05$. Excised tumors from each treatment group at day 15 are shown. (**B**) At day 15 mice were euthanized and tumors were excised, fixed, and sectioned for staining with hematoxylin and eosin (H&E) and detection of CD31 expression by immunohistochemistry (IHC). Representative sections are shown; N denotes areas of necrosis and L denotes live cells.

3. Discussion

Dietary phytochemicals have received unique attention in the search for novel and safer cancer treatment options in light of widely documented findings that many of these natural sourced compounds kill cancer cells but are relatively non-toxic to healthy cells [14,16–19]. In this study, we used MTT assays to show that AF4 suppressed the growth of triple-negative (MDA-MB-231 and MDA-MB-468), estrogen receptor-positive (MCF-7) and HER2 receptor-positive (SKBR3) breast cancer cells but had little effect on the growth of non-malignant mammary epithelial cells (HMECs and MCF-10A), suggesting a pronounced selectivity for neoplastic cells. In contrast, quercetin, which is a minor component of AF4 [12], exhibited less selectivity for breast cancer cells.

MDA-MB-231 cells that were exposed to a low concentration of AF4 tended to accumulate at G_0/G_1, likely as a result of reduced expression of cyclin D3 and CDK4 that promote gene expression needed for G_1 progression [20]. AF4-treated MDA-MB-468 cells also arrested at G_0/G_1. This effect of AF4 on 2 different breast cancer cell lines differed from the G_2/M cell cycle arrest seen in cultures of AF4-treated HepG2 hepatocarcinoma cells [14], suggesting that the anti-proliferative activity of AF4 may be cell type-dependent. Treatment with a higher concentration of AF4 induced MDA-MB-231 cells to undergo apoptosis; however, the viability of non-malignant fibroblasts and MCF-10A mammary epithelial cells was not affected. AF4-induced apoptosis of breast cancer cells was consistent with an earlier report of apoptotic death of liver cancer cells following treatment with AF4 [14]. We demonstrate here, for the first time, that AF4-induced cytotoxicity was at least partially due to the accumulation of intracellular ROS because the antioxidant NAC protected MDA-MB-231 cells from the cytotoxic effect of AF4. In contrast, quercetin-induced apoptosis of MDA-MB-231 cells is reported to be ROS-independent [21], which argues against a major role for quercetin in the cytotoxic effect of AF4. Interestingly, non-malignant MCF-10A cells also showed increased levels of intracellular ROS following AF4 treatment, even though these cells were refractory to the cytotoxic effect of AF4. Multiple mechanisms exist to either prevent oxidative stress or manage the negative consequences of this condition; however, excessive production and accumulation of ROS can overwhelm these defenses [22]. In line with evidence that neoplastic cells are more sensitive to ROS than are their non-malignant counterparts [23], we found that MDA-MB-231 breast cancer cells were more sensitive to ROS than non-malignant MCF-10A mammary epithelial cells. The selective effect of AF4 on breast cancer cells may involve the capacity of healthy cells to defend against endogenous ROS [24]. Although certain components of AF4 possess anti-oxidant capabilities [25], the ability of unfractionated AF4 to protect against oxidative stress has not yet been demonstrated. In any case, a number of natural source antioxidants, at high doses, are capable of causing ROS production in cancer cells [26–28].

Importantly, AF4 inhibited the growth of MCF-7 breast cancer spheroids that, in comparison to monolayer cultures of breast cancer cells, more closely resemble the 3-dimensional structure of solid tumors [29]. In addition, sub-cytotoxic AF4 interfered with the migration of MDA-MB-231 cells in gap closure and trans-well cell migration assays, as well as inhibiting invasion of MDA-MB-231 cells through a fibronectin-coated membrane and suppressing the expression of MMP2. These findings suggest that AF4 may be able to interfere with breast cancer metastasis since tumor cell locomotion and the ability to degrade extracellular matrix components via the synthesis of proteolytic enzymes such as MMP2 play essential roles in the metastatic process [30].

Decreased phosphorylation of Akt in the presence of AF4 may account for its anti-proliferative and cytotoxic effects on MDA-MB-231 cells since the growth, survival, and metabolism of breast cancer cells involves activation of Akt [31]. The important role played by the Akt signaling pathway in the growth and survival of MDA-MB-231 cells was confirmed by the observation that Akt inhibition resulted in apoptosis of MDA-MB-231 cells. Phosphorylation of PTEN, which is a tumor suppressor protein that downregulates Akt signaling [32], was downregulated in AF4-treated MDA-MB-2312 cells. Decreased activation of inhibitory PTEN is consistent with the finding that AF4 did not completely block Akt activation. AF4-induced ROS production is likely to be involved in the effects of AF4 on Akt and PTEN since ROS can directly inhibit Akt via the phosphorylation of thiol groups within the protein, whereas phosphatases such as PTEN are deactivated by ROS [33]. Restoration of Akt and PTEN phosphorylation to control levels when NAC was added to cultures of AF4-treated MDA-MB-231 cells confirmed the involvement of AF4-induced ROS in modulation of the Akt signaling pathway.

Intratumoral administration of AF4 suppressed the growth of MDA-MB-231 xenografts in immune-deficient mice, most likely due to the combination of anti-proliferative and cytotoxic effects of AF4 that were revealed by our in vitro studies. In this regard, AF4-treated tumors contained larger areas of necrosis relative to saline-treated tumors. In addition, decreased expression of the endothelial cell marker CD31 in the periphery and interior of AF-4 treated tumors suggested that AF4 may inhibit angiogenesis. Notably, AF4 did not cause any distress or adverse side effects such as weight loss in treated animals. Injection of AF4 directly into the tumor was employed to eliminate potential issues of AF4 bioavailability following oral dosing. Therefore, it will be important in future studies to assess the effectiveness of oral or intraperitoneal administration of AF4 to tumor-bearing mice. Delivery of an optimal concentration of AF4 to the tumor microenvironment via the oral or intraperitoneal route will likely require a nanoparticle delivery vehicle of the type that has been reported to greatly enhance the bioavailability of other bioactive phytochemicals such as curcumin [34,35]. In this regard, nanoparticles have also been employed to deliver plant extracts with anticancer properties to various types of cancer cells [36]. Identification of the components of AF4 that are responsible for its anticancer activity could allow for the development of nanoparticles containing one or more pure compounds with greater bioactivity relative to the AF4 extract; however, it is important to note that such an approach risks the loss of any potential synergy between major and minor components of AF4. Nevertheless, demonstration of AF4-mediated in vivo tumor suppressor activity, as well as reduced proliferation/survival and motility/invasion of MDA-MB-231 triple-negative breast cancer cells following AF4 treatment, suggests that AF4 and its bioactive components warrant further investigation as potential selective natural-source agents for the treatment of triple-negative breast cancer.

4. Materials and Methods

4.1. Reagents

AF4 was extracted from the peels of the apple cultivar Northern Spy, as previously described [12]. AF4 in ethanol was filter-sterilized and stored at −80 °C. Prior to use in this study, ethanol was evaporated under nitrogen gas and the AF4 residue was dissolved in sterile pyrogen-free water and aliquots of the resulting AF4 stock (10 mg/mL) were stored at −20 °C. Amplex Red reagent, Annexin-V-488, Dulbecco's modified Eagle's medium (DMEM), DMEM/F12, horse serum, fetal calf serum, CM-H_2DCFDA, and PI were from Life Technologies Inc. (Burlington, ON, Canada). Hydroxyethyl piperazineethanesulfonic acid (HEPES)- and bicarbonate-buffered mammary epithelial cell medium, mammary epithelial cell growth supplement, penicillin/streptomycin solution and poly-L-lysine were purchased from ScienCell Research Laboratories Inc. (Carlsbad, CA, USA). DMEM, phenol red-free DMEM, recombinant human insulin, hydrocortisone, phosphatase substrate, Triton X-100, mitomycin C, NAC, MTT, quercetin, MK2206, and SC66 were from Sigma-Aldrich (Oakville, ON, Canada). Paraformaldehyde was from Bioshop Canada Inc. (Burlington, ON, Canada). Fibroblast cell growth medium and supplements were from Lonza Inc. (Walkersville, MD, USA). DNase-free RNase A was from Qiagen Inc. (Mississauga, ON, Canada). Recombinant epidermal growth factor and basic fibroblast growth factor were from PeproTech (Rocky Hill, NJ). Diff-Quik staining kit was from Siemens Healthcare Diagnostics (Los Angeles, CA, USA). Rodent M block, anti-rabbit horse 6 radish peroxidase (HRP)-polymer and HRP/DAB detection system were from Biocare Medical (Markham, ON, Canada). HRP-conjugated anti-β-actin monoclonal antibody (Ab), anti-cyclin D3 monoclonal Ab, anti-CDK4 rabbit Ab, anti-phospho-PTEN (Ser380) monoclonal Ab, anti-PTEN monoclonal Ab, anti-Akt monoclonal Ab, and anti-phospho-Akt (Thr308) monoclonal Ab were from Cell Signaling Technology (Beverly, MA, USA). Anti-MMP2 Ab and anti-CD31 Ab were from Abcam Inc. (Toronto, ON, Canada). HRP-conjugated-goat anti-mouse IgG Ab and HRP-conjugated-donkey anti-rabbit IgG Ab were from Santa Cruz Biotechnology (Santa Cruz, CA, USA).

4.2. Cell Culture

The MDA-MB-231 breast cancer cell line was provided by Dr. S. Drover (Memorial University of Newfoundland, St. John's, NL, Canada). MDA-MB-468, MCF-7, and SKBR3 breast cancer cell lines were from Dr. P. Lee, Dr. K. Goralski and Dr. G. Dellaire, respectively (Dalhousie University, Halifax, NS, Canada). Breast cancer cell lines were authenticated by short tandem repeat analysis conducted by ATCC (Manassas, VA, USA). All breast cancer cell lines were cultured in DMEM supplemented with 10% heat-inactivated fetal calf serum, 5 mM HEPES buffer (pH 7.4), 2 mM L-glutamine, 100 U/mL penicillin, and 100 µg/mL streptomycin, and were maintained at 37 °C in a humidified incubator supplied with 10% CO_2. HMECs from ScienCell Research Laboratories Inc. were grown in serum-free, HEPES- and bicarbonate-buffered mammary epithelial cell medium supplemented with 1% mammary epithelial cell growth supplement and 1% penicillin/streptomycin solution, and maintained for a maximum of seven passages at 37 °C in a humidified incubator supplied with 5% CO_2. The MCF-10A normal mammary epithelial cell line was from Dr. P. Marcato (Dalhousie University, Halifax, NS, Canada). MCF-10A cells were cultured in DMEM/F12 supplemented with 10% heat-inactivated horse serum, 10 µg/mL human insulin, 20 µg/mL EGF, 0.5 µg/mL hydrocortisone, 100 U/mL penicillin, and

100 µg/mL streptomycin. MDF-10A cultures were maintained at 37 °C in a humidified incubator supplied with 10% CO_2. Human dermal fibroblasts from Lonza Inc. (Walkersville, MD, USA) were maintained as per the supplier's instructions.

4.3. MTT (3-(4,5-Dimethythiazol-2-yl)-2,5-Diphenyltetrazolium Bromide) Assay for Cell Viability

Cells were plated in quadruplicate into 96-well flat-bottom plates at a density of 5×10^3 cells/well and cultured in the absence or presence of the indicated concentrations of AF4 for desired time. At the end of culture, MTT was added to each well to a final concentration of 0.5 µg/mL. Plates were then incubated for 2 h at 37 °C, after which supernatant was removed and formazan crystals in each well were solubilized in 100 µL of dimethyl sulfoxide (DMSO). Absorbance was measured at 570 nm using an Asys Expert Microplate Reader (Biochrom Ltd., Cambridge, UK). Results are expressed as % metabolic activity relative to the medium control.

4.4. Acid Phosphatase Assay of Spheroid Growth

MCF-7 cells in F12 medium containing 20 ng/mL basic fibroblast growth factor, 20 ng/mL epidermal growth factor, 100 U/mL penicillin, 100 µg/mL streptomycin and B27 serum-free supplement were cultured for 48 h in ultra-low adherent cell culture plates and then treated with the indicated concentrations of AF4 or vehicle for 72 h. Spheroids were photographed, washed with phosphate-buffered saline, resuspended in 100 µL acid phosphatase assay solution (0.1 M sodium acetate at pH 5.5, 0.1% Triton-X-100, 4 mg/mL phosphatase substrate) and incubated for 2 h at 37 °C in the dark. The reaction was stopped by adding 25 µL 1 N NaOH to each well. Absorbance was measured at 405 nm using an Asys Expert Microplate Reader and % acid phosphatase activity was determined.

4.5. Flow Cytometric Cell Proliferation Assay

MDA-MB-231 cell cultures were synchronized by serum starvation for 20 h and then seeded into 6-well plates and allowed to form monolayers. Cells were stained with 1.25 µM Oregon Green 488 dye in serum-free DMEM and a sample of stained cells was retained for use as a non-proliferative control. The remaining cells were cultured for 72 h in the absence or presence of the indicated concentrations of AF4. Cellular fluorescence was then measured using a FACSCalibur instrument (BD Bioscience, Mississauga, ON, Canada). The fluorescence of control and AF4-treated cells was compared to that of the non-proliferative control and the number of cell divisions (n) was calculated as follows: $MCF_{baseline} = (2^n)(MCF_{sample})$; where n denotes the number of cell divisions and MCF denotes mean channel fluorescence.

4.6. Cell-Cycle Analysis

MDA-MB-231 and MBA-MB-468 cell cultures were synchronized by serum starvation for 20 h and then cultured for 72 h in the absence or presence of the indicated concentrations of AF4. Cells were then collected, washed with ice-cold phosphate-buffered saline, and ice-cold 70% ethanol was added drop-wise to the cells under constant agitation. Cells were then stored at −20°C for 24 h, washed, and resuspended in phosphate-buffered saline containing 0.02 mg/mL PI, 0.1% Triton X-100, and 0.2 mg/mL DNase-free RNase A. After incubation for 30 min at room temperature in the dark, cellular fluorescence was determined using a FACSCalibur instrument. Data were analyzed using ModFitLT V2.0 software (Becton Dickson, CA, US).

4.7. Gap-Closure Assay

MDA-MB-231 cells were seeded at a density of 1×10^4 cells/mL into wells containing culture inserts. After 18 h of culture, cells were treated with 10 µg/mL of mitomycin C in serum-free DMEM for 2 h at 37 °C to prevent cell division. After 12 h, cells were washed with complete DMEM and cultured in the absence or presence of 20 μg/mL AF4. At 0 h and 24 h, culture inserts were removed and the gaps were photographed.

4.8. Trans-Well Migration/Invasion Assay

MDA-MB-231 cells were treated with 20 μg/mL AF4 for 24 h and serum-starved for 6 h, after which 5×10^4 cells in serum-free DMEM were placed into wells of the upper chamber of the trans-well cell migration apparatus. The bottom chamber wells contained DMEM plus 10% fetal calf serum as a chemoattractant. Migration of cells through an 8 μm porous membrane (uncoated or coated with fibronectin) was detected by Diff-Quik staining. Migrated cells were imaged under a light microscope.

4.9. Flow Cytometric Measurement of Apoptosis

MDA-MB-231 cells were seeded at a density of 1×10^5 cells/well into 6-well plates and cultured in the absence or presence of the indicated concentrations of AF4 without or with 5 mM NAC for the desired time. In separate experiments, MDA-MB-231 cells were cultured for 48 h in the absence or presence of the Akt inhibitors MK2206 and SC66. At the end of culture cells were harvested, washed and stained with Annexin-V-488 and PI (1 μg/mL) for 15 min at room temperature. Flow cytometric analysis was performed using a FACSCalibur instrument.

4.10. Reactive Oxygen Species (ROS) Measurements

Measurement of ROS by Amplex Red assay was performed in 96-well flat-bottom plates containing quadruplicate cultures of MDA-MB-231 cells without or with AF4 at 50 μg/mL. In the dark, 100 μL of master mix containing 25 μM Amplex Red reagent and 0.005 U/mL HRP in phenol red-free cDMEM was added to each culture. After incubation at 37 °C for 2 or 24 h, absorbance was measured at 570 nm with an Asys Expert Microplate Reader. Measurement of ROS by fluorescence was performed by staining quadruplicate cultures of MDA-MB-231 cells or MCF-10A cells with 5 μM CM-H_2DCFDA in serum- and phenol-red free DMEM. Cells were then cultured for 2 or 24 h in the absence or presence of the indicated concentrations of AF4 in phenol-red free DMEM containing 1% fetal calf serum. Fluorescence at 529 nm was measured with a Spectramax M2 Microplate Reader (Molecular Devices, San Jose, CA, USA).

4.11. Western Blot Analysis

MDA-MB-231 cells were cultured in the absence or presence of the indicated concentrations of AF4 for 24 h, and then placed in ice-cold lysis buffer (50 mM Tris at pH 7.5, 150 mM NaCl, 50 mM disodium hydrogen phosphate, 0.25% sodium deoxycholate, 0.1% Nonidet P-40, 100 μM Na_3VO_4, 10 mM NaF, 5 mM ethylenediaminetetraacetic acid and 5 mM ethylene glycol tetraacetic acid) containing freshly added protease inhibitors (1 mM phenylmethylsulfonylfluoride, 10 μg/mL aprotinin, 5 μg/mL leupeptin, 10 μM phenylarsine oxide, 1 mM dithiothreitol and 5 μg/mL pepstatin). After 15 min, cell lysates were cleared by centrifugation and the protein concentration was determined by Bradford assay. Equal amounts of protein (20 μg) were loaded into 12% or 15% sodium dodecyl sulfate polyacrylamide gels. Separated proteins were transferred onto nitrocellulose membranes, which were then blocked by 1 h incubation in 5% non-fat milk or 5% bovine serum albumin in Tween-Tris buffered saline (TBS) solution (0.25 M Tris at pH 7.5, 150 mM NaCl, 0.2% Tween-20). Blots were probed overnight at 4 °C with an optimal concentration of primary Ab, and then washed thoroughly with Tween-TBS and probed with HRP-conjugated donkey anti-rabbit IgG Ab or anti-mouse IgG Ab, as appropriate, for 1 h at room temperature. Even protein loading was confirmed by probing the blots with HRP-conjugated rabbit anti-β actin Ab. Proteins of interest were visualized by chemiluminescence.

4.12. Xenograft Breast Cancer Model

Six to eight week-old female NOD-SCID mice were purchased from Charles River Canada (Lasalle, QC, Canada) and housed under sterile conditions and fed a sterilized rodent diet and water supplied ad libitum. Pathogen-free MDA-MB-231 cells (5×10^7) were implanted by subcutaneous injection into the right hind flank. Starting two weeks after xenografting, tumor sizes and body weights were recorded every other day until the last day (day 15) of the experiment. Tumor volume was calculated according to the equation, $(L \times P^2)/2$ where L is tumor length and P is perpendicular to tumor length. Intratumoral injection of AF4 commenced once the tumors reached a volume of 100 mm^3 (recorded as day 1). A total of 5 intratumoral injections of AF4 at 0.5 mg/kg in 20 µL saline (7 mice) or saline alone (10 mice) were administered every other day for 9 days. Mice were monitored for an additional 6 days and their tumor sizes and body weights were recorded. Mice were euthanized at day 15, after which the tumors were excised and photographed. Tumors were fixed in buffered formalin, embedded in paraffin and cut into 5 µm thick sections. Tumor sections were mounted onto glass slides and stained with hematoxylin and eosin for detection of necrotic and live cells. Immunohistochemistry was performed to detect CD31 expression. Ethics approval for animal use was obtained from the Dalhousie University Committee on Laboratory Animals, and was in accordance with Canadian Council on Animal Care guidelines.

Supplementary Materials: The following are available online at http://www.mdpi.com/1420-3049/24/18/3335/s1: Figure S1: AF4 is a more selective but less potent inhibitor of breast cancer cell growth, Figure S2: AF4 induces G_0/G_1 cell cycle arrest in MDA-MB-468 breast cancer cells, Figure S3: AF4 treatment causes ROS accumulation in non-malignant MCF-10A mammary epithelial cells, Figure S4: MDA-MB-231 breast cancer cells are more sensitive than non-malignant MCF-10A mammary epithelial cells to oxidative stress, Figure S5: Akt inhibition causes apoptosis of MDA-MB-231 breast cancer cells.

Author Contributions: Conceptualization, D.W.H. and H.P.V.R.; methodology, C.-Y.L. and W.F.; formal analysis, C.-Y.L. and W.F.; writing-original draft preparation, C.-Y.L. and W.F.; writing-review and editing, D.W.H.; supervision, D.W.H.; project administration, D.W.H. and H.P.V.R.; funding acquisition, D.W.H. and H.P.V.R.

Funding: This research was funded by the Canadian Cancer Society/Canadian Breast Cancer Foundation Endowed Chair in Breast Cancer Research (D.W.H.) and the Natural Sciences and Engineering Research Council of Canada (D.W.H. and H.P.V.R.).

Acknowledgments: W.F. was supported by a trainee award from the Beatrice Hunter Cancer Research Institute with funds provided by the Harvey Graham Cancer Research Fund as part of The Terry Fox Strategic Health Research Training Program in Cancer Research at the Canadian Institutes for Health Research.

Conflicts of Interest: The authors declare no conflict of interest.

References

1. Bamia, C.; Lagiou, P.; Jenab, M.; Aleksandrova, K.; Fedirko, V.; Trichopoulos, D.; Overvad, K.; Tjønneland, A.; Olsen, A.; Clavel-Chapelon, F.; et al. Fruit and vegetable consumption in relation to hepatocellular carcinoma in a multi-centre, European cohort study. *Br. J. Cancer* **2015**, *112*, 1273–1282. [CrossRef] [PubMed]
2. Núñez-Sánchez, M.A.; González-Sarrías, A.; Romo-Vaquero, M.; García-Villalba, R.; Selma, M.V.; Tomás-Barberán, F.A.; García-Conesa, M.-T.; Espín, J.C. Dietary phenolics against colorectal cancer. From promising preclinical results to poor translation into clinical trials: Pitfalls and future needs. *Mol. Nutr. Food Res.* **2015**, *59*, 1274–1291. [CrossRef] [PubMed]
3. Khan, N.; Mukhtar, H. Dietary agents for prevention and treatment of lung cancer. *Cancer Lett.* **2015**, *359*, 155–164. [CrossRef] [PubMed]
4. Liu, H.; Wang, X.-C.; Hu, G.-H.; Guo, Z.-F.; Lai, P.; Xu, L.; Huang, T.-B.; Xu, Y.-F. Fruit and vegetable consumption and risk of bladder cancer. *Eur. J. Cancer Prev.* **2015**, *24*, 508–516. [CrossRef] [PubMed]
5. Bradbury, K.E.; Appleby, P.N.; Key, T.J. Fruit, vegetable, and fiber intake in relation to cancer risk: Findings from the European Prospective Investigation into Cancer and Nutrition (EPIC). *Am. J. Clin. Nutr.* **2014**, *100*, 394S–398S. [CrossRef] [PubMed]
6. Kale, A.; Gawande, S.; Kotwal, S. Cancer phytotherapeutics: Role for flavonoids at the cellular level. *Phytother. Res.* **2008**, *577*, 567–577. [CrossRef]

7. Yao, H.; Xu, W.; Shi, X.; Zhang, Z. Dietary flavonoids as cancer prevention agents. *J. Environ. Sci. Health Part C* **2011**, *29*, 1–31. [CrossRef] [PubMed]
8. Vineetha, V.P.; Girija, S.; Soumya, R.S.; Raghu, K.G. Polyphenol-rich apple (*Malus domestica* L.) peel extract attenuates arsenic trioxide induced cardiotoxicity in H9c2 cells via its antioxidant activity. *Food Funct.* **2014**, *5*, 502–511. [CrossRef]
9. Ribeiro, F.A.P.; Gomes de Moura, C.F.; Aguiar, O.; de Oliveira, F.; Spadari, R.C.; Oliveira, N.R.C.; Oshima, C.T.F.; Ribeiro, D.A. The chemopreventive activity of apple against carcinogenesis. *Eur. J. Cancer Prev.* **2014**, *23*, 477–480. [CrossRef]
10. Balasuriya, N.; Rupasinghe, H.P.V. Antihypertensive properties of flavonoid-rich apple peel extract. *Food Chem.* **2012**, *135*, 2320–2325. [CrossRef]
11. Tow, W.W.; Premier, R.; Jing, H.; Ajlouni, S. Antioxidant and antiproliferation effects of extractable and nonextractable polyphenols isolated from apple waste using different extraction methods. *J. Food Sci.* **2011**, *76*, T163–T172. [CrossRef] [PubMed]
12. Keddy, P.G.W.; Dunlop, K.; Warford, J.; Samson, M.L.; Jones, Q.R.D.; Rupasinghe, H.P.V.; Robertson, G.S. Neuroprotective and anti-inflammatory effects of the flavonoid-enriched fraction AF4 in a mouse model of hypoxic-ischemic brain injury. *PLoS ONE* **2012**, *7*, e51324. [CrossRef] [PubMed]
13. Warford, J.; Jones, Q.R.D.; Nichols, M.; Sullivan, V.; Rupasinghe, H.P.V.; Robertson, G.S. The flavonoid-enriched fraction AF4 suppresses neuroinflammation and promotes restorative gene expression in a mouse model of experimental autoimmune encephalomyelitis. *J. Neuroimmunol.* **2014**, *268*, 71–83. [CrossRef] [PubMed]
14. Sudan, S.; Rupasinghe, H.P.V. Flavonoid-enriched apple fraction AF4 induces cell cycle arrest, DNA topoisomerase II inhibition, and apoptosis in human liver cancer HepG2 cells. *Nutr. Cancer* **2014**, *66*, 1237–1246. [CrossRef] [PubMed]
15. Siegel, R.L.; Miller, K.D.; Jemal, A. Cancer statistics, 2018. *CA Cancer J. Clin.* **2018**, *68*, 7–30. [CrossRef] [PubMed]
16. Cheng, S.; Gao, N.; Zhang, Z.; Chen, G.; Budhraja, A.; Ke, Z.; Son, Y.-O.; Wang, X.; Luo, J.; Shi, X. Quercetin induces tumor-selective apoptosis through downregulation of Mcl-1 and activation of Bax. *Clin. Cancer Res.* **2010**, *16*, 5679–5691. [CrossRef] [PubMed]
17. Matsuo, M.; Sasaki, N.; Saga, K.; Kaneko, T. Cytotoxicity of flavonoids toward cultured normal human cells. *Biol. Pharm. Bull.* **2005**, *28*, 253–259. [CrossRef] [PubMed]
18. Romanouskaya, T.V.; Grinev, V.V. Cytotoxic effect of flavonoids on leukemia cells and normal cells of human blood. *Bull. Exp. Biol. Med.* **2009**, *148*, 57–59. [CrossRef] [PubMed]
19. Yadegarynia, S.; Pham, A.; Ng, A.; Nguyen, D.; Lialiutska, T.; Bortolazzo, A.; Sivryuk, V.; Bremer, M.; White, J.B. Profiling flavonoid cytotoxicity in human breast cancer cell lines: Determination of structure-function relationships. *Nat. Prod. Commun.* **2012**, *7*, 1295–1304. [CrossRef]
20. Takaki, T.; Echalier, A.; Brown, N.R.; Hunt, T.; Endicott, J.A.; Noble, M.E.M. The structure of CDK4/cyclin D3 has implications for models of CDK activation. *Proc. Natl. Acad. Sci. USA* **2009**, *106*, 4171–4176. [CrossRef]
21. Chien, S.Y.; Wu, Y.C.; Chung, J.G.; Yang, J.S.; Lu, H.F.; Tsou, M.F.; Wood, W.G.; Kuo, S.J.; Chen, D.R. Quercetin-induced apoptosis acts through mitochondrial- and caspase-3-dependent pathways in human breast cancer MDA-MB-231 cells. *Hum. Exp. Toxicol.* **2009**, *28*, 493–503. [CrossRef] [PubMed]
22. McEligot, A.J.; Yang, S.; Meyskens, F.L., Jr. Redox regulation by intrinsic species and extrinsic nutrients in normal and cancer cells. *Annu. Rev. Nutr.* **2005**, *25*, 261–295. [CrossRef] [PubMed]
23. Reczek, C.R.; Chandel, N.S. The two faces of reactive oxygen species in cancer. *Annu. Rev. Cancer Biol.* **2017**, *1*, 79–98. [CrossRef]
24. Han, Y.; Chen, J.Z. Oxidative stress induces mitochondrial DNA damage and cytotoxicity through independent mechanisms in human cancer cells. *Biomed. Res. Int.* **2013**, *2013*, 825065. [CrossRef] [PubMed]
25. Rice-Evans, C.A.; Miller, N.J.; Paganga, G. Structure-antioxidant activity relationships of flavonoids and phenolic acids. *Free Radic. Biol. Med.* **1996**, *20*, 933–956. [CrossRef]
26. Polyakov, N.E.; Leshina, T.V.; Konovalova, T.A.; Kispert, L.D. Carotenoids as scavengers of free radicals in a Fenton reaction: Antioxidants or pro-oxidants? *Free Radic. Biol. Med.* **2001**, *31*, 398–404. [CrossRef]
27. Lambert, J.D.; Elias, R.J. The antioxidant and pro-oxidant activities of green tea polyphenols: A role in cancer prevention. *Arch. Biochem. Biophys.* **2010**, *501*, 65–72. [CrossRef]

28. Fernando, W.; Rupasinghe, H.P.V.; Hoskin, D.W. Dietary phytochemicals with anti-oxidant and pro-oxidant activities: A double-edged sword in relation to adjuvant chemotherapy and radiotherapy? *Cancer Lett.* **2019**, *452*, 168–177. [CrossRef]
29. Weigelt, B.; Ghajar, C.M.; Bissell, M.J. The need for complex 3D culture models to unravel novel pathways and identify accurate biomarkers in breast cancer. *Adv. Drug Deliv. Rev.* **2014**, *69–70*, 42–51. [CrossRef]
30. Liotta, L.A. Gene products which play a role in cancer invastion and metastasis. *Breast Cancer Res. Treat.* **1988**, *11*, 113–124. [CrossRef]
31. Dey, N.; De, P.; Leyland-Jones, B. PI3K-AKT-mTOR inhibitors in breast cancers: From tumor cell signaling to clinical trials. *Pharmacol. Ther.* **2017**, *175*, 91–106. [CrossRef] [PubMed]
32. Song, G.; Ouyang, G.; Bao, S. The activation of Akt/PKB signaling pathway and cell survival. *J. Cell. Mol. Med.* **2005**, *9*, 59–71. [CrossRef] [PubMed]
33. Leslie, N.R.; Bennett, D.; Lindsay, Y.E.; Stewart, H.; Gray, A.; Downes, C.P. Redox regulation of PI 3-kinase signalling via inactivation of PTEN. *EMBO J.* **2003**, *22*, 5501–5510. [CrossRef] [PubMed]
34. Camargo, L.E.A.; Brustolin Ludwig, D.; Tominaga, T.T.; Carletto, B.; Favero, G.M.; Mainardes, R.M.; Khalil, N.M. Bovine serum albumin nanoparticles improve the antitumor activity of curcumin in a murine melanoma model. *J. Microencapsul.* **2018**, *35*, 467–474. [CrossRef] [PubMed]
35. Ban, C.; Jo, M.; Park, Y.H.; Kim, J.H.; Han, J.Y.; Lee, K.W.; Kweon, D.H.; Choi, Y.J. Enhancing the oral bioavailability of curcumin using solid lipid nanoparticles. *Food Chem.* **2019**, *302*, 125328. [CrossRef] [PubMed]
36. Armendáriz-Barragán, B.; Zafar, N.; Badri, W.; Galindo-Rodríguez, S.A.; Kabbaj, D.; Fessi, H.; Elaissari, A. Plant extracts: From encapsulation to application. *Expert Opin. Drug Deliv.* **2016**, *13*, 1165–1175. [CrossRef] [PubMed]

Sample Availability: Samples of the compound AF4 are available from the authors.

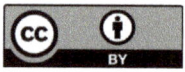

© 2019 by the authors. Licensee MDPI, Basel, Switzerland. This article is an open access article distributed under the terms and conditions of the Creative Commons Attribution (CC BY) license (http://creativecommons.org/licenses/by/4.0/).

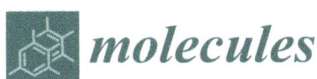

Article

Evaluating the Anti-cancer Efficacy of a Synthetic Curcumin Analog on Human Melanoma Cells and Its Interaction with Standard Chemotherapeutics

Krishan Parashar [1], Siddhartha Sood [1], Ali Mehaidli [1], Colin Curran [1], Caleb Vegh [1], Christopher Nguyen [1], Christopher Pignanelli [1], Jianzhang Wu [2], Guang Liang [2], Yi Wang [2] and Siyaram Pandey [1],*

[1] Department of Chemistry and Biochemistry, University of Windsor, 401 Sunset Avenue, Windsor, ON N9B 3P4, Canada
[2] Chemical Biology Research Center, School of Pharmaceutical Sciences, Whenzhou Medical University, University Town, Chashan, Wenzhou 325035, China
* Correspondence: spandey@uwindsor.ca; Tel.: 519-253-3000 (ext. 3701)

Academic Editor: Kyoko Nakagawa-Goto
Received: 18 June 2019; Accepted: 4 July 2019; Published: 6 July 2019

Abstract: Melanoma is the leading cause of skin-cancer related deaths in North America. Metastatic melanoma is difficult to treat and chemotherapies have limited success. Furthermore, chemotherapies lead to toxic side effects due to nonselective targeting of normal cells. Curcumin is a natural product of *Curcuma longa* (turmeric) and has been shown to possess anti-cancer activity. However, due to its poor bioavailability and stability, natural curcumin is not an effective cancer treatment. We tested synthetic analogs of curcumin that are more stable. One of these derivatives, Compound A, has shown significant anti-cancer efficacy in colon, leukemia, and triple-negative inflammatory breast cancer cells. However, the effects of Compound A against melanoma cells have not been studied before. In this study, for the first time, we demonstrated the efficacy of Compound A for the selective induction of apoptosis in melanoma cells and its interaction with tamoxifen, taxol, and cisplatin. We found that Compound A induced apoptosis selectively in human melanoma cells by increasing oxidative stress. The anti-cancer activity of Compound A was enhanced when combined with tamoxifen and the combination treatment did not result in significant toxicity to noncancerous cells. Additionally, Compound A did not interact negatively with the anti-cancer activity of taxol and cisplatin. These results indicate that Compound A could be developed as a selective and effective melanoma treatment either alone or in combination with other non-toxic agents like tamoxifen.

Keywords: melanoma; curcumin analog; apoptosis; oxidative stress; drug–drug interaction; tamoxifen; taxol; cisplatin

1. Introduction

Melanoma is an aggressive malignancy that emerges from the uncontrolled division of melanocytes and contributes to the larger part of skin cancer deaths [1]. Global incidence of melanoma has increased significantly, with rates rising in Europe and North America [2–4]. Fortunately, melanoma is easily treatable by surgical removal if detected early [5]. Deep melanoma tumors, however, tend to metastasize to lymph nodes and spread to other parts of the body [5,6]. Hence, at advanced stages surgery is not adequate and treatment becomes more difficult. Further treatment options include chemotherapy, radiation, and immunotherapy [7]. Melanoma is known to be highly resistant, thus limiting the effectiveness of these therapies [7,8]. Most chemotherapies are genotoxic or target cytoskeleton structures in cancer cells to induce cell death. However, this targeting is nonselective as it kills normal cells, which leads to severe toxicity.

Recent research has focused on targeting mitochondria, oxidative stress, and metabolic vulnerabilities to induce cancer cell death selectively [9]. Cancer cells shift their metabolism from oxidative phosphorylation to glycolysis, which reduces mitochondrial permeabilization and promotes mitochondrial stability [10–13]. The shift to glycolysis and the up-regulation of anti-apoptotic proteins, enables cancer cells to resist apoptosis [11–13]. Induction of cancer cell death selectively can occur through targeting the unique characteristics of cancerous cells. For example, analogs of the natural compound pancratistatin (PST) were able to induce apoptosis selectively in cancer cells through disrupting the mitochondrial membrane potential and the release of apoptogenic factors [14,15]. Cancer cells also display higher basal levels of reactive oxygen species (ROS), which promotes tumor proliferation and progression [16,17]. However, excessive ROS levels lead to damage of important biomolecules including DNA and protein, thus resulting in cell death [18]. Cancer cells depend on up-regulated expression of antioxidant enzymes to survive. Therefore, external sources of ROS or agents that stimulate oxidative stress may target cancer cells selectively [16]. For example, the natural compound piperlongumine induces cell death selectively through targeting the oxidative pathway [14]. An enhanced cytotoxic effect was observed when piperlongumine was combined with a pancratistatin analog, an activator of the intrinsic pathway of apoptosis through mitochondrial targeting [15].

Curcumin is a natural compound isolated from the *Curcuma longa* plant and has been shown to inhibit cancer growth and induce apoptosis in cancer cells [19,20]. Curcumin is pleiotropic and affects the activity of signaling molecules in a variety of pathways including inflammation [21]. Interestingly, curcumin has been shown to induce cell death through increasing ROS [20,22,23]. Due to poor bioavailability and stability, curcumin is not effective in vivo models and therefore could not advance to clinical success [24]. However, synthetic analogs of natural curcumin could have increased chemical stability and bioavailability. Therefore, these molecules should have the potential to be developed as cancer-selective drugs. Furthermore, a more potent analog could be synthesized that may have very high anti-cancer activity at low concentrations.

We synthesized several novel analogs of curcumin and screened them on various cancer cell lines [24]. Previously, we have demonstrated that two analogs, Compounds A and I, were the most effective in inducing apoptosis selectively in different cancer cell lines including triple-negative breast and p53-negative colorectal cancer cells [24]. Furthermore, these analogs induced cell death at lower doses compared to natural curcumin and the induction of apoptosis was driven by oxidative stress selectively in cancer cells. Compound A was also found to be effective in inhibiting human tumor growth xenografted in nude mice when administered intraperitoneally. This suggested that Compound A is biostable as well as bioavailable. Additionally, Compound A was shown to be well tolerated in mice. However, the anti-cancer activity of Compound A and other analogs of curcumin had yet to be studied in human melanoma cells. The interactions of these compounds with standard chemotherapies have also not been investigated.

Tamoxifen (TAM) is a non-genotoxic drug used to treat and prevent estrogen receptor (ER) positive breast cancer [25]. Though tamoxifen functions as an ER antagonist, it has also been shown to target and disrupt the mitochondria [25,26]. Previous work demonstrated that tamoxifen sensitized cancer cell mitochondria, thereby enhancing the anti-cancer efficacy of PST in ER negative breast cancer, and melanoma cells [27,28]. In a previous study, natural curcumin was combined with tamoxifen, which resulted in a synergistic induction of cell death selective to melanoma cells [29]. Conversely, this combination treatment did not result in significant cell death in noncancerous cells. Cell death was attributed to apoptosis as well as autophagy, a pro-survival or pro-death process, which occurs in response to stress [30,31]. Given that Compound A is more effective than natural curcumin, it is imperative to also investigate the interaction of Compound A with tamoxifen on human melanoma cells.

The objective of this study was to investigate the efficacy of novel synthetic curcumin analogs against human melanoma cells and demonstrate the possible mechanism of induction of apoptosis. We determined the effect of combining Compound A with tamoxifen in melanoma cells. We also investigated the drug–drug interactions of Compound A in combination with the standard chemotherapeutics taxol and cisplatin. Through screening the analogs on melanoma cells, Compound A was determined to be the most effective and selective in reducing cell viability. We have observed the selective induction of apoptosis by Compound A in two different melanoma cell lines. Furthermore, the effective doses of Compound A were well tolerated in normal human fibroblasts. Investigation into the mechanism revealed that cell death was triggered through induction of oxidative stress. The combination treatment of low doses of Compound A and tamoxifen resulted in an enhancement of apoptosis in human melanoma cells. Lastly, Compound A did not interfere with the anti-cancer activity of taxol and cisplatin. In conclusion, in this paper we demonstrate for the first time the anti-cancer activity of Compound A against human melanoma cells. These results may lead to the development of a non-toxic treatment that induces apoptosis selectively in melanoma cells through targeting oxidative vulnerabilities. Additionally, we demonstrate that Compound A has the potential to be developed as an adjuvant with tamoxifen and as a safer and effective melanoma treatment.

2. Results

2.1. Compounds A and I Induce Cell Death Effectively and Selectively in Human Melanoma Cells

The WST-1 colorimetric assay was utilized 48 h post treatment to determine the anti-cancer efficacy of curcumin (Figure 1) and synthetic analogs of curcumin (A-J), on A375 melanoma cells (Figure 2). Overall these analogs were more effective in reducing cell viability in A375 cells than natural curcumin. Natural curcumin was almost ineffective in reducing the viability of A375 cells even up to 20 μM (Figure 3C). However, various synthetic analogs were effective in reducing the viability of these cells at lower doses. The viability data for Compound A, I, and curcumin (for structures see Figure 1) were re-plotted as bar graphs for better comparison (Figure 3A–C). Compounds A and I were the most effective in reducing cell viability as demonstrated by lower IC_{50} values (approximately 1 and 2 μM, respectively; Figure 3A,B). The effective doses of Compounds A and I were tested on noncancerous normal human fibroblasts (NHF) and were well tolerated (Figure 3D,E). Similarly, natural curcumin did not reduce cell viability in NHF cells at different doses as indicated in Figure 3F. These results indicate selective toxicity of Compounds A and I to melanoma cells. It is important to note that Compound H was very effective in killing cancer cells at lower doses but was not taken for further study due to similar toxicity to normal cells, as determined previously [24]. Thus, Compounds A and I were chosen for further investigation with regards to the mode of cell death and mechanism.

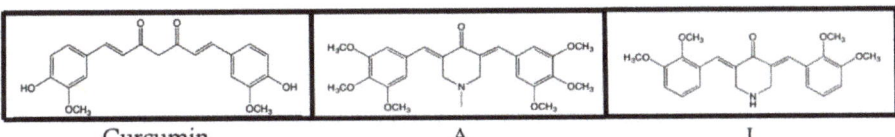

Figure 1. Structures of curcumin and analogs A and I. Previously published in Pignanelli et al. [24].

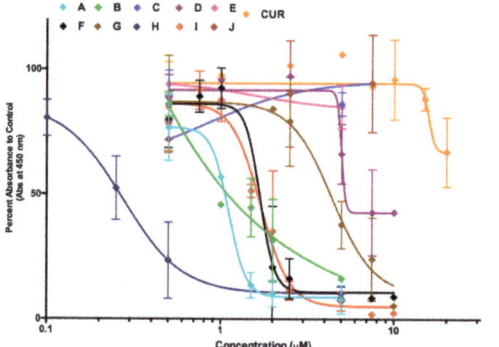

Figure 2. Effect of various curcumin analogs on cell viability of A375 melanoma cells. A375 melanoma cells were treated with natural curcumin (CUR) and curcumin analogs (A-J) for 48 h. The WST-1 assay was performed as described in the materials and methods section. Values are expressed as a mean ± SD from at least three independent experiments. The x-axis represents concentration (μM) and the y-axis represents absorbance (% of control). Graph obtained using the log (inhibitor) vs. response—variable slope (four parameters) curve on GraphPrism6.

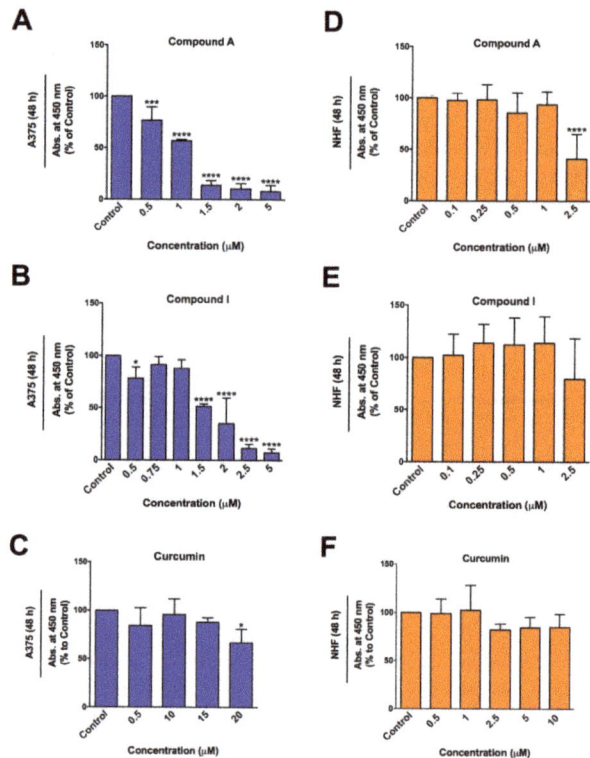

Figure 3. Compounds A and I selectively reduce cell viability in human melanoma cells. (**A–C**) A375 melanoma cells and (**D–F**) noncancerous normal human fibroblasts (NHF) were treated with Compound A, Compound I, and curcumin for 48 h. The WST-1 assay was performed as described in the materials and methods section. A375 cell viability data from Figure 1 were re-plotted as bar graphs to produce Figure 3 (A–C). Values are expressed as a mean ± SD from at least three independent experiments. The x-axis represents concentration (μM) and the y-axis represents absorbance (% of control).

2.2. Compounds A and I Induce Apoptosis Selectively in Human Melanoma Cells

The Annexin V binding assay and propidium iodide (PI) staining was utilized to distinguish early and late stage apoptosis, respectively. A375 (Figure 4A) and NHF (Figure 4B) cells were treated for 48 h with Compound A, Compound I, and curcumin. Compounds A and I induced apoptosis effectively in A375 melanoma cells at significantly lower doses compared to natural curcumin (Figure 4A). As shown in Figure 4A, Compound A induced significant apoptosis at 0.25 µM and 0.5 µM doses whereas limited induction of apoptosis was observed by natural curcumin only at 10 µM dose. Interestingly, the doses of Compound A that were greatly toxic to melanoma cells did not induce apoptosis significantly in noncancerous normal human fibroblasts 48 h following treatment (Figure 4B). However, significant apoptotic induction was observed at higher doses of Compound I (2 µM) and curcumin (10 µM). These results were supported by cellular and nuclear morphology following staining of A375 cells with Hoechst and propidium iodide (Figure 4E). The images revealed morphological changes indicative of apoptosis such as cell shrinkage, nuclear condensation, and PI positive signals (indicating permeability) in cancer cells.

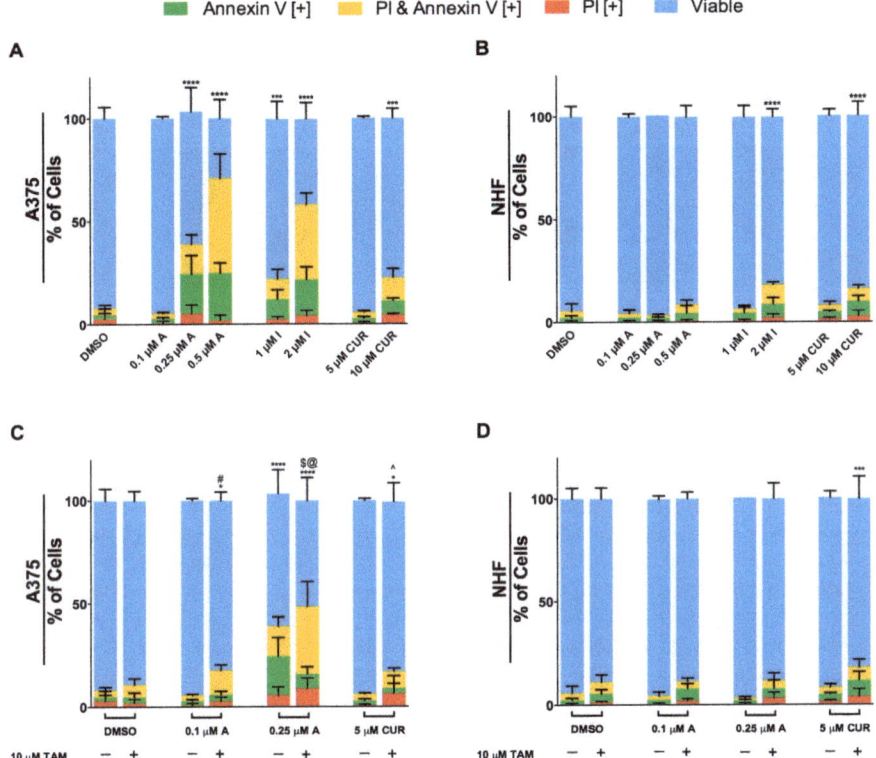

Figure 4. *Cont.*

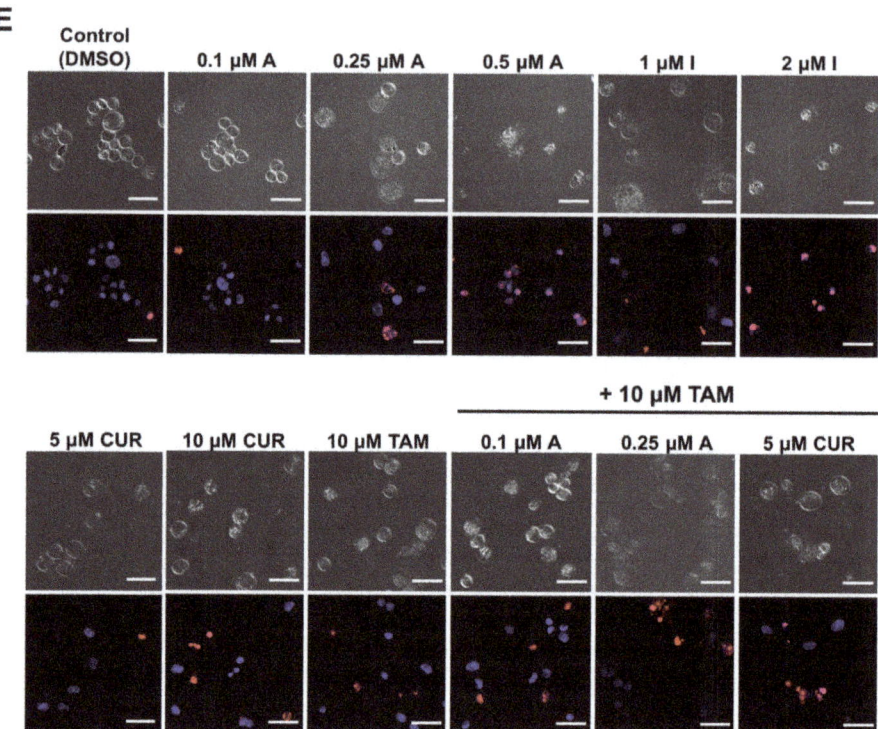

Figure 4. Compounds A and I induce apoptosis selectively and Compound A interacts positively with tamoxifen. (**A**) A375 melanoma cells and (**B**) noncancerous normal human fibroblasts (NHF) were treated with the indicated compounds for 48 h then stained with Annexin V and PI to quantify apoptosis, as described in the materials and methods section. Image based cytometry was utilized to assess apoptosis. The *y*-axis represents the percent of cells positive for Annexin V (green), PI (red), Annexin V and PI (orange), or cells negative for Annexin V and PI (blue). Values are expressed as mean ± SD from three independent experiments. (**C**) A375 melanoma cells and (**D**) NHF cells were treated with Compound A and curcumin alone and in combination with tamoxifen for 48 h. Please note, the data of Compound A and curcumin alone shown in Figure 4A,B were used again in Figure 4C,D, respectively along with the combination treatments for direct comparison. *$p < 0.05$ vs. DMSO control (comparison of viable cells only); **$p < 0.01$ vs. DMSO control (comparison of viable cells only); ***$p < 0.001$ vs. DMSO control (comparison of viable cells only); ****$p < 0.0001$ vs. DMSO control (comparison of viable cells only); #$p < 0.05$ vs. 0.1 µM Compound A alone (comparison of viable cells only); $$p < 0.05$ vs. 0.25 µM Compound A alone (comparison of viable cells only); ^$p < 0.05$ vs. 5 µM CUR alone (comparison of viable cells only); @$p < 0.05$ vs. tamoxifen treatment alone (comparison of viable cells only). (**E**) A375 micrographs at 48 h. Top: Bright field images at 400× magnification. Bottom: Fluorescent images stained with PI (red) and Hoechst (blue). Scale bar = 100 µm. Micrographs are representative of three independent experiments. A = Compound A, I = Compound I, CUR = Curcumin, TAM = Tamoxifen.

2.3. Enhancement of the Anti-cancer Activity of Compound A in Combination with Tamoxifen

Tamoxifen as such does not have strong anti-cancer activity against melanoma cells. Previously it has been reported that tamoxifen in combination with curcumin demostrated sufficient cytotoxicity against melanoma cells [29]. We investigated whether the synthetic curcumin derivative, Compound A would show a similar enhancement wth tamoxifen. A375 cells were treated with Compound A and tamoxifen alone or in combination for 48 h and apoptosis was monitored using Annexin V binding assay and propidium iodide staining. As shown in Figure 4C, there was a clear enhancement of cell death inducing activity of Compound A by tamoxifen particularly at low doses of Compound A (0.1 µM and 0.25 µM). These results were supported by fluorescent micrographs of A375 cells treated with the indicated compounds for 48 h followed by staining with Hoechst and propidium iodide (Figure 4E). On the other hand, the same combination did not show significant toxicity to normal human fibroblasts (Figure 4D).

2.4. Interaction of Compound A with Taxol and Cisplatin in Two Melanoma Cell Lines

We investigated the effect of Compound A on the cell-death-inducing activity of taxol and cisplatin on human melanoma cells. A375 (Figure 5A) and G361 (Figure 5B) cells were treated with a range of taxol and cisplatin doses in the presence or absence of 0.1 µM Compound A. The Annexin V and propidium iodide staining revealed that there was no enhancement of cell death by the combination treatments in A375 cells. In G361 cells, an enhancement was observed when 0.01 µM of taxol was combined with 0.1 µM Compound A, relative to taxol alone. However, there seems to be no enhancement at higher doses of taxol in G361 cells. We did not observe any enhancement of cisplatin when combined with Compound A in G361 cells.

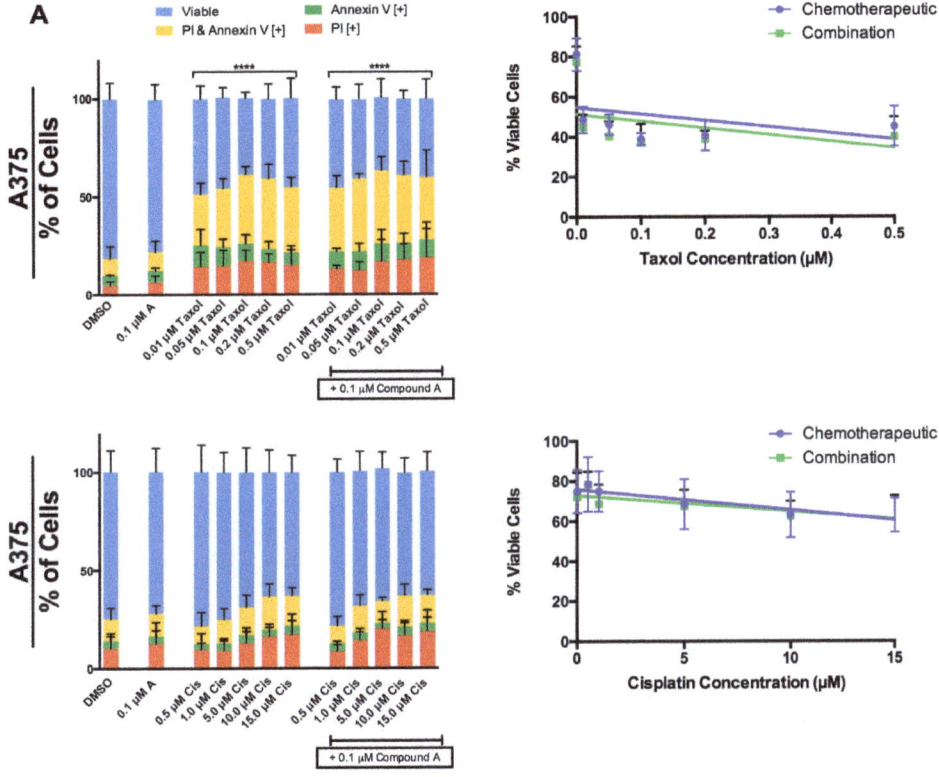

Figure 5. *Cont.*

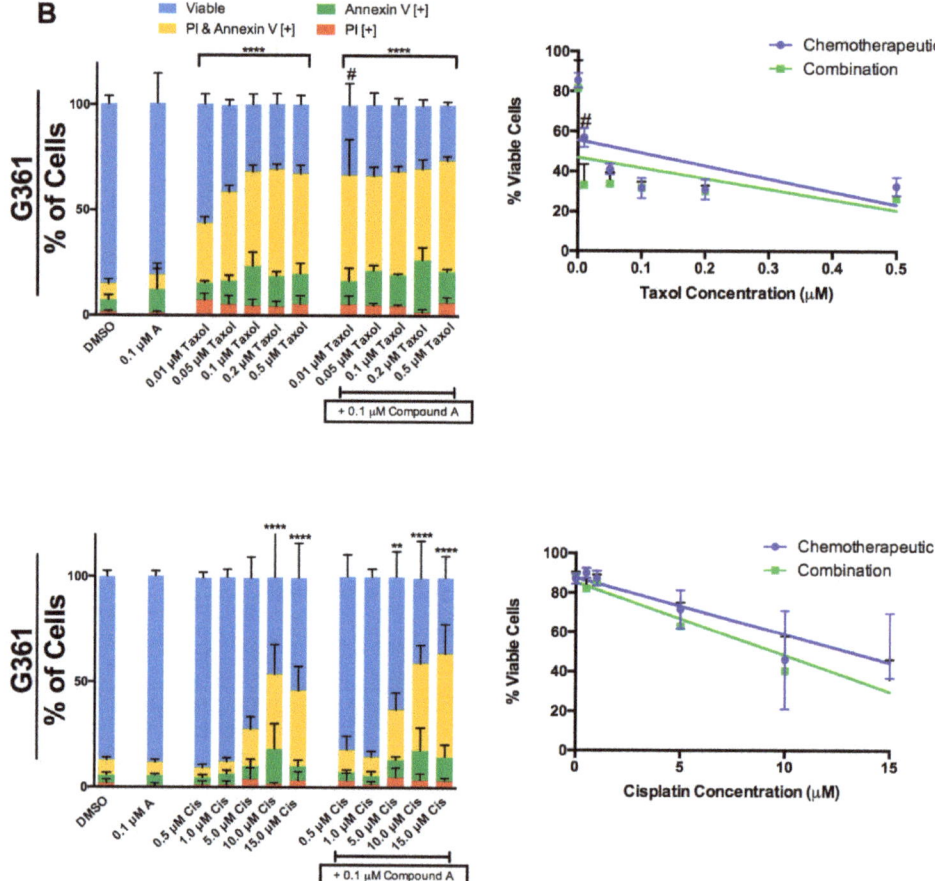

Figure 5. The interaction of Compound A with taxol and cisplatin in two melanoma cell lines. (**A**) A375 and (**B**) G361 melanoma cells were treated with a range of taxol (top panel) and cisplatin concentrations (bottom panel) alone and in combination with a sub lethal dose of Compound A (0.1 μM). Following 48 h of treatment the cells were stained with Annexin V and PI to distinguish early apoptosis and late stage apoptosis, respectively. Image based cytometry was utilized to assess apoptosis. The y-axis represents the percent of cells positive for Annexin V (green), PI (red), Annexin V and PI (yellow), or negative for both Annexin V and PI (blue). All graphical values are expressed as a mean ± SD from three independent experiments. A line graph was constructed using viability values for individual chemotherapeutics in the absence and presence of Compound A (combination). **$p < 0.01$ vs. DMSO control (comparison of viable cells only); ****$p < 0.0001$ vs. DMSO control (comparison of viable cells only); #$p < 0.0001$ vs. 0.01 μM taxol alone (comparison of viable cells only). Cis = Cisplatin.

2.5. Induction of Apoptosis by Compound A is Dependent on the Production of Oxidative Stress

To investigate the role of oxidative stress in apoptosis induction by Compound A we first measured the production of ROS using H_2DCFDA in G361 cells as indicated in the materials and methods section. Paraquat (PQ) was used as positive control for ROS generation [32]. Overall, Compound A and curcumin exhibited pro-oxidant effects and induced ROS production in G361 cells after 3 h of treatment. This was indicated by a significant increase in the percent of cells positive for DCF relative to the control (Figure 6A). Subsequently, we used the antioxidant N-Acetyl-L-cysteine (NAC) to determine if the observed increase in oxidative stress was essential for the induction of apoptosis by

Compound A and curcumin. G361 cells pre-treated with NAC demonstrated a reduction in apoptotic markers indicating that ROS played a critical role in the induction of apoptosis of Compound A and curcumin (Figure 6B).

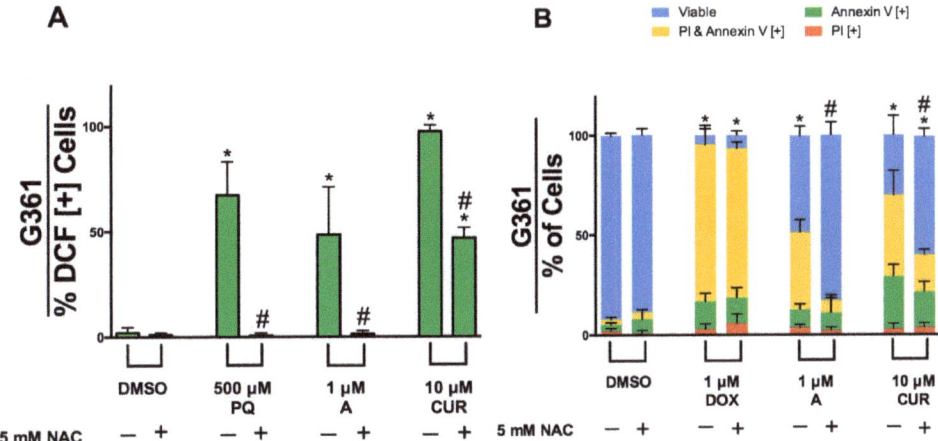

Figure 6. Induction of apoptosis by Compound A is dependent on the production of reactive oxygen species. (**A**) G361 cells were pre-treated with H_2DCFDA and treated with Compound A and curcumin with or without the antioxidant N-Acetyl-L-cysteine (NAC) for 3 h, as described in the materials and methods section. Production of ROS was evaluated through image-based cytometry with the y-axis indicative of the percent of DCF positive cells. *$p < 0.05$ vs. DCF [+] cells of DMSO control; #$p < 0.05$ vs. DCF [+] cells of groups treated without NAC. (**B**) G361 cells were treated with the Compound A and curcumin with or without NAC for 48 h. Subsequently, cells were stained with Annexin V and PI, as described in the materials and methods. Image based cytometry was utilized to assess apoptosis. The y-axis represents the percent of cells positive for Annexin V (green), PI (red), Annexin V and PI (yellow), or negative for both Annexin V and PI (blue). All graphical values are expressed as a mean ± SD from three independent experiments. Doxorubicin (DOX) was used as a positive control. *$p < 0.05$ vs. DMSO control (comparison of viable cells only); #$p < 0.05$ vs. groups treated without NAC (comparison of viable cells only). PQ = Paraquat, A = Compound A, CUR = Curcumin.

2.6. Compound A and Curcumin Induce Mitochondrial Destabilization in Human Melanoma Cells

Increased production of ROS could lead to the collapse of mitochondrial membrane potential in cells undergoing apoptosis. We investigated if G361 cells undergoing apoptosis induced by Compound A and curcumin exhibited mitochondrial destabilization. G361 cells were treated with Compound A and curcumin for 48 h then stained with tetramethylrhodamine methyl ester (TMRM), an indicator of intact mitochondria, as described in the materials and methods. Compound A and curcumin induced mitochondrial collapse as indicated by a decrease in TMRM positive cells (Figure 7).

2.7. Apoptosis Induction by Compound A is Caspase Dependent

Caspases have been shown to be involved in the initiation and execution phases of apoptosis. To determine if Compound A-induced apoptosis is dependent on caspase activity, G361 cells were pre-treated with or without the broad spectrum caspase inhibitor Z-VAD FMK. Subsequently, the cells were treated with Compound A for 48 h then stained with Annexin V and propidium iodide to characterize apoptosis. A decrease in apoptotic indicators was observed in cells treated with Z-VAD FMK (Figure 8). These results indicate that caspase activity is critical for Compound A induced apoptosis.

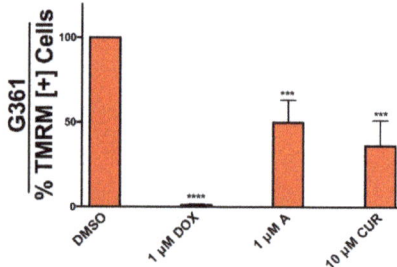

Figure 7. Mitochondrial depolarization in G361 cells undergoing apoptosis. G361 cells were treated with Compound A and curcumin for 48 h followed by incubation with TMRM for 45 min to quantify mitochondrial membrane potential (MMP), as described in the materials and methods section. Results were obtained using image-based cytometry with the y-axis representative of percent of cells positive for TMRM expressed as a mean ± SD from three independent experiments. Doxorubicin (DOX) was used as a positive control. A = Compound A, CUR = Curcumin. ***$p < 0.001$ vs. TMRM [+] cells of DMSO control; ****$p < 0.0001$ vs. TMRM [+] cells of DMSO control.

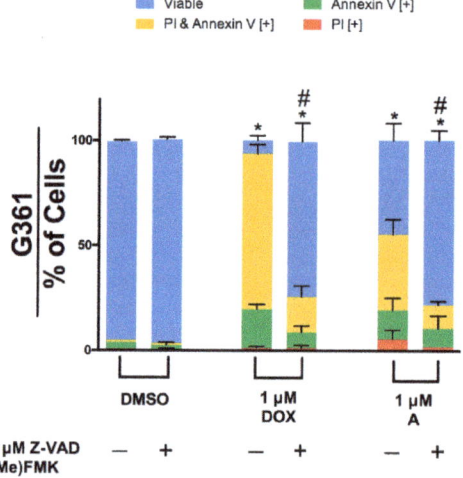

Figure 8. Induction of apoptosis by Compound A is caspase dependent. G361 melanoma cells were pre-treated with or without the caspase inhibitor Z-VAD-FMK for 30 min, followed by treatment with Compound A for 48 h. Cells were stained with Annexin V and propidium iodide to quantify apoptosis. Image based cytometry was utilized to assess apoptosis. The y-axis represents the percent of cells positive for Annexin V (green), PI (red), Annexin V and PI (orange), or cells negative for Annexin V and PI (blue). Values are expressed as mean ± SD from three independent experiments. *$p < 0.05$ vs. DMSO control (comparison of viable cells only); #$p < 0.05$ vs. individual chemotherapeutic treatment (comparison of viable cells only). Doxorubicin (DOX) was used as a positive control. A = Compound A, CUR = Curcumin.

3. Discussion

In this study, we evaluated the anti-cancer efficacy of synthetic derivatives of curcumin against chemo-resistant human melanoma cells. Out of the ten analogs we screened, Compounds A and I (for structures see Figure 1) were the most effective in reducing cell viability. These analogs induced apoptosis effectively and selectively in melanoma cells. We evaluated the interaction of Compound A with tamoxifen and demonstrated a positive interaction on the apoptosis-inducing activity of

Compound A (Figure 4C). We also determined that the induction of apoptosis in cancer cells by Compound A was dependent on the increased production of ROS and caspase activity. Compound A did not interact negatively with taxol and cisplatin in two melanoma cell lines. Overall, we have shown that a novel derivative of natural curcumin, Compound A, targets oxidative vulnerabilities to induce cell death selectively in melanoma cells.

Both melanoma cell lines (A375 and G361) were derived from a primary tumor in malignant melanoma patients. Compounds A and I were found to be very effective at lower doses compared to natural curcumin. Apoptosis is a physiological process important for maintaining homeostasis [30]. Common indicators of apoptosis include DNA condensation or fragmentation, membrane blebbing, and externalization of phosphatidylserine from the inner plasma membrane [30,31]. Analysis of phostatidylserine externalization and permeabilization using the Annexin V binding assay and propidium iodide staining, respectively revealed that these analogs were able to induce apoptosis effectively in A375 cells and at significantly lower concentrations compared to native curcumin. In parallel we tested these compounds on normal human fibroblasts (NHF), a non-transformed noncancerous cell line to investigate the selectivity of Compounds A and I. Importantly, the effective doses of Compounds A and I did not induce apoptosis significantly in NHF cells relative to the DMSO control. Hence, Compounds A and I selectively induce apoptosis in melanoma cells.

Apoptosis can be induced by the extrinsic and intrinsic pathway, which are caused by the activation of a signaling cascade upon binding of an extracellular ligand or a stimulus within the cell, respectively [32]. Both pathways may involve the cleavage and activation of cysteine proteases known as caspases. The intrinsic pathway may be triggered by internal stress, including damage of DNA and oxidative stress [32]. This further causes the mitochondria to lose integrity resulting in the release of apoptogenic factors into the cytoplasm, consequently triggering the induction of apoptosis [33]. Curcumin is a pleiotropic compound with multiple targets and has been characterized to have anti-inflammatory effects [21]. Several researchers have investigated induction of apoptosis targeting mitochondria in cancer cells [34–40]. Curcumin has been shown to induce apoptosis in a caspase dependent [41–43] and independent [44] pathway. We investigated if Compound A induced apoptosis through caspase dependent or independent pathways. Furthermore, the broad caspase inhibitor Z-VAD FMK was able to inhibit Compound A induced apoptosis, indicating a critical role of caspases.

Interestingly, in this study we observed an increased production of ROS following the treatment of melanoma cells with curcumin and Compound A. When curcumin and Compound A were co-treated with the antioxidant NAC, we indeed saw a reduction in ROS generation leading to the inhibition of apoptosis. Thus, Compound A must be targeting oxidative vulnerabilities to induce cell death in melanoma cells. Mitochondrial membrane potential collapse happens at the later stage of apoptosis. Indeed, we observed the collapse of mitochondrial membrane potential (MMP) in melanoma cells following treatment with Compound A and curcumin.

Chemotherapeutic drugs with different targets have the potential to be more effective when combined with a lower chance of resistance [45]. It is integral that we investigate the combined effect of non-toxic, anti-cancer compounds to improve the efficacy of cancer treatments. Tamoxifen is a well-tolerated ER antagonist used for ER positive breast cancer patients and has also been shown to target the mitochondria and induce autophagy [36]. A synergistic induction of apoptosis and autophagy was observed when tamoxifen was combined with an analog of pancratistatin, another mitochondria targeting compound [14]. Likewise, when tamoxifen was combined with curcumin, a synergistic induction of apoptosis and autophagy was observed [29]. We have demonstrated a clear enhancement of Compound A-induced apoptosis by tamoxifen. Importantly, this combination did not exhibit similar toxicity to noncancerous normal human fibroblasts. To our knowledge this is the first time Compound A and tamoxifen have been studied in melanoma cells.

We investigated whether Compound A could be used in conjugation with taxol and cisplatin. Taxol targets the microtubules and causes mitotic arrest [46]. It is used to treat a variety of cancers including melanoma, however is cytotoxic to normal cells [47]. Cisplatin induces apoptosis through DNA damage and is also nonspecific [48]. To determine the drug–drug interactions, we treated A375 and G361 cells with taxol and cisplatin alone or in combination with Compound A. The combination could reveal a positive or negative effect, or no interaction. We did not observe any negative interaction of Compound A with taxol or cisplatin in A375 and G361 cells. However, an enhancement was established at 0.01 µM taxol combined with 0.1 µM Compound A in G361 cells. Overall, Compound A could potentially be combined with taxol and cisplatin, and is safe to use as an adjuvant. Since it is non-toxic compared to other treatments, it could be given over a longer period of time without any adverse side effects.

In conclusion, Compound A is able to induce apoptosis effectively in drug resistant melanoma cells with ten times more efficacy than natural curcumin by targeting oxidative vulnerabilities. The anti-cancer activity of Compound A is enhanced by tamoxifen and the combination treatment was well tolerated by normal cells. Compound A did not interact negatively with taxol and cisplatin. In fact, a positive interaction was observed in G361 cells treated with taxol and Compound A. Compound A could potentially be developed as a safe and effective treatment alone or in combination with tamoxifen. Future work may focus on elucidating the mechanism and targets of Compound A induced cell death, and in vivo models of melanoma should be tested to determine efficacy and stability.

4. Materials and Methods

4.1. Chemical Synthesis of Curcumin Analogs

All chemical reagents were obtained from Sigma–Aldrich, Fluka, and Aladdin (Beijing, China). Synthesis of Compounds A-J has been described previously [24].

4.2. Cell Culture

Malignant melanoma cell line A375 (ATCC, Cat. No. CRL-1619, Manassas, VA, USA) was cultured in RPMI-1640 medium (Sigma–Aldrich Canada, Mississauga, ON, Canada) supplemented with 10% (v/v) fetal bovine serum (FBS) standard (Thermo Scientific, Waltham, MA, USA) and 40 µg/mL gentamicin (Gibco BRL, VWR, Mississauga, ON, Canada).

Malignant melanoma cell line G361 (ATCC, Cat. No. CRL-1424, Manassas, VA, USA) was cultured in McCoy's 5A Medium supplemented with 2 mM L-glutamine, 10% (v/v) FBS (Thermo Scientific, Waltham, MA, USA), and 40 µg/mL gentamicin (Gibco BRL, VWR, Mississauga, ON, Canada).

The noncancerous cell line, normal human skin fibroblast cells (NHF; Coriell Institute for Medical120 Research, Cat. No. AG09309, Camden, NJ, USA) were cultured in Dulbecco's Modified Eagle's Medium (DMEM; ATCC® 30-2002TM) supplemented with 10% (v/v) fetal bovine serum (FBS) and 40 µg/mL gentamicin (Catalog No. 15710-064, Gibco BRL, VWR, Mississauga, ON, CA).

All cultured cells were maintained in an incubator at 37 °C, 5% CO_2, and 95% humidity. The cells were passaged for less than six months.

4.3. Chemicals and Cell Treatment

Human melanoma cells and NHF cells were grown to roughly 70% confluence and then treated with curcumin (CUR; Sigma-Aldrich Canada, Cat. No. 8511, Mississauga, ON, Canada), Compound A and other curcumin analogs (e.g., Compound I) all dissolved in dimethylsulfoxide (DMSO) to make the stock solutions. In parallel, these cells were treated with taxol (Sigma–Aldrich Canada, Cat. No. T7402, Mississauga, ON, Canada), cisplatin (Sigma–Aldrich Canada, Mississauga, ON, Canada), doxorubicin (DOX; Sigma–Aldrich Canada, Cat. No. D1515, Mississauga, ON, Canada), and Z-VAD-FMK (Sigma–Aldrich Canada, Cat. No. V116, Mississauga, ON, Canada). These agents were also dissolved in dimethylsulfoxide (DMSO) to make the stock solutions. N-Acetyl-L-cysteine (NAC; Sigma–Aldrich Canada, Cat. No. A7250) and paraquat (PQ; Sigma–Aldrich Canada, Cat. No.856177, Mississauga, ON, Canada) were dissolved in double distilled water.

4.4. WST-1 Assay for Cell Viability

A WST-1 colorimetric assay was used to quantify cell viability of cells treated with curcumin and its analogs (compound A-J), following a previously published protocol [15]. Briefly, A375 and NHF cells were seeded in ninety-six well clear bottom tissue culture plates then treated with the indicated compounds for 48 h. The cells were then incubated with the WST-1 reagent (Roche Applied Sciences, Indianapolis, IN, USA) for 4 h at 37 °C, 5% CO2, and 95% humidity. The WST-1 reagent is cleaved by viable cells to formazan through its enzymes. Absorbance was read at 450 nm on a Wallac Victor3 1420 Multilabel Counter (PerkinElmer, Waltham, MA, USA) to determine cell viability.

4.5. Analysis of Cell Death

Annexin V binding assay and propidium iodide staining were used to determine early apoptosis and cell permeabilization (found in late apoptotic cells), respectively as described previously [15]. Briefly, melanoma and NHF cells were seeded in six-well plates and after 24 h they were treated with different compounds at various concentrations for 48 h. Cells were washed with phosphate buffer saline (PBS), and then Annexin V Binding buffer (10 mM HEPES, 140 mM NaCl, 2.5 mM CaCl2, pH 7.4) was added, followed by the Annexin V AlexaFluor-488 dye, which fluoresces a green color (1:20; Life Technologies Inc., Cat. No. A13201, Burlington, ON, Canada). Afterwards, 0.01 mg/mL of propidium iodide dye (red fluorescent color) was added (Life Technologies Inc, Cat. No. P3566, Burlington, ON, Canada). Afterwards, the cells were incubated for 15 min at 37 degrees Celsius, 5% CO2, and 95% humidity in the absence of light. A Tali Image-Based Cytometer (Life Technologies Inc., Cat. No. T10796, Burlington, ON, Canada) was used to quantify the percentage of cells stained green (early apoptotic), green and red (late apoptotic), and red (necrotic). Cells from 18 random fields were used to analyze the green (ex. 458 nm; em. 525/20 nm) and red (ex. 530 nm; em. 585 nm) channels. In order to visualize cellular death and apoptosis, a similar protocol was carried out. Cells were stained with propidium iodide and Hoechst 3342 (Molecular Probes, Eugene, OR, USA) at 10 µM during the 15 min incubation. Fluorescent and Brightfield micrographs were taken at 400× magnification using a Leica DMI6000 fluorescent microscope with the LAS AF6000 software.

4.6. Tetramethylrhodamine Methyl Ester Staining

Tetramethylrhodamine methyl ester (TMRM; Thermo Fisher Scientific) stain was used to determine mitochondrial membrane potential (MMP) as outlined in a previously published protocol [24]. G361 cells were cultured and then treated with doxorubicin, Compound A, and curcumin for 48 h. Subsequently, the cells were incubated with 100 nM TMRM for 45 min at 37 °C. Cells were washed with PBS, and then a Tali Image-Based Cytometer (Life Technologies Inc., Cat. No. T10796, Burlington, ON, Canada) was then used to quantify the percentage of red stain from TMRM (stable mitochondrial membrane potential). Cells from 18 random fields were used to analyze the red (ex. 530 nm; em. 585 nm) channel.

4.7. Quantification of Reactive Oxygen Species

The molecule 2′,7′-dicholorofluorescin diacetate (H_2DCFDA) was used to determine whole-cell reactive oxygen species (ROS) generation as outlined in a previously published protocol [24]. The molecule is deacetylated by esterases and oxidized by ROS into a fluorescent green 2′,7′-dicholorofluorescein (DCF; ex. 495 nm; em. 529 nm) once inside the cell. G361 cells were pretreated with a final concentration of 20 µM H_2DCFDA (D6883; Sigma-Aldrich) and then incubated for 30 min at 37 °C and 5% CO_2 in the absence of light. Afterwards, the cells were treated with various drug concentrations for 3 h. The cells were centrifuged at 3000 rpm for 5 min and then suspended in PBS. A Tali Image-Based Cytometer (Life Technologies Inc., Cat. No. T10796, Burlington, ON, Canada) was then used to quantify the percentage of green fluorescent cells from the presence of DCF-positive stain. Cells from 18 random fields were used to analyze the green (ex. 458 nm; em. 525/20 nm) channel. In order to determine the mechanism of action of Compound A and curcumin, G361 cells were pretreated with or without N-Acetyl-L-cysteine (NAC; final concentration 5 mM; Sigma–Aldrich Canada, Cat. No. A7250) and incubated for 30 min. NAC acts as an antioxidant which inhibits the presence of ROS in the cell. H_2DCFDA was utilized to determine ROS generation as mentioned above. Subsequently, the cells were treated with DMSO, paraquat, Compound A, and curcumin. The cells were then read for the presence of green fluorescence at a time point of 3 h following incubation using a Tali Image-Based Cytometer (Life Technologies Inc., Cat. No. T10796, Burlington, ON, Canada).

4.8. Caspase Inhibition

Cell treatment with or without general caspase inhibitor Z-VAD-FMK was used to determine if the apoptotic mechanism of Compound A was caspase dependent or independent. Cells were pretreated with 4 µL Z-VAD-FMK (final concentration 20 µM) for 30 min at 37 °C at 5% CO_2. Cells were then treated with DMSO, doxorubicin (DOX), and Compound A. After incubation for 48 h, cells were collected, washed with phosphate buffer saline (PBS), and apoptosis was quantified using the Annexin V Binding Assay protocol as previously described.

4.9. Statistical Analysis

Statistical analysis was conducted by the GraphPad Prism 6 software. Significance was considered when the p-value was less than 0.05. The type of statistical analysis depended on the experimental variable. Single variable measurements, including quantification of mitochondrial membrane potential, and whole cell ROS, were analyzed by the one-way ANOVA (nonparametric) and the mean of each sample was compared to the mean of the negative control (DMSO) unless otherwise specified. Multi-variable experiments such as the quantification of early and late apoptosis, were analyzed by two-way ANOVA (nonparametric) and the sample of each mean was compared to the mean of the negative control (DMSO) unless otherwise specified.

Author Contributions: K.P. was responsible for the conceptualization, design, and execution of experiments, analysis of data, and preparation of the report. S.S. contributed to the execution of experiments, analysis of data, and preparation of the report. A.M., C.C., C.V., C.N., and C.P. contributed to the execution of the experiments, and analysis of data. Pandey contributed to the conceptualization and design of experiments, analysis of data, preparation and review of the manuscript. J.W. aided in the synthesis of the curcumin analogs. G.L., and Y.W. synthesized and provided the curcumin analogs, provided the chemical stability of curcumin and Compound A.

Funding: Funding for this work was by generous donations by the Windsor Mold Group (Windsor, Ontario), Lotte and John Hecht Foundation, and Natural Science and Engineering Council of Canada. A grant from the National Natural Science Foundation of China (81472307) was used to fund the synthesis of each analog.

Acknowledgments: The authors would like to acknowledge Richa Parashar for revising the paper and providing feedback.

Conflicts of Interest: The authors declare no conflict of interest. The funders had no role in the design of the study; in the collection, analyses, or interpretation of data; in the writing of the manuscript, or in the decision to publish the results.

References

1. Erdei, E.; Torres, S.M. A new understanding in the epidemiology of melanoma. *Expert Rev. Anticancer* **2011**, *10*, 1811–1823. [CrossRef] [PubMed]
2. Langley, A.; Levesque, L.; Baetz, T.; Asai, Y. Brief Report: Increase in Melanoma Incidence in Ontario. *J. Cutan. Med. Surg.* **2018**, *22*, 476–478. [CrossRef] [PubMed]
3. Linos, E.; Swetter, S.M.; Cockburn, M.G.; Colditz, G.A.; Clarke, C.A. Increasing Burden of Melanoma in the United States. *J. Investig. Derm.* **2009**, *129*, 1666–1674. [CrossRef] [PubMed]
4. Erdmann, F.; Lortet-Tieulent, J.; Schuz, J.; Zeeb, H.; Greinert, R.; Breitbart, E.W.; Bray, F. International trends in the incidence of malignant melanoma 1953–2008—Are recent generations at higher or lower risk? *Int. J. Cancer* **2013**, *132*, 385–400. [CrossRef] [PubMed]

5. Balch, C.M.; Buzaid, A.C.; Soong, S.J.; Atkins, M.B.; Cascinelli, N.; Coit, D.G.; Fleming, I.D.; Gershenwald, J.E.; Houghton, A., Jr.; Kirkwood, J.M.; et al. Final version of the American Joint Committee on Cancer staging system for cutaneous melanoma. *J. Clin. Oncol.* **2001**, *19*, 3635–3648. [CrossRef] [PubMed]
6. Vijuk, G.; Coates, A. Survival of patients with visceral metastatic melanoma from an occult primary lesion: A retrospective matched cohort study. *Ann. Oncol.* **1998**, *9*, 419–422. [CrossRef] [PubMed]
7. Soengas, M.S.; Lowe, S.W. Apoptosis and melanoma chemoresistance. *Oncogene* **2003**, *22*, 3138–3151. [CrossRef]
8. Debatin, K.-M. Apoptosis pathways in cancer and cancer therapy. *Cancer Immunol. Immunother.* **2004**, *53*, 153–159. [CrossRef]
9. Martinez-Outschoorn, U.E.; Peiris-Pagés, M.; Pestell, R.G.; Sotgia, F.; Lisanti, M.P. Cancer metabolism: A therapeutic perspective. *Nat. Rev. Clin. Oncol.* **2017**, *14*, 11–31. [CrossRef]
10. Heiden, M.G.V.; Cantley, L.C.; Thompson, C.B. Understanding the Warburg Effect: The Metabolic Requirements of Cell Proliferation. *Science* **2009**, *324*, 1029–1033. [CrossRef]
11. DeBerardinis, R.J.; Lum, J.J.; Hatzivassiliou, G.; Thompson, C.B. The Biology of Cancer: Metabolic Reprogramming Fuels Cell Growth and Proliferation. *Cell Metab.* **2008**, *7*, 11–20. [CrossRef] [PubMed]
12. Gogvadze, V.; Zhivotovsky, B.; Orrenius, S. The Warburg effect and mitochondrial stability in cancer cells. *Mol. Asp. Med.* **2010**, *31*, 60–74. [CrossRef] [PubMed]
13. Plas, D.R.; Thompson, C.B. Cell metabolism in the regulation of programmed cell death. *Trends Endocrinol. Metab.* **2002**, *13*, 75–78. [CrossRef]
14. Ma, D.; Gilbert, T.; Pignanelli, C.; Tarade, D.; Noel, M.; Mansour, F.; Gupta, M.; Ma, S.; Ropat, J.; Curran, C.; et al. Exploiting mitochondrial and oxidative vulnerabilities with a synthetic analog of pancratistatin in combination with piperlongumine for cancer therapy. *FASEB. J.* **2018**, *32*, 417–430. [CrossRef] [PubMed]
15. Ma, D.; Pignanelli, C.; Tarade, D.; Gilbert, T.; Noel, M.; Mansour, F.; Adams, S.; Dowhayko, A.; Stokes, K.; Vshyvenko, S.; et al. Cancer Cell Mitochondria Targeting by Pancratistatin Analogs is Dependent on Functional Complex II and III. *Sci. Rep.* **2017**, *7*, 42957. [CrossRef] [PubMed]
16. Trachootham, D.; Alexandre, J.; Huang, P. Targeting cancer cells by ROS-mediated mechanisms: A radical therapeutic approach? *Nat. Rev. Drug Discov.* **2009**, *8*, 579–591. [CrossRef] [PubMed]
17. Storz, P. Reactive oxygen species in tumor progression. *Front. Biosci.* **2005**, *10*, 1881–1896. [CrossRef] [PubMed]
18. Reuter, S.; Gupta, S.C.; Chaturvedi, M.M.; Aggarwal, B.B. Oxidative stress, inflammation, and cancer: How are they linked? *Free Radic. Biol. Med.* **2010**, *49*, 1603–1616. [CrossRef] [PubMed]
19. Aoki, H.; Takada, Y.; Kondo, S.; Sawaya, R.; Aggarwal, B.B.; Kondo, Y. Evidence That Curcumin Suppresses the Growth of Malignant Gliomas in Vitro and in Vivo through Induction of Autophagy: Role of Akt and Extracellular Signal-Regulated Kinase Signaling Pathways. *Mol. Pharm.* **2007**, *72*, 29–39. [CrossRef]
20. Yoshino, M.; Haneda, M.; Naruse, M.; Htay, H.H.; Tsubouchi, R.; Qiao, S.L.; Li, W.H.; Murakami, K.; Yokochi, T. Prooxidant activity of curcumin: Copper-dependent formation of 8-hydroxy-2′-deoxyguanosine in DNA and induction of apoptotic cell death. *Toxicol. Vitr.* **2004**, *18*, 783–789. [CrossRef]
21. Gupta, S.C.; Patchva, S.; Koh, W.; Aggarwal, B.B. Discovery of curcumin, a component of golden spice, and its miraculous biological activities. *Clin. Exp. Pharm. Physiol.* **2012**, *39*, 283–299. [CrossRef] [PubMed]
22. Kunwar, A.; Jayakumar, S.; Srivastava, A.K.; Priyadarsini, K.I. Dimethoxycurcumin-induced cell death in human breast carcinoma MCF7 cells: Evidence for pro-oxidant activity, mitochondrial dysfunction, and apoptosis. *Arch. Toxicol.* **2012**, *86*, 603–614. [CrossRef] [PubMed]
23. Aggeli, I.-K.; Koustas, E.; Gaitanaki, C.; Aggeli, I.; Beis, I. Curcumin Acts as a Pro–Oxidant Inducing Apoptosis Via JNKs in the Isolated Perfused Rana ridibunda Heart. *J. Exp. Zool. Part A Ecol. Genet. Physiol.* **2013**, *319*, 328–339. [CrossRef] [PubMed]
24. Pignanelli, C.; Ma, D.; Noel, M.; Ropat, J.; Mansour, F.; Curran, C.; Pupulin, S.; Larocque, K.; Wu, J.; Liang, G.; et al. Selective Targeting of Cancer Cells by Oxidative Vulnerabilities with Novel Curcumin Analogs. *Sci. Rep.* **2017**, *7*, 1603. [CrossRef] [PubMed]
25. Howell, A. The endocrine prevention of breast cancer. *Best Pr. Res. Clin. Endocrinol. Metab.* **2008**, *22*, 615–623. [CrossRef] [PubMed]
26. Moreira, P.I.; Custódio, J.; Moreno, A.; Oliveira, C.R.; Santos, M.S. Tamoxifen and Estradiol Interact with the Flavin Mononucleotide Site of Complex I Leading to Mitochondrial Failure. *J. Boil. Chem.* **2006**, *281*, 10143–10152. [CrossRef]

27. Siedlakowski, P.; Mclachlan-Burgess, A.; Griffin, C.; Tirumalai, S.S.; McNulty, J.; Pandey, S. Synergy of pancratistatin and tamoxifen on breast cancer cells in inducing apoptosis by targeting mitochondria. *Cancer Boil.* **2008**, *7*, 376–384. [CrossRef]
28. Chatterjee, S.J.; McNulty, J.; Pandey, S. Sensitization of human melanoma cells by tamoxifen to apoptosis induction by pancratistatin, a nongenotoxic natural compound. *Melanoma Res.* **2011**, *21*, 1–11. [CrossRef]
29. Chatterjee, S.J.; Pandey, S. Chemo-resistant melanoma sensitized by tamoxifen to low dose curcumin treatment through induction of apoptosis and autophagy. *Cancer Boil.* **2011**, *11*, 216–228. [CrossRef]
30. Kroemer, G.; Mariño, G.; Levine, B. Autophagy and the integrated stress response. *Mol. Cell* **2010**, *40*, 280–293. [CrossRef]
31. Dalby, K.N.; Tekedereli, I.; Lopez-Berestein, G.; Ozpolat, B. Targeting the prodeath and prosurvival functions of autophagy as novel therapeutic strategies in cancer. *Autophagy* **2010**, *6*, 322–329. [CrossRef] [PubMed]
32. Cochemé, H.M.; Murphy, M.P. Complex I is the major site of mitochondrial superoxide production by paraquat. *J. Biol. Chem.* **2008**, *283*, 1786–1798. [CrossRef] [PubMed]
33. Canta, A.; Pozzi, E.; Carozzi, V.A. Mitochondrial Dysfunction in Chemotherapy-Induced Peripheral Neuropathy (CIPN). *Toxics* **2015**, *3*, 198–223. [CrossRef] [PubMed]
34. Naksuriya, O.; Okonogi, S.; Schiffelers, R.M.; Hennink, W.E. Curcumin nanoformulations: A review of pharmaceutical properties and preclinical studies and clinical data related to cancer treatment. *Biomaterials* **2014**, *35*, 3365–3383. [CrossRef] [PubMed]
35. Tonnesen, H.H.; Másson, M.; Loftsson, T. Studies of curcumin and curcuminoids. XXVII. Cyclodextrin complexation: Solubility, chemical and photochemical stability. *Int. J. Pharm.* **2002**, *244*, 127–135. [CrossRef]
36. Gupta, S.C.; Patchva, S.; Aggarwal, B.B. Therapeutic roles of curcumin: Lessons learned from clinical trials. *AAPS J.* **2013**, *15*, 195–218. [CrossRef] [PubMed]
37. Kerr, J.F.R.; Wyllie, A.H.; Currie, A.R. Apoptosis: A Basic Biological Phenomenon with Wide-ranging Implications in Tissue Kinetics. *Br. J. Cancer* **1972**, *26*, 239–257. [CrossRef]
38. Fadok, V.A.; Bratton, D.L.; Frasch, S.C.; Warner, M.L.; Henson, P.M. The role of phosphatidylserine in recognition of apoptotic cells by phagocytes. *Cell Death Differ.* **1998**, *5*, 551–562. [CrossRef]
39. Fulda, S.; Debatin, K.-M. Extrinsic versus intrinsic apoptosis pathways in anticancer chemotherapy. *Oncogene* **2006**, *25*, 4798–4811. [CrossRef]
40. Debatin, K.-M.; Poncet, D.; Kroemer, G. Chemotherapy: Targeting the mitochondrial cell death pathway. *Oncogene* **2002**, *21*, 8786–8803. [CrossRef]
41. Mukhopadhyay, A.; Bueso-Ramos, C.; Chatterjee, D.; Pantazis, P.; Aggarwal, B.B. Curcumin downregulates cell survival mechanisms in human prostate cancer cell lines. *Oncogene* **2001**, *20*, 7597–7609. [CrossRef] [PubMed]
42. Gogada, R.; Amadori, M.; Zhang, H.; Jones, A.; Verone, A.; Pitarresi, J.; Jandhyam, S.; Prabhu, V.; Black, J.D.; Chandra, D. Curcumin induces Apaf-1-dependent, p21-mediated caspase activation and apoptosis. *Cell Cycle* **2011**, *10*, 4128–4137. [CrossRef] [PubMed]
43. Sikora, E. Curcumin induces caspase-3-dependent apoptotic pathway but inhibits DNA fragmentation factor 40/caspase-activated DNase endonuclease in human Jurkat cells. *Mol. Cancer* **2006**, *5*, 927–934. [CrossRef] [PubMed]
44. Hilchie, A.L.; Furlong, S.J.; Sutton, K.; Richardson, A.; Robichaud, M.R.J.; Giacomantonio, C.A.; Ridgway, N.D.; Hoskin, D.W. Curcumin-Induced Apoptosis in PC3 Prostate Carcinoma Cells Is Caspase-Independent and Involves Cellular Ceramide Accumulation and Damage to Mitochondria. *Nutr. Cancer* **2010**, *62*, 379–389. [CrossRef] [PubMed]
45. Mokhtari, R.B.; Homayouni, T.S.; Baluch, N.; Morgatskaya, E.; Kumar, S.; Das, B.; Yeger, H. Combination therapy in combating cancer. *Oncotarget* **2017**, *8*, 38022–38043. [CrossRef] [PubMed]
46. Cunha, K.S.; Reguly, M.L.; Graf, U.; Helena, H. Taxanes: The genetic toxicity of paclitaxel and docetaxel in comatic cells of Drosophila melanogaster. *Mutagenesis* **2001**, *16*, 79–84. [CrossRef] [PubMed]
47. Weaver, B.A. How Taxol/paclitaxel kills cancer cells. *Mol. Biol. Cell* **2014**, *25*, 2677–2681. [CrossRef] [PubMed]

48. Dasari, S.; Tchounwou, P.B. Cisplatin in cancer therapy: Molecular mechanisms of action. *Eur. J. Pharm.* **2014**, *740*, 364–378. [CrossRef]

Sample Availability: Samples of the compounds are not available.

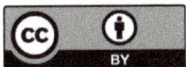 © 2019 by the authors. Licensee MDPI, Basel, Switzerland. This article is an open access article distributed under the terms and conditions of the Creative Commons Attribution (CC BY) license (http://creativecommons.org/licenses/by/4.0/).

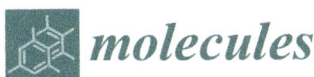

Article

Essential Oil of *Mentha aquatica* var. *Kenting Water Mint* Suppresses Two-Stage Skin Carcinogenesis Accelerated by BRAF Inhibitor Vemurafenib

Chih-Ting Chang [1,2], Wen-Ni Soo [1], Yu-Hsin Chen [3] and Lie-Fen Shyur [1,2,4,*]

1. Agricultural Biotechnology Research Center, Academia Sinica, Taipei 115, Taiwan
2. Department of Biological Science and Technology, National Taiwan University, Taipei 106, Taiwan
3. Taichung District Agricultural Research and Extension Station, Council of Agriculture, Executive Yuan, Taichung 515, Taiwan
4. Graduate Institute of Pharmacognosy, Taipei Medical University, Taipei 110, Taiwan
* Correspondence: lfshyur@ccvax.sinica.edu.tw; Tel.: +886-2-27872102

Academic Editor: Kyoko Nakagawa-Goto
Received: 29 May 2019; Accepted: 22 June 2019; Published: 25 June 2019

Abstract: The v-raf murine sarcoma viral homolog B1 (BRAF) inhibitor drug vemurafenib (PLX4032) is used to treat melanoma; however, epidemiological evidence reveals that it could cause cutaneous keratoacanthomas and squamous cell carcinoma in cancer patients with the most prevalent $HRAS^{Q61L}$ mutation. In a two-stage skin carcinogenesis mouse model, the skin papillomas induced by 7,12-dimethylbenz[a]anthracene (DMBA)/12-O-tetradecanoylphorbol-13-acetate (TPA) (DT) resemble the lesions in BRAF inhibitor-treated patients. In this study, we investigated the bioactivity of *Mentha aquatica* var. *Kenting Water Mint* essential oil (KWM-EO) against PDV cells, mouse keratinocytes bearing $HRAS^{Q61L}$ mutation, and its effect on inhibiting papilloma formation in a two-stage skin carcinogenesis mouse model with or without PLX4032 co-treatment. Our results revealed that KWM-EO effectively attenuated cell viability, colony formation, and the invasive and migratory abilities of PDV cells. Induction of G_2/M cell-cycle arrest and apoptosis in PDV cells was also observed. KWM-EO treatment significantly decreased the formation of cutaneous papilloma further induced by PLX4032 in DT mice (DTP). Immunohistochemistry analyses showed overexpression of keratin14 and COX-2 in DT and DTP skin were profoundly suppressed by KWM-EO treatment. This study demonstrates that KWM-EO has chemopreventive effects against PLX4032-induced cutaneous side-effects in a DMBA/TPA-induced two-stage carcinogenesis model and will be worth further exploration for possible application in melanoma patients.

Keywords: BRAF inhibitor; *Mentha aquatica* var. *Kenting Water Mint*; essential oil; chemoprevention; two-stage skin carcinogenesis

1. Introduction

Cutaneous squamous cell carcinoma (cuSCC) and keratoacanthoma (KA) develop in approximately 20% to 30% of patients who are treated with BRAF (v-raf murine sarcoma viral homolog B1) inhibitors, such as vemurafenib (PLX4032) [1]. Functional studies have demonstrated that these serious side-effects caused during the treatment of PLX4032 are through paradoxical activation of the MAPK signaling pathway of wild-type BRAF cell lines bearing either oncogenic *RAS* mutations or upstream receptor tyrosine kinase activity [2–4]. In a recent study, cuSCC and KAs emerging from patients administrated with BRAF inhibitor were analyzed for oncogenic mutations and activating mutations on *RAS*, especially the *HRAS* isoform was noticed in about 60% of subjects [5]. Among the *RAS* mutants, $HRAS^{Q61L}$ was the most prevalent, and thus, the genetic $HRAS^{Q61L}$ mutation of cells (e.g., keratinocytes PDV) was selected to investigate the pre-clinical pathological mechanisms [6]. Meanwhile, the mouse skin model of multiple-stage chemical carcinogenesis is a representable in vivo model for understanding the development of cuSCC [7,8]. Topical exposure of carcinogens, 7,12-dimethyl[a]anthracene (DMBA), as a tumor initiator results in $HRAS^{Q61L}$ mutation in mouse skin. Subsequently, topical treatment of tumor promoter, 12-O-tetradecanoyl-phorbol-13-acetate (TPA) then leads to the formation of lesions, KAs, and the development of SCC. FVB (Friend Virus B NIH Jackson) mice administrated with DMBA/TPA along with BRAF inhibitor, PLX4720, showed a remarkable acceleration in the appearance of lesions, an increase of incidence, and enhanced progression to KAs and SCC which resemble the papillomas induced by BRAF inhibitors in the clinical setting [5].

Tumor development is correlated with proliferation and expansion of not only cancer cells but also stroma, vessels, and infiltrating inflammatory cells and elements [9]. Neoplastic growth is related to a prolonged inflammatory condition induced by extrinsic or intrinsic pathways. The extrinsic pathways are related to a continued inflammatory condition, while the intrinsic pathways are stimulated by genetic transformations, which result in the activation of oncogenes or inactivation of tumor suppressor genes [10]. Cells with an altered phenotype propagate the secretion of inflammatory mediators, thus triggering the formation of a tumor microenvironment (TME) and development of tumors [11]. Recently, immunoinflammatory cells, such as macrophages, have been identified as critical contributors to malignancies in various tumor types, such as melanoma, lung carcinoma, glioma, gastric cancer, and wound-induced skin cancer [12,13].

Numerous studies have demonstrated that essential oils (EOs) of *Mentha* species have antiviral, antimicrobial, antioxidant, anti-inflammatory, and anti-tumor activities [14–18]. The objective of this study was to investigate the bioefficacy of EO from *Mentha aquatica var. citrata* Kenting Water Mint (KWM-EO) against two-stage skin carcinogenesis, with or without PLX4032 irritation, and the underlying molecular mechanisms. The chemical components of KWM-EO were analyzed using GC×GC-TOF MS, and its effect on *HRAS* mutant PDV keratinocyte activity was further investigated. Our in vitro bioassay results demonstrated that KWM-EO treatment suppressed PDV cell viability, colony formation ability, and induced G_2/M cell-cycle arrest and cell apoptosis in the presence and absence of PLX4032. KWM-EO also inhibited proinflammatory cell infiltration and papilloma formation in DMBA/TPA-induced two-stage skin carcinogenesis facilitated by PLX4032 in mice.

2. Results

2.1. Chemical Compositions of Mentha aquatica var. Kenting Water Mint Essential Oil

KWM-EO was obtained by hydrodistillation of the aerial parts. The chemical profile of KWM-EO was analyzed by GC×GC-TOF MS. Twenty compounds representing 81.86% of the total content were identified in KWM-EO (Table 1). Monoterpene hydrocarbons accounted for 56.01% of KWM-EO with 22.18% β-ocimene as the most abundant component, and β-pinene and α-pinene accounting for 15.41% and 10.49%, respectively. KWM-EO was identified to contain 15.86% oxygenated monoterpenes, of which eucalyptol (12.87%) was the most abundant.

Table 1. Chemical constituents of KWM-EO determined by GC×GC-TOF MS.

	Chemical Compound	CAS no.[a]	RT1[b]	RT2[c]	KI_{exp}[d]	KI_{Lit}[e]	Relative Percentage (%)
1	α-Pinene	7785-70-8	6.27	0.0245	936	929	10.49
2	β-Pinene	127-91-3	7.00	0.0250	981	973	15.41
3	β-Myrcene	123-35-3	7.20	0.0243	992	993	4.86
4	β-Cymene	535-77-3	7.73	0.0253	1027	1031	3.07
5	Eucalyptol	470-82-6	7.93	0.0258	1040	1041	12.87
6	β-Ocimene	3338-55-4	8.07	0.0245	1049	1036	22.18
7	Linalool	78-70-6	8.87	0.0262	1097	1101	0.25
8	Menthone	89-80-5	9.80	0.0325	1160	1154	0.04

Table 1. Cont.

	Chemical Compound	CAS no.[a]	RT1[b]	RT2[c]	KI$_{exp}$[d]	KI$_{Lit}$[e]	Relative Percentage (%)
9	Menthofuran	494-90-6	9.93	0.0267	1169	1169	0.04
10	Levomenthol	2216-51-5	10.07	0.0277	1178	1172	0.05
11	p-Menth-8-en-2-one	5948-4-9	10.60	0.0330	1213	1218	0.07
12	Carveol	1197-07-5	10.73	0.0272	1222	1223	0.13
13	Carvone	6485-40-1	11.13	0.0327	1251	1249	1.59
14	Linalyl acetate	115-95-7	11.20	0.0270	1256	1257	0.08
15	Dihydroedulan I	63335-66-0	11.87	0.0258	1302	1292	0.28
16	β-Bourbonene	5208-59-3	13.13	0.0250	1396	1386	0.78
17	Caryophyllene	87-44-5	13.60	0.0258	1434	1431	2.80
18	Humulene	6753-98-6	14.00	0.0318	1466	1465	0.29
19	Ethyl 4-ethoxybenzoate	23676-09-7	14.73	0.0302	1524	1521	2.37
20	Viridiflorol	552-02-3	15.73	0.0272	1608	1603	3.47
Monoterpene hydrocarbons identified							56.01
Oxygenated monoterpene identified							15.86
Sesquiterpene hydrocarbon identified							3.87
Oxygenated sesquiterpene identified							3.47
Other							2.56
Identified components							81.86

[a] Chemical abstracts service registry number; [b] Retention time of the first column; [c] Retention time of the second column; [d] KI$_{exp}$ = Kovats indices, retention indices relative to C_7–C_{30} n-alkanes based on the retention time of components separated by the 1st dimension Rtx-5MS column; [e] KI$_{Lit}$: Retention indices reported in the literature.

2.2. KWM-EO Effect on PDV Cell Proliferation, Invasion, and Migration

The PDV cell line is a mouse keratinocyte bearing $HRAS^{Q61L}$ mutation, which is the most relevant mutation in BRAF inhibitor-induced cutaneous squamous cell carcinoma. The PDV cell viability after treatment with 0 to 100 μg/mL KWM-EO was determined by MTT assay. The cell viability was decreased when KWM-EO concentration increased. When the PDV cells were treated with up to 100 μg/mL of KWM-EO for 24 h, the cell viability was inhibited to 53.31% (Figure 1A). The long-term colony formation ability of PDV cells was determined by treating with KWM-EO alone or in the presence of PLX4032 (PLX). The MEK (mitogen-activated protein kinase kinase) inhibitor, selumetinib (AZD6244), was used as a reference control. As shown in Figure 1B, 0.5 μM PLX4032 treatment promoted the colony formation of PDV cells compared to the vehicle-treated cells. In the presence or absence of PLX4032, KWM-EO treatment showed a dose-dependent effect, and KWM-EO treatment at the high dose of 40 μg/mL revealed a better effect than 0.5 μM AZD6244 treatment. PDV cell invasive ability was investigated by Matrigel coated-transwell assay. The result showed that PLX4032 treatment facilitated cell invasion relative to vehicle treatment, and KWM-EO suppressed the invasive ability on concentration-dependence (Figure 1C). In wound healing assay representing cell migratory ability, 2 μM PLX4032 treatment significantly and time-dependently increased cell migration. The migratory ability of PDV cells was restricted by 50 μg/mL KWM-EO treatment with or without PLX4032 stimulation (Figure 1D).

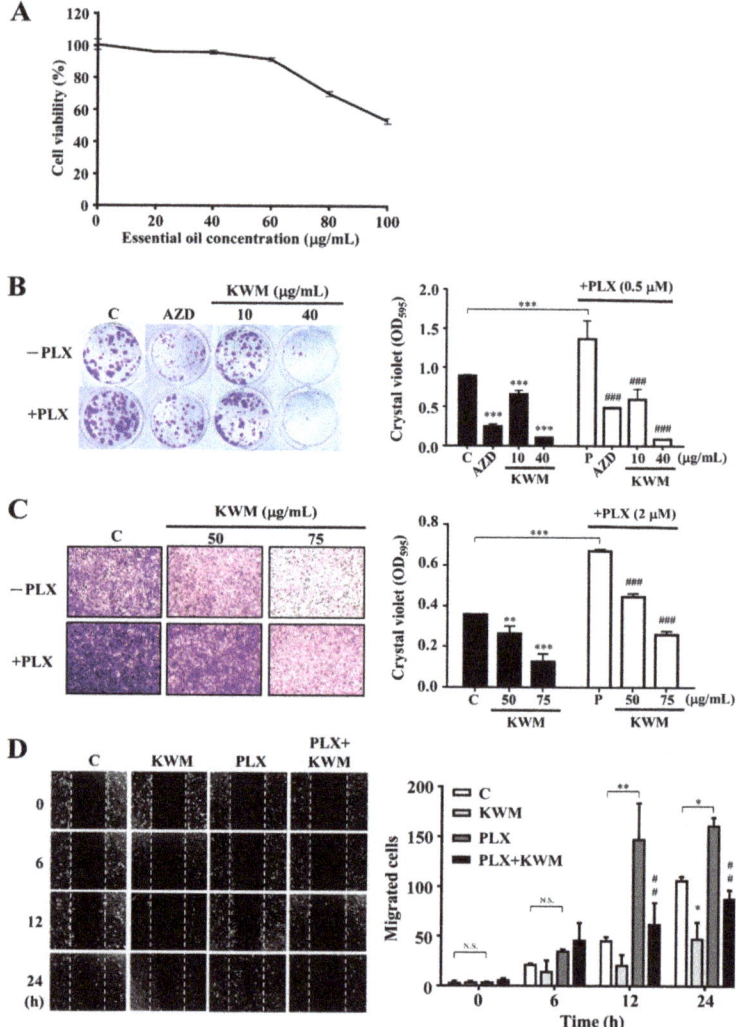

Figure 1. Effect of *Mentha aquatica var. Kenting Water Mint* essential oil (KWM-EO) on PDV cells. (**A**) PDV cells were treated with vehicle or the indicated concentrations of KWM-EO for 24 h. Cell viability (%) was determined by MTT assay. (**B**) PDV cells were incubated with KWM-EO in the presence or absence of 0.5 µM PLX4032 for 6 days, and colony formation was detected by staining cells with crystal violet. (**C**) PDV cells were seeded in Matrigel coated–transwell inserts and incubated with vehicle or KWM-EO in the presence or absence of 2 µM PLX4032 for 24 h. The invasive cells were stained with crystal violet. (**D**) PDV cell migratory ability was examined by wound healing assay. Cells were treated with vehicle or 50 µg/mL KWM-EO in the presence or absence of 2 µM PLX4032, and observed after 0, 6, 12, 24 h. Vehicle controls (C) were obtained from cells treated with 0.5% DMSO. The absorbance at 595 nm was obtained by dissolving crystal violet with 20% acetic acid. The data are representative of three independent experiments and are expressed as mean ± SD. Representative images are shown. $P^* < 0.05$, $P^{**} < 0.01$, $P^{***} < 0.001$ compared to vehicle control; $P^{\#\#} < 0.01$, $P^{\#\#\#} < 0.001$ compared to the PLX4032-treated group (ANOVA). AZD: AZD6244 (MEK inhibitor)

2.3. KWM-EO Induces Cell-Cycle Arrest and Apoptosis in PDV Cells

The KWM-EO effect on the PDV cell-cycle machinery was determined using flow cytometry. The analysis demonstrated that PLX4032 treatment alone had no significant effect on the cell-cycle of PDV cells; however, the cell-cycle profile treated with KWM-EO exhibited G_2/M arrest. After KWM-EO treatment for 24 h, the percentage of cells in the G_2/M phase was raised from 33.0–33.6% to 44.3–45.0%, in the presence or absence of PLX4032 (Figure 2A). According to cell-cycle analysis, an elevated percentage of the sub-G_1 population was also observed with KWM-EO and PLX4032+KWM-EO treatment. Thus cell apoptosis was further examined. Cells were stained with annexin V and propidium iodide and analyzed by flow cytometry. The data demonstrated that treatment with 75 µg/mL KWM-EO strongly induced 86.9% and 80.7% apoptotic cells in the presence or absence of PLX4032, respectively (Figure 2B). Western blotting was further used to explore the protein expression profile related to G_2/M cell-cycle arrest and cell apoptosis. Cyclin B1-cell division cycle protein 2 (cdc2), also known as M-phase promoting factor (MPF), regulates G_2/M transition. Phosphorylation of Thr161 in cdc2 is required for activation of MPF and brings on the onset of mitosis [19]. Treatment with 75 µg/mL KWM-EO for 24 h reduced the protein expression level of cyclin B1 and p-cdc 2 (Thr161), suggesting the inhibition of cell mitosis. Phosphorylation of cdc25C, which is responsible for activation of MPF, was also decreased (Figure 2C). The initiation of apoptotic cell death is needed to activate a group of intracellular cysteine proteases, named caspases. The cleavage of poly(ADP-ribose) polymerase-1 (PARP-1) by caspases is regarded to be a characteristic of cell apoptosis [20]. After treatment with 75 µg/mL KWM-EO for 12 h, both hallmarks of apoptosis, caspase 3 and PARP-1, were cleaved into their activated forms (Figure 2D). Paradoxical MAPK activation is known to be the main reason for cutaneous squamous cell carcinoma induced by BRAF inhibitor in *RAS* mutant cells [21]. KWM-EO (75 µg/mL) treatment for 24 h significantly inhibited ERK and p-ERK expression in PDV cells; while in treatment with 0.5 µM PLX4032, the re-activation of p-MEK and p-ERK was observed, which could be reversed by KWM-EO and MEK inhibitor (Figure 2E).

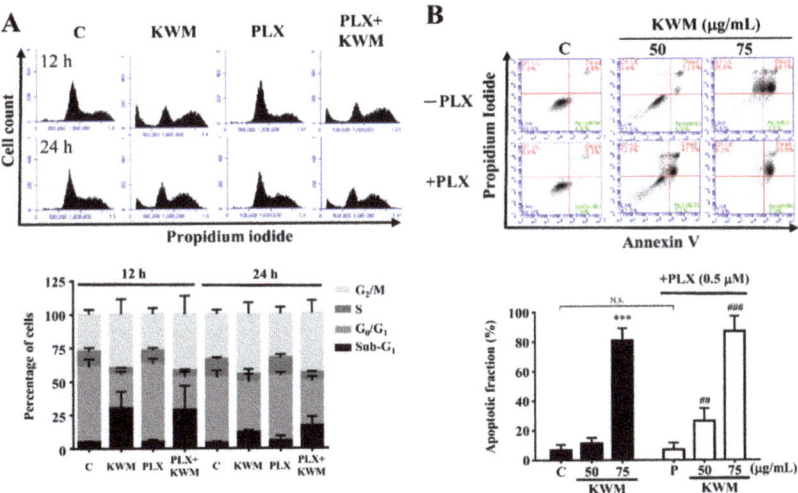

Figure 2. Cont.

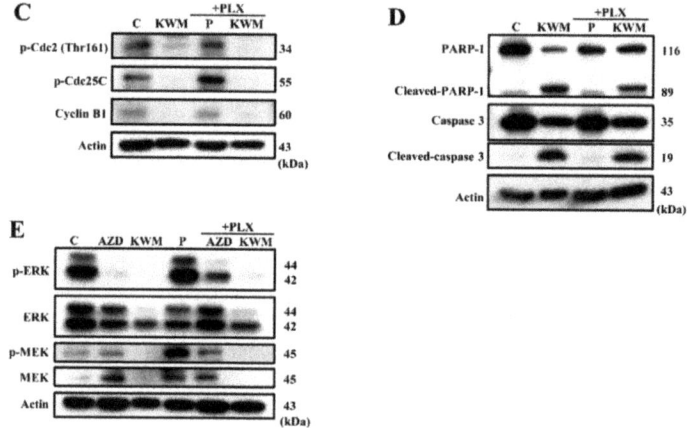

Figure 2. Effect of KWM-EO on cell-cycle and apoptosis in PDV cells. (**A**) PDV cells were exposed to vehicle or 75 μg/mL KWM-EO in the presence or absence of 0.5 μM PLX4032 for 12 or 24 h, then the cell-cycle was analyzed by flow cytometry. (**B**) PDV cells were treated with vehicle or 75 μg/mL KWM-EO in the presence or absence of 0.5 μM PLX4032 for 24 h. Cells were then stained with annexin V and propidium iodide, and the cell apoptosis was detected by flow cytometry. (**C**) PDV cells were treated with 75 μg/mL KWM-EO in the presence or absence of 0.5 μM PLX4032 for 24 h before lysis. The cell lysates were subjected to Western blotting against cell-cycle-related proteins, including p-cdc2 (Thr161), p-cdc25C, and cyclin B1. (**D**) The expression level of apoptosis-related proteins in PDV cells treated with 75 μg/mL KWM-EO in the presence or absence of 0.5 μM PLX4032 for 6 h was examined by Western blotting against PARP-1 and caspase 3. (**E**) Western blotting analysis of MAPK signaling-related proteins (p-ERK, ERK, p-MEK, MEK) in PDV cells treated with 75 μg/mL KWM-EO in the presence or absence of 0.5 μM PLX4032 for 24 h. Actin was used as an internal control in the experiment. Vehicle controls (**C**) were obtained from cells treated with 0.5% DMSO. The data are representative of three independent experiments and are expressed as mean ± SD. N.S. means non significance; $P^{***} < 0.05$ compared to vehicle control; $P^{\#\#} < 0.01$, $P^{\#\#\#} < 0.001$ compared to PLX4032-treated group (ANOVA).

2.4. KWM-EO Inhibits Two-Stage Skin Carcinogenesis in FVB Mice

To investigate the chemopreventive effect of KWM-EO in BRAF inhibitor-induced cutaneous squamous cell carcinoma, a DMBA-initiated and TPA-promoted two-stage skin carcinogenesis model was established, and the study diagram is shown in Supplementary Figure 1. After topical application of 25 μg DMBA and 4 μg TPA (DT) on mouse dorsal skin for 12 weeks, papillomas were successfully induced. If mice were co-treated with 20 mg/kg/BW PLX4032 (DTP), starting at 6 weeks, bigger and more papillomas occurred (Figure 3A). The DT and DTP groups developed papillomas on the skin as early as 5 weeks after TPA treatment. Within 6 to 7 weeks, the tumor incidence in DTP mice was much higher than in DT mice; at 8 weeks, the tumor incidence in the DT and DTP group reached 100%, while KWM-EO treatment delayed and decreased the tumor incidence (Figure 3B). On average, the DT group developed 15.4 papillomas/mouse at 12 weeks, the topical application of 5 mg KWM-EO reduced the average number of papillomas to 7.9/mouse. Under stimulation of PLX4032 in DTP mice, the average number of papillomas was raised to 22.4/mouse which was ameliorated by KWM-EO to 9.1 papillomas/mouse at 12 weeks ($P < 0.05$) (Figure 3C). The dot histogram shows the distribution of papilloma number per mouse and the median in a group (Figure 3D). The papilloma number was significantly decreased by KWM-EO treatment in DTP mice. Mouse body weights were recorded every week during the experimental period, and the results show that the body weights in all treated mice were similar to the sham control mice (Supplementary Figure 2). To examine the toxicology of these applied compounds and essential oil, mouse organ index was calculated, and H&E staining was executed to observe the organ structure and pathology. The mouse organ index was unchanged for the heart, lung, and kidney within the groups; however, the index of the liver organ was lower in the KWM-EO-treated mice, and the index of the spleen organ was increased in PLX4032-treated mice. The H&E staining result on the organs showed that there were no observable differences between the sham and all the treatment groups (Figure 3F).

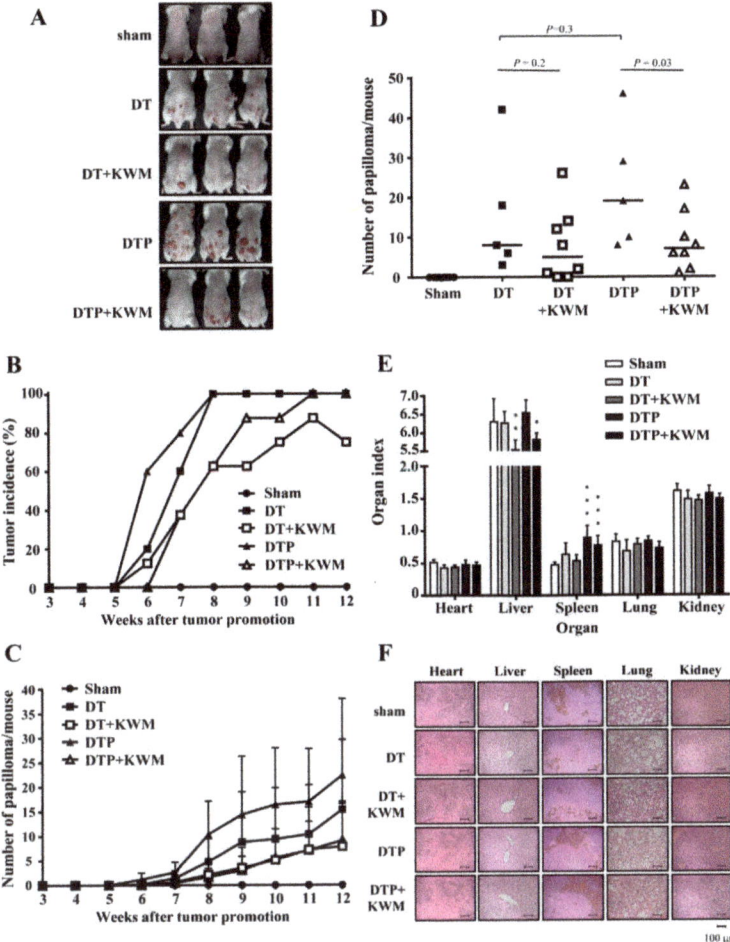

Figure 3. Effect of KWM-EO on two-stage skin carcinogenesis in mice. (**A**) Representative images of mice from each group at week 12 are shown. Tumor incidence (**B**) and mean number of papillomas (**C**) per group during the experimental period are calculated. (**D**) Papilloma numbers per mouse at week 12 are shown in the dot histogram. (**E**) Organ weights were recorded after mice were sacrificed at week 12. Organ index was calculated by the following formula: $organ\ index = (organ\ weight \div body\ weight) \times 100$ empty. $P* < 0.05$, $P** < 0.01$, $P*** < 0.001$ compared to sham group (ANOVA). (**F**) Organ tissues were detected by H&E staining. The DT and DTP groups consisted of 5 mice each. Sham, the DT+KWM, and DTP+KWM groups consisted of 8 mice each. The data are presented as mean ± SD. D: DMBA, T: TPA, P: PLX4032. Scale bar: 100 μm.

2.5. Skin Histology and Epidermal Cell Proliferation in KWM-EO-Treated Mice

Effect of topically applied KWM-EO on chemically induced skin tumorigenesis was further observed by skin histologic changes. The skin structure was first examined by H&E staining. With DMBA and TPA treatment in the presence or absence of PLX4032, the thickness of the epidermis was elevated compared to the sham group (Figure 4A), while the epidermal hyperplasia was attenuated by repeated treatment with KWM-EO for 12 weeks. The main cell type responsible for hyper-proliferative epidermis was further explored by immunofluorescent staining. Ki67 is a representative marker of cell proliferation, and cytokeratin 14 (K14) is the intermediate filament protein of basal keratinocytes. From the microphotographs, the expression level of ki67 showed remarkable upregulation in the DT and DTP group. After merging both ki67 and K14 staining with DAPI, the hyperplasia of the epidermis arising from basal keratinocytes was seen which was alleviated by KWM-EO topical treatment (Figure 4B). In addition, the paradoxical MAPK activation that could lead to cell proliferation in *RAS* mutant cells treated with BRAF inhibitors was also investigated. The IHC staining result revealed considerable p-ERK protein between the dermis and papilloma, especially in the group with PLX4032 stimulation; and this activation was significantly diminished by KWM-EO treatment (Figure 4C).

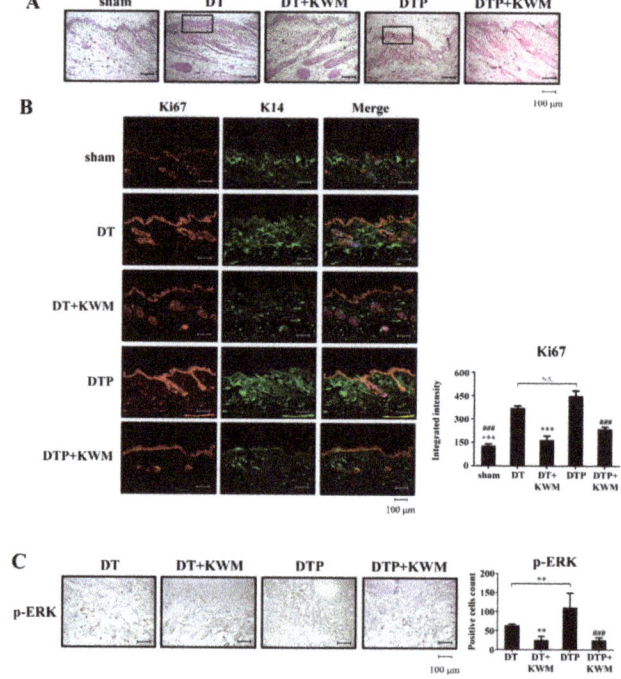

Figure 4. Effect of KWM-EO on skin and papilloma tissue from mice. (**A**) Skin morphology was examined by H&E staining. (**B**) Abnormal epidermal proliferation was detected by immunofluorescent staining of ki67 (red). Basal keratinocytes were stained with K14 (green), and nuclei were stained with DAPI (blue). (**C**) Histological images of papilloma indicated the paradoxical activation of p-ERK. Representative images are shown. The data are representative of three independent experiments and are expressed as mean ± SD. N.S. means non significance; $P^{**} < 0.01$, $P^{***} < 0.001$ compared to DT group; $P^{\#\#\#} < 0.001$ compared to DTP group (ANOVA). Scale bar: 100 µm.

2.6. Anti-Inflammatory Effect of KWM-EO

Inflammation is a vital element in the progression of two-stage skin carcinogenesis. COX-2, a pro-inflammatory enzyme commonly observed in inflamed cells or tissues was counter-stained with pro-inflammatory immune cells, neutrophils (neutrophil elastase+) and macrophages (F4/80+). The overexpression of COX-2 was increased in both DT and DTP mouse dorsal skin. Interestingly, most of the COX-2 proteins were observed colocalized with infiltrated neutrophils, but not macrophages (Figure 5A,B). Upon treatment with KWM-EO, the neutrophil and macrophage infiltration and upregulation of COX-2 were alleviated (Figure 5A,B).

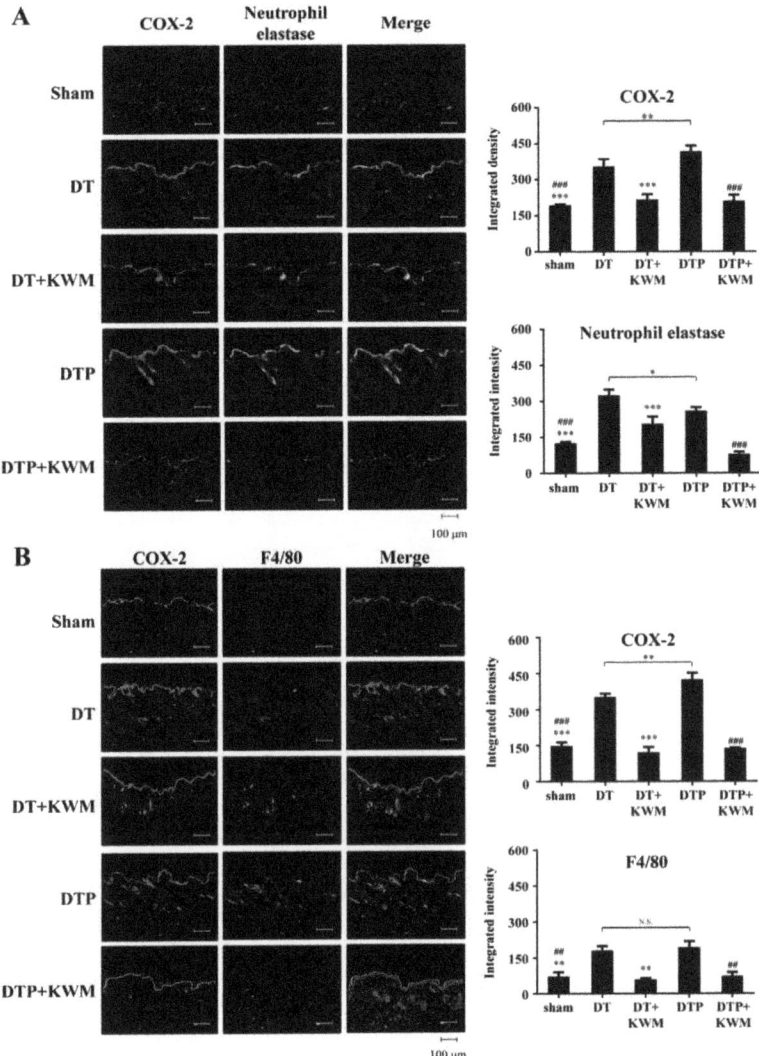

Figure 5. Effect of KWM-EO on the inflammatory immune system in skin tissue from the mice two-stage skin carcinogenesis. Immunofluorescent staining of inflammatory mediator COX-2 (red) with neutrophil elastase (green) (**A**) and macrophage marker, F4/80 (green) (**B**). Nuclei were counterstained with DAPI (blue). Representative images are shown. The data are representative of three independent experiments and are expressed as mean ± SD. N.S. means non significance; $P^* < 0.05$, $P^{**} < 0.01$, $P^{***} < 0.001$ compared to DT group; $P^{\#\#} < 0.01$, $P^{\#\#\#} < 0.001$ compared to DTP group (ANOVA). Scale bar: 100 µm.

3. Discussion

EOs have been utilized as fragrances, food flavorings, and folk medicines, among other applications throughout human history. In recent decades, a large number of studies have reported chemical constituent analysis of EOs and investigated their bio-efficacy and the responsible bioactive compounds. EOs from *Mentha* species have been reported to have anti-inflammatory, anti-oxidant, anti-fungal, and anti-bacterial activities [14–18]. The ethanolic extract of *Mentha×piperita* L., a cross-species of watermint and spearmint, at 50 and 100 µg/mL, suppressed LPS-induced nitric oxide production in macrophages by 18.85% and 41.88% inhibition, respectively [22]. Anti-cancer cell activity has also been reported for mint EOs. For example, *Mentha×piperita* L. extract showed more potent activity against proliferative activity of human MDA-MB-231 breast cancer cells (cell inhibition ratio = 46.53% at 150 µg/mL) than human A375 melanoma cells (cell inhibition ratio = 25.08% at 150 µg/mL) [14]. This study is the first to investigate and observe that KWM-EO can prevent two-stage skin carcinogenesis chemically induced by DMBA/TPA and its acceleration by BRAF inhibitor drug PLX4032. The two-stage skin carcinogenesis mouse model established by DMBA and TPA irritation is considered to be a representative study system through which to explore the pathology and underlying mechanisms of human squamous cell carcinomas [23]. It has also been used to evaluate the BRAF^{V600E} inhibitor drugs, such as vemurafenib-induced cutaneous side-effects, including SCC and KA in patients [3]. We, thus, established this two-stage skin carcinogenesis mouse model, and the bioactivities of KWM-EO were examined. Our results indicated that KWM-EO treatment significantly inhibited papilloma incidence and number in DT and DTP mice. According to the histopathological analysis of skin tissue sections, KWM-EO not only attenuated the abnormal proliferation and hyperplasia of the epidermis but also decreased the inflammatory neutrophil and macrophage infiltration and COX-2 overexpression in neutrophils. Moreover, this study is the first to observe that abnormal epidermis proliferation in DT and DTP mice was mainly contributed by keratinocytes as a co-positively stained marker protein K14 and proliferation marker ki67. Topical administration of KWM-EO can reverse the over proliferation of K14 keratinocytes in DT- or DTP-irritated mouse skins.

A previous review article published by Pandey et al. [24] summarized that EOs of some *Ocimum* species exhibited anti-inflammatory and anti-cancerous properties which contain pinene, β-ocimene, and linalool, the chemical constituents present in KWM-EO. α-Pinene present in KWM-EO by 10.49% was reported to induce cell apoptosis and disrupt mitochondrial potential in B16F10 cells, and it also effectively reduced melanoma lung metastasis [25]. β-Caryophyllene accounted for 2.8% in KWM-EO was a major compound in the EO of *P. missionis*. Pavithra et al. demonstrated that EO from *P. missionis* induced cell death through intrinsic mitochondrial and extrinsic apoptotic pathways in A431 and HaCaT cells [26]. The results from these studies might potentially support part of our observations for the anti-inflammatory and chemopreventive activities of KWM-EO against two-stage skin carcinogenesis.

PDV keratinocytes harboring *HRAS* mutation are commonly found in DT-induced mouse SCC [27]. We adapted this cell model to investigate the in vitro effect and modes of action of KWM-EO. Our data revealed that KWM-EO treatment significantly diminished PDV cell colony formation ability and suppressed reactivation of MEK-ERK signaling stimulated by PLX4032. The PDV cell invasive and migratory abilities were promoted by PLX4032, which were suppressed by KWM-EO treatment. KWM-EO also induced G_2/M arrest in PDV cells through deregulating p-cdc2, p-cdc25C, and cyclin B1 proteins. The cell apoptosis induced by KWM-EO was through activation of caspase 3 and PARP-1 after cells were treated for 6 h. These in vitro data support in part the inhibitory activity of KWM-EO in the DT and DTP mouse skin on keratinocyte proliferation and papilloma formation.

In an open-label phase 2 study using a combination of BRAF inhibitor dabrafenib and MEK inhibitor trametinib in patients, the rate of skin lesions was not significantly reduced although a slight decrease in proliferative skin lesions was observed [28]. A previous study revealed that tumor multiplicity and incidence of skin tumors in DT-induced two-stage skin carcinogenesis accelerated by BRAF inhibitor was decreased when a COX-2 inhibitor celecoxib was orally administered [29]. Our current data show that topical application of KWM-EO attenuated the formation of cutaneous papilloma in mice induced by DMBA/TPA or by DMBA/TPA/PLX4032. The paradoxical MAPK activation induced by PLX4032 in vitro in PDV keratinocytes and in skin of DT and DTP mice was suppressed by KWM-EO. Taken together, the results of this study demonstrate the novel chemopreventive activity of the essential oil of *Mentha aquatica var. citrata Kenting Water Mint* which can be potentially used in preventing BRAF inhibitor drug-induced cutaneous side-effects in cancer patients.

4. Materials and Methods

4.1. Mint Cultivation and Distillation of Essential Oils

A variety of *Mentha aquatica* (Lamiaceae), named *M. aquatica var. Kenting Water Mint* was cultivated in an experimental field at the Taichung District Agricultural Research and Extension Station, Taichung, Taiwan for 2 years. Mature shoots were harvested and subjected to water vapor distillation to collect essential oils. Two kilograms of fresh shoots were distilled with 4 L of water. Mint essential oil was evaporated, passed through a condenser then the oil and hydrosol were collected with a separating funnel. After 1 L of the hydrosol/essential oils were collected, the distillation ended. The hydrosol and essential oil were then separately collected for use in the following experiments. The mint essential oils were stored at −20 °C in sealed vials. Essential oils used in in vitro cell-based assays were diluted into different concentrations with DMSO and those used in in vivo animal studies were diluted in acetone.

4.2. Chemical Profiling of KWM-EO Composition by GC×GC–TOF MS

The samples were analyzed using LECO Pegasus 4D GC×GC–TOF MS (St Joseph, MI, USA). The first dimension capillary column was Restek Rtx-5MS (30 m × 0.25 mm × 0.25 μm) and the second capillary column was Restek Rtx-200 (2 m × 0.25 mm × 0.25 μm). The GC temperature program was set as follows: injection temperature: 280 °C; oven temperature: 40 °C maintained for 1 min, and increased at a rate of 10 °C/min to 310 °C and held constant for 8 min. The helium flow rate was set at 1 mL/min. The mass spectrometry temperature was set at 320 °C. The ion source temperature was 200 °C, and the analysis mass range was 50-800 m/z. KWM-EO was ran in hexane with a dilution of 1 mg/mL. Hexadecane solution, 64.25 μg/mL, was used as an internal standard to monitor the shift of retention time. Compounds were identified by matching the mass spectra fragmentation patterns, and the results were compared with LECO/Fiehn and Wiley Registry 9th Edition mass spectral library and NIST. Linear Kovats index of n-alkanes (C_7-C_{40}, C_7-C_{30}) were calculated for each compound and compared with the literature to identify the compound ID [30].

4.3. Cell Lines and Cell Culture

PDV cells, which harbor the $HRAS^{Q61L}$ mutation were obtained from CLS Cell Lines Service (Eppelheim, Germany). Cells were cultured at 37 °C in DMEM supplemented with 10% FBS, containing 100 units/mL penicillin and 100 μg/mL streptomycin in a humidified 5% CO_2 incubator. Cells were used within 10 passages for this study.

4.4. Measurement of Cell Viability

Cells (5×10^3 cells/well in 96-well plates) were treated with vehicle (0.5% DMSO) or 20, 40, 60, 80, and 100 μg/mL KWM-EO for 24 h. Cell viability was determined by 3-(4,5-Dimethylthiazol-2-yl)-2,5-diphenyl tetrazolium bromide (MTT)-based colorimetric assays according to Scudiero et al. [31]. The viability of the cells treated with vehicle-only was defined as 100% viable. The viability of the cells after treatment with KWM-EO was calculated using the following formula: cell viability (%) = $\left[OD_{570 \text{ (treated cells)}} \div OD_{570 \text{ [vehicle control]}} \right] \times 100$ empty. The data are presented by three independent experiments with six replicates per experiment.

4.5. Colony Formation Assay

Colony formation was obtained by growing PDV cells (250 cells/well in 24-well plates) treated with 10 and 40 μg/mL KWM-EO in the presence or absence of 0.5 μM PLX4032 for 6 days. The culture medium was refreshed once on day 3. Cells were fixed with chilled methanol and stained with 0.1% crystal violet. Cells retaining crystal violet were dissolved with 20% acetic acid and quantified by measuring absorbance at 595 nm [32]. The data are presented by three independent experiments with three replicates per experiment.

4.6. Cell Invasion Assay

The cell invasion assay was performed by Millicell Cell Culture Inserts (Merck Millipore, United States). For invasion assay, 100 μL Matrigel (300 μg/mL) was applied to an 8-mm polycarbonate membrane filter and incubated in 37 °C for 2 h. PDV cells (5×10^4) were seeded to Matrigel-coated filters in 200 μL of serum-free medium in triplicate for 16 h. The bottom chamber of the apparatus contained 1 mL medium with 10% FBS as a chemoattractant and 50 and 75 μg/mL KWM-EO, in the presence or absence of 2 μM PLX4032. Cells were allowed to migrate for 24 h at 37 °C. After incubation for 24 h, the non-migrated cells on the apical side of the membrane were removed with cotton swabs. The migrated cells on the basal side of the membrane were fixed with cold 100% methanol for 20 min and washed 3 times with PBS. The cells were stained with 0.1% crystal violet and then washed with PBS to remove extra dye solution. Images were captured using a reverse-phase microscope (Zeiss Axiovert 200M). Cells retaining crystal violet were dissolved with 20% acetic acid and quantified by measuring absorbance at 595 nm. The data are presented by three independent experiments with three replicates per experiment.

4.7. Wound Healing Assay

The wound healing assay was performed by using Culture-Insert (ibidi GmbH, Germany). Culture-Inserts were inserted in 24-well plates before cells were seeded. PDV cells were seeded in Culture-Inserts at a density of 5×10^5 cells/mL in 70 μL medium. After 16 h, Culture-Inserts were removed which created two cell-free gaps of 500 ± 50 μm. Undetached cells were washed away by PBS, then the remaining attached cells were immersed in 1 mL medium with 50 μg/mL KWM-EO, in the presence or absence of 2 μM PLX4032. Cell migration was observed using a reverse-phase microscope (Zeiss Observer D1) every 6 h. The data are presented by three independent experiments with three replicates per experiment.

4.8. Cell-Cycle Analysis

PDV cells were seeded in 6-well plates at a density of 1×10^5 cells/well with respective medium containing 10% FBS for 16 h. To synchronize the cell-cycle, cells were washed with PBS and incubated with fresh medium containing 5% FBS for 8 h, followed by washing with PBS and incubation with fresh medium containing 0.5% FBS for 24 h. The synchronized PDV cells were then treated with 75 μg/mL KWM-EO, 0.5 μM PLX4032, and 0.5 μM PLX4032+75 μg/mL KWM-EO in the medium containing 10% FBS for 12 and 24 h. Both adherent and floating cells were collected, washed with PBS, and fixed with 500 μL ice-cold 70% ethanol overnight at 4 °C. Cells were stained with 500 μL propidium iodide (PI) solution, which contained 20 μg/mL PI, 20 μg/mL RNase A, 0.1% Triton X-100 for 30 min at room temperature in the dark and then analyzed by flow cytometry (Flow cytometry BD Accuri C6, United States).

4.9. Apoptosis Assay

Cells were seeded in 6-well plates at a density of 1.5×10^5 cells/well for 16 h and then treated with 75 μg/mL KWM-EO, 0.5 μM PLX4032, and 0.5 μM PLX4032+75 μg/mL KWM-EO. After 24 h, both adherent and floating cells were collected and washed with PBS. Apoptotic cells were analyzed by using FITC Annexin V Apoptosis Detection Kit (BD Bioscience, United States) according to the manufacturer's instructions.

4.10. Western Blot Analysis

Cells were treated with KWM-EO at the indicated concentrations in the presence or absence of PLX4032 and lysed in RIPA lysis buffer. Protein concentrations were measured by *DC* protein assay (Bio-Rad, United States). Western blotting was performed as described by Shyur et al. [33]. Primary antibodies ERK 1, cyclin B1, p-cdc2 p34, p-cdc25C, and PARP-1 were purchased from Santa Cruz (Texas, United States). Antibodies phospho-p44/42 MAPK (Erk1/2), MEK1/2, and phospho-MEK1/2 were purchased from Cell Signaling Technology (Massachusetts, United States). Caspase 3 antibody was purchased from GeneTex (Texas, United States).

4.11. Two-Stage Skin Carcinogenesis Study

Female FVB/NJNarl mice (5–6 weeks old) were purchased from the National Laboratory Animal Center (Taipei, Taiwan) and bred in the Laboratory Animal Core Facility (Agricultural Biotechnology Research Center, Academia Sinica, Taiwan). Animals were given a standard laboratory diet and distilled H_2O *ad libitum* and kept on a 12-h light/dark cycle at 22 ± 2 °C with humidity 55 ± 5%. All experimental protocols were approved by the Institutional Animal Care and Utilization Committee (IACUC: Protocol #18-08-1221), Academia Sinica, Taiwan. Mice were randomized and had their back hair shaved three days before topical application of 25 μg DMBA in 200 μL acetone. The first week after tumor initiation, 4 μg of TPA in 200 μL acetone was topically applied twice a week to the shaved dorsal skin for 12 weeks [5]. Mice were treated with the indicated concentration of KWM-EO (in 200 μL acetone) twice a week by topical application the day after TPA treatment for 12 weeks (Supplementary Figure 1). Tumor size of more than 1 mm diameter was counted every week.

4.12. Histopathological and Immunohistochemical Analysis

Tissues were fixed with 10% formalin, hydrated, and embedded in paraffin. Tissue sections were cut at 4 μm thickness, then deparaffinized following rehydration in a descendant ethanol bath. H&E staining, immunohistochemistry, and immunofluorescent staining followed the previously published protocols [30]. An upright microscope (Carl Zeiss Axio Imager, Z1) was used to observe the expression of targeted proteins. Primary antibodies cytokeratin 14 and CD163 were purchased from Proteintech (Illinois, United States). Ki67 and neutrophil elastase were purchased from Abcam (Cambridge, United Kingdom). Antibody against COX-2 was purchased from Cayman (Michigan, United States). Antibody against F4/80 was purchased from Biolegend (California, United States). Antibody against iNOS was purchased from BD transduction Laboratories (California, United States).

4.13. Statistical Analysis

All the data are expressed as mean ± standard deviation (SD). Statistical analyses were conducted by the Predictive Analysis Suite Workstation (PASW Statistics, United States), and the significant difference between different treatment groups was determined by analysis of variance (ANOVA). *P* values of less than 0.05 were considered statistically significant.

5. Conclusions

This study is the first to prove that KWM-EO has potential for prevention of chemically induced two-stage skin carcinogenesis. Topical application of KWM-EO significantly attenuated the number of papillomas in DMBA-initiated and TPA-promoted mouse skin, with or without co-stimulation with PLX4032. KWM-EO suppressed epidermal hyperplasia and over proliferation of keratinocytes in DMBA/TPA and DMBA/TPA/PLX4032 mice. Notably, KWM-EO treatment diminished MAPK pathway reactivation, pro-inflammatory immune cell infiltration, and COX-2 expression in both DMBA/TPA and DMBA/TPA/PLX4032 mouse skin tissues. Overall, the results in this study provide strong support for the development of KWM-EO into chemopreventive agents for squamous cell carcinoma patients or cancer patients taking BRAF inhibitor therapy.

Supplementary Materials: The following are available online at http://www.mdpi.com/1420-3049/24/12/2344/s1, Supplementary Materials Figure 1: The experimental design of two-stage skin carcinogenesis mouse model, Supplementary Materials Figure 2: Mouse body weights recorded every week.

Author Contributions: Conceptualization, L.-F.S.; methodology, L.-F.S., C.-T.C., Y.-H.C. and W.-N.S.; validation, C.-T.C. and L.-F.S.; formal analysis, C.-T.C., W.-N.S. and L.-F.S.; investigation, C.-T.C., W.-N.S., Y.-H.C. and L.-F.S.; resources, L.-F.S.; data curation, C.-T.C. and L.-F.S.; writing—original draft preparation, C.-T.C. and L.-F.S.; writing—review and editing, C.-T.C. and L.-F.S.; visualization, C.-T.C. and L.-F.S.; supervision, L.-F.S.; project administration, L.-F.S.; funding acquisition, L.-F.S.

Funding: This research was funded by an institutional grant from the Agricultural Biotechnology Research Center, Academia Sinica, Taiwan.

Acknowledgments: The authors thank the Metabolomics Core Facility and the Laboratory Animal Facility of Agricultural Biotechnology Research Center, Academia Sinica, Taiwan for their services, and Ms. Miranda Loney, Agricultural Biotechnology Research Center English Editor's Office, Academia Sinica, Taiwan, for English editorial assistance.

Conflicts of Interest: The authors declare no conflict of interest.

References

1. Sosman, J.A.; Kim, K.B.; Schuchter, L.; Gonzalez, R.; Pavlick, A.C.; Weber, J.S.; McArthur, G.A.; Hutson, T.E.; Moschos, S.J.; Flaherty, K.T.; et al. Survial in BRAF V600-mutant advanced melanoma treated vemurafenib. *N. Engl. J. Med.* **2012**, *366*, 707–714. [CrossRef] [PubMed]
2. Gibney, G.T.; Messina, J.L.; Fedorenko, I.V.; Sondak, V.K.; Smalley, K.S.M. Paradoxical oncogenesis-the long-term effects of BRAF inhibition in melanoma. *Nat. Rev. Clin. Oncol.* **2013**, *10*, 390–399. [CrossRef] [PubMed]
3. Zhang, C.; Spevak, W.; Zhang, Y.; Burton, E.A.; Ma, Y.; Habets, G.; Zhang, J.; Lin, J.; Ewing, T.; Matusow, B.; et al. RAF inhibitors that evade paradoxical MAPK pathway activation. *Nature* **2015**, *526*, 583–586. [CrossRef] [PubMed]
4. Doma, E.; Rupp, C.; Varga, A.; Kern, F.; Riegler, B.; Baccarini, M. Skin tumorigenesis stimulated by Raf inhibitors relies upon Raf functions that are dependent and independent of ERK. *Cancer Res.* **2013**, *73*, 6926–6937. [CrossRef] [PubMed]
5. Su, F.; Viros, A.; Milagre, C.; Trunzer, K.; Bollag, G.; Splesis, O.; Reis-Filho, J.S.; Kong, X.; Koya, R.C.; Flasherty, K.T.; et al. RAS mutations in cutaneous squamous-cell carcinomas in patients treated with BRAF inhibitors. *N. Engl. J. Med.* **2012**, *366*, 207–215. [CrossRef] [PubMed]
6. Caulín, C.; Bauluz, C.; Gandarillas, A.; Cano, A.; Quintanilla, M. Changes in keratin expression during malignant progression of transformed mouse epidermal keratinocytes. *Exp. Cell Res.* **1993**, *204*, 11–21. [CrossRef]
7. Abel, E.L.; Angel, J.M; Kiguchi, K.; DiGiovanni, J. Multi-stage chemical carcinogenesis in mouse skin: Fundamentals and applications. *Nat. Protoc.* **2009**, *4*, 1350–1362. [CrossRef]
8. Thomas, G.; Tuk, B.; Song, J.Y.; Truong, H.; Gerritsen, H.C.; Gruijl, F.R.D.; Sterenborg, H.J. Studying skin tumourigenesis and progression in immunocompetent hairless SKH1-h mice using chronic 7,12-dimethylbenz(a)anthracene topical applications to develop a useful experimental skin cancer model. *Lab. Anim.* **2017**, *51*, 24–35. [CrossRef]
9. Gonda, T.A.; Tu, S.; Wang, T.C. Chronic inflammation, the tumor microenvironment and carcinogenesis. *Cell Cycle* **2014**, *8*, 2005–2013. [CrossRef]
10. Korniluk, A.; Koper, O.; Kemona, H.; Dymicka-Piekarska, D. From inflammation to cancer. *Ir. J. Med. Sci.* **2017**, *186*, 57–62. [CrossRef]
11. Mantovani, A.; Allavena, P.; Sica, A.; Balkwill, F. Cancer-related inflammation. *Nature* **2008**, *454*, 436–444. [CrossRef] [PubMed]
12. Pollard, J.W. Trophic macrophages in development and disease. *Nat. Rev. Immunol.* **2009**, *9*, 259–270. [CrossRef] [PubMed]
13. Weber, C.; Telerman, S.B.; Reimer, A.S.; Sequeira, I.; Liakath-Ali, K.; Arwert, E.N.; Watt, F.M. Macrophage infiltration and alternative activation during wound healing promote MEK1-induced skin carcinogenesis. *Cancer Res.* **2016**, *76*, 805–817. [CrossRef] [PubMed]
14. Alexa, E.; Dauciu, C.; Radulov, I.; Obistioiu, D.; Sumalan, R.M.; Morar, A.; Dehelean, C.A. Phytochemical screening and biological activity of *Mentha x piperita* L. and Lavandula angustifolia Mill. Extracts. *Anal. Cell Pathol.* **2018**. [CrossRef] [PubMed]

15. Ogaly, H.A.; Eltablawy, N.A.; Abd-Elsalam, R.M. Antifibrogenic influence of *Mentha piperita* L. essential oil against CCl4-induced liver fibrosis in rats. *Oxid. Med. Cell Longev.* **2018**. [CrossRef]
16. Tsai, M.L.; Wu, C.T.; Lin, T.F.; Lin, W.C.; Huang, Y.C.; Yang, C.H. Chemical composition and biological properties of essential oils of two mint species. *Trop. J. Pharm. Res.* **2013**, *12*, 577–582. [CrossRef]
17. Bouyahya, A.; Et-Touys, A.; Bakri, Y.; Talbaui, A.; Fellah, H.; Abrini, J.; Dakka, N. Chemical composition of Mentha pulegium and Rosmarinus officinalis essential oils and their antileishmanial, antibacterial and antioxidant activities. *Microb. Pathog.* **2017**, *111*, 41–49. [CrossRef]
18. Zu, Y.; Yu, H.; Liang, L.; Fu, Y.; Efferth, T.; Liu, X.; Wu, N. Activities of ten essential oils towards *Propionibacterium acnes* and PC-3, A-549 and MCF-7 cancer cells. *Molecules* **2010**, *15*, 3200–3210. [CrossRef]
19. Hara, M.; Abe, Y.; Tanaka, T.; Yamamto, T.; Okumura, E.; Kishimoto, T. Greatwall kinase and cyclin B-Cdk1 are both critical constituents of M-phase-promoting factor. *Nat. Commun.* **2012**, *3*, 1059–1067. [CrossRef]
20. Gray, D.C.; Mahrus, S.; Wells, J.A. Activation of specific apoptotic caspases with an engineered small-molecule-activated protease. *Cell* **2010**, *142*, 637–646. [CrossRef]
21. Hall-Jackson, C.A; Eyers, P.A; Cohen, P.; Goedert, M.; Boyle, F.T.; Hewitt, N.; Plant, H.; Hedge, P. Paradoxical activation of Raf by a novel Raf inhibitor. *Chem. Biol.* **1999**, *6*, 559–568. [CrossRef]
22. Li, Y.X.; Liu, Y.B.; Ma, A.Q.; Bao, Y.; Wang, M.; Sun, Z.L. In vitro antiviral, anti-inflammatory, and antioxidant activities of the ethanol extract of *Mentha piperita* L. *Food Sci. Biotechnol.* **2017**, *26*, 1675–1683. [CrossRef] [PubMed]
23. Neagu, M.; Caruntu, C.; Constantin, C.; Boda, D.; Zurac, S.; Spandidos, D.A.; Tsatsakis, A.M. Chemically induced skin carcinogenesis: Updates in experimental models (Review). *Oncol. Rep.* **2016**, *35*, 2516–2528. [CrossRef] [PubMed]
24. Pandey, A.K.; Singh, P.; Tripathi, N.N. Chemistry and bioactivities of essential oils of some *Ocimum* species: An overview. *Asian Pac. J. Trop. Biomed.* **2014**, *4*, 682–694. [CrossRef]
25. Matsuo, A.L.; Figueiredo, C.R.; Arruda, D.C.; Pereira, F.V.; Scutti, J.A.B.; Massaoka, M.H.; Travassos, L.R.; Sartorelli, P.; Lago, J.H.G. α-Pinene isolated from Schinus terebinthifolius Raddi (Anacardiaceae) induces apoptosis and confers antimetastatic protection in a melanoma model. *Biochem. Biophys. Res. Commun.* **2011**, *411*, 449–454. [CrossRef] [PubMed]
26. Pavithra, P.S.; Mehta, A.; Verma, R.S. Induction of apoptosis by essential oil from *P. missionis* in skin epidermoid cancer cells. *Phytomedicine* **2018**, *50*, 184–195. [PubMed]
27. Katsanakis, K.D.; Gorgoulis, V.; Papavassiliou, A.G.; Zoumpourlis, V.K. The progression in the mouse skin carcinogenesis model correlates. *Mol. Med.* **2002**, *8*, 624–637. [CrossRef] [PubMed]
28. Flaherty, K.T.; Infante, J.R.; Daud, A.; Gonzalez, R.; Kefford, R.F.; Sosman, J.; Hamid, O.; Schuchter, L.; Cebon, J.; Ibrahim, N. Combined BRAF and MEK inhibition in melanoma with BRAF V600 mutations. *N. Engl. J. Med.* **2012**, *367*, 1694–1703. [CrossRef]
29. Escuin-Ordinas, H.; Atefi, M.; Fu, Y.; Cass, A.; Ng, C.; Huang, R.R.; Yashar, S.; Comin-Anduix, B.; Avramis, E.; Cochran, A.J.; et al. COX-2 inhibition prevents the appearance of cutaneous squamous cell carcinomas accelerated by BRAF inhibitors. *Mol. Oncol.* **2014**, *8*, 250–260. [CrossRef]
30. Schomburg, G.; Dielmann, G. Identification by means of retention parameters. *J. Chromatogr. Sci.* **1973**, *11*, 151–159. [CrossRef]
31. Scudiero, D.A.; Shoemaker, R.H.; Paull, K.D.; Monks, A.; Tierney, S.; Nofziger, T.H.; Currens, M.J.; Seniff, D.; Boyd, M.R. Evaluation of soluble tetrazolium/formazon assay for cell growth sensitivity in culture using human and other tumor cell lines. *Cancer Res.* **1988**, *48*, 4827–4833. [PubMed]
32. Franken, N.A.P.; Rodermond, H.M.; Stap, J.; Haveman, J.; Bree, C.V. Clonogenic assay of cells in vitro. *Nat. Protoc.* **2006**, *1*, 2315–2319. [CrossRef] [PubMed]
33. Apaya, M.K.; Lin, C.Y.; Chiou, C.Y.; Yang, C.C.; Ting, C.Y.; Shyur, L.F. Simvastatin and a plant galactolipid protect animals from septic shock by regulating oxylipin mediator dynamics through the MAPK-cPLA$_2$ signaling pathway. *Mol. Med.* **2016**, *21*, 988–1001. [CrossRef] [PubMed]

Sample Availability: Samples of the compounds are available from the authors.

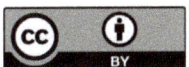

© 2019 by the authors. Licensee MDPI, Basel, Switzerland. This article is an open access article distributed under the terms and conditions of the Creative Commons Attribution (CC BY) license (http://creativecommons.org/licenses/by/4.0/).

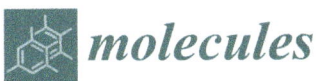

Article

Synthesis and Cytotoxicity Evaluation of DOTA-Conjugates of Ursolic Acid

Michael Kahnt [1], Sophie Hoenke [1], Lucie Fischer [1], Ahmed Al-Harrasi [2] and René Csuk [1,*]

[1] Organic Chemistry, Martin-Luther-University Halle-Wittenberg, Kurt-Mothes-Str. 2, D-06120 Halle (Saale), Germany; michael.kahnt@chemie.uni-halle.de (M.K.); sophie.hoenke@chemie.uni-halle.de (S.H.); lucie.fischer2018@gmx.de (L.F.)

[2] Natural and Medical Sciences Research Center, University of Nizwa, PO Box 33, Birkat Al-Mauz, Nizwa 616, Oman; aharrasi@unizwa.edu.om

[*] Correspondence: rene.csuk@chemie.uni-halle.de; Tel.: +49-345-55-25660

Academic Editor: Kyoko Nakagawa-Goto
Received: 12 May 2019; Accepted: 14 June 2019; Published: 17 June 2019

Abstract: In this study, we report the synthesis of several amine-spacered conjugates of ursolic acid (UA) and 1,4,7,10-tetraazacyclododecane-1,4,7,10-tetraacetic acid (DOTA). Thus, a total of 11 UA-DOTA conjugates were prepared holding various oligo-methylene diamine spacers as well as different substituents at the acetate units of DOTA including *tert*-butyl, benzyl, and allyl esters. Furthermore, three synthetic approaches were compared for the ethylenediamine-spacered conjugate **29** regarding reaction steps, yields, and precursor availability. The prepared conjugates were investigated regarding cytotoxicity using SRB assays and a set of human tumor cell lines. The highest cytotoxicity was observed for piperazinyl spacered compound **22**. Thereby, EC_{50} values of 1.5 µM (for A375 melanoma) and 1.7 µM (for A2780 ovarian carcinoma) were determined. Conjugates **22** and **24** were selected for further cytotoxicity investigations including fluorescence microscopy, annexin V assays and cell cycle analysis.

Keywords: ursolic acid; DOTA; triterpenoids; cytotoxicity

1. Introduction

Despite all medical advances in tumor therapy, cancer is still one of the most prevalent diseases worldwide, with 9.6 million cancer-related deaths counted in 2018 [1]. The research of novel therapeutic approaches and potent chemotherapeutic agents are important contributions in the battle against cancer. However, diagnosis is a prerequisite for successful treatment since an early detection of cancer cells can often significantly reduce the pathogenicity of a tumor and increase the healing rate. One molecule, which made significant impact on the field of diagnostic imaging in the past decades, is the EDTA-related macrocyclic chelator 1,4,7,10-tetraazacyclododecane-1,4,7,10-tetraacetic acid (DOTA, Figure 1) [2,3].

DOTA-derivatives and complexes thereof are widely used for molecular imaging, especially for the medical diagnosis of cancer [2,3]. By variation of the coordinated metal ion or substituents, they are applicable for a number of imaging techniques, such as magnetic resonance imaging (MRI) [2–4], positron emission tomography (PET) [2,3,5,6] and single photon emission computed tomography (SPECT) [2,3,7]. Because of this versatility, a crossover application of DOTA-derivatives as multimodal contrast agents for combined imaging modalities such as PET/MRI or PET/CT is possible and has already been described in the literature [2,3].

Although DOTA and derivatives thereof have a wide range of uses in diagnostic imaging, there are virtually no references for applications in the therapy of cancer. Therefore, we decided to prepare possible cytotoxic DOTA-derivatives by linkage with an ursolic acid backbone. Ursolic acid (UA, Figure 1) is a natural occurring triterpenoic acid with promising pharmacological properties, being widely distributed in various plants and fruits, such as rosemary [8], sage [8], oleander [9], and apples [10,11]. A wide range of biological activities, including antidiabetic, anti-inflammatory, antibacterial, and anticancer effects have been credited to UA and structurally-related derivatives [12–14]. Many structural modifications have been described in the literature starting from ursolic acid with various impacts on cytotoxic properties [12,15–18]. Structure activity investigations concerning modifications at C-3 of UA revealed the presence of an acetyloxy group to be beneficial for obtaining high anti-tumor activity [18]. Furthermore, it has been shown that the modification of C-28 with a piperazine moiety had a positive influence on the cytotoxic properties of ursolic acid [19,20]. Previously, we also have shown oligo-methylene diamine derived carboxamides of ursolic acid to be of high cytotoxicity [21]. Keeping these structure activity relationships in mind, we considered 3-acetyloxy protected and C-28 modified UA derivatives a convenient starting point for the preparation of cytotoxic oligo-methylene diamine spacered DOTA conjugates.

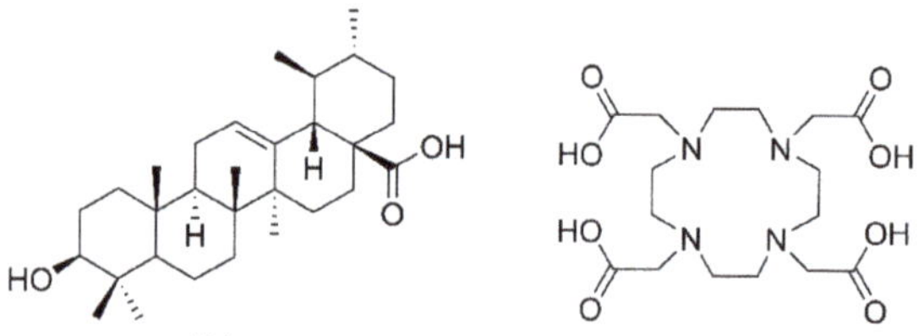

Figure 1. Structures of ursolic acid (UA) and 1,4,7,10-tetraazacyclododecane-1,4,7,10-tetraacetic acid (DOTA).

2. Results and Discussion

The synthesis of UA-DOTA conjugates started with the structural modification of cyclen (**2**) as illustrated in Scheme 1. Treatment of **2** with 3 equiv. of sodium bicarbonate and 3 equiv. of the respective bromoacetic ester (**3–5**) in dry acetonitrile yielded triple substituted cyclen derivatives **6–8**, being ready to be coupled with ursolic acid. We decided to use *tert*-butyl, benzyl and allyl esters as protecting groups. Benzyl, as well as *tert*-butyl bromoacetate, were bought from commercial suppliers. Allyl bromoacetate was prepared from allylic alcohol and bromoacetyl bromide.

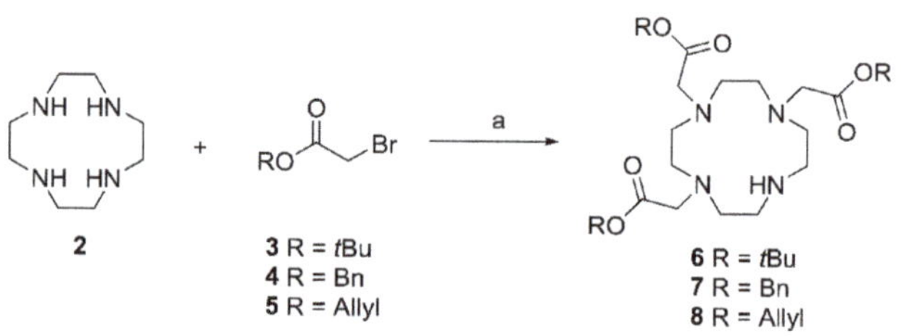

Scheme 1. Synthesis of DOTA precursors **6–8**: (a) NaHCO$_3$, MeCN, 25 °C, 48 h, yield: 50% (**6**), 68% (**7**), 63% (**8**).

Ursolic acid has also been modified before coupling with the DOTA precursors (Scheme 2). Derivatization started with the attachment of a spacer moiety using oxalyl chloride and 1-(2-aminoethyl)piperazine in dry dichloromethane affording compound **10**. The terminal amino moiety was further substituted with chloroacetyl chloride in dry dichloromethane to furnish the ursolic acid precursor **11** in excellent yield. Linkage of both precursors was performed in dry acetonitrile in the presence of potassium carbonate and potassium iodide yielding UA-DOTA conjugates **12–14**. Allylic esters of the acetate groups were removed by treating compound **14** with [(PPh$_3$)$_4$Pd], triphenylphosphane and pyrrolidine in acetonitrile at 25 °C for 3 days; this procedure gave **15** in almost quantitative yield. Purification of **15** was performed by reversed phase chromatography using MeOH/MeCN/TFA as eluent since the compound was difficult to eluate from normal silica phases. Furthermore, a synthetic approach for **15** starting from either **12** or **13** failed. Hydrogenation of **13** employing palladium catalysis retained the benzyl esters, and the deprotection of tert-butyl esters (as in compound **12**) using TFA/DCM resulted in a partial degradation of the triterpenoic backbone.

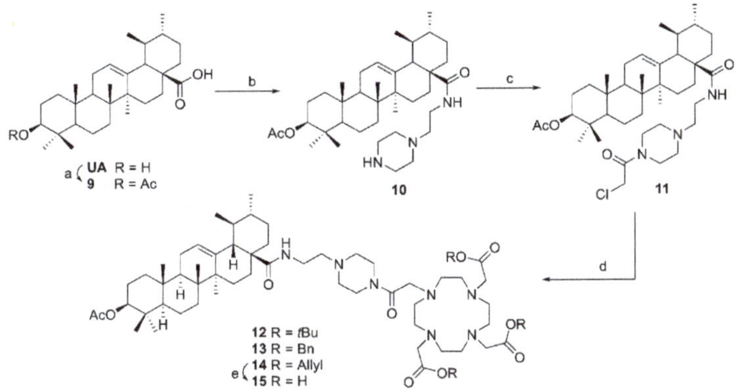

Scheme 2. Synthesis of ursolic acid chelator conjugates **12–15**: (**a**) Ac$_2$O, CH$_2$Cl$_2$, NEt$_3$, 25 °C, 2 days, 82%; (**b**) oxalyl chloride, CH$_2$Cl$_2$, DMF, 0–25 °C, 1 h, then 1-(2-Aminoethyl)piperazine, CH$_2$Cl$_2$, 25 °C, 2 h, yield: 82%; (**c**) chloroacetyl chloride, CH$_2$Cl$_2$, NEt$_3$, 25 °C, 30 min, yield: 91%; (**d**) K$_2$CO$_3$, KI, **6** (for **12**) or **7** (for **13**) or **8** (for **14**), MeCN, 25 °C, 48 h, yield: 54% (**12**), 82% (**13**), and 80% (**14**); (**e**) [(PPh$_3$)$_4$Pd], PPh$_3$, pyrrolidine, MeCN, 25 °C, 3 days, yield: 96%.

The synthetic approach summarized in Scheme 2 can also be applied to various other spacer units. Thus, we decided to alter the amino component. Therefore, ursolic acid was treated with piperazine, ethylene diamine and 2,2'-oxybis(ethylamine), to furnish ursolic carboxamides **16–18** (Scheme 3), respectively. Chloroacetyl derivatives **19–21** and UA-DOTA conjugates **22–27** were prepared analogous to Scheme 2.

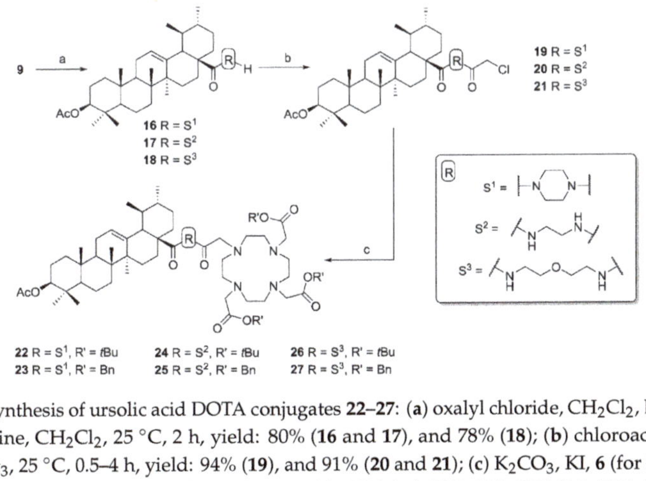

Scheme 3. Synthesis of ursolic acid DOTA conjugates **22–27**: (**a**) oxalyl chloride, CH$_2$Cl$_2$, DMF, 0–25 °C, 1 h, then amine, CH$_2$Cl$_2$, 25 °C, 2 h, yield: 80% (**16** and **17**), and 78% (**18**); (**b**) chloroacetyl chloride, CH$_2$Cl$_2$, NEt$_3$, 25 °C, 0.5–4 h, yield: 94% (**19**), and 91% (**20** and **21**); (**c**) K$_2$CO$_3$, KI, **6** (for **22**, **24** and **26**) or **7** (for **23**, **25** and **27**), MeCN, 25 °C, 5 days, yield: 88% (**22**), 72% (**23**), 73% (**24**), 75% (**25**), 74% (**26**), and 62% (**27**).

Additionally, an alternative synthetic approach was established for the preparation of the ethylene diamine-spacered UA-DOTA conjugate **29** (Scheme 4). Therefore carboxamide **28** was prepared either by deacetylation of **17** or directly from UA by amidation with ethylene diamine using EDC and HOBt in dry DMF. In the next step, DOTA-tris(*tert*-butyl ester) (DOTA-3T) was activated by preparing its HOBt ester. Adding **28** to this freshly prepared ester furnished UA-DOTA conjugate **29**. For comparison, compound **29** was also synthesized from **24** by removing the C-3 acetyloxy moiety. Due to the presence of an unprotected hydroxyl moiety at this position, compound **29** offers the possibility for a set of modifications and is therefore considered to be a good starting material for further modifications.

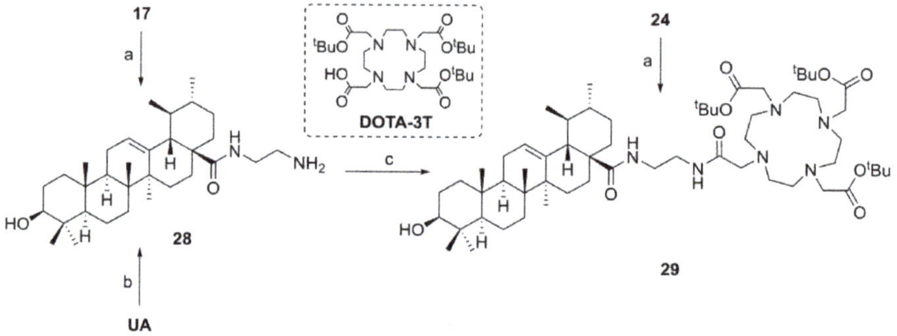

Scheme 4. Synthesis of ursolic acid derivative **29**: (**a**) KOH, MeOH, 25 °C, 48 h (for **28**) or 24 h (for **29**), yield: 85% (**28**) or 86% (**29**); (**b**) ethylene diamine, HOBt·H$_2$O, EDC·HCl, DMF, 25 °C, 24 h, yield: 46% (**c**) DOTA-3T, HOBt·H$_2$O, EDC·HCl, DMF, 25 °C, 5 days, yield: 49%.

Both synthetic approaches for the preparation of **29** (Figure 2) hold advantages but also some disadvantages. Although route A (5 steps) is significantly longer than B, but the former route gave the highest overall yield (44%). Approach B is a rather short and quick way to synthesize **29** (2 steps only), but the overall yield (23%) is barely half as high as in route A. Combining routes A and B, as shown in approach C led to compound **29** in 4 steps with an overall yield of 32%. A major difference between the approaches A and B is the availability and preparation of the DOTA precursors. Both, DOTA-tris(tert-butyl ester) and DO3A-tert-butyl ester (**6**) are available from commercial suppliers, with DOTA-3T being almost twice as expensive as **6**. Most advantageous is the one-step synthesis of **6** starting from cylcen (**2**), since **2** is commercially available for a price, being almost tenfold lower than that of **6**.

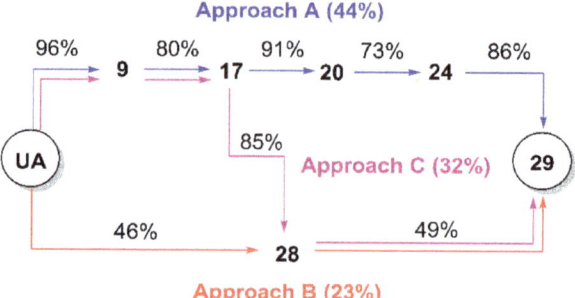

Figure 2. Comparison of synthetic routes **A**, **B**, and **C** for the preparation of UA-DOTA conjugate **29**.

Due to cytotoxicity evaluation, the prepared UA-DOTA conjugates were screened in rhodamine B assays employing a series of human tumor cell lines and non-malignant mouse fibroblasts (NIH 3T3). Results of this investigation are summarized in Table 1.

Table 1. Cytotoxicity of UA-DOTA conjugates (**12–15, 22–27, 29**), DOTA precursors (**6,7**), ursolic acid (UA), and doxorubicin hydrochloride (DRC): EC_{50} values from SRB assays after 72 h of treatment are given in µM (n.d. not detected; n.s. not soluble); the values are averaged from three independent experiments each performed in triplicate; confidence interval CI = 95%.

	A375	A2780	HT29	MCF-7	FaDu	NIH 3T3
UA	n.d.	11.7 ± 0.6	10.6 ± 0.7	12.7 ± 0.1	n.d.	13.1 ± 1.1
6	12.4 ± 2.7	10.5 ± 3.0	8.7 ± 2.7	11.3 ± 2.3	9.5 ± 0.9	17.3 ± 0.1
7	4.7 ± 0.3	3.8 ± 0.3	2.0 ± 0.2	4.1 ± 0.5	3.9 ± 0.7	4.5 ± 0.3
13	n.d.	2.1 ± 0.4	4.0 ± 0.4	3.3 ± 0.2	6.0 ± 0.1	3.6 ± 0.5
15	>60	>60	>60	>60	>60	>60
22	1.5 ± 0.4	1.9 ± 0.3	5.7 ± 0.5	4.4 ± 0.7	3.7 ± 0.6	4.6 ± 1.0
24	2.0 ± 0.1	1.7 ± 0.1	2.3 ± 0.3	1.8 ± 0.1	2.0 ± 0.2	1.4 ± 0.1
29	2.0 ± 0.3	1.6 ± 0.5	1.7 ± 0.4	n.d.	2.9 ± 0.4	2.3 ± 0.7
12, 14, 23, 25–27	n.s.	n.s	n.s	n.s.	n.s.	n.s.
DRC	n.d.	0.01 ± 0.01	0.9 ± 0.2	1.1 ± 0.3	n.d.	0.06 ± 0.03

The DO3A-tert-butyl ester (**6**) showed moderate cytotoxicity as indicated by EC_{50} values between 10 µM and 14 µM, while DO3A-benzyl ester (**7**) showed EC_{50} values lower than 5 µM. Unfortunately, most of the UA-DOTA conjugates were not soluble in solvents suitable for SRB assays. However, combining **7** with ursolic acid gave cytotoxic conjugate **13**, showing EC_{50} values below 6 µM. Removal of ester units (as in **15**) resulted in a complete loss of cytotoxicity (EC_{50} >60 µM for all tumor cells). Compounds **22** and **24**, both holding tert-butyl esters but different spacer units were also highly cytotoxic. Piperazine-spacered conjugate **22** showed the highest cytotoxicity observed in this screening for A375 tumor cells (EC_{50} = 1.5 ± 0.4 µM), while being quite selective, too (SI (NIH 3T3/A375) = 3.07, Table 2). EC_{50} values of ethylenediamine-spacered conjugate **24** were below 2.5 µM for all tumor cell lines. The highest cytotoxicity was observed for ovarian carcinoma (A2780, EC_{50} = 1.7 ± 0.1 µM). Removal of the acetyloxy moiety of **24** (as in **29**) had almost no significant impact on cytotoxicity.

Table 2. Selectivity of selected UA-DOTA conjugates (**13, 22, 24,** and **29**), DOTA precursors (**6, 7**), ursolic acid (UA) and doxorubicin hydrochloride (DRC): Selectivity index (SI) is defined as: SI = EC_{50} (NIH 3T3)/EC_{50} (tumor cell line).

	A375	A2780	HT29	MCF-7	FaDu
UA	-	1.12	1.24	1.03	-
6	1.40	1.65	1.99	1.53	1.82
7	0.96	1.18	2.25	1.10	1.15
13	-	1.71	0.90	1.09	0.60
22	3.07	2.42	0.81	1.05	1.24
24	0.70	0.82	0.61	0.78	0.70
29	1.15	1.44	1.35	-	0.79
DRC	-	6.00	0.07	0.05	-

Because UA-DOTA conjugates **22** and **24** were the most active compounds of this study, these compounds were selected for further cytotoxicity investigations including fluorescence microscopy, annexin V assays, and cell cycle evaluation employing melanoma cells (A375). Microscopic images of A375 cells treated with compound **24** for 24 h showed vital cells (green staining) with some of them having ruptured cell membranes (Figure 3A, white arrows). Further indications of apoptosis have been detected employing flow cytometry and annexin V-FITC/PI staining. After 24 h 63% of the tumor cells treated with **24** were annexin V-FITC-positive, and 51.9% of all cells having died by apoptosis. Additionally, the number of vital cells decreased in comparison to the control from 86.1% to 36.7 % (Figure 3B). An extra investigation of the cell cycle showed a decreased number of cells in G1/G0, G2/M, as well as in S phase. Additionally, a large population of cells has been shifted into the subG1 region (Figure 3C).

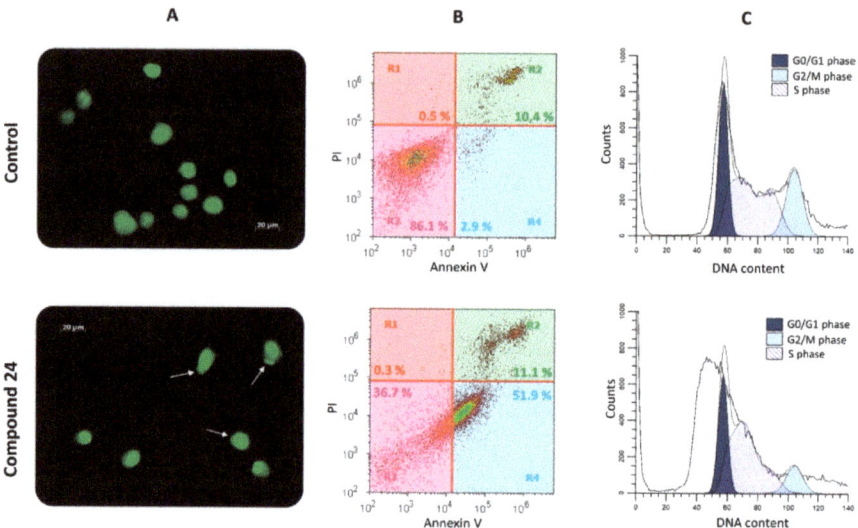

Figure 3. Extended cytotoxicity investigation after treatment of A375 cells with **24** (4.0 µM) for 24 h: (**A**) Fluorescence microscopic images (scale bar 20 µm), AO and PI were used; (**B**) Annexin V-FITC/PI assay. Examples of density plots determined by flow cytometry (Attune® Cytometric Software v 1.2.5), R1: necrotic, R2: secondary necrotic/late stage apoptotic, R3: vital, R4: apoptotic; (**C**) Representative examples for cell cycle evaluation via ModFit LT 5.0.

Fluorescence microscopic images and density plots of A375 cells treated with **22** for 24 h showed no significant differences in comparison to the control (Supplementary material, Figure S1). Therefore, further investigations were performed with a prolonged incubation time of 48 h. After treating A375 cells with compound **22** for 48 h, subsequent fluorescence microscopic investigations using AO/PI staining showed ruptures of the plasma membrane (Figure 4A, white arrows). Additionally, some necrotic/late stage apoptotic cells were observed, indicated by slightly orange stained nuclei (Figure 4 A, orange arrow). The density plot of A375 cells treated with **22** for 48 h showed a decreased number of vital cells (66.3%) compared to the control (86.0%), while 32.9% of the cells were considered annexin V-FITC-positive. Nearly half of them (17.4% of all cells) have died by apoptosis, and the remaining cells (15.5% of all cells) were secondary necrotic/late stage apoptotic (Figure 4 B). During extra investigations of the cell cycle, some differences compared to the control have been observed. Cells treated with **22** for 48 h showed a quite broad and flat DNA distribution. G1/G0, G2/M, and S phase were drastically reduced, while an increased population of cells with reduced DNA content has been observed in the subG1 region (Figure 4C).

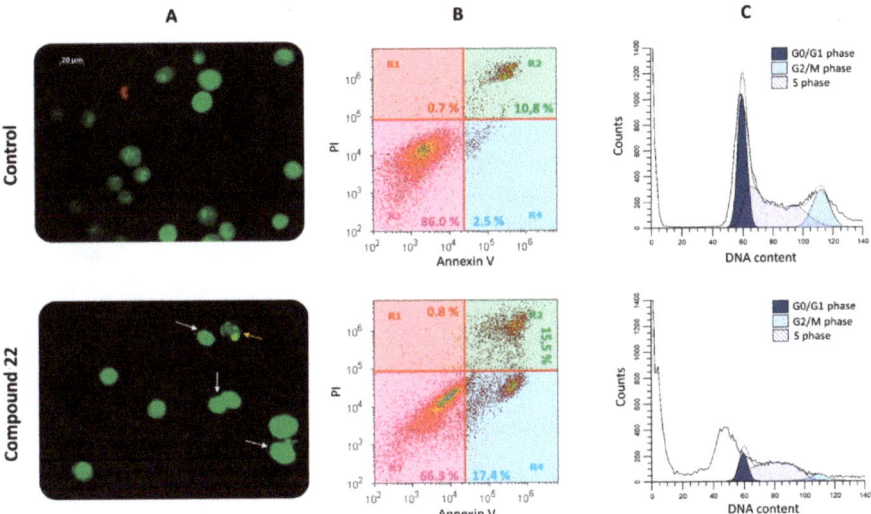

Figure 4. Extended cytotoxicity investigation after treatment of A375 cells with **22** (3.0 μM) for 48 h: (**A**) Fluorescence microscopic images (scale bar 20 μm), AO and PI were used; (**B**) Annexin V-FITC/PI assay. Examples of density plots determined by flow cytometry (Attune® Cytometric Software vl 1.2.5), R1: necrotic, R2: secondary necrotic/late stage apoptotic, R3: vital, R4: apoptotic; (**C**) Representative examples for cell cycle evaluation via ModFit LT 5.0.

3. Conclusions

In this study, a series of overall 11 amine-spacered UA-DOTA conjugates have been prepared starting from the natural occurring triterpenoid ursolic acid (UA). We hereby report a synthetic approach to UA-DOTA conjugates, which is applicable for several amine spacers and other triterpenoic backbones, too. Additionally, we compared three synthetic approaches for the preparation of compound **29** in terms of yield, number of steps and precursor availability. This conjugate offers the possibility for further modifications at the C-3 hydroxylic group, which is known to influence cytotoxicity. All of the prepared DOTA conjugates were screened in SRB assays showing some compounds to be of good cytotoxicity. EC_{50} values were determined to range from 17.3 μM to 1.4 μM. The most active compound of this series was a piperazinyl spacered conjugate **22** showing low EC_{50} values such as 1.5 ± 0.4 μM for A375 tumor cells and 1.9 ± 0.3 μM for A2780 tumor cells, respectively, while showing good selectivity (SI (NIH 3T3(A375) = 3.07), too. Unfortunately, the selectivity of the other screened conjugates was quite low. Additional cytotoxicity investigations such as fluorescence microscopy, annexin V assays, and cell cycle analyses were performed employing the UA-DOTA conjugates **22** and **24** to gain information about their mode of action. The results of these extended biological testing indicate **24** to induce death of A375 cancer cells by apoptosis. These results hold some starting points for further studies. Conjugate **15** and structural related compounds (holding free carboxylic acids at the DOTA unit) are currently subjects of ongoing investigations regarding their ability to form complexes with metal ions or radioactive isotopes like ^{68}Ga to examine possible future uses as tracer or contrast agents in molecular imaging techniques, such as positron emission tomography (PET) [22].

4. Materials and Methods

4.1. General

NMR spectra were recorded using the Varian spectrometers Gemini 2000 or Unity 500 (Varian GmbH, Darmstadt, Germany) δ given in ppm, *J* in Hz; typical experiments: APT, H-H-COSY,

HMBC, HSQC, NOESY), MS spectra were taken on a Finnigan MAT LCQ 7000 (ThermoFisher Scientific, Braunschweig, Germany) electrospray, voltage 4.1 kV, sheath gas nitrogen) instrument. The optical rotations were measured on a Perkin-Elmer polarimeter (Perkin Elmer LAS, Rodgau, Germany) or on a Jasco P-2000 polarimeter (Jasco Germany, Pfungstadt, Germany) at 20 °C; TLC was performed on NP or RP18 silica gel (Macherey-Nagel, detection with cerium molybdate or Dragendorff's reagent). Melting points are uncorrected (*Leica* hot stage microscope, or BUCHI melting point M-565), and elemental analyses were performed on a Foss-Heraeus Vario EL (CHNS, Elementar Analysensysteme GmbH, Langenselbold, Germany) unit. IR spectra were recorded on a Perkin Elmer FT-IR spectrometer Spectrum 1000 or on a Perkin-Elmer Spectrum Two (UATR Two Unit; both instruments from Perkin Elmer LAS, Rodgau, Germany). UV-VIS spectra were taken on a Perkin-Elmer Lambda 14 spectrometer or on a Perkin-Elmer Lambda 750 S (UV/VIS/NIR) spectrometer (both instruments from Perkin Elmer LAS, Rodgau, Germany). The solvents were dried according to usual procedures. The purity of the compounds was determined by HPLC and found to be >96%.

4.2. Cytotoxicity

4.2.1. Cell Lines and Culture Conditions

The cell lines used are human cancer cell lines: A2780 (ovarian carcinoma), HT29 (colon adenocarcinoma), MCF-7 (breast adenocarcinoma), A375 (melanoma), FaDu (pharynx squamous cell carcinoma) and non-malignant mouse fibroblasts NIH 3T3; all cell lines were obtained from the Department of Oncology (Martin-Luther-University Halle-Wittenberg). Cultures were maintained as monolayers in RPMI 1640 medium with L-glutamine (Capricorn Scientific GmbH, Ebsdorfergrund, Germany) supplemented with 10% heat inactivated fetal bovine serum (Sigma-Aldrich Chemie GmbH, Steinheim, Germany) and penicillin/streptomycin (Capricorn Scientific GmbH, Ebsdorfergrund, Germany) at 37 °C in a humidified atmosphere with 5% CO_2.

4.2.2. Cytotoxic Assay (SRB)

The cytotoxicity of the compounds was evaluated using the sulforhodamine-B (Kiton-Red S, ABCR) micro culture colorimetric assay. Cells were seeded into 96-well plates on day 0 at appropriate cell densities to prevent confluence of the cells during the period of experiment. After 24 h, the cells were treated with six different concentrations (1, 3, 7, 12, 20, and 30 µM) minimum. The final concentration of DMSO/DMF never exceeded 0.5%, which was non-toxic to the cells. After a 72-h treatment, the supernatant medium from the 96-well plates was discarded, the cells were fixed with 10% trichloroacetic acid (TCA) and allowed to rest at 4 °C. After 24 h fixation, the cells were washed in a strip washer and dyed with SRB solution (100 µL, 0.4%, in 1% acetic acid) for about 20 min. After dying, the plates were washed four times with 1% acetic acid to remove the excess of the dye and allowed to air-dry overnight. Tris base solution (200 µL, 10 mM) was added to each well and absorbance was measured at λ = 570 nm using a 96 well plate reader (Tecan Spectra, Crailsheim, Germany). The EC_{50} values were averaged from three independent experiments performed each in triplicate calculated from semi logarithmic dose response curves applying a non-linear 4P Hills-slope equation (GraphPad Prism5; variables top and bottom were set to 100 and 0, respectively).

4.2.3. AO/PI Dye Exclusion Test

Morphological characteristics of cell death were analyzed employing an AO/PI assay using human cancer cell line A375. Approx. 2×10^5 cells were seeded in cell culture flasks (25 cm^2), and the cells were allowed to grow up for 24 h. After removing of the used medium, the substance loaded fresh medium was reloaded (or a blank new medium as a control). After 24 h and 48 h, the content of the flask was collected and centrifuged (1200 rpm, 4 °C), the pellet was gently suspended in phosphate-buffered saline (PBS (w/Ca^{2+} and Mg^{2+}), 1 mL) and centrifuged again. The PBS was removed, and the pellet gently suspended in PBS (150 µL) again. The analysis of the cells was performed using a fluorescence microscope after having mixed the cell suspension (10 µL) with a solution of AO/PI (5 µg/mL, 10 µL).

4.2.4. Annexin V-FITC/PI Assay

Approximately 2×10^5 cells (A375) were seeded in cell culture flasks (25 cm^2), and the cells were allowed to grow up for 24 h. After removing of the used medium, the substance loaded fresh medium was reloaded (or a blank fresh medium as a control). After 24 h and 48 h, the cells were harvested, centrifuged (1200 rpm, 4 °C), and washed twice with PBS (w/Ca^{2+} and Mg^{2+}, 1 mL). The cells were counted and approximately 1·10^6 cells were washed with Annexin V binding buffer (BioLegend®, San Diego, USA) and treated with propidium iodide solution (3 µL, 1 mg/mL) and Annexin V-FITC (5 µL, BioLegend®, San Diego, CA, USA) for 15 min in the dark at room temperature. After adding Annexin V binding buffer (400 µL) the suspension was analyzed using Attune® FACS machine. After gating for living cells, the data from detectors BL-1A and BL-3A were collected (20,000 events) in technical triplicates. The assay was performed in duplicates; cell distribution was calculated using Attune® Software (ThermoFisher Scientific, Braunschweig, Germany).

4.2.5. Cell Cycle Investigations

Approximately 2×10^5 cells (A375) were seeded in cell culture flasks (25 cm^2), and the cells were allowed to grow up for 24 h. After removing of the used medium, the substance loaded fresh medium was reloaded (or a blank fresh medium as a control). After 24 h or 48 h, respectively, only the adherent cells were harvested, centrifuged (1200 rpm, 4 °C), and washed twice with PBS ((w/w), 1 mL). The cells were counted and approximately 1×10^6 cells were fixed with ethanol (70%, 4 °C, 24 h). After centrifugation (4500 rpm, 4 °C) the cells were washed with PBS ((w/w), 1 mL) and centrifuged. The pellet was resuspended in 1 mL RNAse A containing PI buffer (100µL RNAse (100 mg/mL), 15 µL PI solution (1 mg/mL)) and after incubating for 30 min at room temperature in the dark, cells were analyzed using the Attune® FACS machine; collecting data from the BL-2A channel. Doublet cells were excluded from the measurements by plotting BL-2A against BL-2H. For each cell cycle distribution 20,000 events were collected in technical triplicates, each sample was measured in duplicates. Cell cycle distribution was calculated using ModFitLT™ (Verity Software House, Topsham, ME, USA).

4.3. Syntheses

4.3.1. General

Ursolic acid (**1**) was obtained from betulinines (Stříbrná Skalice, Czech Republic). 1,4,7,10-Tetraazacyclododecane (cyclen, **2**) was bought from abcr GmbH (Karlsruhe, Germany) in 95% purity. Benzyl bromoacetate (96%) and tert-Butyl bromoacetate (98%) were both purchased from Sigma-Aldrich Chemie GmbH (Steinheim, Germany). DOTA-tris(*tert*-butyl ester) was obtained from TCI Deutschland GmbH (Eschborn, Germany) in 97% purity. Ursolic acid derivatives **10**, **16–18** and **28** have been synthesized as previously reported [20,21]. Experimental procedures and full analytical data of these compounds can be found in the supplementary material [23,24].

4.3.2. General Procedure A for the Synthesis of DOTA Precursors (**6–8**)

To a suspension of cyclen (5.81 mmol) and sodium bicarbonate (17.43 mmol) in dry acetonitrile (100 mL), a solution of the respective bromoacetate (**3–5**, 17.43 mmol) in dry acetonitrile (10 mL) was added dropwise under argon atmosphere. The mixture was stirred for 48 h at 25 °C. After usual aqueous work-up, the solvent was removed under reduced pressure, and the crude products were subjected to column chromatography (silica gel, chloroform/methanol mixtures) affording DOTA precursors **6–8** (50–68%).

4.3.3. General Procedure B for the Synthesis of Carboxamides (**10**, **16–18**)

Compound **9** (0.5 mmol) was dissolved in dry DCM (10 mL), cooled to 0 °C and oxalyl chloride (3.2 mmol) and dry DMF (2 drops) were added. After warming to 25 °C, the mixture was stirred for 1 h. The solvent was removed under reduced pressure, re-evaporated with dry THF (4 × 15 mL), and the residue was immediately resolved in dry DCM (10 mL). This mixture was then added dropwise to a solution of the amine (3.0 mmol) in dry DCM (2 mL) and stirred at 25 °C for 2 h. After usual aqueous work-up, the solvent was removed under reduced pressure, and the crude products were subjected to column chromatography (silica gel, chloroform/methanol mixtures). Compounds **10** and **16–18** were each obtained as colorless solids (78–82%).

4.3.4. General Procedure C for the Alkylation with Chloroacetyl Chloride (**11**, **19–21**)

Chloroacetyl chloride (2.20 mmol) was added dropwise to a solution of the respective carboxamide (**10**, **16–18**; 1.43 mmol) and triethylamine (0.71 mmol) in dry dichloromethane (75 mL). The mixture was stirred at 25 °C for 0.5–4 h. After usual aqueous work-up, the solvent was removed under reduced pressure, and the crude products were subjected to column chromatography (silica gel, chloroform/acetone mixtures). Compounds **11** and **19–21** were each obtained as colorless solids (91%–94%).

4.3.5. General Procedure D for the Synthesis of Ursolic Acid Chelator Conjugates (**12–14**, **22–27**)

To a solution of the respective chloroacetyl derivative (**11**, **19–21**; 0.44 mmol) and freshly grounded potassium carbonate (0.83 mmol) in dry acetonitrile (15 mL) was added potassium iodide (0.35 mmol) and the respective DOTA precursor (**6–8**, 0.41 mmol in 5 mL dry acetonitrile). The mixture was stirred for 2–5 days at 25 °C. After completion of the reaction (as indicated by TLC) the mixture was filtered, and the solvent was removed under reduced pressure. The crude products were subjected to column chromatography (silica gel, chloroform/methanol mixtures) to afford compounds **12–14** and **22–27** (yield: 54–88%), respectively.

Allyl bromoacetate (**5**), To a solution of allyl alcohol (0.62 mol), bromo acetylbromide (0.1 mol) was added dropwise over a period of 30 min at 0 °C under argon atmosphere. The mixture was stirred for 1 h at 0 °C, warmed to 25 °C and stirred for another 3 h. The solvent was removed under reduced pressure and the residue was dissolved in dichloromethane. After usual aqueous work-up, the solvent was removed under reduced pressure, and the crude product was purified by vacuum distillation affording allyl bromoacetate as colorless oil (68%). ^{1}H NMR (400 MHz, CDCl$_3$): δ = 5.88 (*ddt*, *J* = 16.5, 11.0, 5.8 Hz, 1H, C*H*=CH$_2$), 5.38–5.17 (*m*, 2H, CH=C*H*$_2$), 4.61 (*dt*, *J* = 5.8, 1.4 Hz, 2H, C*H*$_2$CH=CH$_2$), 3.82 (*s*, 2H, BrC*H*$_2$) ppm; ^{13}C NMR (101 MHz, CDCl$_3$): δ = 166.8 (C=O), 131.2 (CH=CH$_2$), 119.0 (CH=CH$_2$), 66.6 (CH$_2$CH=CH$_2$), 25.8 (BrCH$_2$) ppm.

Tri-tert-butyl 2,2′,2″-(1,4,7,10-tetraazacyclododecane-1,4,7-triyl)triacetate (**6**), Compound **6** was prepared from **2** according to general procedure A using *tert*-butyl bromoacetate (**3**). Column chromatography (SiO$_2$, CHCl$_3$/MeOH 9:1) gave **6** (yield: 50%); m.p. 180–182 °C (lit.: 181–183 °C [25]); R$_f$ = 0.27 (CHCl$_3$/MeOH 95:5); IR (ATR): ν = 2974*w*, 2943*w*, 2912*w*, 2853*w*, 2736*w*, 1718*s*, 1576*w*, 1466*w*, 1453*w*, 1412*w*, 1392*w*, 1368*m*, 1330*w*, 1255*m*, 1218*w*, 1147*s*, 1117*m*, 1099*m*, 1050*w*, 935*m*, 873*m*, 848*m* cm^{-1}; ^{1}H NMR (400 MHz, CDCl$_3$): δ = 3.36 (*s*, 4H, 2 × CH$_2$ (acetate)), 3.28 (*s*, 2H, CH$_2$ (acetate)), 3.12–3.06 (*m*, 4H, 2 × CH$_2$ (cyclen)), 2.95–2.84 (*m*, 12H, 6 × CH$_2$ (cyclen)), 1.45 (*s*, 18H, 6 × CH$_3$ (*t*-butyl)), 1.45 (*s*, 9H, 3 × CH$_3$ (*t*-butyl)) ppm; ^{13}C NMR (101 MHz, CDCl$_3$): δ = 170.6 (2 × CO, acetate), 169.8 (CO, acetate), 81.9 (C$_q$, *t*-butyl), 81.8 (2 × C$_q$, *t*-butyl), 58.4 (2 × CH$_2$, acetate), 51.5 (2 × CH$_2$, cyclen), 51.4 (2 × CH$_2$, cyclen), 49.4 (2 × CH$_2$, cyclen), 49.0 (CH$_2$, acetate), 47.7 (2 × CH$_2$, cyclen), 28.4 (3 × CH$_3$, *t*-butyl), 28.3 (6 × CH$_3$, *t*-butyl) ppm; MS (ESI, MeOH): *m/z* = 515.3 (100%, [M + H]$^+$), 537.3 (10%, [M + Na]$^+$); analysis calcd for C$_{26}$H$_{50}$N$_4$O$_6$ (514.71): C 60.67, H 9.79, N 10.89; found: C 60.51, H 9.98, N 10.67.

Tribenzyl 2,2',2''-(1,4,7,10-tetraazacyclododecane-1,4,7-triyl)triacetate (**7**). Compound **7** was prepared from **2** according to general procedure A using benzyl bromoacetate (**4**). Column chromatography (SiO$_2$, CHCl$_3$/MeOH 9:1) gave **7** (yield: 68%); R$_f$ = 0.32 (CHCl$_3$/MeOH 95:5); IR (KBr): ν = 2948w, 2857w, 2738w, 1732s, 1586w, 1498w, 1455m, 1418w, 1381w, 1314w, 1169s, 1096m, 1049m, 994m, 739s, 697s cm^{-1}; UV-Vis (CHCl$_3$): λ$_{max}$ (logε) = 251 nm (2.87), 258 nm (2.86), 263 nm (2.76); ^{1}H NMR (400 MHz, CDCl$_3$): δ = 7.40–7.29 (*m*, 15H, 15 × CH (Bn)), 5.13 (*s*, 4H, 2 × CH$_2$ (Bn)), 5.13 (*s*, 2H, CH$_2$ (Bn)), 3.48 (*s*, 4H, 2 × CH$_2$ (acetate)), 3.41 (*s*, 2H, CH$_2$ (acetate)), 3.12–3.05 (*m*, 4H, 2 × CH$_2$ (cyclen)), 2.93–2.79 (*m*, 12H, 6 × CH$_2$ (cyclen)) ppm; ^{13}C NMR (101 MHz, CDCl$_3$): δ = 171.1 (2 × CO, acetate), 170.3 (CO, acetate), 135.5 (C$_i$, Bn), 128.8 (CH, Bn), 128.8 (CH, Bn), 128.7 (CH, Bn), 128.7 (CH, Bn), 128.6 (CH, Bn), 66.8 (CH$_2$, Bn), 57.4 (2 × CH$_2$, acetate), 51.9 (2 × CH$_2$, cyclen), 51.7 (2 × CH$_2$, cyclen), 49.6 (2 × CH$_2$, cyclen), 48.8 (CH$_2$, acetate), 47.5 (2 × CH$_2$, cyclen) ppm; MS (ESI, MeOH): *m/z* = 309.0 (10%, [M + 2H]$^{2+}$), 617.4 (100%, [M + H]$^+$), 639.3 (10%, [M + Na]$^+$); analysis calcd for C$_{35}$H$_{44}$N$_4$O$_6$ (616.76): C 68.16, H 7.19, N 9.08; found: C 67.84, H 7.39, N 8.81.

Triallyl 2,2',2''-(1,4,7,10-tetraazacyclododecane-1,4,7-triyl)triacetate (**8**), Compound **8** was prepared from **2** according to general procedure A using allyl bromoacetate (**5**). Column chromatography (SiO$_2$, CHCl$_3$/MeOH 95:5) gave **8** (yield: 63%); R$_f$ = 0.27 (CHCl$_3$/MeOH 95:5); IR (KBr): ν = 2945w, 2858w, 2743w, 1731s, 1673w, 1648w, 1455w, 1420w, 1364w, 1314w, 1179s, 1095m, 985s, 928s cm^{-1}; ^{1}H NMR (400 MHz, CDCl$_3$): δ = 5.93–5.81 (*m*, 3H, 3 × CH (allyl)), 5.32–5.20 (*m*, 6H, 3 × CH$_2$ (allyl)), 4.60–4.53 (*m*, 6H, 3 × CH$_2$ (allyl)), 3.49 (*s*, 4H, 2 × CH$_2$ (acetate)), 3.41 (*s*, 2H, CH$_2$ (acetate)), 3.12–3.06 (*m*, 4H, 2 × CH$_2$ (cyclen)), 2.96–2.81 (*m*, 12H, 6 × CH$_2$ (cyclen)) ppm; ^{13}C NMR (101 MHz, CDCl$_3$): δ = 170.8 (2 × CO, acetate), 170.0 (CO, acetate), 131.7 (2 × CH, allyl), 131.7 (CH, allyl), 119.2 (CH$_2$, allyl), 119.0 (2 × CH$_2$, allyl), 65.5 (2 × CH$_2$, allyl), 65.4 (CH$_2$, allyl), 57.3 (2 × CH$_2$, acetate), 51.7 (2 × CH$_2$, cyclen), 51.6 (2 × CH$_2$, cyclen), 49.4 (2 × CH$_2$, cyclen), 48.5 (CH$_2$, acetate), 47.4 (CH$_2$, cyclen) ppm; MS (ESI, MeOH): *m/z* = 234.1 (18%, [M + 2H]$^{2+}$), 467.3 (100%, [M + H]$^+$), 489.3 (10%, [M + Na]$^+$); analysis calcd for C$_{23}$H$_{38}$N$_4$O$_6$ (466.6): C 59.21, H 8.21, N 12.01; found: C 59.03, H 8.44, N 11.78.

(3β) 3-Acetyloxy-urs-12-en-28-oic acid (**9**), Compound **1** was prepared from ursolic acid according to the procedure given in the literature [26]. Yield: 96%; m.p. 287–290 °C (lit.: 289–290 °C [27]).

(3β) N-(2-(4-(2-Chloroacetyl)piperazin-1-yl)ethyl)-3-acetyloxy-urs-12-en-28-amide (**11**). Compound **11** was synthesized from **10** according to general procedure C. Column chromatography (SiO$_2$, CHCl$_3$/acetone 4:1) furnished compound **11** (91%); m.p. 124–129 °C; [α]$_D$ = +32.3° (*c* 0.320, CHCl$_3$); R$_f$ = 0.38 (CHCl$_3$/acetone 4:1); IR (KBr): ν = 3423s, 2947s, 1734m, 1654s, 1522m, 1458m, 1370m, 1247s, 1150w, 1027m cm^{-1}; ^{1}H NMR (400 MHz, CDCl$_3$): δ = 6.32 (*t*, *J* = 5.0 Hz, 1H, N*H*), 5.28 (*t*, *J* = 3.6 Hz, 1H, 12-H), 4.49 (*dd*, *J* = 10.4, 5.4 Hz, 1H, 3-H), 4.06 (*s*, 2H, 36-H), 3.72–3.47 (*m*, 4H, 34-H, 34'-H), 3.47–3.36 (*m*, 1H, 31-H$_a$), 3.25–3.15 (*m*, 1H, 31-H$_b$), 2.58–2.39 (*m*, 6H, 33-H, 32-H, 33'-H), 2.04 (*s*, 3H, Ac), 2.02–1.80 (*m*, 5H, 11-H$_a$, 11-H$_b$, 16-H$_a$, 22-H$_a$, 18-H), 1.79–1.70 (*m*, 1H, 16-H$_b$), 1.69–1.21 (*m*, 13H, 15-H$_a$, 1-H$_a$, 2-H$_a$, 2-H$_b$, 9-H, 6-H$_a$, 21-H$_a$, 7-H$_a$, 22-H$_b$, 19-H, 6-H$_b$, 21-H$_b$, 7-H$_b$), 1.09 (*s*, 3H, 27-H), 1.08–1.01 (*m*, 2H, 1-H$_b$, 15-H$_b$), 0.96–0.94 (*m*, 4H, 20-H, 30-H), 0.93 (*s*, 3H, 25-H), 0.89–0.86 (*m*, 3H, 29-H), 0.86 (*s*, 3H, 23-H), 0.85 (*s*, 3H, 24-H), 0.84–0.79 (*m*, 1H, 5-H), 0.78 (*s*, 3H, 26-H) ppm; ^{13}C NMR (101 MHz, CDCl$_3$): δ = 178.1 (C-28), 171.1 (Ac), 165.2 (C-35), 140.0 (C-13), 125.3 (C-12), 80.9 (C-3), 56.7 (C-32), 55.4 (C-5), 54.2 (C-18), 53.0 (C-33), 52.5 (C-33'), 48.0 (C-17), 47.6 (C-9), 46.5 (C-34), 42.6 (C-14), 42.4 (C-34'), 40.9 (C-36), 39.9 (C-19), 39.7 (C-8), 39.3 (C-20) 38.4 (C-1), 37.8 (C-4), 37.5 (C-22), 37.0 (C-10), 35.9 (C-31), 32.8 (C-7), 31.0 (C-21), 28.2 (C-23), 28.0 (C-15), 25.0 (C-16), 23.6 (C-2), 23.6 (C-11), 23.4 (C-27), 21.4 (Ac), 21.3 (C-30), 18.3 (C-6), 17.5 (C-29), 17.1 (C-26), 16.9 (C-24), 15.8 (C-25) ppm; MS (ESI, MeOH): m/z = 686.5 (100%, [M + H]$^+$); analysis calcd for C$_{40}$H$_{64}$ClN$_3$O$_4$ (686.42): C 69.99, H 9.40, N 6.12; found: C 69.70, H 9.63, N 6.02.

Tris-t-butyl 2',2''-[10-[2-[4-[2-(3β-acetyloxy-urs-12-en-28-oylamino)ethyl]piperazin-1-yl]-2-oxoethyl]-1,4,7,10-tetraazacyclododecane-1,4,7-triyl]triacetate (**12**), Compound **12** was synthesized from **6** and **11** according to general procedure D. Column chromatography (SiO$_2$, CHCl$_3$/MeOH 9:1) furnished compound

12 (54%). m.p. 247–250 °C (decomp.); [α]$_D$ = +18.9° (c 0.345, CHCl$_3$); R$_f$ = 0.30 (CHCl$_3$/MeOH 9:1); IR (KBr): ν = 2931m, 1727s, 1644s, 1529w, 1455m, 1425w, 1368s, 1306m, 1228s, 1159s, 1105s, 1005m, 755m cm^{-1}; ^{1}H NMR (400 MHz, CDCl$_3$): δ = 6.38 (s, 1H, NH), 5.26 (t, J = 3.4 Hz, 1H, 12-H), 4.46 (dd, J = 10.5, 5.2 Hz, 1H, 3-H), 3.92–2.04 (m, 36H, 34-H, 34′-H, 36-H, 3 × CH$_2$ (acetate), 31-H$_a$, 31-H$_b$, 8 × CH$_2$ (cyclen), 32-H, 33-H, 33′-H), 2.01 (s, 3H, Ac), 2.00–1.68 (m, 4H, 16-H$_a$, 11-H$_a$, 11-H$_b$, 18-H), 1.69–1.14 (m, 14H, 16-H$_b$, 22-H$_b$, 15-H$_a$, 1-H$_a$, 2-H$_a$, 2-H$_b$, 9-H, 6-H$_a$, 21-H$_a$, 7-H$_a$, 19-H, 6-H$_b$, 21-H$_b$, 7-H$_b$), 1.42 (s, 27H, 9 × CH$_3$ (t-Butyl)), 1.05 (s, 3H, 27-H), 1.11–0.95 (m, 3H, 1-H$_b$, 15-H$_b$, 20-H), 0.91 (d, J = 6.1 Hz, 3H, 30-H), 0.90 (s, 3H, 25-H), 0.85 (d, J = 6.5 Hz, 3H, 29-H), 0.83 (s, 3H, 23-H), 0.82 (s, 3H, 24-H), 0.80–0.75 (m, 1H, 5-H), 0.74 (s, 3H, 26-H) ppm; ^{13}C NMR (100 MHz, CDCl$_3$): δ = 178.0 (C-28), 172.8 (CO, acetate), 171.0 (Ac), 169.8 (C-35), 139.8 (C-13), 125.3 (C-12), 81.9 (C$_q$, t-Butyl), 81.7 (2 × C$_q$, t-Butyl), 80.9 (C-3), 56.8 (C-32), 55.8 (3 × CH$_2$, acetate), 55.3 (C-5), 55.2 (C-36), 53.9 (C-18), 53.4 (8 × CH$_2$, cyclen), 52.2 (C-33, C-33′), 47.8 (C-17), 47.5 (C-9), 44.3 (C-34, C-34′), 42.5 (C-14), 39.8 (C-19), 39.7 (C-8), 39.1 (C-20), 38.4 (C-1), 37.8 (C-4), 37.4 (C-22), 36.9 (C-10), 35.7 (C-31), 32.8 (C-7), 31.0 (C-21), 28.2 (C-23), 28.0 (9 × CH$_3$, t-Butyl), 27.9 (C-15), 24.8 (C-16), 23.6 (C-2), 23.5 (C-11), 23.4 (C-27), 21.4 (Ac), 21.3 (C-30), 18.3 (C-6), 17.4 (C-29), 17.1 (C-26), 16.8 (C-24), 15.7 (C-25) ppm; MS (ESI, MeOH): m/z = 593.9 (100%, [M + Na + H]$^+$), 1186.7 (95%, [M + Na]$^+$); analysis calcd for C$_{66}$H$_{113}$N$_7$O$_{10}$ (1164.67): C 68.06, H 9.78, N 8.42; found: C 67.75, H 9.97, N 8.51.

Tribenzyl 2,2′,2″-[10-[2-[4-[2-(3β-acetyloxy-urs-12-en-28-oylamino)ethyl]piperazin-1-yl]-2-oxoethyl]-1,4,7,10-tetraazacyclododecane-1,4,7-triyl]triacetate (**13**). Compound **13** was synthesized from **7** and **11** according to general procedure D. Column chromatography (SiO$_2$, CHCl$_3$/MeOH 95:5) furnished compound **13** (82%). m.p. 142–146 °C; [α]$_D$ = +14.5° (c 0.300, CHCl$_3$); R$_f$ = 0.50 (CHCl$_3$/MeOH 9:1); IR (KBr): ν = 3440s, 2947m, 1734s, 1641s, 1456m, 1371m, 1310w, 1247m, 1197s, 1105m, 1006w, 750m cm^{-1}; UV-Vis (CHCl$_3$): λ$_{max}$ (logε) = 257 nm (3.99); ^{1}H NMR (400 MHz, CDCl$_3$): δ = 7.36–7.24 (m, 15H, CH$_{Ar}$), 6.36–6.28 (m, 1H, NH), 5.27 (t, J = 3.7 Hz, 1H, 12-H), 5.21–5.13 (m, 4H, 2 × CH$_2$Bn), 5.12–5.05 (m, 2H, CH$_2$Bn), 4.47 (dd, J = 10.7, 5.1 Hz, 1H, 3-H), 3.72–2.81 (m, 12H, 34-H, 34′-H, 36-H, 3 × CH$_2$ (acetate)), 3.40–3.30 (m, 1H, 31-H$_a$), 3.22–3.14 (m, 1H, 31-H$_b$), 2.46–2.33 (m, 6H, 32-H, 33-H, 33′-H), 2.81–2.06 (m, 16H, 8 × CH$_2$ (cyclen)), 2.03 (s, 3H, Ac), 2.00–1.68 (m, 6H, 16-H$_a$, 11-H$_a$, 11-H$_b$, 18-H, 22-H$_a$, 16-H$_b$), 1.68–1.20 (m, 13H, 15-H$_a$, 1-H$_a$, 2-H$_a$, 2-H$_b$, 9-H, 6-H$_a$, 21-H$_a$, 7-H$_a$, 22-H$_b$, 19-H, 6-H$_b$, 21-H$_b$, 7-H$_b$), 1.06 (s, 3H, 27-H), 1.05–0.94 (m, 3H, 1-H$_b$, 15-H$_b$, 20-H), 0.93 (brs, 3H, 30-H), 0.91 (s, 3H, 25-H), 0.85 (d, J = 5.7 Hz, 3H, 29-H), 0.85 (s, 3H, 23-H), 0.83 (s, 3H, 24-H), 0.82–0.77 (m, 1H, 5-H), 0.76 (s, 3H, 26-H) ppm; ^{13}C NMR (101 MHz, CDCl$_3$): δ = 177.9 (C-28), 173.5 (CO, acetate), 170.9 (Ac), 170.0 (C-35), 139.7 (C-13), 135.4 (C$_{Ar}$), 135.3 (C$_{Ar}$), 135.2 (C$_{Ar}$), 128.7 (CH$_{Ar}$), 128.6 (CH$_{Ar}$), 128.5 (CH$_{Ar}$), 128.3 (CH$_{Ar}$), 128.3 (CH$_{Ar}$), 128.2 (CH$_{Ar}$), 125.3 (CH$_{Ar}$), 80.8 (C-3), 67.0 (CH$_2$, Bn), 66.8 (CH$_2$, Bn), 56.7 (C-32), 55.4 (C-36), 55.3 (CH$_2$, acetate), 55.2 (C-5), 53.9 (C-18), 53.4 (CH$_2$, cyclen), 52.7 (C-33, C-33′), 47.7 (C-17), 47.4 (C-9), 42.4 (C-14), 39.7 (C-19), 39.5 (C-8), 39.0 (C-20), 38.3 (C-1), 37.6 (C-4), 37.3 (C-22), 36.8 (C-10), 35.8 (C-31), 32.7 (C-7), 30.9 (C-21), 28.0 (C-23), 27.8 (C-15), 24.8 (C-16), 23.5 (C-2), 23.4 (C-11), 23.2 (C-27), 21.3 (Ac), 21.2 (C-30), 18.1 (C-6), 17.3 (C-29), 17.0 (C-26), 16.7 (C-24), 15.6 (C-25) ppm; MS (ESI, MeOH): m/z = 634 (20%, [M + 2H]$^{2+}$), 645 (100%, [M + H + Na]$^{2+}$), 1289 (62%, [M + Na]$^+$); analysis calcd for C$_{75}$H$_{107}$N$_7$O$_{10}$ (1266.72): C 71.11, H 8.51, N 7.74; found: C 70.73, H 8.70, N 7.49.

Triallyl 2,2′,2″-[10-[2-[4-[2-(3β-acetyloxy-urs-12-en-28-oylamino)ethyl]piperazin-1-yl]-2-oxoethyl]-1,4,7,10-tetraazacyclododecane-1,4,7-triyl]triacetate (**14**). Compound **14** was synthesized from **8** and **11** according to general procedure D. Column chromatography (SiO$_2$, CHCl$_3$/MeOH 95:5) furnished compound **14** (80%); m.p. 159–163 °C (decomp.); [α]$_D$ = +14.8° (c 0.310, CHCl$_3$); R$_f$ = 0.35 (SiO$_2$, CHCl3/MeOH 9:1); IR (KBr): ν = 3342s, 2946m, 2852w, 1734s, 1642s, 1522w, 1456m, 1386w, 1310w, 1246m, 1202m, 1106m, 1026w cm^{-1}; ^{1}H NMR (400 MHz, CDCl$_3$): δ = 6.35 (s, 1H, NH), 5.97 – 5.83 (m, 3H, 3 × CH (allyl)), 5.34–5.19 (m, 7H, 12-H, 3 × CH$_2$ (allyl)), 4.67–4.55 (m, 6H, 3 × CH$_2$ (allyl)), 4.47 (dd, J = 10.6, 5.3 Hz, 1H, 3-H), 3.72–2.97 (m, 14H, 34-H, 34′-H, 36-H, 3 × CH$_2$ (acetate), 31-H$_a$, 31-H$_b$), 2.97–2.14 (m, 22H, 8 × CH$_2$ (cyclen), 32-H, 33-H, 33′-H), 2.03 (s, 3H, Ac), 2.01–1.68 (m, 6H, 16-H$_a$, 11-H$_a$, 11-H$_b$, 18-H, 22-H$_a$, 16-H$_b$), 1.68–1.19 (m, 13H, 15-H$_a$, 1-H$_a$, 2-H$_a$, 2-H$_b$, 9-H, 6-H$_a$, 21-H$_a$, 7-H$_a$, 22-H$_b$, 19-H, 6-H$_b$,

21-H$_b$, 7-H$_b$), 1.07 (s, 3H, 27-H), 1.06–0.94 (m, 3H, 1-H$_b$, 15-H$_b$, 20-H), 0.94 (d, J = 6.5 Hz, 3H, 30-H), 0.92 (s, 3H, 25-H), 0.87 (d, J = 6.5 Hz, 3H, 29-H), 0.85 (s, 3H, 23-H), 0.83 (s, 3H, 24-H), 0.82–0.78 (m, 1H, 5-H), 0.76 (s, 3H, 26-H) ppm; ^{13}C NMR (101 MHz, CDCl$_3$): δ = 178.0 (C-28), 173.4 (2 × CO, acetate), 173.3 (CO, acetate), 171.1 (Ac), 170.0 (C-35), 139.8 (C-13), 131.9 (2 × CH, allyl), 131.7 (CH, allyl), 125.4 (C-12), 119.0 (CH$_2$, allyl), 118.8 (2 × CH$_2$, allyl), 80.9 (C-3), 66.0 (CH$_2$, allyl), 65.9 (2 × CH$_2$, allyl), 56.8 (C-32), 55.4 (C-36), 55.3 (C-5), 55.2 (3 × CH$_2$, acetate), 53.9 (C-18), 53.6 (8 x CH$_2$, cyclen), 52.7 (C-33, C-33′), 47.9 (C-17), 47.5 (C-9), 45.0 (C-34, C-34′), 42.6 (C-24), 39.8 (C-19), 39.7 (C-8), 39.1 (C-20), 38.4 (C-1), 37.8 (C-4), 37.4 (C-22), 37.0 (C-10), 35.9 (C-31), 32.8 (C-7), 31.0 (C-21), 28.2 (C-23), 27.9 (C-15), 24.9 (C-16), 23.6 (C-2), 23.6 (C-11), 23.3 (C-27), 21.4 (Ac), 21.3 (C-30), 18.3 (C-6), 17.4 (C-29), 17.1 (C-26), 16.8 (C-24), 15.7 (C-25) ppm; MS (ESI, MeOH): m/z = 569.8 (100%, [M + Na + H]$^+$), 1138.8 (52%, [M + Na]$^+$); analysis calcd for C$_{63}$H$_{101}$N$_7$O$_{10}$ (1116.54): C 67.77, H 9.12, N 8.78; found: C 67.50, H 9.37, N 8.43.

2,2′,2″-[10-[2-[4-[2-(3β-Acetyloxy-urs-12-en-28-oylamino)ethyl]piperazin-1-yl]-2-oxoethyl]-1,4,7,10-tetraazacyclododecane-1,4,7-triyl]triacetic acid (**15**). Triphenylphosphane (0.038 mmol), [(PPh$_3$)$_4$Pd] (0.013 mmol) and pyrrolidine (0.290 mmol) were added to a solution of compound **14** (0.128 mmol) in acetonitrile (4 mL), and the mixture was stirred for 6 days at 25 °C. After filtration, the solvent was removed under reduced pressure, and the crude product was subjected to column chromatography (RP18, MeCN/MeOH/TFA 60:40:0.1) affording compound **15** as colorless solid (96%); m.p. 206–210 °C (decomp.); [α]$_D$ = +17.1° (c 0.315, MeOH); R$_f$ = 0.35 (RP18, ACN/TFA 100:1); IR (ATR): ν = 2925w, 1634s, 1371m, 1245s, 1199s, 1127s, 1026m, 829m, 800m, 719m cm^{-1}; ^{1}H NMR (400 MHz, CD$_3$OD): δ = 5.35 (t, J = 3.6 Hz, 1H, 12-H), 4.47 (dd, J = 11.0, 5.3 Hz, 1H, 3-H), 3.72–2.93 (m, 14H, 34-H, 34′-H, 36-H, 31-H$_a$, 31-H$_b$, 3 × CH$_2$ (acetate)), 2.91–2.20 (m, 22H, 32-H, 33-H, 33′-H, 8 × CH$_2$ (cyclen)), 2.09–2.06 (m, 1H, 18-H), 2.03 (s, 3H, Ac), 2.02–1.93 (m, 3H, 11-H$_a$, 11-H$_b$, 16-H$_a$), 1.84–1.23 (m, 15H, 15-H$_a$, 22-H$_a$, 1-H$_a$, 16-H$_b$, 2-H$_a$, 2-H$_b$, 9-H, 7-H$_a$, 6-H$_a$, 21-H$_a$, 22-H$_b$, 19-H, 6-H$_b$, 21-H$_b$, 7-H$_b$), 1.15 (s, 3H, 27-H), 1.12–0.96 (m, 3H, 15-H$_b$, 1-H$_b$, 20-H), 0.99 (s, 3H, 25-H), 0.97 (brs, 3H, 30-H), 0.92 (d, J = 6.4 Hz, 3H, 29-H), 0.89 (s, 3H, 24-H), 0.88 (s, 3H, 23-H), 0.87–0.84 (m, 1H, 5-H), 0.83 (s, 3H,26-H) ppm; ^{13}C NMR (101 MHz, CD$_3$OD): δ = 180.1 (C-28), 172.8 (Ac), 172.5 (CO, acetate), 172.1 (2 × CO, acetate), 171.2 (C-35), 140.2 (C-13), 127.0 (C-12), 82.4 (C-3), 59.8 (CH$_2$, acetate), 59.7 (CH$_2$, acetate), 59.1 (CH$_2$, acetate), 57.7 (C-32), 56.7 (C-5), 55.3 (C-36), 54.4 (C-18), 54.2 (8 × CH$_2$, cyclen), 53.8 (C-33, C-33′), 49.0 (C-17), 48.8 (C-9), 46.2 (C-34. C-34′), 43.4 (C-14), 40.9 (C-8), 40.9 (C-19), 40.3 (C-20), 39.4 (C-1), 38.7 (C-4), 38.7 (C-22), 38.1 (C-10), 37.3 (C-31), 34.0 (C-7), 31.9 (C-21), 29.0 (C-15), 28.6 (C-23), 25.4 (C-16), 24.6 (C-2), 24.5 (C-11), 24.0 (C-27), 21.6 (C-30), 21.1 (Ac), 19.3 (C-6), 18.0 (C-26), 17.8 (C-29), 17.2 (C-24), 16.1 (C-25) ppm; MS (ESI, MeOH, positive ion mode): m/z = 1018.6 (27%, [M + Na]$^+$), 1034.7 (100%, [M + K]$^+$); MS (ESI, MeOH, negative ion mode): m/z = 1017.7 (13%, [M − 2H + Na]$^-$), 1032.6 (100%, [M − 2H + K]$^-$); analysis calcd for C$_{54}$H$_{89}$N$_7$O$_{10}$ (996.35): C 65.10, H 9.00, N 9.84; found: C 64.82, H 9.21, N 9.61.

1-(3β-Acetyloxy-urs-12-en-28-oyl)-4-(2-chloroacetyl) piperazine (**19**). Compound **19** has been synthesized from **16** according to general procedure C. Column chromatography (SiO$_2$, CHCl$_3$/acetone/hexanes 95:5:20) furnished compound **19** (94%); m.p. 155–158 °C; [α]$_D$ = +34.3° (c 0.370, CHCl$_3$); R$_f$ = 0.66 (CHCl$_3$/acetone 9:1); IR (ATR): ν = 2924m, 2871w, 1731m, 1658s, 1455m, 1392m, 1370m, 1243s, 1200m, 1145m, 1025m, 985m, 752m cm^{-1}; ^{1}H NMR (400 MHz, CDCl$_3$): δ = 5.21 (t, J = 3.6 Hz, 1H, 12-H), 4.52–4.45 (m, 1H, 3-H), 4.06 (s, 2H, 34-H), 3.73–3.46 (m, 8H, 31-H, 31′-H, 32-H, 32′-H), 2.41 (d, J = 11.6 Hz, 1H, 18-H), 2.24–2.11 (m, 1H, 16-H$_a$), 2.03 (s, 3H, Ac), 1.91 (dd, J = 8.9, 3.6 Hz, 2H, 11-H$_a$, 11-H$_b$), 1.80–1.24 (m, 15H, 15-H$_a$, 16-H$_b$, 22-H$_a$, 1-H$_a$, 2-H$_a$, 2-H$_b$, 22-H$_b$, 9-H, 6-H$_a$, 21-H$_a$, 7-H$_a$, 19-H, 6-H$_b$, 21-H$_b$, 7-H$_b$), 1.07 (s, 3H, 27-H), 1.12–0.98 (m, 3H, 1-H$_b$, 15-H$_b$, 20-H), 0.95 (d, J = 6.2 Hz, 3H, 30-H), 0.93 (s, 3H, 25-H), 0.88 (d, J = 6.4 Hz, 3H, 29-H), 0.85 (s, 3H, 23-H), 0.84 (s, 3H, 24-H), 0.84–0.77 (m, 1H, 5-H), 0.73 (s, 3H, 26-H) ppm; ^{13}C NMR (101 MHz, CDCl$_3$): δ = 175.8 (C-28), 171.1 (Ac), 165.5 (C-33), 138.6 (C-13), 125.5 (C-12), 81.0 (C-3), 55.5 (C-5), 55.1 (C-18), 48.8 (C-17), 47.7 (C-9), 46.3 (C-31), 45.5 (C-31′), 45.1 (C-32), 42.3 (C-32′, C-14), 40.9 (C-34), 39.6 (C-19), 39.6 (C-8), 38.9 (C-20), 38.4 (C-1), 37.8 (C-4), 37.1 (C-10), 34.6 (C-22), 33.1 (C-7), 30.6 (C-21), 28.3 (C-15), 28.2 (C-23), 23.9 (C-27), 23.7 (C-2, C-16), 23.4 (C-11), 21.4 (Ac), 21.4 (C-30), 18.3 (C-6), 17.6 (C-29), 17.0 (C-26), 16.9 (C-24), 15.6 (C-25) ppm; MS

(ESI, MeOH): m/z = 643.5 (100%, [M + H]$^+$), 665.4 (56%, [M + Na]$^+$), 1307.3 78%, [2M + Na]$^+$); analysis calcd for C$_{38}$H$_{59}$ClN$_2$O$_4$ (643.4): C 70.94, H 9.24, N 4.35; found: C 70.72, H 9.51, N 4.09.

(3β) N-(2-(2-Chloroacetyl)aminoethyl)-3-acetyloxy-urs-12-en-28-amide (**20**). Compound **20** was synthesized from **17** according to general procedure C. Column chromatography (SiO$_2$, CHCl$_3$/acetone/hexanes 95:5:20) furnished compound **20** (91%); m.p. 103–107 °C; [α]$_D$ = +25.2° (c 0.300, CHCl$_3$); R$_f$ = 0.40 (CHCl$_3$/acetone 9:1); IR (KBr): ν = 3422br s, 2948s, 2872m, 1734s, 1640s, 1532s, 1456m, 1370m, 1246s, 1148w, 1092w, 1028m, 756m cm^{-1}; ^{1}H NMR (400 MHz, CDCl$_3$): δ = 7.43 (t, J = 5.1 Hz, 1H, NH), 6.28 (t, J = 5.7 Hz, 1H, NH), 5.32 (t, J = 3.6 Hz, 1H, 12-H), 4.48 (dd, J = 9.7, 6.1 Hz, 1H, 3-H), 4.00 (s, 2H, 34-H), 3.56–3.46 (m, 1H, 31-H$_a$), 3.41–3.35 (m, 2H, 32-H), 3.26–3.18 (m, 1H, 31-H$_b$), 2.04 (s, 3H, Ac), 2.03–1.80 (m, 5H, 16-H$_a$, 11-H$_a$, 11-H$_b$, 18-H, 22-H$_a$), 1.80–1.22 (m, 14H, 16-H$_b$, 2-H$_a$, 2-H$_b$, 1-H$_a$, 15-H$_a$, 9-H, 6-H$_a$, 21-H$_a$, 7-H$_a$, 22-H$_b$, 19-H, 6-H$_b$, 21-H$_b$, 7-H$_b$), 1.08 (s, 3H, 27-H), 1.08–0.95 (m, 3H, 1-H$_b$, 15-H$_b$, 20-H), 0.94 (s, 3H, 30-H), 0.93 (s, 3H, 25-H), 0.87 (d, J = 6.5 Hz, 3H, 29-H), 0.86 (s, 3H, 23-H), 0.84 (s, 3H, 24-H), 0.84–0.79 (m, 1H, 5-H), 0.75 (s, 3H, 26-H) ppm; ^{13}C NMR (101 MHz, CDCl$_3$): δ = 180.0 (C-28), 171.1 (Ac), 167.0 (C-33), 139.7 (C-13), 125.9 (C-12), 81.0 (C-3), 55.4 (C-5), 53.8 (C-18), 48.0 (C-17), 47.6 (C-9), 42.6 (C-14), 42.6 (C-34), 41.3 (C-32), 39.9 (C-19), 39.7 (C-8), 39.2 (C-31), 39.2 (C-20), 38.4 (C-1), 37.8 (C-4), 37.4 (C-22), 37.0 (C-10), 32.8 (C-7), 31.0 (C-21), 28.2 (C-23), 27.9 (C-15), 24.9 (C-16), 23.7 (C-2), 23.5 (C-11), 23.4 (C-27), 21.4 (Ac), 21.3 (C-30), 18.3 (C-6), 17.4 (C-29), 17.0 (C-26), 16.8 (C-24), 15.7 (C-25) ppm; MS (ESI, MeOH): m/z = 617.3 (48%, [M + H]$^+$), 639.5 (52%, [M + Na]$^+$), 1255.4 (100%, [2M + Na]$^+$); analysis calcd for C$_{36}$H$_{57}$ClN$_2$O$_4$ (617.31): C 70.04, H 9.31, N 4.54; found: C 69.83, H 9.52, N 4.11.

(3β) N-(2-(2-(2-Chloroacetyl)aminoethoxy)ethyl)-3-acetyloxy-urs-12-en-28-amide (**21**). Compound **21** has been synthesized from **18** according to general procedure C. Column chromatography (SiO$_2$, CHCl$_3$/acetone/hexanes 95:5:20) furnished compound **21** (91%); m.p. 94–97 °C; [α]$_D$ = +33.7° (c 0.335, CHCl$_3$); R$_f$ = 0.35 (CHCl$_3$/acetone 9:1); IR (KBr): ν = 3426br s, 2928m, 2872m, 1734m, 1638s, 1528m, 1458w, 1386w, 1248s, 1124w, 1028m cm^{-1}; ^{1}H NMR (400 MHz, CDCl$_3$): δ = 7.00–6.90 (m, 1H, NH), 6.22 (t, J = 5.0 Hz, 1H, NH), 5.30 (t, J = 3.6 Hz, 1H, 12-H), 4.49 (dd, J = 10.0, 5.7 Hz, 1H, 3-H), 4.06 (s, 2H, 36-H), 3.57–3.47 (m, 7H, 32-H, 31-H$_a$, 33-H, 34-H), 3.31–3.21 (m, 1H, 31-H$_b$), 2.04 (s, 3H, Ac), 2.02–1.76 (m, 5H, 16-H$_a$, 11-H$_a$, 11-H$_b$, 18-H, 22-H$_a$), 1.77–1.21 (m, 14H, 16-H$_b$, 15-H$_a$, 1-H$_a$, 2-H$_a$, 2-H$_b$, 9-H, 6-H$_a$, 21-H$_a$, 7-H$_a$, 22-H$_b$, 19-H, 6-H$_b$, 21-H$_b$, 7-H$_b$), 1.09 (s, 3H, 27-H), 1.08–0.95 (m, 3H, 1-H$_b$, 15-H$_b$, 20-H), 0.94 (d, J = 6.2 Hz, 3H, 30-H), 0.93 (s, 3H, 25-H), 0.88 (d, J = 6.2 Hz, 3H, 29-H), 0.86 (s, 3H, 23-H), 0.85 (s, 3H, 24-H), 0.84–0.80 (m, 1H, 5-H), 0.78 (s, 3H, 26-H) ppm; ^{13}C NMR (101 MHz, CDCl$_3$): δ = 178.4 (C-28), 171.1 (Ac), 166.1 (C-35), 139.9 (C-13), 125.6 (C-12), 80.9 (C-3), 70.0 (C-33), 69.4 (C-32), 55.4 (C-5), 54.0 (C-18), 48.0 (C-17), 47.6 (C-9), 42.8 (C-36), 42.6 (C-14), 39.9 (C-29), 39.8 (C-34), 39.7 (C-8), 39.2 (C-31), 39.2 (C-20), 38.5 (C-1), 37.8 (C-4), 37.4 (C-22), 37.0 (C-10), 32.8 (C-7), 31.0 (C-21), 28.2 (C-23), 28.0 (C-15), 25.0 (C-16), 23.7 (C-2), 23.6 (C-11), 23.4 (C-27), 21.4 (Ac), 21.4 (C-30), 18.3 (C-6), 17.4 (C-29), 17.1 (C-26), 16.9 (C-24), 15.7 (C-25) ppm; MS (ESI, MeOH): m/z = 661.4 (60%, [M + H]$^+$), 685.5 (86%, [M + Na]$^+$), 1343.3 (100%, [2M + Na]$^+$); analysis calcd for C$_{38}$H$_{61}$ClN$_2$O$_5$ (661.37): C 69.01, H 9.30, N 4.24, Cl 5.36; found: C 68.80, H 9.61, N 4.01.

Tri-tert-butyl 2,2′,2″-[10-[2-[4-(3β-acetyloxy-urs-12-en-28-oyl)piperazin-1-yl]-2-oxoethyl]-1,4,7,10-tetraazacyclododecane-1,4,7-triyl]triacetate (**22**). Compound **22** was synthesized from **6** and **19** according to general procedure D. Column chromatography (SiO$_2$, CHCl$_3$/MeOH 95:5) furnished compound **22** (88%); m.p. 237–240 °C (decomp.); [α]$_D$ = +15.0° (c 0.3, CHCl$_3$); R$_f$ = 0.42 (CHCl$_3$/MeOH 9:1); IR (ATR): ν = 2927w, 2928w, 2871w, 2829w, 1726m, 1646m, 1453m, 1424w, 1368s, 1305m, 1227s, 1160s, 1105s, 1004m, 975m, 754m cm^{-1}; ^{1}H NMR (400 MHz, CDCl$_3$): δ = 5.19 (t, J = 3.5 Hz, 1H, 12-H), 4.47 (dd, J = 9.8, 6.0 Hz, 1H, 3-H), 3.93 – 2.05 (m, 32H, 31-H, 31′-H, 32-H, 32′-H, 8 × CH$_2$ (cyclen), 3 × CH$_2$ (acetate), 34-H), 2.40 (d, J = 11.0 Hz, 1H, 18-H), 2.19–2.09 (m, 1H, 16-H$_a$), 2.02 (s, 3H, Ac), 1.93–1.85 (m, 2H, 11-H$_a$, 11-H$_b$), 1.82–1.67 (m, 3H, 15-H$_a$, 16-H$_b$, 22-H$_a$), 1.65–1.21 (m, 12H, 2-H$_a$, 2-H$_b$, 22-H$_b$, 1-H$_a$, 9-H, 21-H$_a$, 6-H$_a$, 7-H$_a$, 19-H, 21-H$_b$, 6-H$_b$, 7-H$_b$), 1.43 (s, 9H, CH$_3$ (tButyl)), 1.42 (s, 9H; CH$_3$ (tButyl)), 1.42 (s, 9H, CH$_3$ (tButyl)), 1.10–0.96 (m, 3H, 1-H$_b$, 15-H$_b$, 20-H), 1.05 (s, 3H, 27-H), 0.92 (d, J = 6.3 Hz, 3H, 30-H), 0.91 (s, 3H, 25-H), 0.86 (d, J = 6.3 Hz, 3H, 29-H), 0.84 (s, 3H, 23-H), 0.82

(s, 3H, 24-H), 0.82–0.76 (m, 1H, 5-H), 0.71 (s, 3H, 26-H) ppm; ^{13}C NMR (101 MHz, CDCl$_3$): δ = 175.9 (C-28), 172.8 (CO, acetate), 172.7 (CO, acetate), 171.0 (Ac), 170.7 (C-33), 138.7 (C-13), 125.1 (C-12), 81.9 (C$_q$, tButyl), 81.7 (C$_q$, tButyl), 81.7 (C$_q$, tButyl), 81.0 (C-3), 55.8 (CH$_2$, acetate), 55.8 (CH$_2$, acetate), 55.7 (CH$_2$, cyclen), 55.4 (C-5), 55.1 (C-18), 48.8 (C-17), 47.6 (C-9), 44.6 (C-31, C-31′, C-32, C-32′), 42.3 (C-14), 41.7 (C-34), 39.5 (C-8), 39.4 (C-19), 38.8 (C-20), 38.3 (C-1), 37.8 (C-4), 37.0 (C-10), 34.4 (C-22), 33.1 (C-7), 30.5 (C-21), 28.3 (C-15), 28.2 (C-23), 28.1 (CH$_3$, tButyl), 28.0 (CH$_3$, tButyl), 23.8 (C-27), 23.6 (C-2, C-16), 23.4 (C-11), 21.4 (Ac), 21.3 (C-30), 18.2 (C-6), 17.5 (C-29), 17.0 (C-26), 16.8 (C-24), 15.6 (C-25) ppm; MS (ESI, MeOH): m/z = 1143.7 (100%, [M + Na]$^+$); analysis calcd for C$_{64}$H$_{108}$N$_6$O$_{10}$ (1121.60): C 68.54, H 9.71, N 7.49; found: C 68.31, H 10.03, N 7.27.

Tribenzyl 2,2′,2″-[10-[2-[4-(3β-acetyloxy-urs-12-en-28-oyl)piperazin-1-yl]-2-oxoethyl]-1,4,7,10-tetraazacyclododecane-1,4,7-triyl]triacetate (**23**). Compound **23** was synthesized from **19** and **7** according to general procedure D. Column chromatography (SiO$_2$, CHCl$_3$/MeOH 95:5) furnished compound **23** (72%); m.p. 157–161 °C; [α]$_D$ = +4.2° (c 0.300, CHCl$_3$); R$_f$ = 0.37 (CHCl$_3$/MeOH 9:1); IR (ATR): ν = 2945w, 2836w, 1730s, 1638m, 1454m, 1424w, 1392m, 1370m, 1302m, 1243s, 1194s, 1105s, 1005m, 966m, 743m, 697s cm^{-1}; UV-Vis (CHCl$_3$): λ$_{max}$ (logε) = 246 nm (3.96), 294 nm (3.47), 364 nm (3.23); ^{1}H NMR (400 MHz, CDCl$_3$): δ = 7.39–7.26 (m, 15H, 15 × CH (Bn)), 5.33–4.97 (m, 7H, 12-H, 3 × CH$_2$ (Bn)), 4.45 (dd, J = 10.1, 5.9 Hz, 1H, 3-H), 4.02–2.05 (m, 34H, 31-H, 31′-H, 32-H, 32′-H, 8 × CH$_2$ (cyclen), 3 × CH$_2$ (acetate), 34-H, 16-H$_a$, 18-H), 2.02 (s, 3H, Ac), 1.95–1.65 (m, 5H, 11-H$_a$, 11-H$_b$, 15-H$_a$, 16-H$_b$, 22-H$_a$), 1.65–1.09 (m, 12H, 2-H$_a$, 2-H$_b$, 22-H$_b$, 1-H$_a$, 9-H, 21-H$_a$, 6-H$_a$, 7-H$_a$, 19-H, 21-H$_b$, 6-H$_b$, 7-H$_b$), 1.03 (s, 3H, 27-H), 1.08–0.95 (m, 3H, 1-H$_b$, 15-H$_b$, 20-H), 0.93 (d, J = 6.0 Hz, 3H, 30-H), 0.85 (d, J = 6.3 Hz, 3H, 29-H), 0.85 (s, 3H, 25-H), 0.82 (s, 3H, 23-H), 0.79 (s, 3H, 24-H), 0.79–0.71 (m, 1H, 5-H), 0.66 (s, 3H, 26-H) ppm; ^{13}C NMR (101 MHz, CDCl$_3$): δ = 175.9 (C-28), 173.6 (CO, acetate), 171.0 (Ac), 170.8 (C-33), 138.6 (C-13), 135.5 (C$_i$, Bn), 135.3 (C$_i$, Bn), 128.7 (CH, Bn), 128.7 (CH, Bn), 128.6 (CH, Bn), 128.6 (CH, Bn), 128.4 (CH, Bn), 128.4 (CH, Bn), 125.1 (C-12), 81.0 (C-3), 67.1 (CH$_2$, Bn), 66.9 (CH$_2$, Bn), 55.7 (CH$_2$, acetate), 55.4 (CH$_2$, cyclen), 55.2 (C-5), 55.1 (C-18), 48.7 (C-17), 47.6 (C-9), 44.8 (C-31, C-31′, C-32, C-32′), 42.2 (C-14), 42.0 (C-34), 39.5 (C-19), 39.5 (C-8), 38.8 (C-20), 38.3 (C-1), 37.7 (C-4), 36.9 (C-10), 34.5 (C-22), 33.1 (C-7), 30.6 (C-21), 28.2 (C-15), 28.1 (C-23), 23.6 (C-2, C-16), 23.5 (C-27), 23.4 (C-11), 21.4 (Ac), 21.3 (C-30), 18.2 (C-6), 17.5 (C-29), 17.0 (C-26), 16.8 (C-24), 15.5 (C-25) ppm; MS (ESI, MeOH): m/z = 1245.8 (100%, [M + Na]$^+$); analysis calcd for C$_{73}$H$_{102}$N$_6$O$_{10}$ (1223.65): C 71.65, H 8.40, N 6.87; found: C 71.42, H 8.69, N 6.56.

Tri-tert-butyl 2,2′,2″-[10-[2-[2-(3β-acetyloxy-urs-12-en-28-oylamino)ethyl]amino-2-oxoethyl]-1,4,7,10-tetraazacyclododecane-1,4,7-triyl]triacetate (**24**). Compound **24** was synthesized from **20** and **6** according to general procedure D. Column chromatography (SiO$_2$, CHCl$_3$/MeOH 95:5) furnished compound **24** (73%); m.p. 254–257 °C (decomp.); [α]$_D$ = +33.8° (c 0.300, CHCl$_3$); R$_f$ = 0.40 (CHCl$_3$/MeOH 9:1); IR (KBr): ν = 2971m, 2929m, 2829w, 1727s, 1668m, 1520m, 1454m, 1426w, 1368s, 1307m, 1228s, 1159s, 1106s, 1027m, 1006m, 975m, 755m cm^{-1}; ^{1}H NMR (400 MHz, CDCl$_3$): δ = 8.03 (s, 1H, NH), 7.08 (s, 1H, NH), 5.46 (t, J = 3.4 Hz, 1H, 12-H), 4.47 (dd, J = 9.8, 6.1 Hz, 1H, 3-H), 3.80–2.05 (m, 28H, 31-H, 32-H, 34-H, 3 × CH$_2$ (acetate), 8 × CH$_2$ (cyclen)), 2.44–2.38 (m, 1H, 18-H), 2.02 (s, 3H, Ac), 2.00–1.67 (m, 6H, 15-H$_a$, 11-H$_a$, 11-H$_b$, 16-H$_a$, 16-H$_b$, 22-H$_a$), 1.66–1.19 (m, 12H, 1-H$_a$, 2-H$_a$, 2-H$_b$, 22-H$_b$, 9-H, 6-H$_a$, 7-H$_a$, 21-H$_a$, 19-H, 6-H$_b$, 21-H$_b$, 7-H$_b$), 1.44 (s, 9H, CH$_3$ (tButyl)), 1.43 (s, 9H, CH$_3$ (tButyl)), 1.43 (s, 9H, CH$_3$ (tButyl)), 1.15–0.98 (m, 3H, 20-H, 1-H$_b$, 15-H$_b$), 1.04 (s, 3H, 27-H), 0.91 (s, 3H, 25-H), 0.90 (d, J = 6.1 Hz, 3H, 30-H), 0.88 (d, J = 6.1 Hz, 3H, 29-H), 0.84 (s, 3H, 23-H), 0.83 (s, 3H, 24-H), 0.82–0.77 (m, 1H, 5-H), 0.74 (s, 3H, 26-H) ppm; ^{13}C NMR (101 MHz, CDCl$_3$): δ = 178.7 (C-28), 172.4 (CO, acetate), 171.7 (C-33), 171.1 (Ac), 139.0 (C-13), 125.5 (C-12), 82.1 (C$_q$, tButyl), 82.1 (C$_q$, tButyl), 82.1 (C$_q$, tButyl), 81.1 (C-3), 56.4 (3 × CH$_2$, acetate), 55.8 (C-34), 55.8 (CH$_2$, cyclen), 55.4 (C-5), 52.3 (C-18), 47.7 (C-9), 47.6 (C-17), 42.2 (C-14), 40.0 (C-32), 39.7 (C-19), 39.7 (C-8), 38.5 (C-20), 38.4 (C-31, C-1), 37.8 (C-4), 37.4 (C-22), 37.0 (C-10), 32.9 (C-7), 31.2 (C-21), 28.2 (C-23), 28.2 (CH$_3$, tButyl), 28.1 (CH$_3$, tButyl), 28.1 (CH$_3$, tButyl), 27.9 (C-15), 24.4 (C-16), 23.7 (C-2), 23.5 (C-27), 23.4 (C-11), 21.5 (C-30), 21.4 (Ac), 18.4 (C-6), 17.2 (C-29), 17.0

(C-26), 16.9 (C-24), 15.7 (C-25) ppm; MS (ESI, MeOH): m/z = 1117.7 (100%, [M + Na]$^+$); analysis calcd for $C_{62}H_{106}N_6O_{10}$ (1095.56): C 67.97, H 9.75, N 7.67; found: C 67.68, H 10.02, N 7.41.

Tribenzyl 2,2',2"-[10-[2-[2-(3β-acetyloxy-urs-12-en-28-oylamino)ethyl]amino-2-oxoethyl]-1,4,7,10-tetraazacyclododecane-1,4,7-triyl]triacetate (**25**). Compound **25** was synthesized from **7** and **20** according to general procedure D. Column chromatography (SiO$_2$, CHCl$_3$/MeOH 95:5) furnished compound **25** (75%); m.p. 142–146 °C; [α]$_D$ = +20.5° (c 0.390, CHCl$_3$); R$_f$ = 0.36 (CHCl$_3$/MeOH 9:1); IR (ATR): ν = 2945w, 2832w, 1732s, 1663m, 1519w, 1454m, 1370m, 1305m, 1245s, 1194s, 1176s, 1105s, 1007m, 965m, 747m, 697s cm^{-1}; UV-Vis (CHCl$_3$): λ$_{max}$ (logε) = 241 nm (3.89), 295 nm (3.29), 364 nm (3.08); ^{1}H NMR (400 MHz, CDCl$_3$): δ = 8.20 (t, J = 4.5 Hz, 1H, NH), 7.39–7.27 (m, 15H, CH (Bn)), 7.01 (t, J = 4.9 Hz, 1H, NH), 5.48 (s, 1H, 12-H), 5.26–5.05 (m, 6H, CH$_2$ (Bn)), 4.47 (dd, J = 10.0, 5.7 Hz, 1H, 3-H), 3.77–2.07 (m, 28H, 31-H$_a$, 31-H$_b$, 32-H, 34-H, 3 × CH$_2$ (acetate),8 × CH$_2$ (cyclen)), 2.41 (d, J = 10.7 Hz, 1H, 18-H), 2.02 (s, 3H, Ac), 2.00–1.64 (m, 6H, 16-H$_a$, 16-H$_b$, 11-H$_a$, 11-H$_b$, 22-H$_a$, 15-H$_a$), 1.64–1.19 (m, 12H, 1-H$_a$, 2-H$_a$, 2-H$_b$, 22-H$_b$, 9-H, 6-H$_a$, 7-H$_a$, 21-H$_a$, 6-H$_b$, 19-H, 21-H$_b$, 7-H$_b$), 1.17–0.97 (m, 3H, 20-H, 1-H$_b$, 15-H$_b$), 1.04 (s, 3H, 27-H), 0.89 (d, J = 6.3 Hz, 6H, 29-H, 30-H), 0.87 (s, 3H, 25-H), 0.83 (s, 3H, 23-H), 0.81 (s, 3H, 24-H), 0.80–0.76 (m, 1H, 5-H), 0.72 (s, 3H, 26-H) ppm; ^{13}C NMR (101 MHz, CDCl$_3$): δ = 178.8 (C-28), 173.2 (CO, acetate), 172.0 (C-33), 171.0 (Ac), 139.0 (C-13), 135.4 (C$_i$, Bn), 135.4 (C$_i$, Bn), 135.3 (C$_i$, Bn), 128.8 (CH, Bn), 128.8 (CH, Bn), 128.7 (CH, Bn), 128.6 (CH, Bn), 125.6 (12-H), 81.0 (3-H), 67.3 (CH$_2$, Bn), 67.3 (CH$_2$, Bn), 67.2 (CH$_2$, Bn), 56.8 (CH$_2$, acetate), 55.4 (C-34), 55.3 (C-5), 55.3 (CH$_2$, cyclen), 52.3 (C-18), 47.7 (C-17), 46.6 (C-9), 42.2 (C-14), 40.1 (C-32), 39.8 (C-19), 39.7 (C-8), 38.5 (C-20), 38.5 (C-31, C-1), 37.8 (C-4), 37.4 (C-22), 37.0 (C-10), 32.9 (C-7), 31.2 (C-21), 28.2 (C-23), 28.0 (C-15), 24.5 (C-16), 23.7 (C-2), 23.5 (C-27), 23.4 (C-11), 21.4 (Ac), 21.4 (C-30), 18.4 (C-6), 17.2 (C-29), 17.1 (C-26), 16.8 (C-24), 15.6 (C-25) ppm; MS (ESI, MeOH): m/z = 1219.8 (100%, [M + Na]$^+$); analysis calcd for $C_{71}H_{100}N_6O_{10}$ (1197.61): C 71.21, H 8.42, N 7.02; found: 70.93, H 8.56, N 6.82.

Tri-tert-butyl 2,2',2"-[10-[2-[2-[2-(3β-acetyloxy-urs-12-en-28-oylamino)ethoxy]ethyl]amino-2-oxoethyl]-1,4,7,10-tetraazacyclododecane-1,4,7-triyl]triacetate (**26**). Compound **26** was synthesized from **6** and **21** according to general procedure D. Column chromatography (SiO$_2$, CHCl$_3$/MeOH 95:5) furnished compound **26** (74%); m.p. 263–266 °C (decomp.); [α]$_D$ = +21.9° (c 0.315, CHCl$_3$); R$_f$ = 0.38 (CHCl$_3$/MeOH 9:1); IR (ATR): ν = 2972m, 2930m, 1726s, 1166m, 1523w, 1453m, 1368s, 1307m, 1228s, 1160s, 1106s, 1026m, 1006m, 975m, 755m cm^{-1}; ^{1}H NMR (400 MHz, CDCl$_3$): δ = 7.82 (t, J = 5.6 Hz, 1H, NH), 6.46 (t, J = 5.1 Hz, 1H, NH), 5.33 (t, J = 3.7 Hz, 1H, 12-H), 4.47 (dd, J = 10.2, 5.9 Hz, 1H, 3-H), 3.56–3.30 (m, 9H, 32-H, 31-H$_a$, 33-H, 36-H, 34-H), 3.28–3.16 (m, 1H, 31-H$_b$), 3.15–2.05 (m, 22H, 3 × CH$_2$ (acetate), 8 × CH$_2$ (cyclen)), 2.02 (s, 3H, Ac), 2.02–1.21 (m, 19H, 18-H, 16-H$_a$, 11-H$_a$, 11-H$_b$, 22-H$_b$, 16-H$_b$, 15-H$_a$, 1-H$_a$, 2-H$_a$, 2-H$_b$, 9-H, 6-H$_a$, 21-H$_a$, 7-H$_a$, 22-H$_b$, 19-H, 6-H$_b$, 21-H$_b$, 7-H$_b$), 1.44 (s, 9H, CH$_3$ (tButyl)), 1.43 (s, 18H, CH$_3$ (tButyl)), 1.06 (s, 3H, 27-H), 1.05–0.94 (m, 3H, 1-H$_b$, 15-H$_b$, 20-H), 0.92 (s, 3H, 25-H), 0.92 (d, J = 6.2 Hz, 3H, 30-H), 0.86 (d, J = 6.5 Hz, 3H, 29-H), 0.84 (s, 3H, 23-H), 0.83 (s, 3H, 24-H), 0.82–0.77 (m, 1H, 5-H), 0.76 (s, 3H, 26-H) ppm; ^{13}C NMR (101 MHz, CDCl$_3$): δ = 178.3 (C-28), 173.0 (CO, acetate), 172.5 (CO, acetate), 172.1 (C-35), 171.1 (Ac), 139.3 (C-13), 125.7 (C-12), 82.1 (C$_q$, tButyl), 82.0 (C$_q$, tButyl), 81.9 (C$_q$, tButyl), 81.0 (C-3), 69.5 (C-33), 69.0 (C-32), 56.5 (C-36), 55.9 (CH$_2$, acetate), 55.8 (CH$_2$, acetate), 55.7 (CH$_2$, cyclen), 55.4 (C-5), 53.4 (C-18), 47.8 (C-17), 47.6 (C-9), 42.4 (C-14), 39.8 (C-19), 39.7 (C-8), 39.2 (C-31), 39.0 (C-34), 39.0 (C-20), 38.4 (C-1), 37.8 (C-4), 37.3 (C-22), 37.0 (C-10), 32.9 (C-7), 31.1 (C-21), 28.2 (CH$_3$, tButyl), 28.0 (CH$_3$, tButyl), 28.0 (C-23), 28.0 (C-15), 24.9 (C-16), 23.7 (C-2), 23.5 (C-11), 23.4 (C-27), 21.4 (Ac), 21.4 (C-30), 18.3 (C-6), 17.3 (C-29), 17.0 (C-26), 16.8 (C-24), 15.7 (C-25) ppm; MS (ESI, MeOH): m/z = 1161.7 (100%, [M + Na]$^+$); analysis calcd for $C_{64}H_{110}N_6O_{11}$ (1139.6): C 67.45, H 9.73, N 7.37; found: C 67.31, H 9.87, N 7.09.

Tribenzyl 2,2',2"-[10-[2-[2-[2-(3β-acetyloxy-urs-12-en-28-oylamino)ethoxy]ethyl]amino-2-oxoethyl]-1,4,7,10-tetraazacyclododecane-1,4,7-triyl]triacetate (**27**). Compound **27** has been synthesized from **7** and **21** according to general procedure D. Column chromatography (SiO$_2$, CHCl$_3$/MeOH 95:5) furnished compound **27** (62%); m.p. 137–141 °C; [α]$_D$ = +15.4° (c 0.350, CHCl$_3$); R$_f$ = 0.35 (CHCl$_3$/MeOH 9:1); IR (ATR): ν = 2945w, 2830w, 1731s, 1662m, 1523w, 1454m, 1390m, 1370m, 1305m, 1245s, 1193s, 1105s,

1026m, 1008m, 967m, 747m, 697m cm^{-1}; UV-Vis (CHCl$_3$): λ_{max} (logε) = 244 nm (3.73), 294 nm (3.36), 363 nm (3.12); ^{1}H NMR (400 MHz, CDCl$_3$): δ = 8.02 (*t*, *J* = 5.4 Hz, 1H, NH), 7.37–7.27 (*m*, 15H, CH (Bn)), 6.48 (*t*, *J* = 5.1 Hz, 1H, NH), 5.32 (*t*, *J* = 3.5 Hz, 1H, 12-H), 5.24–5.14 (*m*, 4H, CH$_2$ (Bn)), 5.14–5.05 (*m*, 2H, CH$_2$ (Bn)), 4.46 (*dd*, *J* = 10.2, 5.7 Hz, 1H, 3-H), 3.59–3.33 (*m*, 9H, 32-H, 33-H, 31-H$_a$, 34-H, 36-H), 3.33–2.01 (*m*, 23H, 31-H$_b$, 8 × CH$_2$ (cyclen), 3 × CH$_2$ (acetate)), 2.02 (*s*, 3H, Ac), 2.00–1.17 (*m*, 19H, 18-H, 16-H$_a$, 11-H$_a$, 11-H$_b$, 22-H$_a$, 16-H$_b$, 15-H$_a$, 1-H$_a$, 2-H$_a$, 2-H$_b$, 9-H, 6-H$_a$, 22-H$_b$, 7-H$_a$, 21-H$_a$, 19-H, 6-H$_b$, 7-H$_b$, 21-H$_b$), 1.05 (*s*, 3H, 27-H), 1.04 – 0.94 (*m*, 3H, 1-H$_b$, 15-H$_b$, 20-H), 0.90 (*s*, 3H, 25-H), 0.90 (*d*, *J* = 5.8 Hz, 3H, 30-H), 0.85 (*d*, *J* = 6.6 Hz, 3H, 29-H), 0.84 (*s*, 3H, 23-H), 0.82 (*s*, 3H, 24-H), 0.81–0.76 (*m*, 1H, 5-H), 0.75 (*s*, 3H, 26-H) ppm; ^{13}C NMR (101 MHz, CDCl$_3$): δ = 178.3 (C-28), 173.3 (CO, acetate), 173.1 (CO, acetate), 172.3 (C-35), 171.1 (Ac), 139.3 (C-13), 135.4 (C$_i$, Bn), 135.3 (C$_i$, Bn), 128.7 (CH, Bn), 128.7 (CH, Bn), 128.7 (CH, Bn), 128.6 (CH, Bn), 128.5 (CH, Bn), 125.7 (C-12), 81.0 (C-3), 69.6 (C-33), 68.9 (C-32), 67.2 (CH$_2$, Bn), 67.2 (CH$_2$, Bn), 56.9 (C-36), 55.4 (3 × CH$_2$, acetate), 55.4 (C-5), 55.3 (8 × CH$_2$, cyclen), 53.3 (C-18), 47.8 (C-17), 47.6 (C-9), 42.4 (C-14), 39.8 (C-19), 39.7 (C-8), 39.2 (C-31, C-34), 38.9 (C-20), 38.4 (C-1), 37.8 (C-4), 37.3 (C-22), 36.9 (C-10), 32.9 (C-7), 31.1 (C-21), 28.2 (C-23), 28.0 (C-15), 24.8 (C-16), 23.6 (C-2), 23.5 (C-11), 23.4 (C-27), 21.4 (Ac), 21.4 (C-30), 18.3 (C-6), 17.3 (C-29), 17.1 (C-26), 16.8 (C-24), 15.7 (C-25) ppm; MS (ESI, MeOH): *m/z* = 1263.9 (100%, [M + Na]$^+$); analysis calcd for C$_{73}$H$_{104}$N$_6$O$_{11}$ (1241.67): C 70.62, H 8.44, N 6.77; found: C 70.41, H 8.69, N 6.41.

(3β) N-(2-Aminoethyl)-3-hydroxy-urs-12-en-28-amide (**28**). Method A: The synthesis was performed according to the procedure given in the Supplementary material in 82%. Method B: Ursolic acid (100 mg, 0.20 mmol), HOBt·H$_2$O (37 mg, 0.24 mmol) and EDC·HCl (46 mg, 0.24 mmol) were dissolved in dry DMF (5 mL), and the mixture was stirred for 30 min at 25 °C. Ethylene diamine (55 μL, 0.82 mmol) was added to the mixture, and stirring was continued for 24 h at 25 °C. Usual aqueous work-up followed by column chromatography (silica gel, CHCl$_3$/MeOH/NH$_4$OH 90:10:0.1) gave **28** (46%). Analytical data of this compound can be found in the supplementary material.

Tri-tert-butyl 2,2',2''-[10-[2-[2-(3β-hydroxy-urs-12-en-28-oylamino)ethyl]amino-2-oxoethyl]-1,4,7,10-tetraazacyclododecane-1,4,7-triyl]triacetate (**29**). Method A: To a solution of DOTA-tris(tert-butyl ester) (58 mg, 0.10 mmol) in dry DMF (8 mL) were added HOBt·H$_2$O (29 mg, 0.19 mmol) and EDC·HCl (29 mg, 0.15 mmol). After stirring for 30 min at 25 °C, a solution of **28** (71 mg, 0.14 mmol) in dry DMF (2 mL) was added and stirring was continued for 5 days. After usual aqueous work-up, the solvent was removed under reduced pressure and the crude product was subjected to column chromatography (silica gel, CHCl$_3$/MeOH 9:1) yielding compound **29** as colorless solid. Yield: 49%. Method B: Compound **24** (50 mg, 0.10 mmol) was dissolved in methanol (7 mL) and a solution of potassium hydroxide (12 mg, 0.21 mmol) in methanol (1 mL) was added. The mixture was stirred at 25 °C for 24 h. After completion of the reaction (as indicated by TLC) and usual work-up, the solvent was removed under reduced pressure, and the residue was subjected to column chromatography (silica gel, CHCl$_3$/MeOH 9:1) affording **29** (yield: 86%); m.p. 136–139 °C; [α]$_D$ = −44.4° (c 0.330, MeOH); R$_f$ = 0.29 (CHCl$_3$/MeOH 9:1); IR (KBr): ν = 3300*br w*, 2973*w*, 2928*m*, 2869*w*, 1728*s*, 1668*m*, 1525*m*, 1455*m*, 1425*w*, 1368*s*, 1307*m*, 1227*s*, 1159*s*, 1121*m*, 1106*s*, 1047*w*, 1006*w* cm^{-1}; ^{1}H NMR (400 MHz, CDCl$_3$): δ = 8.84 (*s*, 1H, NH), 7.55 (*s*, 1H, NH), 5.36 (*t*, *J* = 3.5 Hz, 1H, 12-H), 3.59–2.05 (*m*, 28H, 31-H, 32-H, 33-H, 3 × CH$_2$ (acetate), 8 × CH$_2$ (cyclen)), 3.20 (*dd*, *J* = 11.1, 4.8 Hz, 1H, 3-H), 2.34 (*d*, *J* = 11.0 Hz, 2H, 18-H), 2.03–1.96 (*m*, 1H, 16-H$_a$), 1.95–1.83 (*m*, 3H, 11-H$_a$, 11-H$_b$, 16-H$_b$), 1.83–1.72 (*m*, 1H, 22-H$_a$), 1.64–1.21 (*m*, 13H, 1-H$_a$, 15-H$_a$, 2-H$_a$, 2-H$_b$, 22-H$_b$, 6-H$_a$, 9-H, 7-H$_a$, 21-H$_a$, 19-H, 6-H$_b$, 7-H$_b$, 21-H$_b$), 1.45 (*s*, 9H, CH$_3$ (*t*Butyl)), 1.43 (*s*, 18H, CH$_3$ (*t*Butyl)), 1.05 (*s*, 3H, 27-H), 1.04–0.97 (*m*, 3H, 1-H$_b$, 15-H$_b$, 20-H), 0.97 (*s*, 3H, 23-H), 0.89 (*d*, *J* = 6.3 Hz, 3H, 30-H), 0.89 (*s*, 3H, 25-H), 0.85 (*d*, *J* = 6.4 Hz, 3H, 29-H), 0.76 (*s*, 3H, 24-H), 0.75 (*s*, 3H, 26-H), 0.72–0.68 (*m*, 1H, 5-H) ppm; ^{13}C NMR (101 MHz, CDCl$_3$): δ = 178.4 (C-28), 172.4 (CO, acetate), 171.8 (C-33), 138.9 (C-13), 125.3 (C-12), 82.2 (C$_q$, *t*Butyl), 82.1 (C$_q$, *t*Butyl), 82.1 (C$_q$, *t*Butyl), 79.2 (C-3), 56.0 (CH$_2$, acetate), 55.9 (C-34), 55.8 (CH$_2$, cyclen), 55.3 (C-5), 52.5 (C-18), 47.8 (C-9), 47.5 (C-17), 42.2 (C-14), 40.0 (C-32), 39.7 (C-8), 39.6 (C-19), 38.9 (C-4), 38.7 (C-20), 38.7 (C-31, C-1), 37.4 (C-22), 37.1 (C-10), 33.2 (C-7), 31.3 (C-21), 28.3 (C-23), 28.2 (CH$_3$, *t*Butyl), 28.2 (CH$_3$, *t*Butyl), 28.1 (CH$_3$, tButyl), 28.0 (C-15), 27.4 (C-2), 24.2 (C-16), 23.6 (C-27), 23.5 (C-11), 21.5 (C-30), 18.6 (C-6), 17.2 (C-29), 17.1 (C-26), 15.8 (C-24), 15.7 (C-25) ppm; MS (ESI, MeOH): m/z = 1075.7 (100%, [M + Na]$^+$); analysis calcd for $C_{60}H_{104}N_6O_9$ (1053.53): C 68.40, H 9.95, N 7.98; found: C 60.09, H 10.11, N 7.83.

Supplementary Materials: Supplementary data related to this article including experimental procedures for compounds **10**, **17**, **18**, and **28**, Figure S1: Extended cytotoxicity investigation after treatment of A375 cells with **22** (3.0 µM) for 24 h, representative NMR spectra and calculation of ADMET parameters for compounds **22** and **24** can be found online.

Author Contributions: M.K.; and R.C. conceived and designed the experiments; M.K. performed the experiments; S.H. and L.F. performed the biological assays and experiments; M.K.; A.A-H.; and R.C. analyzed the data and wrote the paper.

Funding: We acknowledge the financial support within the funding program Open Access Publishing by the German Research Foundation (DFG).

Acknowledgments: We would like to thank R. Kluge for measuring the ESI-MS spectra and D. Ströhl and his team for the NMR spectra. Thanks are also due to V. Simon for measuring the IR an UV-VIS spectra and optical rotations. The cell lines were kindly provided by Th. Müller (Dept. of Haematology/Oncology, Martin-Luther Universität Halle-Wittenberg).

Conflicts of Interest: The authors declare no conflict of interest.

References

1. Bray, F.; Ferlay, J.; Soerjomataram, I.; Siegel, R.L.; Torre, L.A.; Jemal, A. Global cancer statistics 2018: GLOBOCAN estimates of incidence and mortality worldwide for 36 cancers in 185 countries. *Ca-Cancer J. Clin.* **2018**, *68*, 394–424. [CrossRef] [PubMed]
2. Stasiuk, G.J.; Long, N.J. The ubiquitous DOTA and its derivatives: The impact of 1, 4, 7, 10-tetraazacyclododecane-1, 4, 7, 10-tetraacetic acid on biomedical imaging. *Chem. Commun.* **2013**, *49*, 2732–2746. [CrossRef] [PubMed]
3. Chilla, S.N.M.; Henoumont, C.; Elst, L.V.; Muller, R.N.; Laurent, S. Importance of DOTA derivatives in bimodal imaging. *Isr. J. Chem.* **2017**, *57*, 800–808. [CrossRef]
4. Magerstädt, M.; Gansow, O.A.; Brechbiel, M.W.; Colcher, D.; Baltzer, L.; Knop, R.H.; Girton, M.E.; Naegele, M. Gd (DOTA): An alternative to Gd (DTPA) as a T1, 2 relaxation agent for NMR imaging or spectroscopy. *Magn. Reson. Med.* **1986**, *3*, 808–812. [CrossRef] [PubMed]
5. Jones-Wilson, T.M.; Deal, K.A.; Anderson, C.J.; McCarthy, D.W.; Kovacs, Z.; Motekaitis, R.J.; Sherry, A.D.; Martell, A.E.; Welch, M.J. The in vivo behavior of copper-64-labeled azamacrocyclic complexes. *Nucl. Med. Biol.* **1998**, *25*, 523–530. [CrossRef]
6. Wu, A.M.; Yazaki, P.J.; Tsai, S.-w.; Nguyen, K.; Anderson, A.-L.; McCarthy, D.W.; Welch, M.J.; Shively, J.E.; Williams, L.E.; Raubitschek, A.A. High-resolution microPET imaging of carcinoembryonic antigen-positive xenografts by using a copper-64-labeled engineered antibody fragment. *Proc. Natl. Acad. Sci. USA* **2000**, *97*, 8495–8500. [CrossRef] [PubMed]
7. Deshpande, S.V.; DeNardo, S.J.; Kukis, D.L.; Moi, M.K.; McCall, M.J.; DeNardo, G.L.; Meares, C.F. Yttrium-90-labeled monoclonal antibody for therapy: Labeling by a new macrocyclic bifunctional chelating agent. *J. Nucl. Med.* **1990**, *31*, 473–479.
8. Razboršek, M.I.; Vončina, D.B.; Doleček, V.; Vončina, E. Determination of Oleanolic, Betulinic and Ursolic Acid in Lamiaceae and Mass Spectral Fragmentation of Their Trimethylsilylated Derivatives. *Chromatographia* **2008**, *67*, 433–440. [CrossRef]
9. Fu, L.; Zhang, S.; Li, N.; Wang, J.; Zhao, M.; Sakai, J.; Hasegawa, T.; Mitsui, T.; Kataoka, T.; Oka, S.; et al. Three New Triterpenes from Nerium oleander and Biological Activity of the Isolated Compounds. *J. Nat. Prod.* **2005**, *68*, 198–206. [CrossRef]
10. Cargnin, S.T.; Gnoatto, S.B. Ursolic acid from apple pomace and traditional plants: A valuable triterpenoid with functional properties. *Food Chem.* **2017**, *220*, 477–489. [CrossRef]
11. Yamaguchi, H.; Noshita, T.; Kidachi, Y.; Umetsu, H.; Hayashi, M.; Komiyama, K.; Funayama, S.; Ryoyama, K. Isolation of Ursolic Acid from Apple Peels and Its Specific Efficacy as a Potent Antitumor Agent. *J. Health Sci.* **2008**, *54*, 654–660. [CrossRef]

12. Chen, H.; Gao, Y.; Wang, A.; Zhou, X.; Zheng, Y.; Zhou, J. Evolution in medicinal chemistry of ursolic acid derivatives as anticancer agents. *Eur. J. Med. Chem.* **2015**, *92*, 648–655. [CrossRef] [PubMed]
13. Hussain, H.; Green, I.R.; Ali, I.; Khan, I.A.; Ali, Z.; Al-Sadi, A.M.; Ahmed, I. Ursolic acid derivatives for pharmaceutical use: A patent review (2012-2016). *Expert Opin. Pat.* **2017**, *27*, 1061–1072. [CrossRef] [PubMed]
14. Seo, D.Y.; Lee, S.R.; Heo, J.-W.; No, M.-H.; Rhee, B.D.; Ko, K.S.; Kwak, H.-B.; Han, J. Ursolic acid in health and disease. *Korean J. Physiol. Pharm.* **2018**, *22*, 235–248. [CrossRef] [PubMed]
15. Zou, J.; Lin, J.; Li, C.; Zhao, R.; Fan, L.; Yu, J.; Shao, J. Ursolic Acid in Cancer Treatment and Metastatic Chemoprevention: From Synthesized Derivatives to Nanoformulations in Preclinical Studies. *Curr. Cancer Drug Targets* **2019**, *19*, 245–256. [CrossRef] [PubMed]
16. Ma, C.-M.; Cai, S.-Q.; Cui, J.-R.; Wang, R.-Q.; Tu, P.-F.; Hattori, M.; Daneshtalab, M. The cytotoxic activity of ursolic acid derivatives. *Eur. J. Med. Chem.* **2005**, *40*, 582–589. [CrossRef] [PubMed]
17. Liu, D.; Meng, Y.-q.; Zhao, J.; Chen, L.-g. Synthesis and Anti-tumor Activity of Novel Amide Derivatives of Ursolic Acid. *Chem. Res. Chin. Univ.* **2008**, *24*, 42–46. [CrossRef]
18. Meng, Y.-Q.; Liu, D.; Cai, L.-L.; Chen, H.; Cao, B.; Wang, Y.-Z. The synthesis of ursolic acid derivatives with cytotoxic activity and the investigation of their preliminary mechanism of action. *Bioorg. Med. Chem.* **2009**, *17*, 848–854. [CrossRef]
19. Liu, M.-C.; Yang, S.-J.; Jin, L.-H.; Hu, D.-Y.; Xue, W.; Song, B.-A.; Yang, S. Synthesis and cytotoxicity of novel ursolic acid derivatives containing an acyl piperazine moiety. *Eur. J. Med. Chem.* **2012**, *58*, 128–135. [CrossRef]
20. Sommerwerk, S.; Heller, L.; Kerzig, C.; Kramell, A.E.; Csuk, R. Rhodamine B conjugates of triterpenoic acids are cytotoxic mitocans even at nanomolar concentrations. *Eur. J. Med. Chem.* **2017**, *127*, 1–9. [CrossRef]
21. Kahnt, M.; Fischer, L.; Al-Harrasi, A.; Csuk, R. Ethylenediamine Derived Carboxamides of Betulinic and Ursolic Acid as Potential Cytotoxic Agents. *Molecules* **2018**, *23*, 2558. [CrossRef] [PubMed]
22. Kim, S.-M.; Jeong, I.H.; Yim, M.S.; Chae, M.K.; Kim, H.N.; Kim, D.K.; Kang, C.M.; Choe, Y.S.; Lee, C.; Ryu, E.K. Characterization of oleanolic acid derivative for colon cancer targeting with positron emission tomography. *J. Drug Target.* **2014**, *22*, 191–199. [CrossRef] [PubMed]
23. Yang, X.; Li, Y.; Jiang, W.; Ou, M.; Chen, Y.; Xu, Y.; Wu, Q.; Zheng, Q.; Wu, F.; Wang, L. Synthesis and biological evaluation of novel ursolic acid derivatives as potential anticancer prodrugs. *Chem. Biol. Drug Des.* **2015**, *86*, 1397–1404. [CrossRef]
24. Bai, K.-K.; Yu, Z.; Chen, F.-L.; Li, F.; Li, W.-Y.; Guo, Y.-H. Synthesis and evaluation of ursolic acid derivatives as potent cytotoxic agents. *Bioorg. Med. Chem. Lett.* **2012**, *22*, 2488–2493. [CrossRef] [PubMed]
25. Rami, M.; Cecchi, A.; Montero, J.-L.; Innocenti, A.; Vullo, D.; Scozzafava, A.; Winum, J.-Y.; Supuran, C.T. Carbonic Anhydrase Inhibitors: Design of Membrane-Impermeant Copper(II) Complexes of DTPA-, DOTA-, and TETA-Tailed Sulfonamides Targeting the Tumor-Associated Transmembrane Isoform IX. *ChemMedChem* **2008**, *3*, 1780–1788. [CrossRef]
26. Loesche, A.; Kahnt, M.; Serbian, I.; Brandt, W.; Csuk, R. Triterpene-Based Carboxamides Act as Good Inhibitors of Butyrylcholinesterase. *Molecules* **2019**, *24*, 948. [CrossRef] [PubMed]
27. Deng, S.-L.; Baglin, I.; Nour, M.; Cavé, C. Synthesis of phosphonodipeptide conjugates of ursolic acid and their homologs. *Heteroat. Chem.* **2008**, *19*, 55–65. [CrossRef]

Sample Availability: Samples of all compounds are available from the authors.

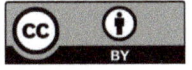

© 2019 by the authors. Licensee MDPI, Basel, Switzerland. This article is an open access article distributed under the terms and conditions of the Creative Commons Attribution (CC BY) license (http://creativecommons.org/licenses/by/4.0/).

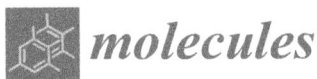

Article

Antiproliferative Aspidosperma-Type Monoterpenoid Indole Alkaloids from *Bousigonia mekongensis* Inhibit Tubulin Polymerization

Yu Zhang [1,2], Masuo Goto [2,*], Akifumi Oda [3], Pei-Ling Hsu [2], Ling-Li Guo [1], Yan-Hui Fu [1], Susan L. Morris-Natschke [2], Ernest Hamel [4], Kuo-Hsiung Lee [2,5,*] and Xiao-Jiang Hao [1,*]

1. Key Laboratory of Phytochemistry and Plant Resources in West China, Kunming Institute of Botany, Chinese Academy of Sciences, Kunming 650201, China; zhangyu@mail.kib.ac.cn (Y.Z.); guolingli@mail.kib.ac.cn (L.-L.G.); fuyanhui80@163.com (Y.-H.F.)
2. Natural Product Research Laboratories, UNC Eshelman School of Pharmacy, University of North Carolina, Chapel Hill, NC 27599, USA; peiling96@livemail.tw (P.-L.H.); susan_natschke@unc.edu (S.L.M.-N.)
3. Graduate School of Pharmacy, Meijo University, 150 Yagotoyama, Tempaku-ku, Nagoya, Aichi 468-8503, Japan; oda@meijo-u.ac.jp
4. Screening Technologies Branch, Developmental Therapeutics Program, Division of Cancer Treatment and Diagnosis, Frederick National Laboratory for Cancer Research, National Cancer Institute, Frederick, MD 21702, USA; hamele@dc37a.nci.nih.gov
5. Chinese Medicine Research and Development Center, China Medical University and Hospital, 2 Yuh-Der Road, Taichung 40447, Taiwan
* Correspondence: goto@med.unc.edu (M.G.); khlee@unc.edu (K.-H.L.); haoxj@mail.kib.ac.cn (X-J.H.); Tel.: +1-919-962-0066 (M.G. and K.-H.L.); +86-871-652-23263 (X-J.H.)

Received: 7 February 2019; Accepted: 28 March 2019; Published: 31 March 2019

Abstract: Monoterpenoid indole alkaloids are structurally diverse natural products found in plants of the family Apocynaceae. Among them, vincristine and its derivatives are well known for their anticancer activity. *Bousigonia mekongensis*, a species in this family, contains various monoterpenoid indole alkaloids. In the current study, fourteen known aspidosperma-type monoterpenoid indole alkaloids (**1–14**) were isolated and identified from a methanol extract of the twigs and leaves of *B. mekongensis* for the first time. Among them, compounds **3**, **6**, **9**, and **13** exhibited similar antiproliferative activity spectra against A549, KB, and multidrug-resistant (MDR) KB subline KB-VIN cells with IC_{50} values ranging from 0.5–0.9 µM. The above alkaloids efficiently induced cell cycle arrest at the G2/M phase by inhibiting tubulin polymerization as well as mitotic bipolar spindle formation. Computer modeling studies indicated that compound **7** likely forms a hydrogen bond (H-bond) with α- or β-tubulin at the colchicine site. Evaluation of the antiproliferative effects and SAR analysis suggested that a 14,15-double bond or 3α-acetonyl group is critical for enhanced antiproliferative activity. Mechanism of action studies demonstrated for the first time that compounds **3**, **4**, **6**, **7**, and **13** efficiently induce cell cycle arrest at G2/M by inhibiting tubulin polymerization by binding to the colchicine site.

Keywords: aspidosperma-type; monoterpenoid indole alkaloids; antiproliferative activity; tubulin inhibitor; *Bousigonia mekongensis*

1. Introduction

Microtubule-binding agents have been developed as an effective therapy in cancer treatment due to the key roles of microtubules in cell proliferation, signal transduction, and cell migration [1]. Currently, many microtubule-binding agents, including taxanes, vinca alkaloids, epothilones, halichondrins, maytansinoids, colchicine-site binding agents, and others, have been discovered from natural products and later progressed to clinical studies and clinical use [2]. However, innate and acquired drug resistance, especially multidrug resistance (MDR), are major obstacles in cancer chemotherapy [3]. Overexpression of P-glycoprotein (P-gp) encoded by the ABCB1 gene leads to poor disease prognosis, and most clinical antimicrotubule drugs, including paclitaxel (PXL), vincristine (VIN), halichondrin B, and their analogs, are P-gp substrates [4]. A recent study indicated that antimitotic agents that target the colchicine site (CS) on the α/β-tubulin dimer were generally active in cells overexpressing βIII-tubulin, which is important in tumor aggressiveness and resistance to chemotherapy [5]. Hence, the discovery of other antimitotic CS-targeting agents might be a valuable approach for effective cancer chemotherapy, especially agents with enhanced tumor specificity and insensitivity to chemoresistance mechanisms.

Monoterpenoid indole alkaloids (MIAs) are secondary metabolites characteristic of plants in the family Apocynaceae [6]. Among them, the vinca alkaloids exhibit significant anticancer activity and vincristine, vinblastine, vinorelbine, vindesine, and vinflunine have been approved for clinical use in the treatment of hematological and lymphatic neoplasms [7]. Previous chemical studies on MIAs mostly focused on the dimeric compounds (vindoline-catharanthine), which generally exhibit superior anticancer activities compared with the corresponding monomeric units. Aspidosperma-type MIAs contain only the vindoline structural unit found in vincristine and are widely distributed in the genera *Tabernaemontana*, *Melodinus*, and *Bousigonia* (family Apocynaceae) [6]. In prior biological activity studies, several aspidosperma-type MIAs, such as jerantinines A, B, and E from *T. corymbose*, displayed significant antiproliferative activity against cancer cells [8]. Further mechanistic studies demonstrated that these alkaloids significantly arrested cells at the G2/M phase by inhibiting tubulin polymerization and, thus, they merit development as potential chemotherapeutic agents [9–11].

The genus *Bousigonia* (family Apocynaceae) contains only two species (*B. mekongensis* and *B. angustifolia*), distributed mainly in Southern China, Laos, and Vietnam [12]. Previous chemical investigation on this genus conducted in our group resulted in a series of new eburnamine-aspidospermine-type bisindole alkaloids and aspidosperma-type MIAs [13–15]. As part of our ongoing work, the present study investigated the antiproliferative activity of aspidosperma-type MIAs (**1–14**) against five cancer cell lines, A549, MDA-MB-231, KB, P-gp-overexpressing KB subline KB-VIN, and MCF-7, as well as a primary structure activity relationship (SAR) analysis including computer modeling. The detailed mechanisms of action of these alkaloids (Figure 1) were also further investigated and are described herein.

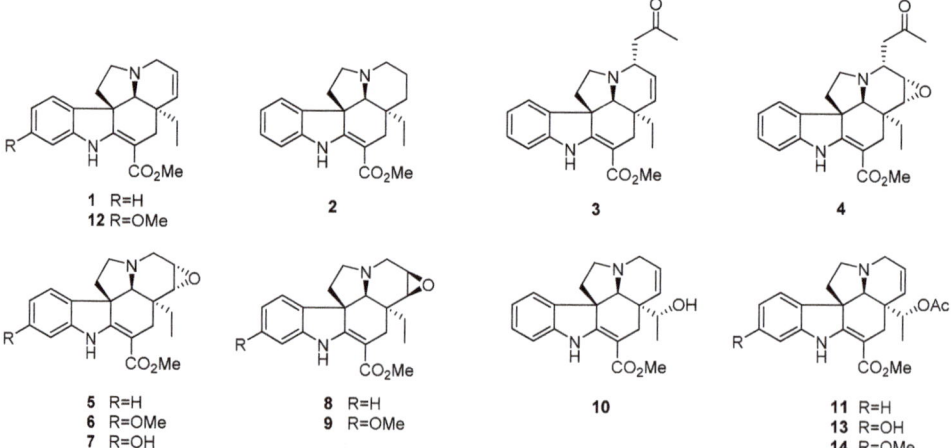

Figure 1. Structures of aspidosperma-type MIAs (**1–14**) from *B. mekongensis*.

2. Results and Discussion

2.1. Chemistry

Fourteen aspidosperma-type monoterpenoid indole alkaloids, tabersonine (1) [16], vincadifformine (2) [16], 3α-acetonyl-tabersonine (3) [17], melodinine S (4) [18], lochnericine (5) [19], 14,15-α-epoxy-11-methoxytabersonine (6) [20], 11-hydroxylochnericine (7) [20], pachysiphine (8) [21], lochnerinine (9) [22], 19-(R)-hydroxytabersonine (10) [23], 19-(R)-acetoxytabersonine (11) [24], 11-methoxytabersonine (12) [16], 19-(R)-acetoxy-11-hydroxytabersonine (13) [24], 19-(R)-acetoxy-11-methoxytabersonine (14) [24] were isolated and identified from the methanol extract of *B. mekongensis* for the first time by a combination of chromatographic and spectroscopic methods (Figure 1, Tables S1–S3). The effects of the substituents at positions C-3, C-11, C-14/C-15, and C-19 were evaluated by considering the hydrophilic or hydrophobic properties.

2.2. Antiproliferative Activity of Compounds 1–14

We tested the fourteen known aspidosperma-type alkaloids (1–14) against chemosensitive KB (originally isolated from epidermoid carcinoma of the nasopharynx) and P-gp over-expressing multidrug-resistant (MDR) KB subline KB-VIN, as well as three additional human cancer cell lines, A549 (lung carcinoma), MDA-MB-231 (triple negative breast cancer), and MCF-7 (estrogen receptor-positive breast cancer), using a sulforhodamine B (SRB) assay (Table 1). Vincristine (VIN), paclitaxel (PXL), and a CS agent combretastatin A-4 (CA-4) were also tested as positive controls.

Table 1. Antiproliferative activity and effect on tubulin assembly.

Compound	IC$_{50}$ (μM) [a]					Tubulin Assay	
	A549	MDA-MB-231	KB	KB-VIN	MCF-7	ITA[d] (μM)	ICB[e] (%)
1	6.9 ± 0.1	5.9 ± 0.0	5.5 ± 0.0	7.4 ± 0.3	7.2 ± 0.4	NT[b]	NT
2	>40	>40	>40	>40	>40	NA[c]	NA
3	0.6 ± 0.0	0.9 ± 0.0	0.6 ± 0.0	0.6 ± 0.1	2.2 ± 0.2	NT	NT
4	5.6 ± 0.0	8.2 ± 0.8	5.8 ± 0.3	6.3 ± 0.2	10.0 ± 0.9	NT	NT
5	>40	>40	>40	>40	>40	NA	NA
6	0.5 ± 0.0	0.8 ± 0.0	0.5 ± 0.0	0.5 ± 0.0	0.8 ± 0.0	0.7 ± 0.0	54 ± 0.8
7	5.6 ± 0.1	9.8 ± 0.9	5.4 ± 0.3	6.1 ± 0.4	10.8 ± 0.8	4.6 ± 0.1	35 ± 1
8	27.7 ± 0.1	34.5 ± 0.2	>40	>40	>40	NA	NA
9	0.8 ± 0.0	6.0 ± 0.8	0.9 ± 0.0	0.7 ± 0.0	10.2 ± 0.5	NT	NT
10	>40	>40	>40	>40	>40	NA	NA
11	>40	>40	26.5 ± 2.5	>40	>40	NA	NA
12	5.2 ± 0.1	6.8 ± 1.1	5.4 ± 0.4	5.8 ± 0.1	8.2 ± 0.9	NT	NT
13	0.7 ± 0.1	0.9 ± 0.0	0.7 ± 0.0	0.7 ± 0.0	6.7 ± 0.1	NT	NT
14	>40	>40	>40	>40	>40	NA	NA
VIN (nM)	22.9 ± 2.4	32.0 ± 0.5	4.4 ± 0.1	2479.2 ± 28.2	7.3 ± 0.2	NT	NT
PXL (nM)	4.5 ± 0.9	7.0 ± 0.9	3.7 ± 1.1	2357.7 ± 59.5	8.8 ± 1.0	NT	NT
CA-4 (nM)	5.5 ± 0.1	8.2 ± 0.5	3.6 ± 0.1	3.8 ± 0.1	487.4 ± 11	0.7 ± 0.0	100 ± 0.4

[a] Antiproliferative activity as IC$_{50}$ values for each cell line, the concentration of compound that caused a 50% reduction relative to untreated cells determined by the SRB assay. [b] NT, not tested. [c] NA, not active (IC$_{50}$ > 40 μM). [d] Inhibition of purified tubulin assembly, EC$_{50}$ (μM) values of 50% inhibition (ITA). [e] Percent inhibition of 5 μM [^{3}H] colchicine binding to 1 μM tubulin in the presence of 5 μM test compound (ICB).

2.3. Biological Activity Comparison

While six alkaloids (2, 5, 8, 10, 11, and 14) were essentially inactive, the remaining eight alkaloids (1, 3, 4, 6, 7, 9, 12, and 13) exhibited antiproliferative activity against all cell lines tested in this study, including the MDR subline KB-VIN (Table 1). Particularly, alkaloids 3, 6, 9, and 13 showed substantial potency against KB-VIN cells with IC$_{50}$ values ranging from 0.5–0.7 μM. Notably, all eight active alkaloids were effective against both chemosensitive and MDR cells, as compared with well-known P-gp substrates VIN and PXL, which required 600-fold higher concentration against KB-VIN cells.

The results indicate that the tested alkaloids are not substrates of P-gp and, thus, could be effective against tumors expressing the MDR phenotype.

Alkaloids **1–14** have the same carbon skeleton but differ in the substituents or oxidation state at various positions. Based on the antiproliferative activity data, a 14,15-double bond is critical for activity as alkaloids **2**, **5**, and **8** with a 14,15-single bond lost potency. Addition of a 3α-acetonyl group led to greatly increased potency (compare **3** versus **1**, **4** versus **5**). Potency was lost when the α-carbon of the ethyl group attached at C-19 of **1** was substituted with a hydroxyl (**10**) or acetoxy (**11**) moiety. The presence of a hydroxyl group at C-11 had a significant effect on potency (compare **7** versus **5**, **13** versus **11**), while a methoxy group at the same position led to both increased (~60-fold rise between **5** and **6**, **8** and **9**) and negligible (compare **1** versus **12**, **14** and **11**) potency.

Taken together, a 14,15-double bond or 3α-acetonyl group was required for antiproliferative activity against human cancer cell lines, including the MDR subline KB-VIN. A hydroxyl group at C-11 is necessary, while the effect of a methoxy group at C-11 was dependent on the parent skeleton. The compatibility of the synergistic groups will be considered in subsequent SAR studies.

2.4. Mechanisms of Action of 3, 4, 6, 7, and 13 in KB-VIN Cells

Bioactive analogs **6** and **7** were tested for inhibitory effects on tubulin assembly as well as inhibition of [^{3}H] colchicine binding to tubulin in a cell-free system, using highly purified bovine brain tubulin (Table 1). The results showed that alkaloid **6** strongly inhibited tubulin assembly with an EC_{50} (50% effective concentration for inhibiting tubulin assembly) value of 0.7 μM and inhibited the binding of colchicine to tubulin by 54%, while **7** showed moderate inhibition of tubulin assembly with an EC_{50} value of 4.6 μM. The data for **6** and **7** indicate that both alkaloids bind to tubulin and inhibit its assembly, and these effects are closely related to their antiproliferative activities against tumor cells. Thus, we further investigated whether the inhibition of tubulin polymerization was the major action of these alkaloids.

CA-4, a colchicine site (CS) agent, and other tubulin polymerization inhibitors induce cell cycle arrest at G2/M. Accordingly, we investigated whether the MIAs affected the cell cycle progression. KB-VIN cells were treated with compounds **3**, **4**, **6**, **7**, and **13** at their IC_{50} (1 × IC_{50}) or three-fold IC_{50} (3 × IC_{50}) concentration, and the cell cycle progression was analyzed by flow cytometer (Figure 2A). Expectedly, the accumulation of cells in the G2/M phase was observed in cells treated with alkaloids **3**, **4**, **6**, **7**, and **13**, as compared with CA-4 and vincristine (VIN).

To determine whether the cell cycle arrest was due to an antimicrotubule effect, cells treated with compounds were analyzed by immunocytochemistry using antibodies to α-tubulin for microtubules and mitotic spindles, Ser10-phosphorylated histone H3 (pH3) for the condensed chromatins and 4′,6-diamidino-2-phenylindole (DAPI) for DNA. In cells treated with alkaloids **3**, **4**, **6**, **7**, and **13**, dotted tubulin aggregations without spindles were seen in the pH3-positive mitotic cells, while microtubules were undetectable in pH3-negative interphase cells (Figure 2B). These observations demonstrated that the tested alkaloids inhibited tubulin polymerization in both interphase and mitosis for bipolar spindle formation, inducing cell cycle arrest at G2/M, probably at prometaphase. In addition, alkaloid **7** was less active than **6**, which corresponded to the inhibitory activity observed in cell-based proliferation and cell-free tubulin assembly assays. Thus, we concluded that these alkaloids are tubulin polymerization inhibitors. Furthermore, the immunocytochemical data suggest that alkaloids **3**, **4**, **6**, **7**, and **13** probably interact with tubulin in a biological manner similar to that of CA-4. These results agreed with those in a recent study on aspidosperma-type MIAs, such as jerantinine A, which potentially inhibit tubulin polymerization by binding to the CS on tubulin dimers [25].

Accordingly, we performed molecular docking studies to predict how alkaloid **7** binds to the tubulin dimer. An inactive alkaloid **5** was used as a comparison compound. In the tubulin binding assay described above (Table 1), CA-4 totally inhibited colchicine binding to tubulin, while **5** or **7** inhibited binding with 0 or 35% ICB value, respectively. Thus, compared with CA-4, alkaloid **5** and its hydroxyl analog **7** might bind differently to the CS. As expected, an overview of the predicted binding modes of **5** and **7** in the crystal structure of the α/β-tubulin dimer revealed considerable differences (Figures 3 and 4). The docked model of **5** showed an H-bond between the carbonyl oxygen and the side chain of Val181 on α-tubulin (αVal181), while that of **7** showed an H-bond between the C-11 hydroxyl group and the side chain of Val315 on β-tubulin (βVal315). Interestingly, in a cell-free tubulin assembly assay, compound **7** (EC_{50} 4.6 μM) was more potent than **5** (EC_{50} > 40 μM). These analyses suggested that the binding mode of **5** was insufficient to inhibit tubulin assembly. The docking model also predicted that active compound **13** (IC_{50} 0.6~6.7 μM) forms an H-bond with βAsn249, while less active compounds **4** (IC_{50} 5.6~10.0 μM) and **11** (IC_{50} > 26.5 μM) form H-bonds with αThr179 and αSer178, respectively (Supplementary Figure S2). However, H-bonding with αVal181 may also be important and depends on a steric hindrance due to the parent skeleton (compare **3** versus **5**). This docking model suggested that the force of the H-bond between βVal315 or βAsn249 and the C-11 hydroxyl group of **7** might be critical for greater inhibition of tubulin assembly, which is also reflected in greater antiproliferative activity.

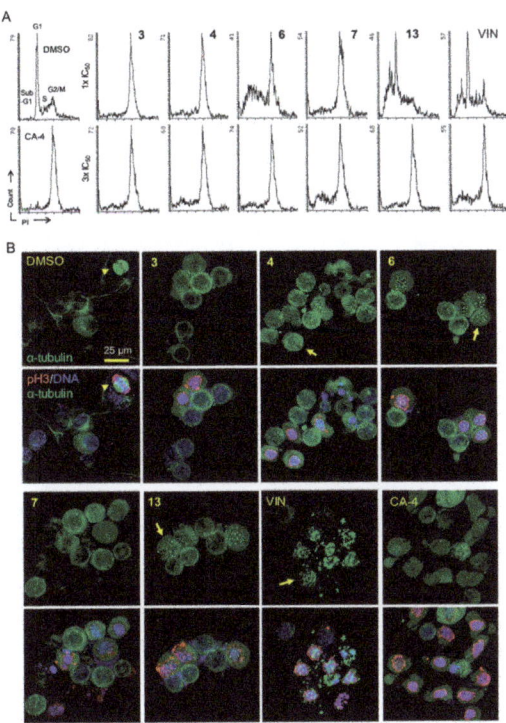

Figure 2. Mitotic defects in KB-VIN cells treated by compounds. (**A**) Vincristine-resistant subline KB-VIN cells were treated with compounds for 24 h at a concentration of one- or three-fold IC_{50} (1× IC_{50} or 3 × IC_{50}). CA-4 at 0.2 μM was used as a colchicine-type tubulin polymerization inhibitor. Cell cycle distributions (sub-G1, G1, S, G2/M) were analyzed using flow cytometry after staining cells with propidium iodide (PI). (**B**) KB-VIN cells were treated with compounds for 24 h at a concentration of 3 × IC_{50}. CA-4 was used at 0.2 μM. Fixed cells were stained with antibodies to α-tubulin (green) and phospho-histone H3 (pH3, red), and DAPI was used for DNA (blue). Stained cells were observed by confocal fluorescence microscope. The represented image is a projection of 15~20 optical sections acquired at 0.5~1 μm intervals. Normal mitotic spindle formation (arrow head) in control (DMSO) and dotted tubulin aggregations without spindles (**4, 6, 13**) or with multipolar spindles (VIN) were observed (arrows). Bar, 0.025 mm. Additional images are available in Supplementary Figure S1.

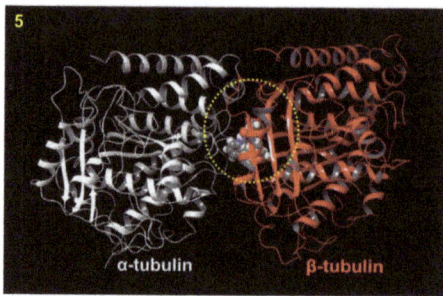
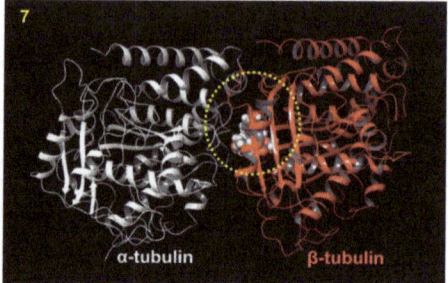

Figure 3. Predicted docking models for **5** and **7** binding to tubulin. Top 1 ranked docking models of **5** and **7** (sphere in 3D with gray in carbon, proton in white, oxygen in red, nitrogen in blue) in the colchicine site (CS, yellow circle) of the tubulin crystal structure (α and β tubulin heterodimer: α- (white) and β-tubulin (red)) (PDB: 1SA0) are shown as a ribbon diagram.

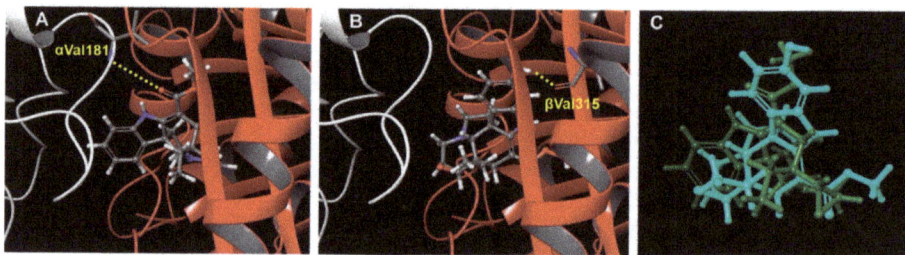

Figure 4. Predicted docking models for **5** and **7** binding in the CS. The crystal structures (PDB: 1SA0) of α- (white) and β-tubulin (red) are shown as ribbon diagrams. The distances calculated to be less than 5 Å between heavy atoms are represented by dashed lines. Docking models of compounds (gray skeleton with oxygen in red and nitrogen in blue) **5** (**A**) and **7** (**B**) in the CS are shown. Superimposition of docked compound **5** or **7** shows H-bonds with the side chain of αVal181 or βVal315, respectively. (**C**) Comparison of docking mode of **5** (green) with that of **7** (blue) in CS.

3. Materials and Methods

3.1. General Experimental Procedures

All chemicals and solvents were used as purchased. ESIMS data were obtained on a Finnigan MAT 90 spectrometer. NMR spectra were recorded on Bruker DRX-500 and Avance III -600 NMR spectrometers using TMS as an internal standard. All chemical shifts are reported in ppm, and apparent scalar coupling constants J are given in Hertz. Silica gel (300–400 mesh, Qingdao Marine Chemical Inc., Shandong, China), silica gel H (10–40 μm, Qingdao Marine Chemical Inc.), Lichroprep RP-18 gel (40–63 μm, Merck, Darmstadt, Germany), and Sephadex LH-20 (40–70 μm, Amersham Biosciences, Waltham, MA, USA) were used for column chromatography (CC). All target compounds were characterized and determined to be at least >95% pure by ^{1}H NMR and analytical HPLC.

3.2. Plant Material

The twigs and leaves of *B. mekongensis* were collected during April 2010 from Mengla County, Yunnan Province, PR China and identified by Mr. Jing-Yun Cui, Xishuangbanna Tropical Plant Garden. A voucher specimen (No. CUI20100419) has been deposited at the State Key Laboratory of Phytochemistry and Plant Resources in West China, Kunming Institute of Botany, Chinese Academy of Science (CAS).

3.3. Extraction and Isolation

The dried twigs and leaves of *B. mekongensis* (12 kg) were extracted with CH_3OH, the crude extract was dissolved in aqueous solution, and then the pH was adjusted to 2 by adding saturated tartaric acid with adequate stirring. The acidic mixture was defatted with petroleum ether (PE) and then extracted with $CHCl_3$. The aqueous phase was basified to pH~10 with saturated Na_2CO_3 and then extracted with $CHCl_3$ to obtain crude alkaloids. The crude alkaloids (60 g) were separated on a silica gel column (200–300 mesh; $CHCl_3/CH_3OH$, 1:0 → 0:1), yielding five major fractions (Fr 1–5). Fraction 1 (12.8 g) was chromatographed with a series of silica gel columns ($CHCl_3$/acetone and $CHCl_3/CH_3OH$) to afford compounds **3** (21 mg) and **4** (16 mg). Fraction 2 (11.2 g) was further chromatographed on a reversed-phase C_{18} silica gel medium-pressure column (CH_3OH/H_2O, 1:1 → 1:0) to give four fractions (Fr 2A–2D). Fraction 2C (3.2 g) was separated on a silica gel column (300–400 mesh; PE/acetone, 3:1), yielding three fractions (Fr 2C1–2C3). Compound **1** (16 mg) was separated from fraction 2C2 (760 mg) by semipreparative HPLC using a Waters XBridge C_{18} (10 × 250 mm, 5 µm) column with 70% CH_3CN/H_2O with added 0.1 v/v diethylamine. Compound **11** (36 mg) was obtained from fraction 2C3 (368 mg) by semipreparative HPLC using a Waters XBridge C_{18} (10 × 250 mm, 5 µm) column with 70% CH_3OH/H_2O with added 0.1 v/v diethylamine. Fraction 3 (9.8 g) was further chromatographed over a reversed-phase C_{18} silica gel medium-pressure column (CH_3OH/H_2O, 1:1 → 1:0) to give four fractions (Fr 3A–3D). Fraction 3A (480 mg) was separated by semipreparative HPLC using a Waters XBridge C_{18} (10 × 250 mm, 5 µm) column with 45% CH_3OH/H_2O to give compounds **5** (21 mg), **10** (4.0 mg) and **12** (28 mg). Fraction 3C (780 mg) was purified using a Sephadex LH-20 column eluted with CH_3OH, followed by semipreparative HPLC using a Waters XBridge C_{18} (19 × 250 mm, 5 µm) column with 70% CH_3OH/H_2O to afford compounds **8** (22 mg) and **14** (48 mg). Fraction 4 (9.8 g) was further chromatographed over a reversed-phase C_{18} silica gel medium-pressure column (CH_3OH/H_2O, 1:1 → 1:0) to give four fractions (Fr 4A–4D). Fr 4A (518 mg) was separated by semipreparative HPLC using a Waters XBridge C_{18} (10 × 250 mm, 5 µm) column with 40% CH_3OH/H_2O to afford compounds **2** (9 mg), **6** (28 mg), **7** (20 mg), and **9** (12 mg). Fr 4B (300 mg) was further purified using a Sephadex LH-20 column eluted with CH_3OH to afford **13** (35 mg).

3.4. Antiproliferative Activity Assay

Antiproliferative activity was determined by the sulforhodamine B (SRB) colorimetric assay as previously described [26]. In brief, human tumor cell lines were cultured in RPMI-1640 medium containing 2 mM l-glutamine and 25 mM HEPES (Gibco), supplemented with 10% fetal bovine serum (Speciality Media), 100 µg/mL streptomycin, 100 IU/mL penicillin, and 0.25 µg/mL amphotericin B (Corning). MDR stock cells (KB-VIN) were maintained in the presence of 100 nM vincristine (VIN) (Sigma-Aldrich, Saint Louis, MI, USA).

Freshly trypsinized cell suspensions were seeded in 96-well microtiter plates at densities of 4000–11,000 cells per well (based on the cell lines) with compounds. After 72 h in culture with test compounds, cells were fixed in 10% trichloroacetic acid followed by staining with 0.04% sulforhodamine B (Sigma-Aldrich). The bound SRB was solubilized in 10 mM Tris-base and the absorbance at 515 nm was measured using a Microplate Reader (ELx800, Bio-Tek Instruments, Winooski, VT, USA) operated by Gen5 software (BioTek) after solubilizing the protein-bound dye with 10 mM Tris base. The mean IC_{50} is the concentration of agent that reduced cell growth by 50% compared with vehicle (DMSO) control under the experimental conditions and is the average from at least three independent experiments with duplicate samples.

The following human tumor cell lines were used in the assay: A549 (lung carcinoma), MDA-MB-231 (triplen-egative breast cancer), KB (originally isolated from epidermoid carcinoma of the nasopharynx), KB-VIN (VIN-resistant KB subline showing MDR phenotype by overexpressing P-gp), MCF-7 (estrogen receptor (ER)-positive, HER2-negative breast cancer). It should be noted that we confirmed the KB and KB-VIN cell lines were identical to AV-3 (ATCC number, CCL-21) as a HeLa (cervical carcinoma) contaminant by short tandem repeat (STR) profiling. All cell lines were obtained from the Lineberger Comprehensive Cancer Center (UNC-CH) or from ATCC (Manassas, VA), except KB-VIN, which was a generous gift from Professor Y.-C. Cheng (Yale University). Paclitaxel was purchased from Sigma-Aldrich.

3.5. Tubulin Assays

Inhibitory effects of compounds on tubulin assembly were evaluated using electrophoretically homogeneous bovine brain tubulin as described previously [27,28] using 1.0 mg/mL (10 µM) tubulin. The turbidity development as tubulin assembly was initiated by adding 0.4 mM GTP and followed for 20 min at 30 °C following a rapid temperature jump. Compound concentrations as EC_{50} values that inhibited the increase in turbidity by 50% relative to a control sample were determined. In colchicine inhibition assays, tubulin (1.0 µM) was incubated with 5.0 µM [^{3}H] colchicine and 5.0 µM test compound at 37 °C for 10 min, when about 40–60% of maximum colchicine binding occurs in control samples.

3.6. Cell Cycle Analysis

KB-VIN cells were seeded in 12-well plates at a density of 1×10^5 per well and incubated overnight. After 24 h of treatment with tested compounds at a concentration of one- or three-fold IC_{50}, the cells were harvested and fixed in 70% EtOH at −20 °C overnight followed by staining with propidium iodide (PI) containing RNase (BD Pharmingen, Franklin Lakes, NJ, USA) for 30 min at 37 °C. The DNA contents of stained cells were analyzed by flow cytometer (LSRFortessa, BD Biosciences) controlled by FACSDiva software (BD Biosciences). Paclitaxel (PXL) was used at 3 or 6 µM. Combretastatin A-4 (CA-4) was purchased from Sigma-Aldrich and used at 0.2 µM. Experiments were repeated a minimum of two times.

3.7. Immunofluorescence Staining

Immunocytochemical analysis was performed as previously described [26]. KB-VIN cells were grown on an 8-well chamber slide (Lab-Tech) for 24 h prior to treatment with the compound at a concentration of three-fold IC_{50}. CA-4 was used at 0.2 µM (Figure 2A and Supporting Information, Supplementary Figure S1). After treatment of cells with the agent for 24 h, cells were fixed with 4% paraformaldehyde in PBS and permeabilized with 0.5% Triton X-100 in PBS. Fixed cells were labeled with mouse monoclonal antibody to α-tubulin (B5-1-2, Sigma) and rabbit IgG to Ser10-phosphorylated histone H3 (p-H3) (#06570, EMD Millipore), followed by FITC-conjugated antibody to mouse IgG (Sigma) and Alexa Fluor 549-conjugated antibody to rabbit IgG (Life Technologies). Nuclei were labeled with DAPI (Sigma). Fluorescently-labeled cells were observed using a confocal microscope (Zeiss, LSM700) with ZEN (black edition) software (Zeiss). The 15~20 optical sections acquired at 0.5~1 µm intervals were stacked and reconstructed using ZEN (black edition) software. Experiments were repeated at least twice for each compound. Final images were prepared using Adobe Photoshop CS3.

3.8. Computer Modeling

GOLD 5.1 software with default settings was used to predict the three-dimensional (3D) structures of tubulin-ligand complexes [29]. The human tubulin 3D structure (TUBA1A and TUBB2B) used in this study was built from a Protein Data Bank entry (PDB ID: 1SA0) [30]. Absent hydrogen atoms in the crystal structure were added computationally by Hermes software 5.1 version. The active site radius was set to 10.0 Å, and the active site center was defined as the ligand center in 1SA0. The docking calculations used the quantum chemically-optimized ligand structures as the initial structures. Structural optimizations of ligands were performed with B3LYP/6-311+G (df, p) using Gaussian 09, Revision B.01 [31].

4. Conclusions

Fourteen aspidosperma-type monoterpenoid indole alkaloids (1–14) were isolated from a methanol extract of the twigs and leaves of *Bousigonia mekongensis*. All isolates were evaluated for antiproliferative activity against five human tumor cell lines, including the MDR subline KB-VIN. Alkaloids **3**, **4**, **6**, **7**, and **13** showed significant antiproliferative effects against all five tumor cell lines. Because activity was retained against KB-VIN, the active alkaloids are not P-gp substrates and, thus, could be effective against tumors expressing the MDR phenotype. SAR studies suggested that the presence of a 14,15-double bond or 3α-acetonyl group is critical for antiproliferative activity. Furthermore, mechanistic studies revealed for the first time that the five active alkaloids cause significant arrest of the cell cycle progression at the G2/M cell cycle phase via inhibition of tubulin polymerization. In addition, the compounds interact with tubulin in a manner distinct from that of CA-4.

Supplementary Materials: The following are available online at http://www.mdpi.com/1420-3049/24/7/1256/s1, Figure S1: Inhibition of tubulin polymerization by compounds, Figure S2: Predicted docking models for **3**, **4**, **11**, and **13** binding in the CS; Tables S1–S3: ^{1}H and ^{13}C NMR data (δ) for compounds **1–14**.

Author Contributions: Conceptualization, Y.Z. and M.G.; Methodology, M.G., P.-L.H. and E.H.; Software, A.O.; Formal Analysis, Y.Z. and M.G.; Resources, Y.-H.F. and L.-L.G.; Data Curation, Y.Z. and M.G.; Writing—Original Draft Preparation, Y.Z.; Writing—Review & Editing, M.G., S.L.M.-N. and K.-H.L.; Supervision, K.-H.L. and X.-J.H.; Project Administration, Y.Z. and X.-J.H.; Funding Acquisition, Y.Z.

Funding: This research was financially supported by the National Natural Science Foundation of China (No. 81874295) to Y.Z., Yunnan Applied Basic Research Projects (No. 2018FA049) to Y.Z., CAS "Light of West China" Program to Y.Z., the Youth Innovation Promotion Association of CAS (2015323), and the Young Academic and Technical Leader Raising Foundation of Yunnan Province (to Y.Z.). This study was also supported in part by NIH Grant CA177584 from the National Cancer Institute awarded to KH Lee and the Eshelman Institute for Innovation, Chapel Hill, North Carolina, awarded to M.G.

Acknowledgments: We wish to thank the Microscopy Service Laboratory (UNC-CH) for its expertise in the confocal microscopy studies.

Disclaimer: The content of this paper is solely the responsibility of the authors and does not necessarily reflect the official views of the National Institutes of Health.

Conflicts of Interest: The authors declare no conflict of interest.

References

1. Dumontet, C.; Jordan, M.A. Microtubule-binding agents: A dynamic field of cancer therapeutics. *Nat. Rev. Drug Discov.* **2010**, *9*, 790–803. [CrossRef]
2. Perez, E.A. Microtubule inhibitors: Differentiating tubulin-inhibiting agents based on mechanisms of action, clinical activity, and resistance. *Mol. Cancer Ther.* **2009**, *8*, 2086–2095. [CrossRef]
3. Szakács, G.; Hall, M.D.; Gottesman, M.M.; Boumendjel, A.; Kachadourian, R.; Day, B.J.; Baubichon-Cortay, H.; Pietro, A.D. Targeting the Achilles heel of multidrug-resistant cancer by exploiting the fitness cost of resistance. *Chem. Rev.* **2014**, *114*, 5753–5774. [CrossRef]
4. Eckford, P.D.; Sharom, F.J. ABC efflux pump-based resistance to chemotherapy drugs. *Chem. Rev.* **2009**, *109*, 2989–3011. [CrossRef] [PubMed]
5. Kavellaris, M. Microtubules and resistance to tubulin-binding agents. *Nat. Rev. Cancer* **2010**, *10*, 194–204. [CrossRef] [PubMed]
6. Dewick, P.M. Alkaloids. In *Medicinal Natural Products: A Biosynthetic Approach*, 3rd ed.; John Wiley & Sons Ltd.: Chichester, UK, 2009; pp. 369–380. ISBN 978-0-470-74168-9.
7. Martino, E.; Casamassima, G.; Castiglione, S.; Cellupica, E.; Pantalone, S.; Papagni, F.; Rui, M.; Siciliano, A.M.; Collina, S. Vinca alkaloids and analogues as anti-cancer agents: Looking back, peering ahead. *Bioorg. Med. Chem. Lett.* **2018**, *28*, 2816–2826. [CrossRef] [PubMed]
8. Lim, K.H.; Hiraku, O.; Komiyama, K.; Kam, T.S. Jerantinines A–G, cytotoxic Aspidosperma alkaloids from *Tabernaemontana corymbosa*. *J. Nat. Prod.* **2008**, *71*, 1591–1594. [CrossRef] [PubMed]
9. Frei, R.; Staedler, D.; Raja, A.; Franke, R.; Sasse, F.; Gerber-Lemaire, S.; Waser, J. Total synthesis and biological evaluation of Jerantinine E. *Angew. Chem. Int. Ed.* **2013**, *52*, 13373–13376. [CrossRef]

10. Raja, V.J.; Lim, K.H.; Leong, C.O.; Kam, T.S.; Bradshaw, T.D. Novel antitumor indole alkaloid, Jerantinine A, evokes potent G2/M cell cycle arrest targeting microtubules. *Invest New Drugs* **2014**, *32*, 838–850. [CrossRef] [PubMed]
11. Qazzaz, M.E.; Raja, V.J.; Lim, K.H.; Kam, T.S.; Lee, J.B.; Gershkovich, P.; Bradshaw, T.D. In vitro anticancer properties and biological evaluation of novel natural alkaloid jerantinine B. *Cancer Lett.* **2016**, *370*, 185–197. [CrossRef] [PubMed]
12. Li, B.T.; Leeuwenberg, J.M.; Middleton, D.J. *Flora of China*; Science Press: Beijing, China, 1995; Volume 16, p. 150.
13. Fu, Y.H.; He, H.P.; Di, Y.T.; Li, S.L.; Zhang, Y.; Hao, X.J. Mekongenines A and B, two new alkaloids from *Bousigonia mekongensis*. *Tetrahedron Lett.* **2012**, *53*, 3642–3646. [CrossRef]
14. Fu, Y.H.; Di, Y.T.; He, H.P.; Li, S.L.; Zhang, Y.; Hao, X.J. Angustifonines A and B, cytotoxic bisindole alkaloids from *Bousigonia angustifolia*. *J. Nat. Prod.* **2014**, *77*, 56–62. [CrossRef]
15. Fu, Y.H.; Li, S.L.; Li, S.F.; He, H.P.; Di, Y.T.; Zhang, Y.; Hao, X.J. Cytotoxic eburnamine-aspidospermine type bisindole alkaloids from *Bousigonia mekongensis*. *Fitoterapia* **2014**, *98*, 45–52. [CrossRef]
16. Baassou, S.; Mehri, H.; Plat, M. Plants of New Caledonia. Part 49. Alkaloids of *Melodinus aeneus*. *Phytochemistry* **1978**, *17*, 1449–1450. [CrossRef]
17. Fahn, W.; Kaiser, V.; Schübel, H.; Stöckigt, J.; Danieli, B. *Catharanthus roseus* enzyme mediated synthesis of 3-hydroxyvoafrine A and B—A simple route to the voafrines. *Phytochemistry* **1990**, *29*, 129–133. [CrossRef]
18. Liu, Y.P.; Li, Y.; Cai, X.H.; Li, X.Y.; Kong, L.M.; Cheng, G.G.; Luo, X.D. Melodinines M-U, cytotoxic alkaloids from *Melodinus suaveolens*. *J. Nat. Prod.* **2012**, *75*, 220–224. [CrossRef]
19. Nair, C.P.N.; Pillay, P.P. Lochnericine. A new alkaloid from *Lochnera rosea*. *Tetrahedron* **1959**, *6*, 89–93. [CrossRef]
20. Guo, L.W.; Zhou, Y.L. Alkaloids from *Melodinus hemsleyanus*. *Phytochemistry* **1993**, *34*, 563–566. [CrossRef]
21. Men-Olivier, L.L.; Richard, B.; Men, J.L. Alcaloïdes des grains du *Pandaca retusa*. *Phytochemistry* **1993**, *34*, 563–566.
22. Feng, T.; Li, Y.; Cai, X.H.; Gong, X.; Liu, Y.P.; Zhang, R.T.; Zhang, X.Y.; Tan, Q.G.; Luo, X.D. Monoterpenoid indole alkaloids from *Alstonia yunnanensis*. *J. Nat. Prod.* **2009**, *72*, 1836–1841. [CrossRef]
23. Langlois, N.; Andriamialisoa, R.Z. Studies on vindolinine. 6. Partial synthesis of aspidospermane-type alkaloids. *J. Org. Chem.* **1979**, *44*, 2468–2471. [CrossRef]
24. Kutney J., P.; Choi, L.S.L.; Kolodziejczyk, P.; Sleigh, S.K.; Stuart, K.L.; Worth, B.R.; Kurz, W.G.W.; Chatson, K.B.; Constabel, F. Alkaloid production in *Catharanthus roseus* cell cultures: Isolation and characterization of alkaloids from one cell line. *Phytochemistry* **1980**, *19*, 2589–2595. [CrossRef]
25. Smedley, C.J.; Stanley, P.A.; Qazzaz, M.E.; Prota, A.E.; Olieric, N.; Collins, H.; Eastman, H.; Barrow, A.S.; Lim, K.H.; Kam, T.S.; et al. Sustainable syntheses of (-)-jerantinines A & E and structural characterisation of the jerantinine-tubulin complex at the colchicine binding Site. *Sci. Rep.* **2018**, *8*, 10617. [PubMed]
26. Nakagawa-Goto, K.; Oda, A.; Hamel, E.; Ohkoshi, E.; Lee, K.H.; Goto, M. Development of a novel class of tubulin inhibitor from desmosdumotin B with a hydroxylated bicyclic B-ring. *J. Med. Chem.* **2015**, *58*, 2378–2389. [CrossRef]
27. Hamel, E. Evaluation of antimitotic agents by quantitative comparisons of their effects on the polymerization of purified tubulin. *Cell Biochem. Biophys.* **2003**, *38*, 1–22. [CrossRef]
28. Verdier-Pinard, P.; Lai, J.Y.; Yoo, H.D.; Yu, J.; Marquez, B.; Nagle, D.G.; Nambu, M.; White, J.D.; Falck, J.R.; Gerwick, W.H.; et al. Structure−activity analysis of the interaction of curacin A, the potent colchicine site antimitotic agent, with tubulin and effects of analogs on the growth of MCF-7 breast cancer cells. *Mol. Pharmacol.* **1998**, *53*, 62–76. [CrossRef] [PubMed]
29. Jones, G.; Willett, P.; Glen, R.C. Molecular recognition of receptor sites using a genetic algorithm with a description of desolvation. *J. Mol. Biol.* **1995**, *245*, 43–53. [CrossRef]
30. Ravelli, R.B.; Gigant, B.; Curmi, P.A.; Jourdain, I.; Lachkar, S.; Sobel, A.; Knossow, M. Insight into tubulin regulation from a complex with colchicine and a stathmin-like domain. *Nature* **2004**, *428*, 198–202. [CrossRef]
31. Frisch, M.J.; Trucks, G.W.; Schlegel, H.B.; Scuseria, G.E.; Robb, M.A.; Cheeseman, J.R.; Scalmani, G.; Barone, V.; Mennucci, B.; Petersson, G.A.; et al. *Gaussian 09 (Revision B.01)*; Gaussian, Inc.: Wallingford, CT, USA, 2010.

Sample Availability: Samples of the compounds **1–14** are available from the authors.

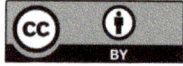

© 2019 by the authors. Licensee MDPI, Basel, Switzerland. This article is an open access article distributed under the terms and conditions of the Creative Commons Attribution (CC BY) license (http://creativecommons.org/licenses/by/4.0/).

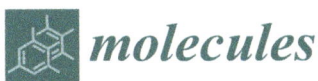

Article

Synthesis and Biological Evaluation of Phaeosphaeride A Derivatives as Antitumor Agents

Victoria Abzianidze [1,*], Petr Beltyukov [2], Sofya Zakharenkova [1], Natalia Moiseeva [3], Jennifer Mejia [4], Alvin Holder [4], Yuri Trishin [5], Alexander Berestetskiy [6] and Victor Kuznetsov [1]

1. Laboratory of Chemical Modeling, Research Institute of Hygiene, Occupational Pathology and Human Ecology, Federal Medical Biological Agency, p/o Kuz'molovsky, 188663 Saint Petersburg, Russia; sofya.zakharenkova@gmail.com (S.Z.); kuznetsov_va1956@bk.ru (V.K.)
2. Laboratory of Molecular Toxicology and Experimental Therapy, Research Institute of Hygiene, Occupational Pathology and Human Ecology, Federal Medical Biological Agency, p/o Kuz'molovsky, 188663 Saint Petersburg, Russia; biochem2005@rambler.ru
3. N.N. Blokchin National Medical Research Center of Oncology, 115478 Moscow, Russia; n.i.moiseeva@gmail.com
4. Department of Chemistry and Biochemistry, Old Dominion University, 4541 Hampton Boulevard, Norfolk, VA 23529, USA; jmatt024@odu.edu (J.M.); aholder@odu.edu (A.H.)
5. Saint Petersburg State University of industrial technologies and design, Ivana Chernyh str., 4, 198095 Saint Petersburg, Russia; trish@yt4470.spb.edu
6. All-Russian Institute of Plant Protection, Russian Academy of Agricultural Sciences, Pushkin, 196608 Saint Petersburg, Russia; aberestski@yahoo.com
* Correspondence: vvaavv@mail.ru; Tel.: +7-981-249-0902

Received: 19 October 2018; Accepted: 16 November 2018; Published: 21 November 2018

Abstract: New derivatives of phaeosphaeride A (PPA) were synthesized and characterized. Anti-tumor activity studies were carried out on the HCT-116, PC3, MCF-7, A549, K562, NCI-H929, Jurkat, THP-1, RPMI8228 tumor cell lines, and on the HEF cell line. All of the compounds synthesized were found to have better efficacy than PPA towards the tumor cell lines mentioned. Compound **6** was potent against six cancer cell lines, HCT-116, PC-3, K562, NCI-H929, Jurkat, and RPMI8226, showing a 47, 13.5, 16, 4, 1.5, and 7-fold increase in anticancer activity comparative to those of etoposide, respectively. Compound **1** possessed selectivity toward the NCI-H929 cell line (IC_{50} = 1.35 ± 0.69 µM), while product **7** was selective against three cancer cell lines, HCT-116, MCF-7, and NCI-H929, each having IC_{50} values of 1.65 µM, 1.80 µM and 2.00 µM, respectively.

Keywords: natural phaeosphaeride A; antitumor activity; human tumor cell lines; HEF cell line; acute toxicity

1. Introduction

Modern chemotherapeutic treatment of malignant tumors is widely considered to have begun approximately 75 years ago when researchers found that nitrogen mustard displayed anti-tumor activity [1]. In more recent decades, leading research approaches have focused on the development of new antitumor agents for targeted therapy, as well as combined treatment with immunotherapeutic and chemotherapeutic agents [2]. Diversity, and in many cases, the genetic uniqueness of tumors, does not allow for the development of universal and specific therapeutic treatment. As a result, the use of non-specific chemotherapeutic treatment is still the principal therapeutic option used in patients. Despite advances in cancer treatments, the disabling side effects and relative effectivity of these broad antitumor drugs plagues scientists to urgently develop improved chemotherapeutic agents.

Many chemotherapeutic agents used in clinical practice are developed from natural compounds or their derivatives and analogs, e.g., etoposide, eribulin, paclitaxel, vincristine, vinblastine, topotecan, cytarabine, doxorubicin, dactinomycin, and bleomycin [3–5]. These also include medicines developed and introduced into clinical practice from the 1950s–1960s (vincristine, vinblastine, cytarabine, etc.), as well as modern agents developed in the 2000's (topotecan, eribulin). Many chemotherapeutic agents based on natural analogs continue to undergo clinical studies to evaluate their effectiveness in the treatment of various types of tumors, as drugs developed from natural compounds often show lower toxicity and have higher target values towards malignant tumor cells [3]. While scientists continue to research these compounds, these naturally derived drugs are already relevant in the market today, with close to 40% of antitumor drugs approved by the FDA being of natural origin or semi-synthetic derivatives of natural compounds. When we reexamine this number and consider only the use of synthetic drugs, the analogues of natural compounds, the proportion of these antitumor agents are estimated at 70% [6]. Clearly, nature remains an inexhaustible source of new substances and has vast potential to aid in the fight against various tumors.

Here, phaeosphaeride A, produced by endophytic fungi from the genus *Phaeosphaeria*, was chosen for its ability to inhibit the Signal Transducer and Activator of Transcription 3 (STAT3) signaling pathway. The stereochemical configuration of this natural product had been established by total synthesis of ent-phaeosphaeride A and phaeosphaeride A [7,8] and by X-ray diffraction [9]. High incidence of STAT3 protein is characteristic of several oncological diseases like leukemia, multiple myeloma, cancers of the breast and lung, as well as multiple carcinomas such as renal, prostate, hepatocellular, ovarian, and pancreatic [10,11]. STAT3 also is shown to play an important role in regulating cell growth and viability [10,12–15]. Therefore, phaeosphaeride A, and its derivatives, are potentially promising anticancer agents for targeted therapy and combined treatments [10,11].

The results of the study in this article include information on the methods for the synthesis of the phaeosphaeride A derivatives and their biological evaluation, including the measurements of the cytotoxic effects and a preliminary assessment of acute toxicity in mice.

2. Results and Discussion

2.1. Chemistry

The synthesis of target compounds **1–8** is presented in Scheme 1. Mesylation of PPA with MeSO$_2$Cl and Et$_3$N in CH$_2$Cl$_2$ gave the mesylate as a sole product, which was used in the next step without purification.

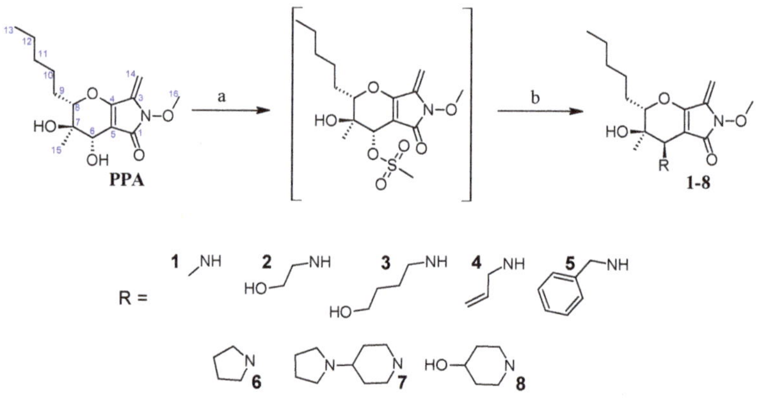

Scheme 1. Synthesis of compounds **1–8**. *Reagents and conditions*: (**a**) MsCl, TEA, CH$_2$Cl$_2$, 0 °C, 1 h; (**b**) cyclic or primary amine, with or without TEA, acetonitrile or THF, room temperature or 70–75 °C.

Treatment of the mesylate with cyclic amines and (or without) TEA in acetonitrile (or THF) at room temperature (or at 70–75 °C) or with primary amines in acetonitrile at room temperature gave the corresponding amino derivatives in 11–27% yield with inversion occurring on the C-6 atom. The ROESY spectra of the products showed a correlation between the methyl protons (H-15) and the H-6 proton confirming the inversion of configuration of the C-6 atom (see Supplementary Material). Product **6** was synthesized by our research group in 2017 with the present method doubling the total yield [16]. Previously it was impossible to obtain the desired derivatives through chloroacetyl PPA derivative from primary amines as those reactions proceeded solely at the exocyclic double bond (unpublished data) [17].

2.2. Biological Evaluation

2.2.1. Cytotoxicity Assay Using 9 Tumor Cell Lines and HEF Cell Line

All newly synthesized PPA derivatives **1–8** were evaluated for their anti-proliferative activity against human breast cancer MCF-7, human prostate adenocarcinoma PC-3, human colorectal cancer HCT-116, human lung cancer A549, human chronic myelogenous leukemia K562, human acute monocytic leukemia THP-1, human multiple myeloma RPMI8226, human acute T-cell leukemia Jurkat, human multiple myeloma NCI-H929, and human embryonic fibroblasts HEF cell lines by MTT assays. All cells were incubated with different concentrations of PPA derivatives for 72 h, with etoposide and PPA used as reference compounds. The anticancer activity of the tested compounds was described as the concentration of drug inhibiting 50% cell growth IC_{50} (Tables 1 and 2).

Table 1. IC_{50} values for the respective compounds when studied on the adhesive cell lines. Data was expressed as the inhibitory ratio ± SD based on three independent experiments ($n = 3$).

Compound	Adhesive Cell Cultures, IC_{50} (µM)				
	HCT-116	PC-3	MCF-7	A549	HEF
PPA	24.21 ± 0.75	32.14 ± 0.77	20.30 ± 0.8	41.10 ± 2.6	19.05 ± 0.25
1	3.68 ± 0.81	3.35 ± 0.92	4.10 ± 0.44	12.73 ± 0.40	22.30 ± 0.44
2	4.63 ± 0.04	5.55 ± 1.48	3.23 ± 1.07	15.14 ± 0.45	16.20 ± 0.26
3	2.90 ± 0.98	4.50 ± 1.56	3.05 ± 1.20	11.41 ± 0,19	15.19 ± 1.02
4	8.40 ± 0.24	6.37 ± 0.18	4.13 ± 0.23	12.65 ± 0.27	5.03 ± 0.15
5	12.93 ± 0.30	24.67 ± 1.24	35.71 ± 0.65	37.51 ± 1.33	53.11 ± 1.06
6	0.47 ± 0.01	0.20 ± 0.07	3.25 ± 0.64	10.11 ± 0.5	4.00 ± 0.17
7	1.65 ± 0.63	3.65 ± 0.64	1.80 ± 0.44	12.22 ± 0.2	22.30 ± 0.33
8	2.64 ± 0.05	4.53 ± 0.40	3.20 ± 0.52	9.40 ± 0.14	6.70 ± 0.23
Etoposide	22.00 ± 1.10	2.70 ± 0.05	9.60 ± 0.27	>100	>100

Table 2. IC_{50} values for the respective compounds when studied on the suspension cell lines. Data were expressed as inhibitory ratio ± SD based on three independent experiments ($n = 3$).

Compound	Suspension Cell Cultures, IC_{50} (µM)				
	K562	NCI-H929	Jurkat	THP-1	RPMI8228
PPA	20.47 ± 1.46	6.50 ± 0.30	9.70 ± 0.42	19.10 ± 0.45	9.15 ± 0.64
1	3.25 ± 0.64	1.35 ± 0.69	2.75 ± 0.21	2.25 ± 0.21	3.97 ± 0.68
2	5.50 ± 0.57	2.05 ± 0.35	2.60 ± 0.99	2.30 ± 0.57	3.50 ± 0.82
3	6.70 ± 0.28	1.95 ± 0.21	3.15 ± 1.77	2.60 ± 0.57	2.70 ± 0.28
4	10.48 ± 0.41	2.35 ± 0.09	3.27 ± 0.07	3.32 ± 0.10	6.00 ± 0.13
5	14.13 ± 0.48	7.73 ± 0,25	10.10 ± 0.44	15.11 ± 0.36	16 ± 0.16
6	0.54 ± 0.03	0.23 ± 0.02	0.55 ± 0.29	2.05 ± 0.21	0.63 ± 0.23
7	6.03 ± 0.91	2.00 ± 0.26	2.73 ± 1.53	3.45 ± 0.21	3.35 ± 1.48
8	4.90 ± 2.40	1.87 ± 0.25	2.60 ± 1.13	2.10 ± 0.28	1.40 ± 0.28
Etoposide	8.47 ± 0.95	0.92 ± 0.03	0.88 ± 0.74	0.83 ± 0.21	4.60 ± 0.28

Compound **6** was found to be the most potent against six cancer cell lines (0.47 µM for HCT-116, 0.2 µM for PC-3, 0.54 µM for K562, 0.23 µM for NCI-H929, 0.55 µM for Jurkat and 0.63 µM for

RPMI8226), which was 51, 160, 37, 28, 17.5, and 14.5-fold stronger than those of the reference compound PPA, respectively (Figure 1).

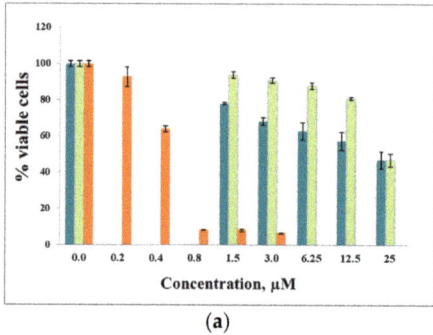 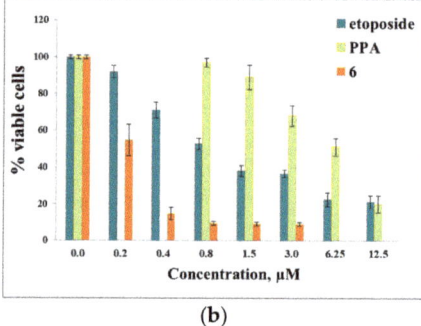

(a) (b)

Figure 1. (a) The in vitro effects of compound **6** on the cell viability of human HCT-116 cell line; (b) The in vitro effects of compound **6** on the cell viability of human NCI-H929 cell line.

Compound **1** showed selectivity toward the NCI-H929 cell line (IC_{50} = 1.35 ± 0.69 µM) while product **7** was selective against three cancer cell lines (IC_{50} was 1.65 µM, 1.80 µM and 2.00 µM towards HCT-116, MCF-7 and NCI-H929, respectively). The results obtained indicate product **6** to be more toxic than the positive control, etoposide, against HCT-116 (47-fold), PC-3 (13.5-fold), K562 (16-fold), NCI-H929 (4-fold), Jurkat (1.5-fold) and RPMI8226 (7-fold) cancer cell lines. Human embryonic fibroblasts were used as a control.

2.2.2. Acute Intraperitoneal Toxicity Study

No adverse effects were found from compound **6** on body weight and food consumption. There was no indication of morbidity, mortality, or lethal effects during the 14 days after i.p. administration (intraperiotenal) in mice of two low doses (8.25 and 82.5 mg/kg). LD50 was not reached in all experiments. Mortality (two of eight mice) was observed in the highest dose group (one was found deceased on Day 2 and one on Day 3). No effect was observed on mean body weight or mass coefficients (spleen, liver, heart, kidney, lung, thymus, and adrenal). No gross abnormalities were observed in the organs tested. Maximum tolerated dose of **6** after i.p. injection in mice was equal to or more than 82.5 mg/kg. Median lethal dose (LD50) of **6** has not been determined but is believed to be more than 200 mg/kg. It can be concluded that compound **6** is less toxic comparative to etoposide. Intraperitoneal LD50 of etoposide for mice is 64 mg/kg (RTECS # KC0190000).

3. Materials and Methods

3.1. Materials and Instruments

^{1}H-NMR spectra were acquired on an AVANCE III 400 MHz NMR spectrometer (Bruker, Rheinstetten, Germany) in CDCl$_3$. Optical rotations were acquired on a Polaar 3005 Polarimeter (Optical Activity, Huntingdon, Great Britain) using a 2.5 cm cell with a Na 589 nm filter and the concentration of samples was denoted as *c*. Mass spectra data were acquired on a TSQ Quantum Access Max Mass spectrometer (Thermo Fisher Scientific, Waltham, MA, USA). High-resolution mass spectra (HRMS) were acquired on a LTQ Orbitrap Velos spectrometer (Thermo Scientific) and on a Bruker MicrOTOF. FTIR spectra were acquired on an IR Affinity-1 spectrometer (Shimadzu, Thermo Scientific). Organic solvents used were dried by standard methods when necessary. Commercially available reagents were used without further purification. All reactions were monitored by TLC with silica gel coated plates (EMD/Merck KGaA, Darmstadt, Germany), with visualization by UV light and by charring with 0.1% ninhydrin in EtOH. Column chromatography was performed using Merck 60 Å

70–230 mesh silica gel. The optical density was determined using a Multiskan FC spectrophotometer (Thermo Scientific) at a wavelength of 540 nm when using the MTT assay.

3.2. Chemical Syntheses

3.2.1. Synthesis of (2*S*,3*S*,4*S*)-3-Hydroxy-6-methoxy-3-methyl-7-methylene-5-oxo-2-pentyl-2,3,4,5,6,7-hexahydropyrano[2,3-*c*]pyrrol-4-yl methanesulfonate

PPA (1 mmol) was dissolved in CH_2Cl_2 (2 mL) and cooled to 0 °C. Triethylamine (3.5 mmol) was added followed by the dropwise addition of methanesulfonyl chloride (2.5 mmol). The mixture was stirred at 0 °C for 1 h. The reaction was quenched by the addition of saturated $NaHCO_3$ solution and the mixture was extracted with dichloromethane (3 × 20 mL). The organic layer was washed with water and brine, dried over magnesium sulfate, and concentrated in vacuo after filtration. Mesylate was used in the next step without further purification. HRMS revealed an $[M + H]^+$ ion with exact mass 376.14219, corresponding to the molecular formula $C_{16}H_{26}NO_7S$.

3.2.2. General Procedure for the Synthesis of Compounds **1–5**

A mixture of the crude (2*S*,3*S*,4*S*)-3-hydroxy-6-methoxy-3-methyl-7-methylene-5-oxo-2-pentyl-2,3,4,5,6,7-hexahydropyrano[2,3-*c*]pyrrol-4-yl methanesulfonate (1 mmol) and an appropriate primary amine (2 mmol) was stirred in dry acetonitrile (2 mL) at room temperature until consumption of the starting material was complete as judged by TLC analysis (24–48 h). The reaction mixture was diluted with ether (20 mL) and transferred to a separatory funnel. The layers were separated and the aqueous layer was extracted with ether (3 × 20 mL). The organic extracts were combined, washed with brine (2 × 20 mL), dried over magnesium sulfate, and concentrated in vacuo. The crude product was purified by flash chromatography (DCM:methanol = 60:1).

(2S,3R,4R)-3-Hydroxy-6-methoxy-3-methyl-4-(methylamino)-7-methylene-2-pentyl-3,4,6,7-tetrahydro-pyrano [2,3-c]pyrrol-5(2H)-one (**1**): Yield 17%, yellow oil. $[\alpha]_D^{20.0} = -120.36$ (c 0.28, CH_2Cl_2). ^{1}H-NMR ($CDCl_3$) δ 5.56 (m, 2H), 5.12 (s, 1H), 5.07 (s, 1H), 4.05 (m, 1H), 3.93 (s, 3H), 3.41 (m, 1H), 2.75 (s, 3H), 1.93 (m, 1H), 1.63 (m, 2H), 1.43–1.33 (m, 5H), 1.15 (s, 3H), 0.90 (m, 3H). ^{13}C-NMR ($CDCl_3$) δ 165.87 (s), 159.47 (s), 136.05 (s), 99.07 (s), 93.27 (s), 81.54 (s), 68.97 (s), 64.70 (s), 57.32 (s), 33.50 (s), 31.58 (s), 27.62 (s), 25.99 (s), 22.53 (s), 19.45 (s), 14.05 (s). IR (KBr) 3319, 2955, 2930, 2859, 1721, 1667, 1633, 1438, 1379, 1266, 1196, 1166, 1085, 979, 915 cm^{-1}. HRMS $[M + H]^+$ calcd for $C_{16}H_{27}N_2O_4$ 311.19653, found 311.1953.

(2S,3R,4R)-3-Hydroxy-4-[(2-hydroxyethyl)amino]-6-methoxy-3-methyl-7-methylene-2-pentyl-3,4,6,7-tetra-hydropyrano[2,3-c]pyrrol-5(2H)-one (**2**): Yield 25%, yellow oil. $[\alpha]_D^{20.0} = -99.54$ (c 0.22, CH_2Cl_2). ^{1}H-NMR ($CDCl_3$) δ 5.09 (s, 1H), 5.04 (s, 1H), 3.93 (m, 4H), 3.61 (m, 2H), 3.12 (s, 1H), 3.06–2.91 (m, 2H), 1.94 (m, 1H), 1.65–1.58 (m, 2H), 1.35 (m, 6H), 1.06 (s, 3H), 0.91 (s, 3H). ^{13}C-NMR ($CDCl_3$) δ 167.38 (s), 157.36 (s), 136.27 (s), 104.10 (s), 92.86 (s), 82.53 (s), 69.28 (s), 64.71 (s), 61.07 (s), 54.14 (s), 52.07 (s), 31.66 (s), 27.47 (s), 26.28 (s), 22.57 (s), 18.58 (s), 14.08 (s). IR (KBr) 3322, 2954, 2927, 2857, 1718, 1633, 1547, 1458, 1437, 1378, 1263, 1191, 1117, 1081, 978, 914 cm^{-1}. HRMS $[M + H]^+$ calcd for $C_{17}H_{29}N_2O_5$ 341.20710, found 341.2060.

(2S,3R,4R)-3-Hydroxy-4-[(4-hydroxybutyl)amino]-6-methoxy-3-methyl-7-methylene-2-pentyl-3,4,6,7-tetra-hydropyrano[2,3-c]pyrrol-5(2H)-one (**3**): Yield 20%, yellow oil. $[\alpha]_D^{20.0} = -89.80$ (c 0.51, CH_2Cl_2). ^{1}H-NMR ($CDCl_3$) δ 5.11 (d, *J* = 1.2 Hz, 1H), 5.05 (d, *J* = 1.3 Hz, 1H), 4.94 (m, 3H), 4.05 (m, 1H), 3.93 (s, 3H), 3.80–3.50 (m, 2H), 3.36 (s, 1H), 3.27–3.12 (m, 1H), 3.06–2.87 (m, 1H), 1.95 (m, 1H), 1.78 (m, 2H), 1.69–1.55 (m, 4H), 1.45–1.33 (m, 5H), 1.12 (s, 3H), 0.90 (m, 3H). ^{13}C-NMR ($CDCl_3$) δ 166.37 (s), 158.18 (s), 136.38 (s), 102.16 (s), 92.59 (s), 82.14 (s), 68.78 (s), 64.64 (s), 62.26 (s), 55.97 (s), 48.77 (s), 31.64 (s), 30.14 (s), 27.61 (s), 26.12 (s), 22.57 (s), 19.15 (s), 14.08 (s). IR (KBr) 3292, 2927, 2858, 1712, 1632, 1548, 1438, 1379, 1191, 1083, 989, 914 cm^{-1}. HRMS $[M + H]^+$ calcd for $C_{19}H_{33}N_2O_5$ 369.23840, found 369.2373.

(2S,3R,4R)-4-(Allylamino)-3-hydroxy-6-methoxy-3-methyl-7-methylene-2-pentyl-3,4,6,7-tetrahydropyrano-[2,3-c]pyrrol-5(2H)-one (**4**): Yield 14%, yellow oil. $[\alpha]_D^{20.0} = -157.50$ (c 0.31, CH_2Cl_2). ^{1}H-NMR ($CDCl_3$) δ

5.89 (ddt, *J* = 12.2, 10.1, 6.1 Hz, 1H), 5.25 (dd, *J* = 17.2, 1.3 Hz, 1H), 5.12 (m, 1H), 5.03 (d, *J* = 1.3 Hz, 1H), 4.99 (d, *J* = 1.3 Hz, 1H), 3.93 (s, 3H), 3.78–3.66 (m, 1H), 3.58–3.49 (m, 1H), 3.44 (ddd, *J* = 13.8, 4.6, 1.2 Hz, 1H), 3.03 (s, 1H), 1.94 (m, 1H), 1.60 (m, 2H), 1.43–1.35 (m, 5H), 1.06 (s, 3H), 0.91 (m, 3H). ^{13}C-NMR (CDCl$_3$) δ 166.68 (s), 156.86 (s), 136.78 (s), 136.06 (s), 117.05 (s), 105.17 (s), 91.79 (s), 82.65 (s), 68.23 (s), 64.59 (s), 54.92 (s), 52.14 (s), 31.69 (s), 27.63 (s), 26.29 (s), 22.57 (s), 18.72 (s), 14.09 (s). IR (KBr) 3314, 2955, 2928, 2858, 1720, 1668, 1634, 1437, 1367, 1232, 1192, 1087, 992, 919 cm^{-1}. HRMS [M + H]$^+$ calcd for C$_{18}$H$_{29}$N$_2$O$_4$ 337.21218, found 337.2111.

(2S,3R,4R)-4-(benzylamino)-3-hydroxy-6-methoxy-3-methyl-7-methylene-2-pentyl-3,4,6,7-tetrahydro-pyrano [2,3-c]pyrrol-5(2H)-one (**5**): Yield 17%, yellow oil. $[\alpha]_D^{20.0}$ = −137.81 (c 0.43, CH$_2$Cl$_2$). ^{1}H-NMR (CDCl$_3$) δ 7.39–7.26 (m, 5H), 5.04 (d, *J* = 1.4 Hz, 1H), 5.00 (d, *J* = 1.4 Hz, 1H), 4.30 (d, *J* = 12.3 Hz, 1H), 3.94 (m, 4H), 3.53 (m, 1H), 3.12 (s, 1H), 1.93 (m, 1H), 1.61 (m, 2H), 1.34 (m, 5H), 1.06 (s, 3H), 0.90 (m, 3H). ^{13}C-NMR (CDCl$_3$) δ 166.78 (s), 156.89 (s), 139.35 (s), 136.81 (s), 128.61 (d, *J* = 8.7 Hz), 127.47 (s), 105.30 (s), 91.89 (s), 82.70 (s), 68.26 (s), 64.63 (s), 55.37 (s), 53.62 (s), 31.68 (s), 27.63 (s), 26.27 (s), 22.56 (s), 18.82 (s), 14.07 (s). IR (KBr) 3309, 2955, 2927, 2858, 1720, 1633, 1454, 1436, 1378, 1232, 1192, 1086, 978, 914 cm^{-1}. HRMS [M + H]$^+$ calcd for C$_{22}$H$_{31}$N$_2$O$_4$ 387.22783, found 387.2262.

3.2.3. General Procedure for the Synthesis of Compounds 6–8

A mixture of the crude (2*S*,3*S*,4*S*)-3-hydroxy-6-methoxy-3-methyl-7-methylene-5-oxo-2-pentyl-2,3,4,5,6,7-hexahydropyrano[2,3-*c*]pyrrol-4-yl methanesulfonate (1 mmol), the corresponding cyclic amine (1.5 mmol) and triethylamine (3 mmol) was stirred in dry acetonitrile (2 mL) at room temperature until consumption of the starting material was complete as judged by TLC analysis (24–48 h). The reaction mixture was quenched with water and extracted with EtOAc (2 × 20 mL). The organic extract was washed with brine, dried over magnesium sulfate, and concentrated in vacuo. The crude product was purified by flash chromatography (DCM/methanol).

3.2.4. Alternative General Procedure for the Synthesis of Compounds 6–8

A mixture of the crude (2*S*,3*S*,4*S*)-3-hydroxy-6-methoxy-3-methyl-7-methylene-5-oxo-2-pentyl-2,3,4,5,6,7-hexahydropyrano[2,3-*c*]pyrrol-4-yl methanesulfonate (1 mmol) and the corresponding cyclic amine (5 mmol) in dry THF (2 mL) was heated at 70–75 °C in a sealed tube for 18 h. The mixture was cooled to room temperature, filtered, and the THF solution was diluted with saturated sodium bicarbonate solution (20 mL). The resulting mixture was extracted with DCM (3 × 20 mL). The organic extracts were washed with water, dried with magnesium sulfate, and concentrated in vacuo. The crude product was purified by flash chromatography (DCM/methanol).

(2S,3R,4R)-3-Hydroxy-6-methoxy-3-methyl-7-methylene-2-pentyl-4-pyrrolidin-1-yl-3,4,6,7-tetrahydro-pyrano [2,3-c]pyrrol-5(2H)-one (**6**): Yield 27%, yellow oil. $[\alpha]_D^{20.0}$ = −176.52 (c 0.40, CH$_2$Cl$_2$). ^{1}H-NMR (CDCl$_3$) δ 5.40 (s, 1H), 5.02 (d, *J* = 1.4 Hz, 1H), 4.98 (d, *J* = 1.4 Hz, 1H), 3.92 (s, 3H), 3.64 (d, *J* = 9.9 Hz, 1H), 3.31 (s, 1H), 3.10–2.55 (m, 4H), 2.03–1.89 (m, 1H), 1.84–1.70 (m, 4H), 1.69–1.52 (m, 2H), 1.45–1.29 (m, 5H), 1.05 (s, 3H), 0.91 (t, *J* = 6.7 Hz, 3H). ^{13}C-NMR (CDCl$_3$) δ 167.11 (s), 158.44 (s), 137.00 (s), 101.65 (s), 91.38 (s), 83.60 (s), 68.00 (s), 64.41 (s), 59.55 (s), 31.73 (s), 28.21 (s), 26.43 (s), 23.91 (s), 22.55 (s), 19.66 (s), 14.04 (s). IR (KBr) 3430, 2957, 2930, 2860, 1722, 1633, 1438, 1190, 1144 cm^{-1}. HRMS [M + H]$^+$, calcd. for C$_{19}$H$_{31}$N$_2$O$_4$ 351.227834, found 351.22733.

(2S,3R,4R)-3-Hydroxy-6-methoxy-3-methyl-7-methylene-2-pentyl-4-(4-pyrrolidin-1-ylpiperidin-1-yl)-3,4,6,7-tetrahydropyrano[2,3-c]pyrrol-5(2H)-one (**7**): Yield 11%, yellow oil. $[\alpha]_D^{20.0}$ = −115.82 (c 0.41, CH$_2$Cl$_2$). ^{1}H-NMR (CDCl$_3$) δ 5.05 (s, 1H), 5.00 (s, 1H), 3.91 (s, 3H), 3.56 (m, 1H), 3.29–2.91 (m, 8H), 2.81 (m, 1H), 2.27 (t, *J* = 10.9 Hz, 1H), 2.11–1.83 (m, 9H), 1.69–1.48 (m, 2H), 1.35 (s, 5H), 1.02 (s, 3H), 0.91 (s, 3H). ^{13}C-NMR (CDCl$_3$) δ 167.08 (s), 158.19 (s), 136.87 (s), 101.35 (s), 91.69 (s), 83.39 (s), 68.22 (s), 64.49 (s), 62.51 (s), 61.35 (s), 55.67 (s), 51.39 (s), 49.52 (s), 32.19 (s), 31.74 (s), 28.29 (s), 26.44 (s), 23.20 (s), 22.57 (s), 19.96 (s), 14.08 (s). IR (KBr) 3213, 2928, 2857, 2782, 1724, 1669, 1635, 1437, 1377, 1354, 1321, 1193, 1150, 1126, 1085, 979 cm^{-1}. HRMS [M + H]$^+$ calcd for C$_{24}$H$_{40}$N$_3$O$_4$ 434.30133, found 434.3009.

(2S,3R,4R)-3-Hydroxy-4-(4-hydroxypiperidin-1-yl)-6-methoxy-3-methyl-7-methylene-2-pentyl-3,4,6,7-tetrahydropyrano[2,3-c]pyrrol-5(2H)-one (**8**): Yield 16%, yellow oil. $[\alpha]_D^{20.0} = -111.11$ (c 0.36, CH_2Cl_2). ^{1}H-NMR ($CDCl_3$) δ 5.17 (s, 1H), 5.03 (d, *J* = 1.1 Hz, 1H), 5.00 (d, *J* = 1.1 Hz, 1H), 3.93 (s, 3H), 3.68 (s, 1H), 3.59 (m, 1H), 3.02 (s, 1H), 2.87 (s, 2H), 2.35 (s, 1H), 2.03–1.85 (m, 3H), 1.68–1.50 (m, 6H), 1.35 (m, 5H), 1.05 (s, 3H), 0.91 (m, 3H). ^{13}C-NMR ($CDCl_3$) δ 167.01 (s), 158.15 (s), 136.85 (s), 101.35 (s), 91.75 (s), 83.35 (s), 68.20 (s), 64.53 (s), 62.45 (s), 35.20 (s), 31.79 (s), 28.35 (s), 26.48 (s), 22.58 (s), 20.00 (s), 14.09 (s). IR (KBr) 3213, 2926, 2855, 1720, 1671, 1634, 1547, 1438, 1375, 1139, 1066, 1045 cm^{-1}. HRMS $[M + H]^+$ calcd for $C_{20}H_{33}N_2O_5$ 381.23840, found 381.2377.

3.3. Bio-Evaluation Methods

3.3.1. In-Vitro Cytotoxicity Study (MTT Assay)

MCF-7 (breast cancer), PC-3 (prostate adenocarcinoma), HCT-116 (colorectal cancer cell), A549 (lung cancer), K562 (chronic myelogenous leukemia), THP-1 (acute monocytic leukemia), and RPMI8226 (multiple myeloma), Jurkat (acute T-cell leukemia), HEF (human embryonic fibroblasts) was purchased from the Russian Academy of Sciences Cells Bank (Institute of Cytology of the Russian Academy of Sciences, Saint Petersburg, Russian Federation). Multiple myeloma cell line NCI-H929 was purchased from ATCC (USA). The MCF-7, A549 and HEF (human embryonic fibroblasts) were cultured in DMEM medium. Other cell lines were cultured in RPMI1640 medium, (PanEco, Russia) supplemented with 10% fetal bovine serum (GE Healthcare LifeSciences, São Paulo, Brazil), and gentamicin at a concentration of 40 µg/mL and cultured at 37 °C in a humidified atmosphere containing 5% CO_2. All experiments were performed with cells at passages 3 to 7 in the logarithmic phase of growth.

Cells were seeded into 96-well plates of 5×10^3 for adhesive cultures and 20×10^3 for suspension cultures per well in 90 µL and 135 µL of culture medium, respectively. The test substances were dissolved in DMSO to a concentration of 1×10^{-2} M. For subsequent dilution of the substances, a serum-free culture medium was used as the diluent. Final concentration of DMSO in wells was no more than 1%. It was found that this concentration of DMSO didn't affect the cells. Substances were added to the cells in 3–4 replicates after 24 h for adhesive cultures and immediately for suspension cultures. 10–15 µL of serum-free medium was added to the control wells with non-exposed cells. Cells were cultured for 72 h at 37 °C in an atmosphere of 5% CO_2.

3.3.2. Experimental Animals

Six to eight-week-old outbreed male mice were purchased from the Rappolovo Animal Farm of the Russian Academy of Sciences. Animals were group housed in solid bottom polycarbonate cages (3–5 animals/cage) and provided with sterilized pelleted food and pure water ad libitum.

3.3.3. Ethical Guidelines

Animal care and protocols of the study were conducted in compliance with ethical standards and recommendations for the human treatment of animals used in experimental and other scientific purposes according to the European Convention for the Protection of Vertebrate Animals used for Experimental and other Scientific Purposes (and protocol of amendment ETS No 170), the National Standard of the Russian Federation GOST R-53434-2009, "Principles of Good Laboratory Practice," and by the order of the Ministry of Health of the Russian Federation 01.04.2016, No 199n «On approval of the rules of good laboratory practice».

3.3.4. Acute Intraperitoneal Toxicity Study

Thirty mice were randomly assigned to the acute toxicity study. Animals in experimental groups (8 per/group) received a dose formulation containing compound **6** solution in 5% DMSO at various dosages (8.25, 82.5 and 200 mg/kg) via single i.p. injection. Mice in the control group treated with vehicle (5% DMSO). The location of the i.p. injection was in the lower left abdominal quadrant. Volume of injection did not exceed 250 µL. After treatments, the following parameters and end points were evaluated for 14 days: mortality, clinical signs, body weight, food consumption, locomotion, salivation, diarrhea, and lethargy. The maximum tolerated dose in this study is defined as the highest dose that will be tolerated and not produce major life-threatening toxicity for the study duration [18]. All experimental procedures were performed according to the principles and guidelines for the care and use of laboratory animals. The animals were sacrificed by carbon dioxide asphyxiation and cervical dislocation. All efforts were made to minimize suffering. Post mortem evaluation included gross examination for all animals at terminal necropsy and calculation of organ mass coefficients. No histopathological examinations were performed.

4. Conclusions

In summary, a series of PPA derivatives were synthesized via mesylation and amination. Some of these derivatives represent a promising class of cytotoxic agents with potential therapeutic values. Compound **6** demonstrated the highest cytotoxicity and was less toxic when used in vivo compared with the clinically used etoposide.

Supplementary Materials: ^{1}H-NMR, ^{13}C-NMR, ^{1}H-^{1}H ROESY and HRMS of these compounds are available in the supplementary materials.

Author Contributions: V.A. performed the research, analyzed the data and wrote the paper. S.Z. carried out the synthesis of the target compounds. P.B. and N.M. performed the biological assay of the products. J.M. and A.H. analyzed data and revised the manuscript. Y.T. and V.K. conceived the work, gave critical comments. P.B. performed animal studies. A.B. isolated phaeosphaeride A from a fungal strain.

Funding: This research received no external funding.

Conflicts of Interest: The authors declare no conflict of interest.

References

1. Goodman, L.S.; Wintrobe, M.M.; Dameshek, W.; Goodman, M.J.; Gilman, A.Z.; McLennan, M.T. Nitrogen mustard therapy. Use of methyl-bis(beta-chloroethyl)amine hydrochloride and tris(beta-chloroethyl)amine hydrochloride for hodgkin's disease, lymphosarcoma, leukemia and certain allied and miscellaneous disorders. *J. Am. Med. Assoc.* **1946**, *132*, 126–132. [CrossRef] [PubMed]
2. Wilson, A.L.; Plebanski, M.; Stephens, A.N. New trends in anti-cancer therapy: Combining conventional chemotherapeutics with novel immunomodulators. *Curr. Med. Chem.* **2017**. [CrossRef] [PubMed]
3. Bhavana, V.; Sudharshan, S.J.S.; Madhu, D. Natural anticancer compounds and their derivatives in clinical trials. In *Anticancer Plants: Clinical Trials and Nanotechnology*; Akhtar, M., Swamy, M., Eds.; Springer: Singapore, 2017; pp. 51–104.
4. Cragg, G.M.; Newman, D.J. Plants as a source of anti-cancer agents. *J. Ethnopharmacol.* **2005**, *100*, 72–79. [CrossRef] [PubMed]
5. Cragg, G.M.; Newman, D.J. Natural products: A continuing source of novel drug leads. *Biochim. Biophys. Acta.* **2013**, *1830*, 3670–3695. [CrossRef] [PubMed]
6. Newman, D.J.; Cragg, G.M. Natural products as sources of new drugs from 1981 to 2014. *J. Nat. Prod.* **2016**, *79*, 629–661. [CrossRef] [PubMed]
7. Kobayashi, K.; Kobayashi, Y.; Nakamura, M.; Tamura, O.; Kogen, H. Establishment of Relative and Absolute Configurations of Phaeosphaeride A: Total Synthesis of ent-Phaeosphaeride A. *J. Org. Chem.* **2015**, *80*, 1243–1248. [CrossRef] [PubMed]
8. Kobayashi, K.; Tanaka, K., III; Kogen, H. Total Synthesis and Biological Evaluation of Phaeosphaerides. *Catalysts* **2018**, *8*, 206–215. [CrossRef]
9. Abzianidze, V.V.; Poluektova, E.V.; Bolshakova, K.P.; Panikorovskii, T.L.; Bogachenkov, A.S.; Berestetskiy, A.O. Crystal structure of natural phaeosphaeride A. *Acta Crystallogr. E: Crystallogr. Commun.* **2015**, *71*, 625–626. [CrossRef] [PubMed]

10. Wake, M.S.; Watson, C.J. STAT3 the oncogene–still eluding therapy? *FEBS J.* **2015**, *282*, 2600–2611. [CrossRef] [PubMed]
11. Johnston, P.A.; Grandis, J.R. STAT3 signaling: Anticancer strategies and challenges. *Mol. Interv.* **2011**, *11*, 18–26. [CrossRef] [PubMed]
12. Maloney, K.N.; Hao, W.; Xu, J.; Gibbons, J.; Hucul, J.; Roll, D.; Brady, S.F.; Schroeder, F.C.; Clardy, J. Phaeosphaeride A, an inhibitor of STAT3-dependent signaling isolated from an endophytic fungus. *Org. Lett.* **2006**, *8*, 4067–4070. [CrossRef] [PubMed]
13. Shao, H.; Cheng, H.Y.; Cook, R.G.; Tweardy, D.J. Identification and characterization of signal transducer and activator of transcription 3 recruitment sites within the epidermal growth factor receptor. *Cancer Res.* **2003**, *63*, 3923–3930. [PubMed]
14. Chatzimpaloglou, A.; Yavropoulou, M.P.; Rooij, K.E.; Biedermann, R.; Mueller, U.; Kaskel, S.; Sarli, V. Total Synthesis and Biological Activity of the Proposed Structure of Phaeosphaeride A. *J. Org. Chem.* **2012**, *77*, 9659–9667. [CrossRef] [PubMed]
15. Chatzimpaloglou, A.; Kolosov, M.; Eckols, T.K.; Tweardy, D.J.; Sarli, V. Synthetic and Biological Studies of Phaeosphaerides. *J. Org. Chem.* **2014**, *79*, 4043–4054. [CrossRef] [PubMed]
16. Abzianidze, V.V.; Efimova, K.P.; Poluektova, E.V.; Trishin, Y.G.; Kuznetsov, V.A. Synthesis of natural phaeosphaeride A and semi-natural phaeosphaeride B derivatives. *Mendeleev Commun.* **2017**, *27*, 490–492. [CrossRef]
17. Efimova, K.P. Synthesis of Natural Phaeosphaeride A Derivatives with Antitumor and Herbicidal Activity. Master's Thesis, Saint-Petersburg State University of Industrial Technologies and Design, Saint Petersburg, Russia, July 2017.
18. Robinson, S.; Delongeas, J.L.; Donald, E.; Dreher, D.; Festag, M.; Kervyn, S.; Lampo, A.; Nahas, K.; Nogues, V.; Ockert, D.; et al. A European pharmaceutical company initiative challenging the regulatory requirement for acute toxicity studies in pharmaceutical drug development. *Regul. Toxicol. Pharmacol.* **2008**, *50*, 345–352. [CrossRef] [PubMed]

Sample Availability: Samples of compounds **1–8** are available from the authors.

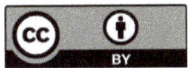

© 2018 by the authors. Licensee MDPI, Basel, Switzerland. This article is an open access article distributed under the terms and conditions of the Creative Commons Attribution (CC BY) license (http://creativecommons.org/licenses/by/4.0/).

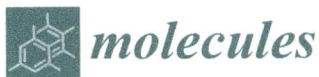

Review

Anticancer Potential of Resveratrol, β-Lapachone and Their Analogues

Danielly C. Ferraz da Costa [1,†], Luciana Pereira Rangel [2,†], Mafalda Maria Duarte da Cunha Martins-Dinis [3,†], Giulia Diniz da Silva Ferretti [3,†], Vitor F. Ferreira [4] and Jerson L. Silva [3,*]

1. Departamento de Nutrição Básica e Experimental, Instituto de Nutrição, Universidade do Estado do Rio de Janeiro, Rio de Janeiro 20550-013, Brazil; danielly.costa@uerj.br
2. Faculdade de Farmácia, Universidade Federal do Rio de Janeiro, Rio de Janeiro 21941-902, Brazil; lprangel@pharma.ufrj.br
3. Programa de Biologia Estrutural, Instituto de Bioquímica Médica Leopoldo de Meis, Instituto Nacional de Ciência e Tecnologia de Biologia Estrutural e Bioimagem, Universidade Federal do Rio de Janeiro, Rio de Janeiro 21941-902, Brazil; mafaldamariamartins@gmail.com (M.M.D.d.C.M.-D.); giuliadiniz@hotmail.com (G.D.d.S.F.)
4. Departamento de Tecnologia Farmacêutica, Faculdade de Farmácia, Universidade Federal Fluminense, Rio de Janeiro 24241-000, Brazil; vitorferreira@id.uff.br
* Correspondence: jerson@bioqmed.ufrj.br
† These authors contributed equally to this work.

Received: 31 December 2019; Accepted: 13 February 2020; Published: 18 February 2020

Abstract: This review aims to explore the potential of resveratrol, a polyphenol stilbene, and beta-lapachone, a naphthoquinone, as well as their derivatives, in the development of new drug candidates for cancer. A brief history of these compounds is reviewed along with their potential effects and mechanisms of action and the most recent attempts to improve their bioavailability and potency against different types of cancer.

Keywords: resveratrol; β-lapachone; cancer

---

1. Introduction

Cancer is a critical public health problem worldwide, with more than 18 million new cases and 9.6 million deaths estimated in 2018 [1]. Cancer therapeutics involves multiple combined approaches and requires the development of strategies based on the design and synthesis of promising compounds to improve treatment response. The search for new molecules with antitumor activity is still necessary and pursued by the pharmaceutical industry and many different research groups. Natural compounds have long been used for this purpose, leading to the development of new drugs, or as templates for new molecules with similar structures and effects [2]. Historically, bioactive compounds derived from animals and plants have been extensively used to treat diseases, which explain the scientific interest in natural products for drug discovery [3]. Both resveratrol and β-lapachone have been used with this purpose, leading to the development of new derivatives and the production of delivery systems aimed at improving the bioavailability of these compounds. In this review, we describe the potential of resveratrol, a polyphenol stilbene, and β-lapachone, a napthoquinone (Figure 1), as well as their derivatives, in the development of new drug candidates for cancer. We begin with a brief history of these compounds and move further to the discussion of their potential effects and mechanisms of action and the most recent attempts to improve their bioavailability and potency against different types of cancer.

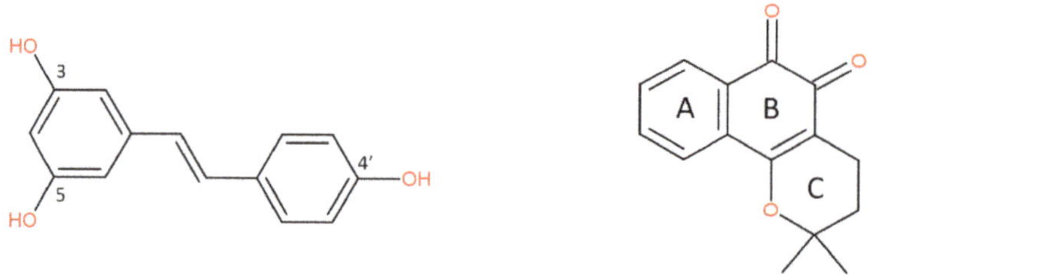

Resveratrol
(3,4′,5-trihydroxy-trans-stilbene)

β-Lapachone
(3,4-dihydro-2,2-dimethyl-2H-naphthol[1,2-b]pyran-5,6-dione)

Figure 1. Structures of resveratrol and β-lapachone.

2. Resveratrol and Stilbene-Based Compounds

Stilbenes are phytochemicals with small molecular weights (approximately 200–300 g/mol) found in a wide range of plants and dietary supplements [4]. Stilbene-based compounds have become of particular interest because of their wide range of biological activities. Among them, resveratrol (3,4′,5-trihydroxy-*trans*-stilbene) is a natural nonflavonoid polyphenol, classified as a phytoalexin, which can be naturally produced by more than 70 plant species (including grapes, blueberries, raspberries, mulberries and peanuts) in response to stressful conditions, such as fungal infection and ultraviolet radiation. In plants, the molecule exists as *trans*-resveratrol and *cis*-resveratrol isomers, and their glucosides, *trans*-piceid and *cis*-piceid. Since resveratrol is efficiently extracted from grape skin during the wine-making process, red wine is the most important dietary source of this bioactive compound [5–7]. Resveratrol has attracted scientific attention since 1997, when Jang et al. first demonstrated its ability to modulate in vivo carcinogenesis by inhibiting tumor initiation, promotion and progression in mice [8]. After that, the number of published papers regarding the role of resveratrol in blocking the multistep process of carcinogenesis increased substantially [9,10].

Currently, resveratrol is well characterized as a potent chemopreventive and chemotherapeutic agent in different cancer experimental models and clinical trials (for a review, see our recent publication) [11]. Several cell processes are targeted by this phytoalexin by upregulation or downregulation of multiple molecular pathways involved in cancer. Resveratrol modulates xenobiotic metabolism by inhibiting phase I cytochrome P450 enzymes responsible for carcinogen activation and by inducing phase II carcinogen detoxifying enzymes; reduces oxidative stress and inflammation by decreasing reactive oxygen species (ROS) generation and downregulating cyclooxygenase (COX) and inflammatory cytokines; promotes cell proliferation arrest by modulating cell cycle regulatory machinery such as cyclins and cyclin-dependent kinases (CDKs); induces apoptosis of damaged or transformed cells by different mechanisms, including upregulation of the p53 tumor suppressor protein and BAX and downregulation of Bcl2 and survivin; suppresses angiogenesis, invasion and metastasis by inhibiting hypoxia-induced factor-1α (HIF-1α) and matrix metalloproteinases; targets hormone signaling due to its relevant antiestrogenic activity in hormone-dependent cancers; and reduces the risk of multidrug resistance (MDR) via multiple targets related to carcinogenesis and chemo/radioresistance [12,13]. Resveratrol has also been proposed as a pro-oxidant agent depending on the concentration, exposure time and cell type. The oxidative damage caused by this compound represents one of the cytotoxic mechanisms involved in tumor cell death [14,15].

Mutant p53 is associated with aggregation, which results in negative dominance and gain-of-function effects [16–19]. Novel compounds can directly target the interaction of p53 mutant aggregates with their p63 and p73 paralogues and with other transcription factors [17,20]. New compounds capable of intervening in the formation of aggregates can range from natural molecules such as resveratrol analogues, synthetic molecules such as Michael acceptors, small synthetic peptides, aptamers of nucleic acids and glycosaminoglycans [17]. These new drugs have great potential to represent radical innovation. In our recently published paper, we demonstrated that resveratrol inhibits the aggregation of p53 mutants *in vitro*, in tumor cells and in xenotransplants implanted in nude mouse models (Figure 2) [21]. However, very high doses were required to exert the effect. We intend to use synthetic chemistry to produce resveratrol analogs with higher potency that can be used as pharmaceuticals.

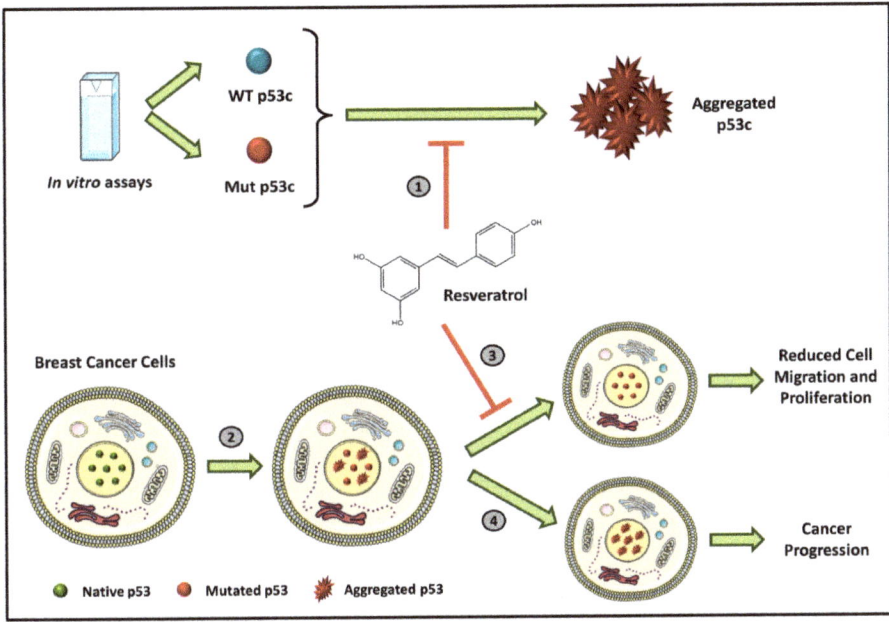

Figure 2. Schematic representation of p53 inhibition by resveratrol. In (**1**), the resveratrol in vitro capacity of inhibition of both WT and mutant p53 aggregation is described. (**2**) When mutations in the TP53 gene appear, the protein produced is less stable and forms aggregates. These aggregates are related to a direct effect in cancer proliferation and migration that is inhibited by treatment with resveratrol (**3**). Otherwise, cancer progression occurs (**4**). Extracted from Ferraz da Costa, 2018 [21].

In another study, we described that transient transfection of the wild-type p53 gene causes H1299 cells (null to p53) to become more sensitive and responsive to the pro-apoptotic properties of resveratrol, similar to what was observed in MCF-7 cells. It was proposed that resveratrol could be used therapeutically in combination with other methods of promoting p53 activity in cells, such as gene therapy using the wild-type (WT) p53 gene or chemicals that restore p53 function [22].

In mammalian experimental models, resveratrol is extensively metabolized and quickly eliminated, resulting in poor bioavailability. After oral administration, resveratrol is absorbed by passive diffusion or by membrane transporters at the intestinal level and is then released in the bloodstream, where it can be detected as an unmodified or metabolized molecule [13,23]. Although 75% of resveratrol is absorbed through the oral route, only 1% is detected in the blood plasma after the whole metabolism [24]. In recent years, different methodological approaches and synthetic derivatives have been developed to improve resveratrol bioavailability. Many studies have been performed to synthesize new and more effective resveratrol analogs that display better pharmacokinetic properties, low toxicity and minimum side effects. The methoxylated, hydroxylated and halogenated resveratrol derivatives are more explored due to their beneficial biological activities and increased oral bioavailability [25]. Previous studies showed that methoxylation increases metabolic stability and the time length required for the molecules to reach the plasma concentration peak. Moreover, the substitution of hydroxyl groups of resveratrol to methoxyl groups substantially potentiated its therapeutic versatility. It was also reported that the introduction of additional hydroxyl groups significantly increased the biological activity of resveratrol analogs [23,25]. In this review, we collect and present recent evidence in the literature regarding resveratrol derivatives and their anticancer effects, with an emphasis on the molecular mechanisms involved.

2.1. Methoxylated Resveratrol Derivatives

2.1.1. Pterostilbene

Pterostilbene (*trans*-3,5-dimethoxy-40-hydroxystilbene) is a naturally occurring stilbene, found mainly in blueberries and grapes. It is a dimethylated derivative of resveratrol with comparable antioxidant, anti-inflammatory and anticarcinogenic properties [26]. Substituting its hydroxyl for a methoxyl group enhances the lipophilicity of pterostilbene, adding to its in vivo bioavailability and, thus, improving the biological activity of this compound compared to resveratrol [27]. A study designed to compare the bioavailability, pharmacokinetics and metabolism of resveratrol and pterostilbene following equimolar oral dosing administered in rats showed that resveratrol and pterostilbene were approximately 20% and 80% bioavailable, respectively [28]. Cumulative experimental data have noted that pterostilbene exerts multiple effects against a variety of cancer models through modulation of the cell cycle, induction of cell death, and inhibition of invasion and metastasis [26,29].

The first evidence of the anticancer properties of pterostilbene was demonstrated in a colon tumorigenesis model. Pterostilbene was shown to decrease the expression of inflammatory genes, such as iNOS in the colonic crypts and aberrant crypt foci (ACF) in rats, thus suggesting that its anti-inflammatory properties may be critical in colon cancer prevention [30]. Additionally, this compound inhibits preneoplastic lesions and adenomas in mouse colon by suppressing GSK3β phosphorylation and Wnt/β-catenin signaling pathway and reduces the expression of cyclin D1, vascular endothelial growth factor (VEGF) and matrix metalloproteinases (MMPs) [31]. It was also reported that pterostilbene showed significant dose-dependent antiproliferative and cytotoxic effects and inhibited Myc, beta-catenin and cyclin D gene expression in human colon cancer Caco-2 cells [32]. In gastric adenocarcinoma cells, pterostilbene inhibits cellular proliferation and leads cells to apoptosis by different pathways, such as caspase cascade activation and modulation of cell-cycle regulating proteins [33]. In a human model of hepatocellular carcinoma, pterostilbene suppresses tumor growth by interfering in the signal transduction pathways of NF-κB and on the expression of VEGF, matrix metalloproteinase-9 (MMP-9), AP-1 and mitogen-activated protein kinase (MAPK) [34,35]. Breast cancer stem cells isolated from MCF-7, which expresses the surface antigen CD44+/CD24−, were selectively eliminated by pterostilbene. Furthermore, this compound induces necrosis and inhibits mammosphere formation, increases the activity of paclitaxel, decreases CD44 expression, induces β-catenin phosphorylation through the inhibition of hedgehog/Akt/GSK3β signaling and decreases the expression of c-Myc and cyclin D1 [36]. More recent studies showed that pterostilbene is a promising agent against human papillomavirus (HPV) E6+ tumors tested in vitro and in vivo. In vitro, this compound downregulates the viral oncogene E6. On the other hand, in mouse TC1 tumors, in addition to inhibiting E6, pterostilbene suppressed VEGF and tumor development [37]. In acute lymphoblastic leukemia cell lines Jurkat and Molt-4, the potential of pterostilbene to modulate Fas, a member of the death-inducing family of tumor necrosis factor (TNF), was investigated. Pterostilbene increased both Fas mRNA and its cell surface levels, thus leading to apoptosis [38].

2.1.2. Trimethoxystilbene

Trimethoxystilbene (*trans*-3,4′,5-trimethoxystilbene) is also a methylated resveratrol derivative, described as a potent chemopreventive agent, which promotes the induction of cell cycle arrest, reduces angiogenesis, inhibits cancer cell proliferation, increases apoptosis and decreases metastasis [25]. In MCF-7 breast cancer cells, this compound acts by inhibiting epithelial–mesenchymal transition (EMT), negatively modulating β-catenin nuclear translocation and phosphatidylinositol 3-kinase (PI3K)/protein kinase B (AKT) signaling [39]. Its anticancer mechanisms on lung cancer cells involve apoptosis induction by activation of caspases 3 and 9 and poly (ADP-ribose) polymerase interruption [40]. Additionally, in human lung cancer (A549), trimethoxystilbene promotes a decrease in invasive, migratory and adhesive characteristics of these cells and modulates the mRNA levels that encode for MMP-2 protein [41]. When evaluating the effect of this resveratrol derivative in rat C6 and human T98G glioma cells, a massive accumulation of cells at the G2/M phase of the cell cycle and apoptosis via caspase-3 related to p53 tumor suppressor protein induction were observed [42]. Trimethoxystilbene is a more effective derivative than resveratrol in suppressing the growth of HepG2 hepatocellular carcinoma cells via induction of G2/M cell cycle arrest (by upregulation of cyclin B1) and apoptosis (by downregulation of Bcl-2) [43].

2.1.3. Tetramethoxystilbene

The modification of the resveratrol structure that generates its analogue tetramethoxystilbene improved its bioactivity by suppressing cell growth in prostate, colon, ovarian and hepatocellular cancer cells. This analogue demonstrates a higher activity on human melanoma A375 by decreasing cell proliferation after treatment using a lower dose (IC_{50} = 0.7 µM) than resveratrol (IC_{50} = 100 µM) [44]. Compared with the *trans* form of the 3,4,5,4′-tetramethoxystilbene resveratrol derivative compound, the *cis* form is ten times more potent at decreasing the growth of human WI38VA virally transformed fibroblasts [45]. Using a xenograft of human ovarian cancer (A2780 and SKOV-3) as a model to study the effect of *trans*-3,4,5,4′-tetramethoxystilbene, it was observed that treatment with this derivative is able to reduce tumor cell growth [46,47]. For breast cancer, it was demonstrated that proapoptotic proteins and voltage-dependent anion channel 1 (VDAC-1) expression were increased after treatment [48]. As a new approach to treat osteosarcoma cells resistant to paclitaxel and cisplatin, the use of tetramethoxystilbene decreases, in vitro and in vivo, the viability of resistant cells and induces massive apoptosis [49].

2.1.4. Pentamethoxystilbene

Pentamethoxystilbene is a hybrid molecule chemically synthesized and, similar to resveratrol, has low oral bioavailability but presents high intravenous bioavailability. In breast carcinoma cells (MCF-7), this derivative is a good antiproliferative candidate that acts through different pathways as a G1 cell cycle regulator, modulating cyclins E and D and retinoblastoma protein (pRb). It is a better suppressor agent for breast cancer cells than resveratrol or other methoxylated derivatives. At the IC_{50} concentration of this derivative (37.8 µM), treatment with resveratrol only reduces cell survival 20% [50]. In colon cancer, a better response was reached with this compound, with activation of apoptosis through cell cycle arrest in G2/M phase, polymerization of microtubules and finally caspase-induced apoptosis. Beyond apoptosis, the compound may decrease iNOS, β-catenin and cell proliferation [51,52]. No further studies have been published with this derivative since 2012.

2.2. Hydroxylated Resveratrol Derivatives

2.2.1. Dihydroxystilbene

The resveratrol analogue 4,4′-dihydroxy-*trans*-stilbene (4,4′-DHS) was designed to improve resveratrol efficiency, both as an antioxidant and antiproliferative agent. 4,4′-DHS exhibits remarkably higher cytotoxicity than resveratrol against human promyelocytic leukemia (HL-60) cells [53]. 4,4′-DHS also inhibits the clonogenic efficiency of fibroblasts nine times more potently than resveratrol, although with a different mechanism. 4,4′-DHS predominantly induces an accumulation of cells in G1 phase, whereas resveratrol disturbs the G1/S phase transition. Furthermore, 4,4′-DHS increases p21 and p53 protein levels, whereas resveratrol leads to phosphorylation of the S-phase checkpoint protein Chk1 [54]. In a mouse lung cancer model, 2,3- and 4,4′-dihydroxystilbene (at 10 and 25 mg/kg, administered twice daily) inhibited tumor growth and metastasis. The antitumor and antimetastatic effects of these compounds were partly due to anti-lymphangiogenesis and the regulation of M2 macrophage activation and differentiation [55]. The cytotoxic action of 4,4′-DHS was also investigated in vitro in human neuroblastoma cell lines and in a mouse xenograft model of human neuroblastoma. The pharmacological action of 4,4′-DHS in the human neuroblastoma IMR32 cells was mediated by the destabilization of mitochondrial and lysosomal membranes, associated with modulation of several related pro- and anti-apoptotic cascades of proteins. Additionally, in the animal model, the oral administration of 4,4′-DHS for one month was well tolerated and demonstrated a greater therapeutic potential than resveratrol [56]. More recently, Saha et al. demonstrated that in melanoma cells, 4,4′-DHS acts by inducing apoptosis and cell cycle arrest in G1 phase and inhibiting cell proliferation. A significant reduction of melanoma tumors in a preclinical murine model was observed, and the antimetastatic effect of 4,4′-DHS was shown in a melanoma-mediated lung metastasis model in vivo [57]. In vivo assays performed in different mouse models of tumor xenografts demonstrated that 4,4′-DHS was able to disrupt the DNA replication pathway, leading to the apoptosis of pancreatic, ovarian and colorectal cancer cells [58].

2.2.2. Tetrahydroxystilbene

Tetrahydroxystilbene is a natural resveratrol analogue with multiple biological activities. In SK-Mel-28 melanoma cells, treatment with this compound induced apoptosis and inhibited cell proliferation [59,60]. In prostate cancer, its anticancer mechanisms involve JAK1 leading to STAT3 activation, which leads to a cytokine signal transduction pathway [61]. In liver and colon cancer cells, tetrahydroxystilbene arrests the cell cycle at G1 phase by modulating the cyclins pathway [62,63]. In human leukemia cells (U937), this compound induces massive apoptosis and leads to cell cycle arrest in G1 phase by regulating Bcl-2 and cIAP-2 (anti-apoptotic proteins). In cervix cancer, it acts by modulating p53 protein, thus leading cells to apoptosis [64,65]. In the last year, the 2,3,5,4′-tetrahydroxystilbene-2-O-β-D-glucoside (THSG) derivative was the major compound studied. In HT-29 colon adenocarcinoma cells, treatment with this compound reduced cell migration, invasion and adhesion, thus inhibiting metastasis. This is possible because THSG inhibits NF-κB pathway activation and consequently suppresses proteins involved in migration and invasion, such as MMP-2 and p-VE-cadherin, and ICAM-1 proteins involved in cell adhesion [66]. In vivo assays with THSG, using azoxymethane-induced colorectal cancer in rats, induced a 50% reduction in total colonic aberrant crypt foci by the inhibition of NF-κB pathway activation [67]. In MCF-7 breast cancer cells exposed to adriamycin and THSG, the vascular endothelial growth factor/phosphatidylinositol 3-kinase/Akt pathway was inhibited, triggering apoptosis by modulating Bcl-2 and caspase-3 [68].

2.2.3. Hexahydroxystilbene

Hexahydroxystilbene is a synthetic resveratrol derivative with higher biological activity [69]. When tested in breast cancer cells, hexahydroxystilbene induced apoptosis and inhibited cell proliferation by p53 protein accumulation and downregulation of mitochondrial superoxide dismutase [70]. In human colon cancer cells (HT-29), treatment with this compound leads to apoptosis and cell cycle arrest [71]. Similar results were observed in leukemia cells, with apoptosis induction by caspase activation pathways [72]. In vivo assays in a melanoma mouse model also demonstrate the induction of apoptosis pathway by upregulation of p21, downregulation of CDK-2 and cell cycle arrest at the G2/M phase [73]. Hexahydroxystilbene demonstrates an antiproliferative effect and accelerates senescence in cultured human peritoneal mesothelial cells by an oxidative stress-dependent mechanism. Treatment with 10 µM hexahydroxystilbene promoted an increase in 8-OHdG levels, a product of DNA oxidation, and a time-dependent increase in ROS release was also reported. On the other hand, soluble factors released by human peritoneal mesothelial cells that senesced prematurely in response to treatment promoted the growth of colorectal and pancreatic carcinomas in vitro [74]. No further studies have used this compound since 2013.

Although many studies have reported that stilbene compounds could play essential roles as chemotherapeutic agents by regulating multiple mechanisms and acting on different targets, further translational research is required to determine if the preclinical anticancer properties of these compounds, either alone or as part of combined therapies, are applicable in a clinical setting. The IC_{50} values for resveratrol and its derivatives vary in a wide range, as indicated in Table 1.

Table 1. IC_{50} values of resveratrol and derivatives in different study models.

Compound	2D Structure	IC_{50}	Study Model	References
Resveratrol and Resveratrol Methoxylated Derivatives				
Resveratrol		15–145 µM	Breast (MCF-7, MDA-MB-231, MDA-MB-468, MDA-MB-453), lung (A549, H460), pancreatic (Colo-357, Panc-1), prostate (LNCap, DU145) and colon (HCT116, Caco2) cancer cells; cervix carcinoma (HeLa); hepatocarcinoma (HepG2); melanoma (A357, SK-MEL-31); glioma (C6, T98G)	[22,42,75–78]
Pterostilbene		4.1–108 µM	Acute lymphoblastic leukemia (Molt-4), acute T cell leukemia (Jurkat), breast (MDA-MB-231), colon (COLO 205, HCT-116, HT-29) and endometrial (HEC-1A, ECC-1) cancer cells; melanoma (A357); hepatocarcinoma (HepG2); cervix carcinoma (HeLa, SiHa); epidermoid carcinoma (CaSki);	[27,38,79–81]
Trimethoxystilbene		0.08–80.3 µM	Colon (Caco2, SW480), head and neck (KB), lymphoma (TK6) and breast (MCF-7) cancer cells; glioma (C6, T98G)	[39,42,82]
Tetramethoxystilbene		4-60-µM	Leukemia (HL-60) and breast (BT-459) cancer cells, melanoma (SK-MEL); cervix carcinoma (HeLa)	[83]
Pentamethoxystilbene		29.2–37.8 µM	Breast (MCF-7) and colon (Colon26) cancer cells	[50,52]
Hydroxylated Resveratrol Derivatives				
Dihydroxystilbene		2.3–6.5 µM	Leukemia (HL-60), colon (HCT-116) and breast (MDA-MB-231) cancer cells; osteosarcoma (U2OS)	[57]
Tetrahydroxystilbene		58.4–620.6 µM	Acute T cell leukemia (Jurkat), breast (MCF-7), lung (H1299, A549) and prostate (LNC) cancer cells;	[68,72,84]
Hexahydroxystilbene		6.25–127.8 µM	Breast (T47D, ZR-75-1, MDA-MB-231), colon (HT-29), leukemia (HL-60) cancer cells; melanoma (M24met)	[69–71,73]

3. β-Lapachone and Its Derivatives: The South American Promise for Cancer

Quinones are widely distributed in nature, products of the secondary metabolism of several different species, with an incredible variety of biological responses [85,86]. Quinones may act as vitamins, antioxidants and are capable of stimulating antibacterial, antiallergic and anticancer effects, among others [87], which motivate their investigation as a therapeutic tool. Quinones can be cytotoxic through several mechanisms of action, including redox cycles, arylation of the thiol groups of proteins, intercalation, induction of breaks in the DNA chain, generation of free radicals and other ROS and bioreductive alkylation of critical cellular proteins and DNA via the formation of quinone methide. Besides basic research studies, quinone-based compounds are already used in the clinic. For instance, in cancer, doxorubicin, mitoxantrone and mitomycin C are used, among others [88,89]. Among all naphthoquinones described to date, three of them are widely known, mostly due to their anticancer effects and the story of their discovery—lapachol, β-lapachone and α-lapachone—of which lapachol (2-hydroxy-3-(3-methyl-2-butenyl-)-1,4-naphthoquinone, $C_{15}H_{14}O_3$), with a molecular weight of 242.2738 g/mol, was isolated first from the heartwood of *Tabebuia impetiginosa*, a widespread tree species in Brazil and other South American countries [90]. No antitumor properties were reported for lapachol until Rao et al., in 1962, described a potent anticancer effect in rats [91]. Since then, a great interest in the research of the anticancer properties of lapachol and its derivatives, or structural isomers, α- and β-lapachone, has risen [92].

β-lapachone (3,4-dihydro-2,2-dimethyl-2H-naphthol[1,2-b]pyran-5,6-dione, $C_{15}H_{14}O_3$), molecular weight 242.2738 g/mol, is an isomer of lapachol and has been described to promote several biological effects, such as anti-inflammatory, antibacterial and anti-*Trypanosoma* [93,94], and most important for this review, anticancer properties in different cancer types such as pancreatic cancer [95], breast cancer [96], hepatocellular carcinoma [97] and others. Several derivatives have been developed throughout the years, and it is noteworthy that a β-lapachone pro-drug, with commercial name ARQ-761, is in phase I/II of clinical studies for solid tumors [98].

3.1. Anticancer Effects

As mentioned previously, there is a plethora of studies that demonstrate the ability of β-lapachone to induce cell death in several cancer cell lines, [95–97,99–101], but depending on the type of cancer, it is able to induce different types of cell death. Many studies demonstrate that β-lapachone is capable of inducing apoptosis [96,101,102] in cells such as HepG2, a hepatocellular carcinoma cell line [103], but, on the other hand, others demonstrate an ability to induce cell death via necroptosis, which is a type of organized necrosis [104–106]. As another example, Park et al., 2014 [97], showed that β-lapachone is capable of inducing this type of cell death in SK-Hep1, another hepatocellular carcinoma cell line.

Most anti-neoplastic drugs demonstrate a cytostatic effect, meaning that they are able to inhibit cell proliferation, and the ability of β-lapachone to prevent the proliferation of cancer cells has long been described [107]. IC_{50} values vary in a wide range, depending on the model tested (Table 2). As observed for the type of cell death that is induced by β-lapachone, the mode of cell cycle arrest is also dependent on the cell type under study. Dias et al. (2018) demonstrated that lapachone and its iodine derivatives induce cell cycle arrest in G2/M in human oral squamous cell carcinoma cells, and Lai et al. (1998) [108] showed cell cycle arrest in the S phase for a hepatoma cell line (HepA2).

There is also evidence of antitumoral effects of β-lapachone in preclinical studies. Wu et al. reported the promotion of heat shock protein 90 cleavage by β-lapachone, mediated by oxidative stress in NQO1-expressing cell lines. In the same work, in a mouse xenotransplant model, human lung cancer xenograft growth and angiogenesis were inhibited by β-lapachone treatment [109]. Kee et al. also demonstrated that β-lapachone is able to suppress lung metastasis of melanoma in an experimental mouse model [102].

Table 2. IC$_{50}$ values of β-lapachone and derivatives in different study models.

Compound	2D Structure	IC$_{50}$	Study Model	References
Lapachol		16.04–72.3 µM	Human chronic myelogenous leukemia (K562, Lucena), Burkitt's lymphoma (Daudi), Breast cancer (MCF-7, SK-BR3)	[110,111]
ß-lapachone		0.03–70.13 µM	Lung cancer cells (A549 cell line); Tongue squamous cell carcinoma (HSC-3, SCC4, SCC9, SCC15, SCC25), hepatocellular carcinoma (HEPG2), HL-60, K562, Gastric adenocarcinoma (AGP-01, ACP-02, ACP-03), colon adenocarcinoma (HT-29, HCT-116).	[112,113]
α-lapachone		38–69 µM	K562, Lucena, Daudi, MCF-7	[111]
3-iodo-ß-lapachone		0.02–5.61 µM	Tongue squamous cell carcinoma (HSC-3, SCC4, SCC9, SCC15, SCC25), hepatocellular carcinoma (HEPG2), HL-60, K562, Gastric adenocarcinoma (AGP-01, ACP-02, ACP-03), colon adenocarcinoma (HT-29, HCT-116).	[113]
3-I-α-lapachone		0.77–14.65 µM		
naphtho[2,1-d]oxazole-4,5-diones		4.6–20 µM *	Lung cancer cells (A549 cell line)	[112]

* IC$_{50}$ values range for all derivatives shown in reference [112].

3.2. Mechanisms of Action

3.2.1. ROS and NQO1

The primary mechanism of action of β-lapachone and its derivatives is the formation of ROS [92] through its processing by NAD(P)H quinone oxidoreductase 1 (NQO1). This enzyme is able to catalyze a futile redox cycle, leading to the formation of unstable hydroquinone, which is rapidly oxidized back to the original quinone under aerobic conditions [114]. The continuous redox cycles eventually oxidize a large number of reduced pyridine nucleotides, which form ROS [115]. This effect is quite robust, since one mol of β-lapachone is capable of generating 120 mol of superoxide in two min, consuming 60 mol of NAD(P)H [106], which results in a rapid depletion of intracellular NAD+ pool over 20 to 30 min [116]. This abnormal production of ROS leads to an increase in Ca^{++}, depolarization of the mitochondrial membrane and a decrease in ATP synthesis. Therefore, in a general way, the activation of β-lapachone by NQO1 leads to cell death by apoptosis [117,118]. There are several studies that show that β-lapachone leads to the formation of ROS in cancer cells, such as Park et al., in 2014, who report that the increase of ROS is capable of inducing cell death of hepatocellular carcinoma cells (SK-Hep1) [97]. In 2011, the same group showed that ROS were involved in β-lapachone-induced autophagy in glioma cells (U87 MG). Bey et al. (2013) showed that H_2O_2 is the primary obligate ROS species necessary for β-lapachone breast cancer cell cytotoxicity through lipid peroxidation, which damages cellular membranes and organelles [106].

It is important to note that several types of solid tumors, such as cholangiocarcinoma [119], lung [120], pancreas [121], breast [122] and squamous cell carcinoma of the uterine cervix [123], have high expression of NQO1, and there are studies that demonstrate a β-lapachone preferential tropism for NQO1-positive cells [124].

Liver tumors are a very interesting case, since normal hepatocytes do not express NQO1 [125,126], but preneoplastic lesions and hepatic tumors demonstrate the presence of this enzyme [127,128]. Thus, this differentiated expression may be very important in the development of targeted therapies since it induces cell death of neoplastic or preneoplastic cells, greatly reducing side effects on healthy liver cells. Additionally, hyperthermia has been reported as an enhancer of β-lapachone effects due to the increase in NQO1 levels after heat shock and its stabilization by HSP70 [129–132]. Finally, it is noteworthy that NQO1-positive breast cancer cells correlate with the malignancy of the disease and could be used as a prognostic biomarker for breast cancer [124].

3.2.2. Topoisomerase Inhibition

One of the first mechanisms of action reported for β-lapachone was its role as a topoisomerase I modulator. Earlier thought of as a topoisomerase activator [133–135], it was later shown to act as an inhibitor, through the demonstration that β-lapachone inhibits the catalytic activity of topoisomerase I (purified from calf thymus and human cells), through its direct binding, since the incubation of topoisomerase I with β-lapachone (before adding DNA) considerably increased its inhibition, but the incubation of topoisomerase I with DNA prior to the treatment did not show any effect [136]. Other studies refer to similar effects in cell lines of different cancers, such as prostate cancer, breast cancer and leukemia [96,137,138].

3.2.3. p53

A number of studies have demonstrated β-lapachone effects on p53 independently of the cell p53 status (no expression or expression of wild-type or mutant p53); in all cases, cells can be sensitive to the effects of β-lapachone [107,139,140]. Huang Pardee, in 1999 [107], reported that β-lapachone had the ability to drastically reduce levels of mutant p53 in colon cancer cells, although it did not alter the expression levels of wild-type p53. In addition, p53 can also be regulated by β-lapachone through its phosphorylation and consequent activation, with no modification in its expression levels [141]. Finally, Pink et al. (2000) reported the β-lapachone-mediated activation of a cysteine-protease capable of digesting several cellular proteins, including p53 [142].

3.2.4. Other Cellular or Molecular Pathways

Yu et al. demonstrated the anti-tumor effect of β-lapachone on breast cancer tumors with a variation in the phosphorylation of AKT, 4EBP-1 and S6, which are related to the mTOR pathway and is also related to the apoptotic activity of this compound in gastric carcinoma cells [101]. Additionally, Wu et al., in 2016 [109], demonstrated that the effect of β-lapachone on reducing the growth of lung cancer cell tumors is related to AKT. In addition to the mTOR pathway, E-cadherin was altered in tumors, and Kim et al. (2007) [102] suggested that β-lapachone inhibits the progression and metastasis of hepatocellular carcinoma by increasing the expression of this protein and other proteins of the mTOR pathway. Additionally, the inactivation of the Akt/mTOR pathway was again attributed to β-lapachone, promoting the inhibition of EMT transition in NQO1-positive cells.

3.3. Strategies to Overcome β-Lapachone Bioavailability and Toxicity Issues: Drug Delivery and Derivatives Synthesis

Even though β-lapachone is a promising anticancer drug, its low bioavailability represents a limitation for clinical use due to low solubility in water and gastrointestinal fluids [143]. There is also a concern with the low concentration reached in the target cells and systemic toxicity, since β-lapachone displays a general distribution pattern and a dose limitation because of the risk of methemoglobinemia through the generation of nonspecific ROS at high doses [116,143].

As mentioned before, β-lapachone (Table 2) has a molecular weight of 242.29 g/mol; it is a small molecule, nonionized in the intestinal system, with pH-independent solubility. The experimental solubility value is very similar to the theoretical value of 48.33 µg/mL [112,144]. β-lapachone has the potential to be orally administered; its estimated oral fraction absorbed and intestinal effective permeability value is 85% [145]; however, a bioavailability of 15.5% through oral administration was shown in rats, probably due to broad metabolic first-pass degradation in the liver, intestines and low solubility in water, with a slow dissolution rate in the intestinal tissue [144]. Moreover, preclinical studies demonstrate that, to promote a better absorption of β-lapachone, different formulations would be necessary, and due to these findings, along with its first-pass metabolism, it was considered a difficult drug for oral administration [144,146].

Due to the low availability and unspecific toxicity of β-lapachone, there is a constant need for the development of new drug delivery systems to increase bioavailability to promote its use. There are two classical systems of β-lapachone delivery, cyclodextrin inclusion complexes and liposomes, although most studies are concerned with physical–chemical and absorption properties without any cancer therapy approach. A thorough review on this subject was written by Ferreira et al., 2016 [147]. Here, we focus on anticancer approaches.

The intricate structure of cyclodextrin allows the formation of β-lapachone/cyclodextrin inclusion complexes because of its hydrophobic core [145,148]. These inclusion complexes are capable of increasing drug bioavailability, altering their permeability, dissolution properties or both [149]. Seoane et al. (2013) used a methylated-β-cyclodextrin/poloxamer 407 mixture to create a delivery system of β-lapachone and evaluated its antitumoral activity. This system has the particularity of forming a gel above 29 °C, which facilitates intratumoral and extended drug delivery. MCF-7 tumor-bearing mice treated with this system, by intratumoral injection, showed a reduction of tumor volume without apparent liver and kidney toxicity [150].

Liposomes (one or multiple layers of phospholipids) are very interesting delivery systems because they can be used for both hydrophobic and hydrophilic drugs and display remote drug loading, homogeneous particle size, long-circulating stability, specific release and the ability to lower drug toxicity [151]. Liposomes with β-lapachone, in different mixed micellar formulations of phosphatidylcholine, sodium deoxycholate and sodium lauryl sulfate (SLS), showed the ability to increase gastrointestinal absorption at different sites (particularly in the large intestines) due to β-lapachone solubilization and interaction with the intestinal membrane [152].

Recently, there has been an increased exploration of nanosystems or nanoparticle delivery systems to surpass the limitations of these delivery systems and increase specificity and cytotoxicity to cancer cells. Dai et al. (2019) [153] developed a nanosystem with a charge-reversal ability and self-amplifiable drug release system that encapsulated β-lapachone in a pH/ROS cascade-responsive polymeric prodrug micelle. They showed that this system is capable of effectively increasing cell uptake and specific delivery through acidity-activating charge conversion and ROS-response drug release. Upon the uptake of β-lapachone, ROS formation was increased (NQO1-mediated), which lowered the cell ATP levels and consequently reduced P-gp-mediated drug efflux, decreasing multidrug resistance (MDR). This caused a massive reduction of MCF-7 tumors treated with this β-lapachone delivery system and low systemic toxicity [153].

Another strategy to increase the therapeutic efficacy of β-lapachone, through the reduction of MDR, is to promote its codelivery with another drug, such as doxorubicin. This was an option used by Li et al., demonstrating that a nanostructured lipid carrier (NLC) codelivering β-lapachone and doxorubicin had a higher therapeutic efficacy in breast cancer tumor-bearing mice, leading the authors to propose this as a possible strategy to overcome MDR in breast cancer [154].

A nanoparticle developed by Yin et al., a ROS-responsive block copolymer prodrug that self-assembles into polymeric micelles that encapsulate β-lapachone, increased tumor-specific ROS formation after intravenous administration in tumor-bearing mice. This increased ROS level and triggered drug release, allowing maximization of therapeutic efficacy, suppression of tumor growth and minimization of systemic toxicity [155].

There are three main strategies to develop β-lapachone derivatives or analogues—A- and C-ring modifications and redox center modifications—which can be obtained by copper-catalyzed azide-alkalyne cycloaddition, palladium-catalyzed cross couplings and heterocyclization reactions [156]. The great progress seen in this field is due to essential contributions from Brazilian research groups, such as Vitor Francisco Ferreira and Eufrânio Nunes da Silva Júnior [156–161]. However, most studies of β-lapachone derivatives or analogues are composed of a series of compounds with different modifications and analysis of the possible anticancer effect in cancer cell lines [89,156,161]. Nevertheless, there are more in-depth studies that attempt to understand the mechanisms of action of the compounds and eventually test them on experimental tumor models.

Recently, Dias et al. (2018) [113] showed that β-lapachone and its 3-iodine derivatives (3-I-α-lapachone and 3-I-β-lapachone) were able to induce significant cytotoxicity against different types of cancer cells (Table 2), with cell cycle arrest in G2/M, DNA fragmentation, increase in apoptosis protein levels and morphology, and production of ROS. This work also demonstrated that these compounds were able to reduce tumor burden for mice xenotransplanted with breast adenocarcinoma cells, without any alteration of biochemical, hematological or histological parameters of the treated mice, showing a nonsignificant systemic toxicity. Li et al. described a new class of β-lapachone derivatives, naphtho[2,1-d]oxazole-4,5-diones (Table 2), with higher solubility and comparable activities, both in vitro and in vivo (xenotransplants), against NQO1-positive A549 lung cancer cells [112]. The compounds β-lap-dC3 and -dC6 are prodrug diester derivatives of β-lapachone. When encapsulated in PEG-β-PLA micelles, they were described to be more efficient in loading micelles than β-lapachone itself, and β-lap-dC3 improved the survival rate of NSCLC xenograft-bearing mice, increasing β-lapachone concentration in the target tissues, which makes it a promising therapy to be developed against NQO1-positive cells [162].

Finally, the sensitization of cells promoted by different energy sources, such as light or radiation, in combination with β-lapachone and its derivatives has also been described. Lamberti et al. (2018) showed the synergism between halogenated derivatives of β-lapachone and photodynamic therapy in melanoma cells with positive results due to the upregulation of NQO1 expression [163]. Ionizing radiation at low doses was applied in combination with sublethal doses of β-lapachone in non-small-cell lung cancer (NSCLC) cell lines and in xenograft models in vivo [164]. Additionally, the massive release of ROS promoted by ionizing radiation was applied together with nontoxic β-lapachone doses to head and neck patient samples [165]. These results suggested the use of this combination to increase the efficacy of radiotherapy in NQO1-positive tumors and shall be tested in clinical trials in the near future.

4. Conclusions

Both of the molecules reviewed here, β-lapachone and resveratrol, are paradoxical. While they are naturally occurring products, or at least derived from natural sources, they can be radically improved by human manipulation. They represent a case study for natural products that can be enhanced by structural manipulation and/or delivery systems. In this paper, we intended to compile the available information about β-lapachone and resveratrol, with a special focus on what has been found in recent years and on the possible impact in cancer therapy, also showing how a bioactive compound/molecule can be found in natural resources, which are a possible reservoir of new therapies. However, it is essential not to be dismissive of the importance of manipulating natural molecules to increase their efficiency and specificity. The results obtained with β-lapachone, resveratrol and their analogues for cancer therapy are promising, especially if we manage to improve their specificity for cancer cells, with less systemic toxicity (a major problem for most chemotherapies) and their delivery, particularly by making them orally bioavailable for patient comfort. The similarities and differences between the two groups of compounds can be observed through the comparison between the values shown in Tables 1 and 2 and the properties listed in the supplementary material tables (Tables S1–S4).

Supplementary Materials: The following are available online, Table S1: Bioactivity prediction (druglikeness*) of β-lapachone and its derivatives for specific biological activities; Table S2: Bioactivity prediction (druglikeness*) of resveratrol and its derivatives for specific biological activities; Table S3: Chemical and pharmacological properties of Lapachol, β-lapachone and derivatives; Table S4: Chemical and pharmacological properties of resveratrol and derivatives.

Author Contributions: D.C.F.d.C., L.P.R., V.F.F. and J.L.S. wrote and edited the text. M.M.D.d.C.M.-D. and G.D.d.S.F. wrote the text. All authors have read and agreed to the published version of the manuscript.

Funding: We thank Conselho Nacional de Desenvolvimento Científico e Tecnológico (CNPq), Fundação Carlos Chagas Filho de Amparo à Pesquisa do Estado do Rio de Janeiro (FAPERJ), Fundação do Câncer and Coordenação de Aperfeiçoamento de Pessoal de Nível Superior (CAPES) for the support.

Conflicts of Interest: The authors declare no conflict of interest.

References

1. The International Agency for Research on Cancer (IARC). *Latest Global CANCER Data: Cancer Burden Rises to 18.1 Million New Cases and 9.6 Million Cancer Deaths in 2018*; IARC: Lyon, France, 2018.
2. Newman, D.J.; Cragg, G.M. Natural products as sources of new drugs over the 30 years from 1981 to 2010. *J. Nat. Prod.* **2012**, *75*, 311–335. [CrossRef] [PubMed]
3. Harvey, A.L.; Edrada-Ebel, R.; Quinn, R.J. The re-emergence of natural products for drug discovery in the genomics era. *Nat. Rev. Drug Discov.* **2015**, *14*, 111–129. [CrossRef] [PubMed]
4. Roupe, K.; Remsberg, C.; Yanez, J.; Davies, N. Pharmacometrics of Stilbenes: Seguing Towards the Clinic. *Curr. Clin. Pharmacol.* **2008**, *1*, 81–101. [CrossRef] [PubMed]
5. Siemann, E.H.; Creasy, L.L. Concentration of the phytoalexin resveratrol in wine. *Am. J. Enol. Vitic.* **1992**, *43*, 49–52.
6. Signorelli, P.; Ghidoni, R. Resveratrol as an anticancer nutrient: Molecular basis, open questions and promises. *J. Nutr. Biochem.* **2005**, *16*, 449–466. [CrossRef] [PubMed]
7. Ali, K.; Maltese, F.; Choi, Y.H.; Verpoorte, R. Metabolic constituents of grapevine and grape-derived products. *Phytochem. Rev.* **2010**, *9*, 357–378. [CrossRef]
8. Jang, M.; Cai, L.; Udeani, G.O.; Slowing, K.V.; Thomas, C.F.; Beecher, C.W.W.; Fong, H.H.S.; Farnsworth, N.R.; Kinghorn, A.D.; Mehta, R.G.; et al. Cancer chemopreventive activity of resveratrol, a natural product derived from grapes. *Science* **1997**, *275*, 218–220. [CrossRef]
9. Baur, J.A.; Sinclair, D.A. Therapeutic potential of resveratrol: The in vivo evidence. *Nat. Rev. Drug Discov.* **2006**, *5*, 493–506. [CrossRef]
10. Pezzuto, J.M. Resveratrol as an inhibitor of carcinogenesis. *Pharm. Biol.* **2008**, *46*, 443–573. [CrossRef]
11. Da Costa, D.C.F.; Fialho, E.; Silva, J.L. Cancer chemoprevention by resveratrol: The P53 tumor suppressor protein as a promising molecular target. *Molecules* **2017**, *22*, 1014. [CrossRef]
12. Kundu, J.K.; Surh, Y.J. Cancer chemopreventive and therapeutic potential of resveratrol: Mechanistic perspectives. *Cancer Lett.* **2008**, *269*, 243–261. [CrossRef] [PubMed]
13. Varoni, E.M.; Lo Faro, A.F.; Sharifi-Rad, J.; Iriti, M. Anticancer Molecular Mechanisms of Resveratrol. *Front. Nutr.* **2016**, *3*, 8. [CrossRef] [PubMed]
14. De la Lastra, C.A.; Villegas, I. Resveratrol as an antioxidant and pro-oxidant agent: Mechanisms and clinical implications. *Biochem. Soc. Trans.* **2007**, *35*, 1156–1160. [CrossRef]

15. Martins, L.A.M.; Coelho, B.P.; Behr, G.; Pettenuzzo, L.F.; Souza, I.C.C.; Moreira, J.C.F.; Borojevic, R.; Gottfried, C.; Guma, F.C.R. Resveratrol Induces Pro-oxidant Effects and Time-Dependent Resistance to Cytotoxicity in Activated Hepatic Stellate Cells. *Cell Biochem. Biophys.* **2014**, *68*, 247–257. [CrossRef] [PubMed]
16. Silva, J.L.; Vieira, T.C.R.G.; Gomes, M.P.B.; Ano Bom, A.P.; Lima, L.M.T.R.; Freitas, M.S.; Ishimaru, D.; Cordeiro, Y.; Foguel, D. Ligand binding and hydration in protein misfolding: Insights from studies of prion and p53 tumor suppressor proteins. *Acc. Chem. Res.* **2010**, *43*, 271–279. [CrossRef] [PubMed]
17. Silva, J.L.; Cino, E.A.; Soares, I.N.; Ferreira, V.F.; De Oliveira, G. Targeting the Prion-like Aggregation of Mutant p53 to Combat Cancer. *Acc. Chem. Res.* **2018**, *51*, 181–190. [CrossRef]
18. Ano Bom, A.P.D.; Rangel, L.P.; Costa, D.C.F.; De Oliveira, G.A.P.; Sanches, D.; Braga, C.A.; Gava, L.M.; Ramos, C.H.I.; Cepeda, A.O.T.; Stumbo, A.C.; et al. Mutant p53 aggregates into prion-like amyloid oligomers and fibrils: Implications for cancer. *J. Biol. Chem.* **2012**, *287*, 28152–28162. [CrossRef]
19. Silva, J.L.; Gallo, C.V.D.M.; Costa, D.C.F.; Rangel, L.P. Prion-like aggregation of mutant p53 in cancer. *Trends Biochem. Sci.* **2014**, *39*, 260–267. [CrossRef]
20. Xu, J.; Reumers, J.; Couceiro, J.R.; De Smet, F.; Gallardo, R.; Rudyak, S.; Cornelis, A.; Rozenski, J.; Zwolinska, A.; Marine, J.C.; et al. Gain of function of mutant p53 by coaggregation with multiple tumor suppressors. *Nat. Chem. Biol.* **2011**, *7*, 285–295. [CrossRef]
21. Ferraz Da Costa, D.C.; Campos, N.P.C.; Santos, R.A.; Guedes-Da-Silva, F.H.; Martins-Dinis, M.M.D.C.; Zanphorlin, L.; Ramos, C.; Rangel, L.P.; Silva, J.L. Resveratrol prevents p53 aggregation in vitro and in breast cancer cells. *Oncotarget* **2018**, *9*, 29112–29122.
22. Ferraz da Costa, D.C.; Casanova, F.A.; Quarti, J.; Malheiros, M.S.; Sanches, D.; dos Santos, P.S.; Fialho, E.; Silva, J.L. Transient Transfection of a Wild-Type p53 Gene Triggers Resveratrol-Induced Apoptosis in Cancer Cells. *PLoS ONE* **2012**, *7*, e48746. [CrossRef] [PubMed]
23. Chimento, A.; De Amicis, F.; Sirianni, R.; Sinicropi, M.S.; Puoci, F.; Casaburi, I.; Saturnino, C.; Pezzi, V. Progress to improve oral bioavailability and beneficial effects of resveratrol. *Int. J. Mol. Sci.* **2019**, *20*, 1381. [CrossRef] [PubMed]
24. Walle, T. Bioavailability of resveratrol. *Ann. N. Y. Acad. Sci.* **2011**, *1215*, 9–15. [CrossRef] [PubMed]
25. Nawaz, W.; Zhou, Z.; Deng, S.; Ma, X.; Ma, X.; Li, C.; Shu, X. Therapeutic versatility of resveratrol derivatives. *Nutrients* **2017**, *9*, 1188. [CrossRef] [PubMed]
26. McCormack, D.; McFadden, D. Pterostilbene and cancer: Current review. *J. Surg. Res.* **2012**, *173*, e53–e61. [CrossRef]
27. Kosuru, R.; Rai, U.; Prakash, S.; Singh, A.; Singh, S. Promising therapeutic potential of pterostilbene and its mechanistic insight based on preclinical evidence. *Eur. J. Pharmacol.* **2016**, *789*, 229–243. [CrossRef]
28. Kapetanovic, I.M.; Muzzio, M.; Huang, Z.; Thompson, T.N.; McCormick, D.L. Pharmacokinetics, oral bioavailability, and metabolic profile of resveratrol and its dimethylether analog, pterostilbene, in rats. *Cancer Chemother. Pharmacol.* **2011**, *68*, 593–601. [CrossRef]
29. Ma, Z.; Zhang, X.; Xu, L.; Liu, D.; Di, S.; Li, W.; Zhang, J.; Zhang, H.; Li, X.; Han, J.; et al. Pterostilbene: Mechanisms of its action as oncostatic agent in cell models and in vivo studies. *Pharmacol. Res.* **2019**, *145*, 104265. [CrossRef]
30. Suh, N.; Paul, S.; Hao, X.; Simi, B.; Xiao, H.; Rimando, A.M.; Reddy, B.S. Pterostilbene, an active constituent of blueberries, suppresses aberrant crypt foci formation in the azoxymethane-induced colon carcinogenesis model in rats. *Clin. Cancer Res.* **2007**, *13*, 350–355. [CrossRef]
31. Chiou, Y.S.; Tsai, M.L.; Wang, Y.J.; Cheng, A.C.; Lai, W.M.; Badmaev, V.; Ho, C.T.; Pan, M.H. Pterostilbene inhibits colorectal aberrant crypt foci (ACF) and colon carcinogenesis via suppression of multiple signal transduction pathways in azoxymethane-treated mice. *J. Agric. Food Chem.* **2010**, *58*, 8833–8841. [CrossRef]
32. Wawszczyk, J.; Kapral, M.; Hollek, A.; Węglarz, L. In vitro evaluation of antiproliferative and cytotoxic properties of pterostilbene against human colon cancer cells. *Acta Pol. Pharmacol.* **2014**, *71*, 1051–1055.
33. Pan, M.H.; Chang, Y.H.; Badmaev, V.; Nagabhushanam, K.; Ho, C.T. Pterostilbene induces apoptosis and cell cycle arrest in human gastric carcinoma cells. *J. Agric. Food Chem.* **2007**, *55*, 7777–7785. [CrossRef] [PubMed]
34. Pan, M.H.; Chiou, Y.S.; Chen, W.J.; Wang, J.M.; Badmaev, V.; Ho, C.T. Pterostilbene inhibited tumor invasion via suppressing multiple signal transduction pathways in human hepatocellular carcinoma cells. *Carcinogenesis* **2009**, *30*, 1234–1242. [CrossRef]

35. Huang, C.S.; Ho, C.T.; Tu, S.H.; Pan, M.H.; Chuang, C.H.; Chang, H.W.; Chang, C.H.; Wu, C.H.; Ho, Y.S. Long-term ethanol exposure-induced hepatocellular carcinoma cell migration and invasion through lysyl oxidase activation are attenuated by combined treatment with pterostilbene and curcumin analogues. *J. Agric. Food Chem.* **2013**, *61*, 4326–4335. [CrossRef] [PubMed]
36. Wu, C.H.; Hong, B.H.; Ho, C.T.; Yen, G.C. Targeting cancer stem cells in breast cancer: Potential anticancer properties of 6-shogaol and pterostilbene. *J. Agric. Food Chem.* **2015**, *63*, 2432–2441. [CrossRef] [PubMed]
37. Chatterjee, K.; Mukherjee, S.; Vanmanen, J.; Banerjee, P.; Fata, J.E. Dietary polyphenols, resveratrol and pterostilbene exhibit antitumor activity on an HPV E6-positive cervical cancer model: An in vitro and in vivo analysis. *Front. Oncol.* **2019**, *9*, 352. [CrossRef] [PubMed]
38. Ramezani, G.; Pourgheysari, B.; Shirzad, H.; Sourani, Z. Pterostilbene increases Fas expression in T-lymphoblastic leukemia cell lines. *Res. Pharmacol. Sci.* **2019**, *14*, 55.
39. Tsai, J.H.; Hsu, L.S.; Lin, C.L.; Hong, H.M.; Pan, M.H.; Way, T.D.; Chen, W.J. 3,5,4′-Trimethoxystilbene, a natural methoxylated analog of resveratrol, inhibits breast cancer cell invasiveness by downregulation of PI3K/Akt and Wnt/β-catenin signaling cascades and reversal of epithelial-mesenchymal transition. *Toxicol. Appl. Pharmacol.* **2013**, *272*, 746–756. [CrossRef]
40. Weng, C.J.; Yang, Y.T.; Ho, C.T.; Yen, G.C. Mechanisms of apoptotic effects induced by resveratrol, dibenzoylmethane, and their analogues on human lung carcinoma cells. *J. Agric. Food Chem.* **2009**, *57*, 5235–5243. [CrossRef]
41. Yang, Y.T.; Weng, C.J.; Ho, C.T.; Yen, G.C. Resveratrol analog-3,5,4′-trimethoxy-*trans*-stilbene inhibits invasion of human lung adenocarcinoma cells by suppressing the MAPK pathway and decreasing matrix metalloproteinase-2 expression. *Mol. Nutr. Food Res.* **2009**, *53*, 407–416. [CrossRef]
42. Zielińska-Przyjemska, M.; Kaczmarek, M.; Krajka-Kuźniak, V.; Łuczak, M.; Baer-Dubowska, W. The effect of resveratrol, its naturally occurring derivatives and tannic acid on the induction of cell cycle arrest and apoptosis in rat C6 and human T98G glioma cell lines. *Toxicol. In Vitro* **2017**, *43*, 69–75. [CrossRef] [PubMed]
43. Wang, G.; Guo, X.; Chen, H.; Lin, T.; Xu, Y.; Chen, Q.; Liu, J.; Zeng, J.; Zhang, X.K.; Yao, X. A resveratrol analog, phoyunbene B, induces G2/M cell cycle arrest and apoptosis in HepG2 liver cancer cells. *Bioorg. Med. Chem. Lett.* **2012**, *22*, 2114–2118. [CrossRef] [PubMed]
44. Androutsopoulos, V.P.; Fragiadaki, I.; Spandidos, D.A.; Tosca, A. The resveratrol analogue, 3,4,5,4′-trans-tetramethoxystilbene, inhibits the growth of A375 melanoma cells through multiple anticancer modes of action. *Int. J. Oncol.* **2016**, *49*, 1305–1314. [CrossRef] [PubMed]
45. Gosslau, A.; Pabbaraja, S.; Knapp, S.; Chen, K.Y. Trans- and cis-stilbene polyphenols induced rapid perinuclear mitochondrial clustering and p53-independent apoptosis in cancer cells but not normal cells. *Eur. J. Pharmacol.* **2008**, *587*, 25–34. [CrossRef]
46. Piotrowska, H.; Myszkowski, K.; Abraszek, J.; Kwiatkowska-Borowczyk, E.; Amarowicz, R.; Murias, M.; Wierzchowski, M.; Jodynis-Liebert, J. DMU-212 inhibits tumor growth in xenograft model of human ovarian cancer. *Biomed. Pharmacol.* **2014**, *68*, 397–400. [CrossRef]
47. Piotrowska-Kempisty, H.; Rucinski, M.; Borys, S.; Kucinska, M.; Kaczmarek, M.; Zawierucha, P.; Wierzchowski, M.; Lazewski, D.; Murias, M.; Jodynis-Liebert, J. 3′-hydroxy-3,4,5,4′-tetramethoxystilbene, the metabolite of resveratrol analogue DMU-212, inhibits ovarian cancer cell growth in vitro and in a mice xenograft model. *Sci. Rep.* **2016**, *6*, 32627. [CrossRef]
48. Hong, M.; Park, N.; Chun, Y.J. Role of annexin A5 on mitochondria-dependent apoptosis induced by tetramethoxystilbene in human breast cancer cells. *Biomol. Ther.* **2014**, *22*, 519–524. [CrossRef]
49. Xu, H. (Z)-3,4,3′,5′-Tetramethoxystilbene, a natural product, induces apoptosis and reduces viability of paclitaxel-And cisplatin-resistant osteosarcoma cells. *J. Cancer Res. Ther.* **2016**, *12*, 1261. [CrossRef]
50. Pan, M.H.; Lin, C.L.I.; Tsal, J.H.; Ho, C.T.; Chen, W.J. 3,5,3′,4′,5′-Pentamethoxystilbene (MR-5), a synthetically methoxylated analogue of resveratrol, inhibits growth and induces G1 cell cycle arrest of human breast carcinoma MCF-7 Cells. *J. Agric. Food Chem.* **2010**, *58*, 226–234. [CrossRef]
51. Li, H.; Wu, W.K.K.; Zheng, Z.; Che, C.T.; Yu, L.; Li, Z.J.; Wu, Y.C.; Cheng, K.W.; Yu, J.; Cho, C.H.; et al. 2,3′,4,4′,5-Pentamethoxy-*trans*-stilbene, a resveratrol derivative, is a potent inducer of apoptosis in colon cancer cells via targeting microtubules. *Biochem. Pharmacol.* **2009**, *78*, 1224–1232. [CrossRef]
52. Li, H.; Wu, W.K.K.; Li, Z.J.; Chan, K.M.; Wong, C.C.M.; Ye, C.G.; Yu, L.; Sung, J.J.Y.; Cho, C.H.; Wang, M. 2,3′,4,4′,5′-Pentamethoxy-*trans*-stilbene, a resveratrol derivative, inhibits colitis-associated colorectal carcinogenesis in mice. *Br. J. Pharmacol.* **2010**, *160*, 1352–1361. [CrossRef]

53. Fan, G.J.; Liu, X.D.; Qian, Y.P.; Shang, Y.J.; Li, X.Z.; Dai, F.; Fang, J.G.; Jin, X.L.; Zhou, B. 4,4′-Dihydroxy-*trans*-stilbene, a resveratrol analogue, exhibited enhanced antioxidant activity and cytotoxicity. *Bioorg. Med. Chem.* **2009**, *17*, 2360–2365. [CrossRef]
54. Savio, M.; Coppa, T.; Bianchi, L.; Vannini, V.; Maga, G.; Forti, L.; Cazzalini, O.; Lazzè, M.C.; Perucca, P.; Prosperi, E.; et al. The resveratrol analogue 4,4′-dihydroxy-*trans*-stilbene inhibits cell proliferation with higher efficiency but different mechanism from resveratrol. *Int. J. Biochem. Cell Biol.* **2009**, *41*, 2493–2502. [CrossRef]
55. Kimura, Y.; Sumiyoshi, M.; Baba, K. Antitumor and antimetastatic activity of synthetic hydroxystilbenes through inhibition of lymphangiogenesis and M2 macrophage differentiation of tumor-associated macrophages. *Anticancer Res.* **2016**, *36*, 137–148.
56. Saha, B.; Patro, B.S.; Koli, M.; Pai, G.; Ray, J.; Bandyopadhyay, S.K.; Chattopadhyay, S. *trans*-4,4′-Dihydroxystilbene (DHS) inhibits human neuroblastoma tumor growth and induces mitochondrial and lysosomal damages in neuroblastoma cell lines. *Oncotarget* **2017**, *8*, 73905. [CrossRef]
57. Saha, B.; Pai, G.B.; Subramanian, M.; Gupta, P.; Tyagi, M.; Patro, B.S.; Chattopadhyay, S. Resveratrol analogue, *trans*-4,4′-dihydroxystilbene (DHS), inhibits melanoma tumor growth and suppresses its metastatic colonization in lungs. *Biomed. Pharmacol.* **2018**, *107*, 1104–1114. [CrossRef]
58. Chen, C.W.; Li, Y.; Hu, S.; Zhou, W.; Meng, Y.; Li, Z.; Zhang, Y.; Sun, J.; Bo, Z.; DePamphilis, M.L.; et al. DHS (trans−4,4′-dihydroxystilbene) suppresses DNA replication and tumor growth by inhibiting RRM2 (ribonucleotide reductase regulatory subunit M2). *Oncogene* **2019**, *38*, 2364–2379. [CrossRef]
59. Larrosa, M.; Tomás-Barberán, F.A.; Espín, J.C. Grape polyphenol resveratrol and the related molecule 4-hydroxystilbene induce growth inhibition, apoptosis, S-phase arrest, and upregulation of cyclins A, E, and B1 in human SK-Mel-28 melanoma cells. *J. Agric. Food Chem.* **2003**, *51*, 4576–4584. [CrossRef]
60. Larrosa, M.; Tomás-Barberán, F.A.; Espín, J.C. The grape and wine polyphenol piceatannol is a potent inducer of apoptosis in human SK-Mel-28 melanoma cells. *Eur. J. Nutr.* **2004**, *43*, 275–284. [CrossRef]
61. Barton, B.E.; Karras, J.G.; Murphy, T.F.; Barton, A.; Huang, H.F.S. Signal transducer and activator of transcription 3 (STAT3) activation in prostate cancer: Direct STAT3 inhibition induces apoptosis in prostate cancer lines. *Mol. Cancer Ther.* **2004**, *3*, 11–20.
62. Wolter, F.; Clausnitzer, A.; Akoglu, B.; Stein, J. Piceatannol, a Natural Analog of Resveratrol, Inhibits Progression through the S Phase of the Cell Cycle in Colorectal Cancer Cell Lines. *J. Nutr.* **2002**, *132*, 298–302. [CrossRef]
63. Kuo, P.L.; Hsu, Y.L. The grape and wine constituent piceatannol inhibits proliferation of human bladder cancer cells via blocking cell cycle progression and inducing Fas/membrane bound Fas ligand-mediated apoptotic pathway. *Mol. Nutr. Food Res.* **2008**, *52*, 408–418. [CrossRef]
64. Liu, W.H.; Chang, L. Sen Piceatannol induces Fas and FasL up-regulation in human leukemia U937 cells via Ca2+/p38α MAPK-mediated activation of c-Jun and ATF-2 pathways. *Int. J. Biochem. Cell Biol.* **2010**, *42*, 1498–1506. [CrossRef]
65. Füllbeck, M.; Huang, X.; Dumdey, R.; Frommel, C.; Dubiel, W.; Preissner, R. Novel curcumin- and emodin-related compounds identified by in silico 2D/3D conformer screening induce apoptosis in tumor cells. *BMC Cancer* **2005**, *5*, 97. [CrossRef] [PubMed]
66. CL, L.; SL, H.; Leung, W.; JH, J.; GC, H.; CT, L.; CC, W. 2,3,5,4′-tetrahydroxystilbene-2-O-β-D-glucoside suppresses human colorectal cancer cell metastasis through inhibiting NF-κB activation. *Int. J. Oncol.* **2016**, *49*, 629–638.
67. Lin, C.L.; Jeng, J.H.; Wu, C.C.; Hsieh, S.L.; Huang, G.C.; Leung, W.; Lee, C.T.; Chen, C.Y.; Lee, C.H. Chemopreventive Potential of 2,3,5,4′-Tetrahydroxystilbene-2-O-β-D-glucoside on the Formation of Aberrant Crypt Foci in Azoxymethane-Induced Colorectal Cancer in Rats. *Biomed Res. Int.* **2017**, *2017*, 3634915. [CrossRef]
68. Shen, J.; Zhang, Y.; Shen, H.; Pan, H.; Xu, L.; Yuan, L.; Ding, Z. The synergistic effect of 2,3,5,4′-Tetrahydroxystilbene-2-O-β-D-glucoside combined with Aadriamycin on MCF-7 breast cancer cells. *Drug Des. Dev. Ther.* **2018**, *12*, 4083–4094. [CrossRef]
69. Szekeres, T.; Saiko, P.; Fritzer-Szekeres, M.; Djavan, B.; Jäger, W. Chemopreventive effects of resveratrol and resveratrol derivatives. *Ann. N. Y. Acad. Sci.* **2011**, *1215*, 89–95. [CrossRef]

70. Murias, M.; Luczak, M.W.; Niepsuj, A.; Krajka-Kuzniak, V.; Zielinska-Przyjemska, M.; Jagodzinski, P.P.; Jäger, W.; Szekeres, T.; Jodynis-Liebert, J. Cytotoxic activity of 3,3′,4,4′,5,5′-hexahydroxystilbene against breast cancer cells is mediated by induction of p53 and downregulation of mitochondrial superoxide dismutase. *Toxicol. In Vitro* **2008**, *22*, 1361–1370. [CrossRef]
71. Saiko, P.; Pemberger, M.; Horvath, Z.; Savinc, I.; Grusch, M.; Handler, N.; Erker, T.; Jaeger, W.; Fritzer-Szekeres, M.; Szekeres, T. Novel resveratrol analogs induce apoptosis and cause cell cycle arrest in HT29 human colon cancer cells: Inhibition of ribonucleotide reductase activity. *Oncol. Rep.* **2008**, *19*, 1621–1626.
72. Kucinska, M.; Piotrowska, H.; Luczak, M.W.; Mikula-Pietrasik, J.; Ksiazek, K.; Wozniak, M.; Wierzchowski, M.; Dudka, J.; Jäger, W.; Murias, M. Effects of hydroxylated resveratrol analogs on oxidative stress and cancer cells death in human acute T cell leukemia cell line: Prooxidative potential of hydroxylated resveratrol analogs. *Chem. Biol. Interact.* **2014**, *209*, 96–110. [CrossRef] [PubMed]
73. Paulitschke, V.; Schicher, N.; Szekeres, T.; Jäger, W.; Elbling, L.; Riemer, A.B.; Scheiner, O.; Trimurtulu, G.; Venkateswarlu, S.; Mikula, M.; et al. 3,3′,4,4′,5,5′-hexahydroxystilbene impairs melanoma progression in a metastatic mouse model. *J. Investig. Dermatol.* **2010**, *130*, 1668–1679. [CrossRef] [PubMed]
74. Mikuła-Pietrasik, J.; Sosińska, P.; Wierzchowski, M.; Piwocka, K.; Ksiazek, K. Synthetic resveratrol analogue, 3,3′,4,4′,5,5′-hexahydroxy-*trans*-stilbene, accelerates senescence in peritoneal mesothelium and promotes senescence-dependent growth of gastrointestinal cancers. *Int. J. Mol. Sci.* **2013**, *14*, 22483–22498. [CrossRef]
75. Kotha, A.; Sekharam, M.; Cilenti, L.; Siddiquee, K.; Khaled, A.; Zervos, A.S.; Carter, B.; Turkson, J.; Jove, R. Resveratrol inhibits Src and Stat3 signaling and induces the apoptosis of malignant cells containing activated Stat3 protein. *Mol. Cancer Ther.* **2006**, *5*, 621–629. [CrossRef]
76. Fouad, M.A.; Agha, A.M.; Merzabani, M.A.; Shouman, S.A. Resveratrol inhibits proliferation, angiogenesis and induces apoptosis in colon cancer cells: Calorie restriction is the force to the cytotoxicity. *Hum. Exp. Toxicol.* **2013**, *32*, 1067–1080. [CrossRef]
77. Li, P.; Yang, S.; Dou, M.; Chen, Y.; Zhang, J.; Zhao, X. Synergic effects of artemisinin and resveratrol in cancer cells. *J. Cancer Res. Clin. Oncol.* **2014**, *140*, 2065–2075. [CrossRef]
78. Wu, Z.; Liu, B.; Cailing, E.; Liu, J.; Zhang, Q.; Liu, J.; Chen, N.; Chen, R.; Zhu, R. Resveratrol inhibits the proliferation of human melanoma cells by inducing G1/S cell cycle arrest and apoptosis. *Mol. Med. Rep.* **2015**, *11*, 400–404. [CrossRef]
79. Shin, H.J.; Han, J.M.; Choi, Y.S.; Jung, H.J. Pterostilbene suppresses both cancer cells and cancer stem-like cells in cervical cancer with superior bioavailability to resveratrol. *Molecules* **2020**, *25*, 228. [CrossRef]
80. Wen, W.; Lowe, G.; Roberts, C.M.; Finlay, J.; Han, E.S.; Glackin, C.A.; Dellinger, T.H. Pterostilbene, a natural phenolic compound, synergizes the antineoplastic effects of megestrol acetate in endometrial cancer. *Sci. Rep.* **2017**, *7*, 1–10. [CrossRef]
81. Cheng, T.C.; Lai, C.S.; Chung, M.C.; Kalyanam, N.; Majeed, M.; Ho, C.T.; Ho, Y.S.; Pan, M.H. Potent anti-cancer effect of 39-hydroxypterostilbene in human colon xenograft tumors. *PLoS ONE* **2014**, *9*, e111814. [CrossRef]
82. Schneider, Y.; Chabert, P.; Stutzmann, J.; Coelho, D.; Fougerousse, A.; Gossé, F.; Launay, J.F.; Brouillard, R.; Raul, F. Resveratrol analog (Z)-3,5,4′-trimethoxystilbene is a potent anti-mitotic drug inhibiting tubulin polymerization. *Int. J. Cancer* **2003**, *107*, 189–196. [CrossRef]
83. Zaki, M.A.; Balachandran, P.; Khan, S.; Wang, M.; Mohammed, R.; Hetta, M.H.; Pasco, D.S.; Muhammad, I. Cytotoxicity and modulation of cancer-related signaling by (Z)- and (E)-3,4,3′,5′-tetramethoxystilbene isolated from *Eugenia rigida*. *J. Nat. Prod.* **2013**, *76*, 679–684. [CrossRef]
84. Xu, M.; Wang, C.; Zhu, M.; Wang, X.; Zhang, L.; Zhao, J. 2, 3, 5, 4-tetrahydroxy diphenylethylene-2-O-glucoside inhibits the adhesion and invasion of A549 human lung cancer cells. *Mol. Med. Rep.* **2017**, *16*, 8900–8906.
85. Bolton, J.L.; Trush, M.A.; Penning, T.M.; Dryhurst, G.; Monks, T.J. Role of quinones in toxicology. *Chem. Res. Toxicol.* **2000**, *13*, 135–160. [CrossRef]
86. El-Najjar, N.; Gali-Muhtasib, H.; Ketola, R.A.; Vuorela, P.; Urtti, A.; Vuorela, H. The chemical and biological activities of quinones: Overview and implications in analytical detection. *Phytochem. Rev.* **2011**, *10*, 353. [CrossRef]
87. Tseng, C.H.; Cheng, C.M.; Tzeng, C.C.; Peng, S.I.; Yang, C.L.; Chen, Y.L. Synthesis and anti-inflammatory evaluations of β-lapachone derivatives. *Bioorg. Med. Chem.* **2013**, *21*, 523–531. [CrossRef]

88. Bolton, J.L.; Dunlap, T. Formation and biological targets of quinones: Cytotoxic versus cytoprotective effects. *Chem. Res. Toxicol.* **2017**, *30*, 13–37. [CrossRef]
89. Cardoso, M.F.C.; Rodrigues, P.C.; Oliveira, M.E.I.M.; Gama, I.L.; Da Silva, I.M.C.B.; Santos, I.O.; Rocha, D.R.; Pinho, R.T.; Ferreira, V.F.; De Souza, M.C.B.V.; et al. Synthesis and evaluation of the cytotoxic activity of 1,2-furanonaphthoquinones tethered to 1,2,3-1H-triazoles in myeloid and lymphoid leukemia cell lines. *Eur. J. Med. Chem.* **2014**, *84*, 708–717. [CrossRef]
90. Thomson, R.H. Distribution and Biogenesis. In *Naturally Occurring Quinones*; Elsevier: Amsterdam, The Netherlands, 1971.
91. Rao, K.V.; Mcbride, T.J.; Oleson, J.J. Recognition and Evaluation of Lapachol as an Antitumor Agent. *Cancer Res.* **1968**, *28*, 1952–1954.
92. Hussain, H.; Green, I.R. Lapachol and lapachone analogs: A journey of two decades of patent research (1997–2016). *Expert Opin. Ther. Pat.* **2017**, *27*, 1111–1121. [CrossRef]
93. Salas, C.; Tapia, R.A.; Ciudad, K.; Armstrong, V.; Orellana, M.; Kemmerling, U.; Ferreira, J.; Maya, J.D.; Morello, A. *Trypanosoma cruzi*: Activities of lapachol and α- and β-lapachone derivatives against epimastigote and trypomastigote forms. *Bioorg. Med. Chem.* **2008**, *16*, 668–674. [CrossRef]
94. Boveris, A.; Stoppani, A.O.M.; Docampo, R.; Cruz, F.S. Superoxide anion production and trypanocidal action of naphthoquinones on *Trypanosoma cruzi*. *Comp. Biochem. Physiol. Part C Comp.* **1978**, *61*, 327–329. [CrossRef]
95. Silvers, M.A.; Deja, S.; Singh, N.; Egnatchik, R.A.; Sudderth, J.; Luo, X.; Beg, M.S.; Burgess, S.C.; DeBerardinis, R.J.; Boothman, D.A.; et al. The NQO1 bioactivatable drug, β-lapachone, alters the redox state of NQO1 pancreatic cancer cells, causing perturbation in central carbon metabolism. *J. Biol. Chem.* **2017**, *292*, 18203–18216. [CrossRef]
96. Wuerzberger, S.M.; Pink, J.J.; Planchon, S.M.; Byers, K.L.; Bornmann, W.G.; Boothman, D.A. Induction of apoptosis in MCF-7: WS8 breast cancer cells by β-Lapachone. *Cancer Res.* **1998**, *58*, 1876–1885. [PubMed]
97. Park, E.J.; Min, K.J.; Lee, T.J.; Yoo, Y.H.; Kim, Y.S.; Kwon, T.K. β-Lapachone induces programmed necrosis through the RIP1-PARP-AIF-dependent pathway in human hepatocellular carcinoma SK-Hep1 cells. *Cell Death Dis.* **2014**, *5*, e1230. [CrossRef] [PubMed]
98. Gerber, D.E.; Beg, M.S.; Fattah, F.; Frankel, A.E.; Fatunde, O.; Arriaga, Y.; Dowell, J.E.; Bisen, A.; Leff, R.D.; Meek, C.C.; et al. Phase 1 study of ARQ 761, a β-lapachone analogue that promotes NQO1-mediated programmed cancer cell necrosis. *Br. J. Cancer* **2018**, *119*, 928. [CrossRef]
99. Don, M.J.; Chang, Y.H.; Chen, K.K.; Ho, L.K.; Chau, Y.P. Induction of CDK inhibitors (p21WAF1 and p27Kip1) and BAK in the β-lapachone-induced apoptosis of human prostate cancer cells. *Mol. Pharmacol.* **2001**, *59*, 784–794. [CrossRef]
100. Liu, T.J.; Lin, S.Y.; Chau, Y.P. Inhibition of poly(ADP-ribose) polymerase activation attenuates β-lapachone-induced necrotic cell death in human osteosarcoma cells. *Toxicol. Appl. Pharmacol.* **2002**, *182*, 116–125. [CrossRef]
101. Yu, H.Y.; Kim, S.O.; Jin, C.Y.; Kim, G.Y.; Kim, W.J.; Yoo, Y.H.; Choi, Y.H. β-lapachone-induced apoptosis of human gastric carcinoma AGS cells is caspase-dependent and regulated by the PI3K/Akt pathway. *Biomol. Ther.* **2014**, *22*, 184. [CrossRef]
102. Kee, J.Y.; Han, Y.H.; Kim, D.S.; Mun, J.G.; Park, S.H.; So, H.S.; Park, S.J.; Park, R.; Um, J.Y.; Hong, S.H. β-Lapachone suppresses the lung metastasis of melanoma via the MAPK signaling pathway. *PLoS ONE* **2017**, *12*, e0176937. [CrossRef]
103. Woo, H.J.; Park, K.Y.; Rhu, C.H.; Lee, W.H.; Choi, B.T.; Kim, G.Y.; Park, Y.M.; Choi, Y.H. β-lapachone, a quinone isolated from Tabebuia avellanedae, induces apoptosis in HepG2 hepatoma cell line through induction of Bax and activation of caspase. *J. Med. Food* **2006**, *9*, 161–168. [CrossRef]
104. Bey, E.A.; Bentle, M.S.; Reinicke, K.E.; Dong, Y.; Yang, C.R.; Girard, L.; Minna, J.D.; Bornmann, W.G.; Gao, J.; Boothman, D.A. An NQO1- and PARP-1-mediated cell death pathway induced in non-small-cell lung cancer cells by β-lapachone. *Proc. Natl. Acad. Sci. USA* **2007**, *104*, 11832–11837. [CrossRef]
105. Huang, X.; Dong, Y.; Bey, E.A.; Kilgore, J.A.; Bair, J.S.; Li, L.S.; Patel, M.; Parkinson, E.I.; Wang, Y.; Williams, N.S.; et al. An NQO1 substrate with potent antitumor activity that selectively kills by PARP1-induced programmed necrosis. *Cancer Res.* **2012**, *72*, 3038–3047. [CrossRef] [PubMed]
106. Bey, E.A.; Reinicke, K.E.; Srougi, M.C.; Varnes, M.; Anderson, V.E.; Pink, J.J.; Li, L.S.; Patel, M.; Cao, L.; Moore, Z.; et al. Catalase abrogates β-lapachone-induced PARP1 hyperactivation-directed programmed necrosis in NQO1-positive breast cancers. *Mol. Cancer Ther.* **2013**, *12*, 2110–2120. [CrossRef] [PubMed]

107. Huang, L.; Pardee, A.B. β-lapachone induces cell cycle arrest and apoptosis in human colon cancer cells. *Mol. Med.* **1999**, *5*, 711–720. [CrossRef] [PubMed]
108. Lai, C.; Liu, T.; Ho, L.; Don, M.; Chau, Y. Beta-lapachone induced cell death in human hepatoma (HepA2) cells. *Histol. Histopathol.* **1998**, *13*, 89–97. [PubMed]
109. Wu, Y.; Wang, X.; Chang, S.; Lu, W.; Liu, M.; Pang, X. β-lapachone induces NAD(P)H:quinone oxidoreductase-1- and oxidative stress-dependent heat shock protein 90 cleavage and inhibits tumor growth and angiogenesiss. *J. Pharmacol. Exp. Ther.* **2016**, *357*, 466–475. [CrossRef]
110. Silva, E.O.; de Carvalho, T.C.; Parshikov, I.A.; dos Santos, R.A.; Emery, F.S.; Furtado, N.A.J.C. Cytotoxicity of lapachol metabolites produced by probiotics. *Lett. Appl. Microbiol.* **2014**, *59*, 108–114. [CrossRef]
111. Salustiano, E.J.S.; Netto, C.D.; Fernandes, R.F.; Da Silva, A.J.M.; Bacelar, T.S.; Castro, C.P.; Buarque, C.D.; Maia, R.C.; Rumjanek, V.M.; Costa, P.R.R. Comparison of the cytotoxic effect of lapachol, α-lapachone and pentacyclic 1,4-naphthoquinones on human leukemic cells. *Investig. New Drugs* **2010**, *28*, 139–144. [CrossRef]
112. Li, X.; Bian, J.; Wang, N.; Qian, X.; Gu, J.; Mu, T.; Fan, J.; Yang, X.; Li, S.; Yang, T.; et al. Novel naphtho[2,1-d]oxazole-4,5-diones as NQO1 substrates with improved aqueous solubility: Design, synthesis, and in vivo antitumor evaluation. *Bioorg. Med. Chem.* **2016**, *24*, 1006–1013. [CrossRef]
113. Dias, R.B.; de Araújo, T.B.S.; de Freitas, R.D.; Rodrigues, A.C.B.D.C.; Sousa, L.P.; Sales, C.B.S.; de Valverde, L.F.; Soares, M.B.P.; dos Reis, M.G.; Coletta, R.D.; et al. β-Lapachone and its iodine derivatives cause cell cycle arrest at G2/M phase and reactive oxygen species-mediated apoptosis in human oral squamous cell carcinoma cells. *Free Radic. Biol. Med.* **2018**, *126*, 87–100.
114. Ross, D.; Siegel, D. Functions of NQO1 in cellular protection and CoQ10 metabolism and its potential role as a redox sensitive molecular switch. *Front. Physiol.* **2017**, *8*, 595. [CrossRef] [PubMed]
115. Siegel, D.; Yan, C.; Ross, D. NAD(P)H:quinone oxidoreductase 1 (NQO1) in the sensitivity and resistance to antitumor quinones. *Biochem. Pharmacol.* **2012**, *83*, 1033–1040. [CrossRef] [PubMed]
116. Chakrabarti, G.; Moore, Z.R.; Luo, X.; Ilcheva, M.; Ali, A.; Padanad, M.; Zhou, Y.; Xie, Y.; Burma, S.; Scaglioni, P.P.; et al. Targeting glutamine metabolism sensitizes pancreatic cancer to PARP-driven metabolic catastrophe induced by ß-lapachone. *Cancer Metab.* **2015**, *3*, 12. [CrossRef] [PubMed]
117. Tagliarino, C.; Pink, J.J.; Reinicke, K.E.; Simmers, S.M.; Wuerzberger-Davis, S.M.; Boothman, D.A. μ-calpain activation in β-lapachone-mediated apoptosis. *Cancer Biol. Ther.* **2003**, *2*, 141–152. [CrossRef] [PubMed]
118. Li, L.S.; Bey, E.A.; Dong, Y.; Meng, J.; Patra, B.; Yan, J.; Xie, X.J.; Brekken, R.A.; Barnett, C.C.; Bornmann, W.G.; et al. Modulating endogenous NQO1 levels identifies key regulatory mechanisms of action of β-lapachone for pancreatic cancer therapy. *Clin. Cancer Res.* **2011**, *17*, 275–285. [CrossRef] [PubMed]
119. Buranrat, B.; Chau-In, S.; Prawan, A.; Puapairoj, A.; Zeekpudsa, P.; Kukongviriyapan, V. NQO1 expression correlates with Cholangiocarcinoma prognosis. *Asian Pac. J. Cancer Prev.* **2012**, *13*, 131–136.
120. Siegel, D.; Franklin, W.A.; Ross, D. Immunohistochemical detection of NAD(P)H:Quinone oxidoreductase in human lung and lung tumors. *Clin. Cancer Res.* **1998**, *4*, 2065–2070.
121. Awadallah, N.S.; Dehn, D.; Shah, R.J.; Russell Nash, S.; Chen, Y.K.; Ross, D.; Bentz, J.S.; Shroyer, K.R. NQO1 expression in pancreatic cancer and its potential use as a biomarker. *Appl. Immunohistochem. Mol. Morphol.* **2008**, *16*, 24–31. [CrossRef]
122. Yang, Y.; Zhang, Y.; Wu, Q.; Cui, X.; Lin, Z.; Liu, S.; Chen, L. Clinical implications of high NQO1 expression in breast cancers. *J. Exp. Clin. Cancer Res.* **2014**, *33*, 14. [CrossRef]
123. Ma, Y.; Kong, J.; Yan, G.; Ren, X.; Jin, D.; Jin, T.; Lin, L.; Lin, Z. NQO1 overexpression is associated with poor prognosis in squamous cell carcinoma of the uterine cervix. *BMC Cancer* **2014**, *14*, 414. [CrossRef]
124. Yang, Y.; Zhou, X.; Xu, M.; Piao, J.; Zhang, Y.; Lin, Z.; Chen, L. β-Lapachone suppresses tumour progression by inhibiting epithelial-to-mesenchymal transition in NQO1-positive breast cancers. *Sci. Rep.* **2017**, *7*, 2681. [CrossRef] [PubMed]
125. Siegel, D.; Ross, D. Immunodetection of NAD(P)H:quinone oxidoreductase 1 (NQO1) in human tissues. *Free Radic. Biol. Med.* **2000**, *29*, 246–253. [CrossRef]
126. Strassburg, A.; Strassburg, C.P.; Manns, M.P.; Tukey, R.H. Differential gene expression of NAD(P)H:Quinone oxidoreductase and NRH:Quinone oxidoreductase in human hepatocellular and biliary tissue. *Mol. Pharmacol.* **2002**, *61*, 320–325. [CrossRef]
127. Schor, N.A.; Morris, H.P. The activity of the D T diaphorase in experimental hepatomas. *Cancer Biochem. Biophys.* **1977**, *2*, 5–9.

128. Cresteil, T.; Jaiswal, A.K. High levels of expression of the NAD(P)H:Quinone oxidoreductase (NQO1) gene in tumor cells compared to normal cells of the same origin. *Biochem. Pharmacol.* **1991**, *42*, 1021–1027. [CrossRef]
129. Hori, T.; Kondo, T.; Lee, H.; Song, C.W.; Park, H.J. Hyperthermia enhances the effect of β-lapachone to cause γh2AX formations and cell death in human osteosarcoma cells. *Int. J. Hyperth.* **2011**, *27*, 53–62. [CrossRef]
130. Dong, G.Z.; Youn, H.; Park, M.T.; Oh, E.T.; Park, K.H.; Song, C.W.; Kyung Choi, E.; Park, H.J. Heat shock increases expression of NAD(P)H:quinone oxidoreductase (NQO1), mediator of β-lapachone cytotoxicity, by increasing NQO1 gene activity and via Hsp70-mediated stabilisation of NQO1 protein. *Int. J. Hyperth.* **2009**, *25*, 477–487. [CrossRef]
131. Song, C.W.; Chae, J.J.; Choi, E.K.; Hwang, T.S.; Kim, C.; Lim, B.U.L.; Park, H.J. Anti-cancer effect of bio-reductive drug β-lapachon is enhanced by activating NQO1 with heat shock. *Int. J. Hyperth.* **2008**, *24*, 161–169. [CrossRef]
132. Park, H.J.; Choi, E.K.; Choi, J.; Ahn, K.J.; Kim, E.J.; Ji, I.M.; Kook, Y.H.; Ahn, S.D.; Williams, B.; Griffin, R.; et al. Heat-induced up-regulation of NAD(P)H:quinone oxidoreductase potentiates anticancer effects of β-lapachone. *Clin. Cancer Res.* **2005**, *11*, 8866–8871. [CrossRef]
133. Boothman, D.A.; Trask, D.K.; Pardee, A.B. Inhibition of Potentially Lethal DNA Damage Repair in Human Tumor Cells by β-Lapachone, an Activator of Topoisomerase I. *Cancer Res.* **1989**, *49*, 605–612.
134. Jones, J.C.; Stevnsner, T.; Mattern, M.R.; Bohr, V.A. Effect of specific enzyme inhibitors on replication, total genome DNA repair and on gene-specific DNA repair after UV irradiation in CHO cells. *Mutat. Res. Repair* **1991**, *255*, 155–162. [CrossRef]
135. Katz, E.J.; Vick, J.S.; Kling, K.M.; Andrews, P.A.; Howell, S.B. Effect of topoisomerase modulators on cisplatin cytotoxicity in human ovarian carcinoma cells. *Eur. J. Cancer Clin. Oncol.* **1990**, *26*, 724–727. [CrossRef]
136. Li, C.J.; Averboukh, L.; Pardee, A.B. β-Lapachone, a novel DNA topoisomerase I inhibitor with a mode of action different from camptothecin. *J. Biol. Chem.* **1993**, *268*, 22463–22468.
137. Li, C.J.; Wang, C.; Pardee, A.B. Induction of Apoptosis by β-Lapachone in Human Prostate Cancer Cells. *Cancer Res.* **1995**, *55*, 3712–3715. [PubMed]
138. Furuya, Y.; Ohta, S.; Ito, H. Apoptosis of androgen-independent mammary and prostate cell lines induced by topoisomerase inhibitors: Common pathway of gene regulation. *Anticancer Res.* **1997**, *17*, 2089–2093.
139. Planchon, S.M.; Wuerzberger, S.; Boothman, D.A.; Church, D.R.; Wilding, G.; Frydman, B.; Witiak, D.T.; Hutson, P. β-Lapachone-mediated Apoptosis in Human Promyelocytic Leukemia (HL-60) and Human Prostate Cancer Cells: A p53-independent Response. *Cancer Res.* **1995**, *55*, 3706–3711.
140. Li, Y.; Sun, X.; LaMont, J.T.; Pardee, A.B.; Li, C.J. Selective killing of cancer cells by β-lapachone: Direct checkpoint activation as a strategy against cancer. *Proc. Natl. Acad. Sci. USA* **2003**, *100*, 2674–2678. [CrossRef]
141. Choi, Y.H.; Ho, S.K.; Yoo, M.A. Suppression of human prostate cancer cell growth by β-lapachone via down-regulation of pRB phosphorylation and induction of Cdk inhibitor P21 WAF1/CIP1. *J. Biochem. Mol. Biol.* **2003**, *36*, 223–229. [CrossRef]
142. Pink, J.J.; Wuerzberger-Davis, S.; Tagliarino, C.; Planchon, S.M.; Yang, X.H.; Froelich, C.J.; Boothman, D.A. Activation of a cysteine protease in MCF-7 and T47D breast cancer cells during β-lapachone-mediated apoptosis. *Exp. Cell Res.* **2000**, *255*, 144–145. [CrossRef]
143. Ough, M.; Lewis, A.; Bey, E.A.; Gao, J.; Ritchie, J.M.; Bornmann, W.; Boothman, D.A.; Oberley, L.W.; Cullen, J.J. Efficacy of β-lapachone in pancreatic cancer treatment: Exploiting the novel, therapeutic target NQO1. *Cancer Biol. Ther.* **2005**, *4*, 102–109. [CrossRef]
144. Kim, I.; Kim, H.; Ro, J.; Jo, K.; Karki, S.; Khadka, P.; Yun, G.; Lee, J. Preclinical pharmacokinetic evaluation of β-lapachone: Characteristics of oral bioavailability and first-pass metabolism in rats. *Biomol. Ther.* **2015**, *23*, 296. [CrossRef] [PubMed]
145. Mangas-Sanjuan, V.; Gutiérrez-Nieto, J.; Echezarreta-López, M.; González-Álvarez, I.; González-Álvarez, M.; Casabó, V.G.; Bermejo, M.; Landin, M. Intestinal Permeability of β-Lapachone and Its Cyclodextrin Complexes and Physical Mixtures. *Eur. J. Drug Metab. Pharmacokinet.* **2016**, *41*, 795–806. [CrossRef] [PubMed]
146. Blanco, E.; Bey, E.A.; Khemtong, C.; Yang, S.G.; Setti-Guthi, J.; Chen, H.; Kessinger, C.W.; Carnevale, K.A.; Bornmann, W.G.; Boothman, D.A.; et al. β-lapachone micellar nanotherapeutics for non-small cell lung cancer therapy. *Cancer Res.* **2010**, *70*, 3896–3904. [CrossRef] [PubMed]

147. Ferreira, V.; Nicoletti, C.; Ferreira, P.; Futuro, D.; da Silva, F. Strategies for Increasing the Solubility and Bioavailability of Anticancer Compounds: β-Lapachone and Other Naphthoquinones. *Curr. Pharm. Des.* **2016**, *22*, 5899–5914. [CrossRef]
148. Szejtli, J. *Cyclodextrin Technology*; Springer: Berlin, Germany, 2013; ISBN 9788578110796.
149. Dahan, A.; Lennernäs, H.; Amidon, G.L. The fraction dose absorbed, in humans, and high jejunal human permeability relationship. *Mol. Pharm.* **2012**, *9*, 1847–1851. [CrossRef]
150. Seoane, S.; Díaz-Rodríguez, P.; Sendon-Lago, J.; Gallego, R.; Pérez-Fernández, R.; Landin, M. Administration of the optimized β-Lapachone-poloxamer-cyclodextrin ternary system induces apoptosis, DNA damage and reduces tumor growth in a human breast adenocarcinoma xenograft mouse model. *Eur. J. Pharm. Biopharm.* **2013**, *84*, 497–504. [CrossRef]
151. Allen, T.M.; Cullis, P.R. Liposomal drug delivery systems: From concept to clinical applications. *Adv. Drug Deliv. Rev.* **2013**, *65*, 36–48. [CrossRef]
152. Jang, S.B.; Kim, D.; Kim, S.Y.; Park, C.; Jeong, J.H.; Kuh, H.J.; Lee, J. Impact of micellar vehicles on in situ intestinal absorption properties of β-lapachone in rats. *Korean J. Physiol. Pharmacol.* **2013**, *17*, 9–13. [CrossRef]
153. Dai, L.; Li, X.; Duan, X.; Li, M.; Niu, P.; Xu, H.; Cai, K.; Yang, H. A pH/ROS Cascade-Responsive Charge-Reversal Nanosystem with Self-Amplified Drug Release for Synergistic Oxidation-Chemotherapy. *Adv. Sci.* **2019**, *6*, 1801807. [CrossRef]
154. Li, X.; Jia, X.; Niu, H. Nanostructured lipid carriers co-delivering lapachone and doxorubicin for overcoming multidrug resistance in breast cancer therapy. *Int. J. Nanomed.* **2018**, *13*, 4107–4119. [CrossRef]
155. Yin, W.; Ke, W.; Chen, W.; Xi, L.; Zhou, Q.; Mukerabigwi, J.F.; Ge, Z. Integrated block copolymer prodrug nanoparticles for combination of tumor oxidative stress amplification and ROS-responsive drug release. *Biomaterials* **2019**, *195*, 63–74. [CrossRef]
156. Da Silva Júnior, E.N.; Jardim, G.A.M.; Jacob, C.; Dhawa, U.; Ackermann, L.; de Castro, S.L. Synthesis of quinones with highlighted biological applications: A critical update on the strategies towards bioactive compounds with emphasis on lapachones. *Eur. J. Med. Chem.* **2019**. [CrossRef]
157. Di Rosso, M.E.; Barreiro Arcos, M.L.; Elingold, I.; Sterle, H.; Baptista Ferreira, S.; Ferreira, V.F.; Galleano, M.; Cremaschi, G.; Dubin, M. Novel o-naphthoquinones induce apoptosis of EL-4 T lymphoma cells through the increase of reactive oxygen species. *Toxicol. In Vitro* **2013**, *27*, 2094–2104. [CrossRef]
158. Araújo, A.J.; de Souza, A.A.; da Silva Júnior, E.N.; Marinho-Filho, J.D.B.; de Moura, M.A.B.F.; Rocha, D.D.; Vasconcellos, M.C.; Costa, C.O.; Pessoa, C.; de Moraes, M.O.; et al. Growth inhibitory effects of 3′-nitro-3-phenylamino nor-beta-lapachone against HL-60: A redox-dependent mechanism. *Toxicol. In Vitro* **2012**, *26*, 585–594. [CrossRef]
159. Da Rocha, D.R.; De Souza, A.C.G.; Resende, J.A.L.C.; Santos, W.C.; Dos Santos, E.A.; Pessoa, C.; De Moraes, M.O.; Costa-Lotufo, L.V.; Montenegro, R.C.; Ferreira, V.F. Synthesis of new 9-hydroxy-α- and 7-hydroxy-β-pyran naphthoquinones and cytotoxicity against cancer cell lines. *Org. Biomol. Chem.* **2011**, *9*, 4315–4322. [CrossRef]
160. Bortolot, C.S.; da S.M. Forezi, L.; Marra, R.K.F.; Reis, M.I.P.; Sá, B.V.F.; Filho, R.I.; Ghasemishahrestani, Z.; Sola-Penna, M.; Zancan, P.; Ferreira, V.F.; et al. Design, Synthesis and Biological Evaluation of 1H-1,2,3-Triazole-Linked-1H-Dibenzo[b,h]xanthenes as Inductors of ROS-Mediated Apoptosis in the Breast Cancer Cell Line MCF-7. *Med. Chem.* **2018**, *15*, 119–129.
161. Da Cruz, E.H.G.; Silvers, M.A.; Jardim, G.A.M.; Resende, J.M.; Cavalcanti, B.C.; Bomfim, I.S.; Pessoa, C.; De Simone, C.A.; Botteselle, G.V.; Braga, A.L.; et al. Synthesis and antitumor activity of selenium-containing quinone-based triazoles possessing two redox centres, and their mechanistic insights. *Eur. J. Med. Chem.* **2016**, *122*, 1–16. [CrossRef]
162. Ma, X.; Huang, X.; Moore, Z.; Huang, G.; Kilgore, J.A.; Wang, Y.; Hammer, S.; Williams, N.S.; Boothman, D.A.; Gao, J. Esterase-activatable β-lapachone prodrug micelles for NQO1-targeted lung cancer therapy. *J. Control. Release* **2015**, *200*, 201–211. [CrossRef]
163. Lamberti, M.J.; Morales Vasconsuelo, A.B.; Chiaramello, M.; Ferreira, V.F.; Macedo Oliveira, M.; Baptista Ferreira, S.; Rivarola, V.A.; Rumie Vittar, N.B. NQO1 induction mediated by photodynamic therapy synergizes with β-Lapachone-halogenated derivative against melanoma. *Biomed. Pharmacother.* **2018**, *108*, 1553–1564. [CrossRef]

164. Motea, E.A.; Huang, X.; Singh, N.; Kilgore, J.A.; Williams, N.S.; Xie, X.J.; Gerber, D.E.; Beg, M.S.; Bey, E.A.; Boothman, D.A. NQO1-dependent, tumor-selective radiosensitization of non-small cell lung cancers. *Clin. Cancer Res.* **2019**, *25*, 2601–2609. [CrossRef]
165. Li, L.S.; Reddy, S.; Lin, Z.H.; Liu, S.; Park, H.; Chun, S.G.; Bornmann, W.G.; Thibodeaux, J.; Yan, J.; Chakrabarti, G.; et al. NQO1-Mediated tumor-selective lethality and radiosensitization for head and neck cancer. *Mol. Cancer Ther.* **2016**, *15*, 1757–1767. [CrossRef] [PubMed]

© 2020 by the authors. Licensee MDPI, Basel, Switzerland. This article is an open access article distributed under the terms and conditions of the Creative Commons Attribution (CC BY) license (http://creativecommons.org/licenses/by/4.0/).

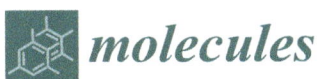

Review

Molecular Mechanisms of the Anti-Cancer Effects of Isothiocyanates from Cruciferous Vegetables in Bladder Cancer

Tomhiro Mastuo, Yasuyoshi Miyata *, Tsutomu Yuno, Yuta Mukae, Asato Otsubo, Kensuke Mitsunari, Kojiro Ohba and Hideki Sakai

Department of Urology, Nagasaki University Graduate School of Biomedical Sciences, Nagasaki 852-8501, Japan; tomozo1228@hotmail.com (T.M.); t.yuno@nagasaki-u.ac.jp (T.Y.); ytmk_n2@yahoo.co.jp (Y.M.); a.06131dpsc@gmail.com (A.O.); ken.mitsunari@gmail.com (K.M.); ohba-k@nagasaki-u.ac.jp (K.O.); hsakai@nagasaki-u.ac.jp (H.S.)
* Correspondence: yasu-myt@nagasaki-u.ac.jp; Tel.: +81 95 819 7340; Fax: +81 95 819 7343

Received: 10 January 2020; Accepted: 28 January 2020; Published: 29 January 2020

Abstract: Bladder cancer (BC) is a representative of urological cancer with a high recurrence and metastasis potential. Currently, cisplatin-based chemotherapy and immune checkpoint inhibitors are used as standard therapy in patients with advanced/metastatic BC. However, these therapies often show severe adverse events, and prolongation of survival is unsatisfactory. Therefore, a treatment strategy using natural compounds is of great interest. In this review, we focused on the anti-cancer effects of isothiocyanates (ITCs) derived from cruciferous vegetables, which are widely cultivated and consumed in many regions worldwide. Specifically, we discuss the anti-cancer effects of four ITC compounds—allyl isothiocyanate, benzyl isothiocyanate, sulforaphane, and phenethyl isothiocyanate—in BC; the molecular mechanisms underlying their anti-cancer effects; current trends and future direction of ITC-based treatment strategies; and the carcinogenic potential of ITCs. We also discuss the advantages and limitations of each ITC in BC treatment, furthering the consideration of ITCs in treatment strategies and for improving the prognosis of patients with BC.

Keywords: allyl isothiocyanate; benzyl isothiocyanate; sulforaphane; phenethyl isothiocyanate; bladder cancer

1. Introduction

Bladder cancer (BC) is recognized as a representative of urological cancer (UC), but it has specific pathological characteristics and treatment strategies. BC shows a high recurrence and metastasis potential, even if radical operation is performed [1,2]. Regarding treatment strategies, only two regimens have been approved as effective methods: platinum-based chemotherapy, including gemcitabine and cisplatin combination therapy and MVAC therapy, and immune checkpoint inhibitors, such as pembrolizumab [3–5]. Unfortunately, these regimens have shown relatively severe adverse events, including renal dysfunction, neutropenia, and immunogenic abnormalities, and it is currently difficult to predict therapeutic effects [3,4,6]. Although there is an improved prognosis of BC patients undergoing these therapies, prolongation of survival is far from satisfactory, especially in patients with advanced/metastatic disease. Currently, new anti-cancer drugs for UC are under development, some of which are expected to be approved for the treatment of advanced/metastatic BC in the near feature [7,8]. However, there is little information on the safety and adverse events of these new drugs.

Based on these facts, as well as the artificially produced anti-cancer drugs, treatment strategies employing natural compounds have garnered special interest for various types of malignancies. There is a general consensus that considering treatment strategies using natural product(s) is important for improving the quality of life and prognosis of cancer patients. In fact, there is a report that curcumin, a natural occurring polyphenol derived from turmeric (*Curcuma longa*), had anti-cancer effects via suppression of cancer cell proliferation, invasion, and metastasis in lung cancer cells [9]. The authors also showed that regulation of microRNA expression plays important roles in the curcumin-induced anti-cancer effects [9]. Furthermore, Yiqi Huayu Jiedu decoction, which comprises various Chinese herbs and natural compounds, was reported to increase the anti-cancer effects of standard chemotherapy in patients with stage III gastric cancer after radical gastrectomy and improve the quality of life of patients [10]. In addition to these reports, several reviews and *in vivo* and *in vitro* studies have demonstrated that a variety of natural products possess anti-cancer potential and can avoid the undesirable effects of standard therapies of malignancies [11–14].

Regarding BC, multiple studies showed that a variety of natural products have anti-cancer effects and maintain quality of life, including *Evodia rutaecarpa* or curcumin [15,16]. Several reports also demonstrated the relationship between natural products and prevention of carcinogenesis, clinicopathological features, and anti-cancer effects in BC [17,18]. In previous studies, we showed the anti-cancer effects, clinical usefulness, and pathological mechanisms of green tea polyphenol or royal jelly in urological cancers, including BC [19–25]. Although green tea and royal jelly are eaten in some parts of Asia and Western countries, this is not the case globally. In contrast, cruciferous vegetables, such as broccoli, kale, cauliflower, bock choy, and horseradish, are widely cultivated in many regions and are commonly eaten worldwide. Isothiocyanates (ITCs) are naturally occurring products of cruciferous vegetables, and researchers have investigated their health benefits and efficacy in the treatment of various diseases, including malignancies. Although some reviews mentioned the anti-cancer effects of ITCs in BC, there is relatively little comprehensive information on the molecular mechanisms of the ITC anti-cancer effects in BC cells [26–28]. In addition, comprehensive information on each ITC member, including allyl isothiocyanate (AITC), benzyl isothiocyanate (BITC), sulforaphane (SFN), and phenethyl isothiocyanate (PEITC), is limited. Therefore, in this review, we discuss the anti-cancer effects and efficacy of ITCs in BC cells obtained by *in vivo* and *in vitro* studies. In particular, we focus on the changes in malignant behaviors and cancer-related molecules by ITC members in BC cells. Furthermore, we provide future direction of ITC-based therapy for patients with BC.

2. Isothiocyanates in Cruciferous Vegetables

Cruciferous vegetables are classified in the family Brassicaceae/Cruciferae. Several *in vivo*, *in vitro*, and epidemiological studies have shown that cruciferous vegetables inhibit carcinogenesis of BC [27,29,30]. However, in contrast to these reports, a study suggested that cruciferous vegetable intake is not significantly associated with reduced BC risk [31]. Thus, there are controversial results regarding the relationship between cruciferous vegetables and cancer risk in UC. Additionally, there is limited knowledge on the molecular mechanisms of the anti-cancer effects of cruciferous vegetables.

ITCs are naturally present in cruciferous vegetables and are produced by the hydrolysis of glucosinolates [32]. There is a general agreement that ITCs are beneficial for human health via various mechanisms, such as their anti-microbial activity, prevention of cardiovascular disease, and improvement of fasting glucose levels [33,34]. ITCs are also reported to exhibit anti-carcinogenic activities in various cancer types, including BC [27,33,35,36]. ITCs include the compounds AITC, BITC, SFN, and PEITC (Figure 1), each of which has multiple activities, including anti-cancer effects [37]. In the following sections, we will present the changes in malignant aggressiveness and molecular expression/activity in BC by each ITC member.

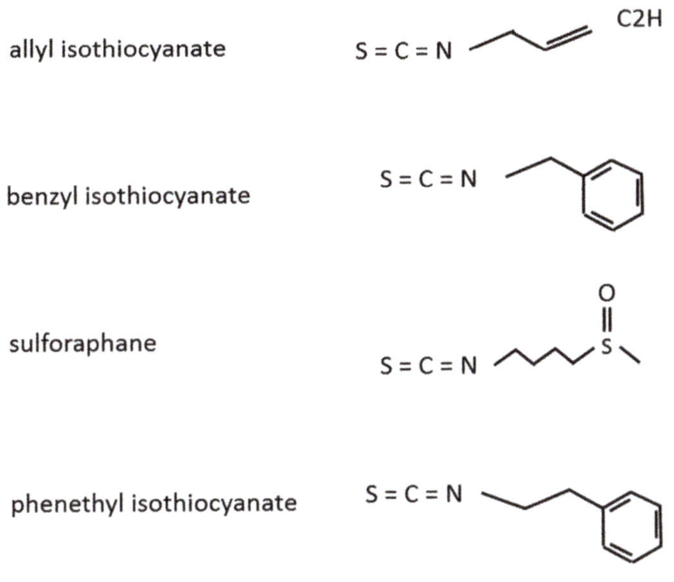

Figure 1. Structures of the isothiocyanate members.

2.1. Allyl Isothiocyanate

AITC is a volatile and water-insoluble compound derived from various cruciferous vegetables that exhibits multiple functions, such as anti-inflammation, neuroprotection, and anti-bacterial activity [38,39]. In addition, AITC is reported to have anti-cancer effects in various types of malignancies [40–42]. However, a study showed that AITC had no significant inhibitory effects on cell proliferation or stimulation of apoptosis in the human breast cancer cell line MDA-MB-231 [43]. Nevertheless, other studies have highlighted the potential advantages of AITC in BC treatment, as the major route of excretion of orally administered AITC is through urine, demonstrating relatively high bioavailability in urine and bladder tissue compared with other organs [44,45]. In this section, we will introduce the anti-cancer effects of AITC in BC and provide future direction for novel treatment strategies using AITC.

2.1.1. In Vitro Studies

The anti-cancer effects of AITC and its molecular mechanisms have been investigated in various BC cell lines; for instance, AITC was found to lead to morphological changes and inhibit the cell proliferation of the human BC cell lines RT4 and T24 [46]. AITC was also reported to affect cell cycle arrest and apoptosis of RT4 and T24 cells [44]. Moreover, the cytotoxic effects of AITC were confirmed in another BC cell line (UM-UC-3 cells) [47], and the percentages of apoptotic cells increased in an AITC dose-dependent manner in three different BC cell lines (UM-UC-3, UM-UC-6, and T24) [48]. This same study demonstrated that AITC-induced apoptosis is mediated by a mitochondrion-mediated system, including activation of caspase-9, caspase-3, lamin B1, and poly ADP-ribose polymerase (PARP) as well as Bcl-2 phosphorylation at Ser-70 by c-Jun N-terminal kinase (JNK) [48].

These anti-cancer effects, such as anti-proliferation and pro-apoptosis, of AITC are speculated to be independent from TP53—an important regulator of cell death—because RT4 cells possess wild-type TP53, while T24 and UM-UC-3 cells possess mutated TP53 [49]. Moreover, the anti-cancer effects of AITC involved different molecular mechanisms between RT4 and T24 cells. In RT4 cells, AITC treatment increased S100P and Bax levels and decreased Bcl-2 levels; meanwhile, Bax, Bcl-2, and anillin levels increased while S100P levels decreased in T24 cells [46]. The Bax/Bcl-2 pathway is speculated to be a key modulator of AITC in RT4 cells, with anillin and S100P mainly functioning in this system [46].

Thus, these *in vitro* studies demonstrated that the anti-cancer effects of AITC in BC cells are dependent on the pathological and molecular characteristics of cancer cells.

Molecular mechanisms of the AITC-induced anti-cancer effect in BC cells are shown in Table 1. To our knowledge, there are only two *in vitro* studies on this topic, warranting further research to discuss treatment strategies using ITCs.

Table 1. *In vitro* molecular mechanism of the anti-cancer effects of allyl isothiocyanate.

Anti-Cancer Effect	Underlying Molecular Mechanisms	Reference
Cell growth ↓	Increased S100P and Bax expression and decreased Bcl-2 expression in RT4 cells	Sávio et al., 2015 [46]
Cell growth ↓	Increased Bcl-2, Bax, and anillin expression and decreased S100P expression in T24 cells	Sávio et al., 2015 [46]
Apoptosis ↑	Regulation of mitochondrion-mediated mechanisms and Bcl-2 phosphorylation	Geng et al., 2011 [48]

Bcl, B-cell lymphoma-2; Bax, Bcl-2-associated X protein.

2.1.2. N-acetylcysteine Conjugate Allyl Isothiocyanate

AITC is mainly excreted in urine as *N*-acetylcysteine conjugate (NAC-AITC). In human and rat BC cells (UM-UC-3 and AY-27 cells, respectively), NAC-AITC inhibits cell proliferation and regulates cell cycle arrest and apoptosis [50]. The anti-cancer effects of NAC-AITC were found associated with downregulation of α-tubulin, β-tubulin/ and vascular endothelial growth factor and activation of caspase-3. Moreover, the authors conclude that the anti-cancer effects of NAC-AITC, including prevention and treatment of cancer are superior to AITC in terms of pharmacokinetic and physical properties. Similar anti-tumor growth activity was found in an orthotopic rat BC model, wherein bladder tumor weight in the NAC-AITC group is significantly lower than that in control ($p = 0.0213$) [50]. In addition, NAC-AITC suppressed muscle invasion of BC cells (NAC-AITC group = 30%; control = 79%). Similar to the BC cell lines, α- and β-tubulin, vascular endothelial growth factor, and cleaved caspase-3 were found associated with the *in vivo* anti-cancer effects [50].

2.1.3. In Vivo Studies

Dietary administration of a freeze-dried, aqueous extract of broccoli sprouts that included AITC was found to reduce the incidence, multiplicity, and size of BC in an *N*-butyl-*N*-(4-hydroxybutyl) nitrosamine (BBN)-induced rat BC model [51]. However, the detailed molecular mechanisms of this anti-cancer effect were not clearly defined. Another study showed that oral intake of AITC-rich mustard seed powder inhibits tumor growth and muscle invasion in an orthotopic rat BC model via regulation of apoptosis, cell cycle, and angiogenic potential [52]; downregulation of vascular endothelial growth factor and cyclin B1 and upregulation of caspase-3 and cleavage of PARP were found associated with these anti-cancer effects [52].

When AITC is stably stored as its glucosinolate precursor (sinigrin) in mustard seed powder (MSP-1), a study revealed that sinigrin itself is not bioactive, whereas hydrated MSP-1 leads to apoptosis and G2/M phase arrest in bladder cancer cell lines *in vitro*. In an orthotopic rat bladder cancer model, oral MSP-1 inhibited bladder cancer growth by 34.5% ($P < 0.05$) and blocked muscle invasion by 100%. The anti-cancer activity of AITC delivered as MSP-1 appears to be more robust than that of pure AITC. Therefore, MSP-1 may be an attractive delivery vehicle for AITC, as it strongly inhibits bladder cancer development and progression [52].

2.1.4. Combination Therapy of Allyl Isothiocyanate and Conventional Anti-cancer Agents

The cyclooxygenase (COX)-2-plastaglandin (PG) E2-system is an important pathological mechanism of carcinogenesis, tumor growth, and progression in UC [53–55]. Therefore, COX-2 inhibitors have been suggested as chemoprotective and therapeutic agents in a variety of cancers [56–58]. The synergistic effects of a combination of COX-2 inhibitors and other standard therapy have also been reported [59,60]. Celecoxib, a selective COX-2 inhibitor, is used for various pathological conditions worldwide. Thus, to clarify the anti-cancer effects of a combination of celecoxib and AITC, *in vitro* studies employing AY-27 bladder cancer cells and *in vivo* studies with the F344/AY-27 rat bladder urothelial cell carcinoma model were performed [61]. *In vitro*, AITC first showed no significant impact on COX-2 expression, and PGE2 production was confirmed. However, when the growth inhibitory effects of AITC and celecoxib were analyzed, growth inhibition of AY-27 cells by AITC was not altered by celecoxib addition. The authors thus speculated that the COX-2-mediated anti-tumor growth effects of celecoxib did not reach detectable levels due to excessive dilution of PGE2 in the culture medium. On the other hand, *in vivo* studies employing an animal model with orthotopic BC showed that combination therapy of AITC (1 mg/Kg) and celecoxib (10 mg/Kg) suppresses tumor growth and muscle invasion and that these anti-cancer effects are stronger compared with those of AITC or celecoxib alone. Inhibition of tumor-related angiogenesis regulated by vascular endothelial growth was found to play a crucial role in these anti-cancer effects.

Another combination therapy employed AITC and cisplatin, a standard anti-cancer drug for patients with BC [62]. *In vitro* studies with lung cancer cells (HOP62) and ovarian cancer cells (2008) showed that the variabilities of both cancer cell lines are significantly inhibited by a combination of AITC and cisplatin, whose inhibitory effects are stronger compared with those of AITC or cisplatin alone. The anti-proliferative effects were confirmed by colony formation assays, and when relationships between cell death and the combination therapy were examined, levels of pro-apoptotic molecules (caspase-3) were found increased and anti-apoptotic molecules (Bcl-2 and survivin) decreased; thus, this combination can suppress tumor growth *in vitro*. Mechanistically, regulation of cell cycle, β-tubulin depletion, and microtubule dysfunction are associated with the anti-cancer effects of AITC and cisplatin. Finally, the combination index of ATIC and cisplatin in lung cancer cells indicates a synergistic interaction. Indeed, *in vivo* studies with A549-derived lung cancer xenograft tumor models showed decreases in tumor volumes after combination therapy (AITC = 50 mg/Kg and cisplatin = 6 mg/kg), whereas tumor volumes increased after AITC (50 mg/Kg) or cisplatin (6 mg/kg) monotherapy. Overall, the anti-cancer effect parameters (i.e., maximum tumor growth inhibition, tumor doubling time, and frequency of partial response and complete response) are remarkably better after combination therapy than after either monotherapy. Furthermore, AITC + cisplatin therapy exhibits no toxicity, including maximum weight loss of pretreatment bodyweight.

2.1.5. Clinical Trials and Future Direction of Allyl Isothiocyanate-Based Therapy

Recently, an *in vitro* study employing the macrophage cell line RAW 264.7 and human BC cell line HT1376 was conducted to clarify the anti-inflammatory activity and anti-cancer effect of AITC nanoparticles [63]. The results showed that AITC nanoparticles inhibit cancer cell proliferation and migration; however, these anti-cancer effects are dependent on AITC concentration; inhibition of cancer cell proliferation and migration is achieved at 70 mg L^{-1} and 8.75 mg L^{-1} of AITC nanoparticles, respectively. AITC nanoparticles were also found to suppress production of lipopolysaccharide-induced tumor necrosis factor (TNF)-α, interleukin (IL)-6, nitric oxide (NO), and inducible NO synthase in macrophage cells, and their anti-inflammatory effects are stronger than those of AITC or nanoparticles alone. The authors thus suggested that AITC nanoparticles can be a valuable treatment strategy for BC via their regulation of inflammation, immunity, and oxidative stress.

Other novel strategies employing AITC are currently under development. For example, the anti-cancer effects of AITC-conjugated silicon quantum dots were examined in human umbilical vein endothelial cells (HUVECs) and human hepatocellular carcinoma cells (HepG2) [64]. Interestingly, high doses of AITC (40–320 μM) were found to significantly inhibit HepG2 cell viability, whereas low doses (5 μM) significantly stimulated cancer cell viability. Similar trends were confirmed for cancer cell migration (inhibition at 20 μM AITC and stimulation at 2.5 μM) and angiogenesis (HUVEC tube formation ability is suppressed at > 5 µM but stimulated at even lower doses of 1.25 and 2.5 µM AITC). Thus, there is a possibility that the anti-cancer effects of AITC are dependent on its concentration and that low concentrations of AITC may have detrimental effects via increased cancer cell proliferation, migration, and angiogenesis in hepatocellular carcinoma. The authors further showed that AITC-conjugated silicon quantum dots overcame the limitation of AITC in the same analysis. Therefore, AITC-conjugated silicon quantum dots are suggested as a useful drug delivery system for AITC in cancer patients. Although there are no data in BC, AITC is also predicted to have biphasic effects of anti-cancer effects and angiogenesis. Therefore, we suggest additional *in vivo* and *in vitro* studies of the silicon quantum dot system in BC to elucidate new treatment strategies for patients.

2.2. Benzyl Isothiocyanate

Similar to other ITC members, BITC has immunomodulatory, anti-microbial, and anti-oxidative activities under various pathological conditions [34,65,66] Several studies have also shown that BITC possesses anti-cancer and chemopreventive effects in various types of malignancies [67–69]. However, there is limited information on its anti-cancer effects and molecular mechanisms in UC.

2.2.1. In Vitro Studies

Similar to AITC, BITC has shown anti-proliferative and pro-apoptotic activity in BC cells [70,71]; however, the pro-apoptotic activity of BITC is stronger compared with that of other ITC members, including AITC and SFN. Moreover, caspase-9 is the main regulator of BITC-induced apoptosis in UM-UC-3 cells, although all ITC members exhibit pro-apoptotic activities via activation of caspase-3, 8, and 9 [70,72]. Additionally, mitochondrial activities are targets of BITC, and BITC-induced changes are regulated by various members of the Bcl-2 family, including Bcl-2, Bax, Bak, and Bcl-xl [70].

As previously mentioned, ITCs are primarily disposed and concentrated in the urine as NAC conjugates. UC originates from urothelial cells and is constantly exposed to urine in the urinary tract. Therefore, studies have focused on the anti-cancer effects of NAC-conjugated BITC in BC cells [71] and found that it suppresses BC cell growth through anti-proliferative and pro-apoptotic activities. Activation of caspase-3, 8, and 9; cell cycle arrest in phases S and G2/M; and regulation of Cdc25C were associated with the anti-proliferative function of NAC-conjugated BITC. The authors confirmed, however, that longer treatment durations or higher doses of NAC-conjugated BITC are necessary to exert similar effects as those of BITC.

miRNAs are major modulators of carcinogenesis, malignant aggressiveness, and outcome in UC [73,74] and several miRNAs are closely associated with cisplatin sensitivity of BC cells [75]. miR-99a-5p, a tumor suppressor, exhibits anti-proliferative and pro-apoptotic activities in UC [76–78]. One study demonstrated that BITC treatment upregulates miR-99a-5p expression in the BC cell lines 5637 and T24 [76], which leads to decreased mRNA and protein levels of IGF-1R, FGF-R3, and mTOR in both BC cell lines. The authors also demonstrated a molecular mechanism associated with regulation of BC cell survival and apoptosis by BITC. Taken together, these findings indicate that BITC exhibits anti-cancer effects via regulation of cell survival in UC. Another study elucidated the anti-cancer effects of BITC-induced miR-99a expression in BC cells [79] and reported that BITC enhances miR-99a expression in 5637 and T24 BC cells, which is associated with ERK activation and nuclear transcriptional activation of c-Jun/(activator protein) AP-1. Thus, the authors suggested that BITC stimulates miR-99a expression via regulation of the ERK/AP-1 pathway in BC and demonstrated the anti-cancer effects of miR-99a in UC. Nevertheless, there is a general consensus that the anti-carcinogenic and anti-cancer effects of miR-99a represent a complex mechanism in BC cells [80–82]. Therefore, this information is useful for understanding the biological function of BITC in BC. The molecular mechanisms of the anti-cancer effects of BITC are shown in Table 2.

Table 2. *In vitro* molecular mechanisms of the anti-cancer effects of benzyl isothiocyanate.

Anti-Cancer Effect	Underlying Molecular Mechanisms	Reference
Cell growth ↓	Suppression of IGF1R, FGFR3, and mTOR activation by miR-99a-5p upregulation	Liu et al., 2019 [76]
Apoptosis ↑	Via caspase-9, a major regulator, and Bcl-2, Bax, Bak, and Bcl-xl	Tang & Zhang, 2005 [70]
Apoptosis ↑	Stimulation of caspase-3, 8, and 9 and cell cycle arrest in the same phases by Cdc25C	Tang et al., 2006 [71]

IGF1R, insulin-like growth factor 1 receptor; FGFR, fibroblast growth factor receptor; mTOR, mechanistic target of rapamycin; Bcl, B-cell lymphoma-2; Bax, Bcl-2-associated X protein; Bak, BCL2-antagonist/killer.

2.2.2. In Vivo Studies

In a rat model of BBN-induced BC, oral intake of BITC suppressed the incidence of neoplastic pathological changes, such as dysplasia, papilloma, and carcinoma, and multiplicities in a dose-dependent manner (10, 100, or 1,000 ppm BITC) [83]. Notably, epithelial hyperplasia of the bladder was found in rats treated with 100 or 1,000 ppm BITC without BBN [83]. The same researchers also demonstrated the carcinogenic potential of BITC in this BC animal model [84]. Therefore, the toxicity and risk of BITC in BC treatment should be considered; this is further detailed later in the text (see Section 2.1).

2.2.3. Combination Therapy of Benzyl Isothiocyanate and Cisplatin

As mentioned in Section 2.4, combination therapy of ITCs and cisplatin is expected to have better anti-cancer effects than those of ITCs or cisplatin alone. Indeed, several reports showed that BITC enhances the anti-cancer effects of cisplatin in lung cancer cells (NCI-H596), head and neck squamous cell carcinoma cells (HN12, HN8, and HN30), and leukemia cells (HL-60) [85–87]; there are no similar studies in BC cells, however.

2.3. Sulforaphane

SFN can be found in cruciferous vegetables, such as broccoli, cauliflower, brussel sprouts, cabbage, kale, and kohlrabi [88]. SFN is reported to regulate cancer cell survival via inhibition of cell proliferation and stimulation of apoptosis in a variety of cancers [89,90]. Among the ITC members, SFN has been the most widely investigated regarding its pathological roles and molecular mechanisms both *in vivo* and *in vitro*.

2.3.1. In Vitro Studies: Cell Cycle-, Caspase- and Bcl-2-Related Molecules

Regarding the relationships between SFN and cell survival, including cell proliferation, cell cycle, and death, various mechanisms have been suggested. For example, SFN was reported to induce growth arrest and apoptosis in a BC cell line (5637 cells) [91]. Moreover, induction and stimulation of cyclin B1 and Cdk1 were found associated with the anti-proliferative effects of SFN, whereas activation of caspase-3, 8, and 9 and PARP corresponded to its pro-apoptotic effects; these SFN-induced anti-cancer effects are speculated to be regulated via reactive oxygen species (ROS)-dependent mechanisms [91]. Another study showed that SFN treatment suppresses cell viability in a dose-dependent manner and induces apoptosis in T24 human BC cells via regulation of caspase-3, caspase-9, and PARP [92]. Moreover, the SFN-induced apoptosis of BC cells is mediated by dysregulation of mitochondria function, cytochrome *c* release, and Bcl-2-related pathways [92].

Other studies focused on the relationships between cell cycle-related molecules and SFN. For instance, after 10–40 μM SFN treatment for 24 or 48 h, T24 cell viability is significantly suppressed with IC50 values of 26.9 ± 1.12 μM (24 h) or 15.9 ± 0.76 μM (48 h) [93]. Conversely, 20 μM SFN treatment for 24 or 48 h resulted in apoptotic features, such as cell shrinkage, condensed chromatin, and apoptotic bodies, in the same BC cells; increased numbers of apoptotic cells were confirmed by flow cytometry [93]. SFN is also associated with blocking cell cycle progression at G0/G1 phase. In addition to its pro-apoptotic activities, upregulation of the cyclin-dependent kinase inhibitor p27 plays crucial roles in the 20 µM SFN-induced anti-cancer effects in BC cells, whereas p16 or cyclin D1 expression does not [93]. Thus, regulation of cell cycle-related molecules and mitochondrial function, caspases, and the Bcl-2 protein family represent the molecular mechanisms of SFN-induced anti-proliferative and pro-apoptotic activities in BC cells.

2.3.2. In Vitro Studies: Oxidative Stress, Endoplasmic Reticulum Stress, and Growth Factors

As mentioned above, many investigators believe that the anti-cancer effects of SFN in BC are mainly associated with caspase- and mitochondria-related pathways. Nevertheless, there are other cancer-related factors involved. For instance, SFN can inhibit DNA damage induced by chemical carcinogens in BC T24 cells [94]. Moreover, SFN-induced oxidative stress through ROS has been suggested as a key modulator [91,92]. Nuclear factor erythroid 2-related factor-2 (Nrf2) regulation and endoplasmic reticulum (ER) stress are also associated with SFN and carcinogenesis, pathological behavior, and cell survival in UC [28,92]. Notably, these Nrf2 and ER signaling pathways are important factors in the response to oxidative stress and anti-oxidative activities [28,92,95]. A study showed that enhanced insulin-like growth-factor-binding protein-3 (IGFBP-3) and suppressed nuclear factor-kappa B (NF-κB) expression by SFN are associated with the anti-proliferative effect of SFN in the BC cell line BIU87. Interestingly, the authors also found that SFN stimulates apoptosis and cell cycle arrest at the G2/M phase, resulting from IGFBP-3 and NF-κB regulation [96]. As IGFBP-3 and NF-κB are known to possess pro-apoptotic and anti-apoptotic functions, respectively, in various malignancies [97,98], this stimulation of apoptosis by SPN via increased IGFBP-3 and decreased NF-κB levels are in agreement with established findings. Another report on the relationship between SFN-induced anti-cancer effects and growth factors demonstrated that 20 µM SFN leads to a 2.6-, 3.0-, or 3.1-fold increase in the G2/M phase compared with that of controls in three BC cell lines (RT4, J82, and UM-UC-3, respectively) [99]. In addition, SFN induces apoptosis in RT4 and UM-UC-3 cells. Thus, these findings indicate that upregulation of caspase-3/7 and PARP activity and downregulation of survivin, EGFR, and HER2/neu are the underlying molecular mechanisms.

TNF-related apoptosis-inducing ligand (TRAIL) is recognized as an initiator of apoptosis. Its dysregulation has been identified in various malignant cells, including BC [100,101]. As a result, resistance to TRAIL is associated with high malignant potential and worse prognosis for patients with BC [102]. SFN treatment however, has been reported to reverse the pro-apoptotic activity of TRAIL in TRAIL-resistant BC cells [103]; the SFN-induced mechanisms were found associated with apoptosis-related molecules (e.g., caspases, mitochondrial membrane potential, Bid, and death receptor 5) and oxidative stress-related factors (e.g., ROS and Nrf2).

The anti-cancer effects of SFN under hypoxic conditions in BC cell lines have also been reported [88]; in RT112 cells, 20 µM SFN inhibited cancer cell proliferation by 26.1 ± 4.1% and 39.7 ± 5.2% under normoxia and hypoxia, respectively (P < 0.05), with similar results observed for RT4 cells (normoxia, 29.7 ± 4.6%; hypoxia, 48.3 ± 5.2%). Tumor tissues, especially those within the center, are generally under hypoxic conditions due to the oxygen consumption of the tumor to support its growth. Thus, these findings indicate that SFN can suppress cell proliferation under hypoxic conditions in BC with rapid tumor growth compared with that under normoxia and relatively slow growth. Interestingly, the same study also showed that SFN suppresses glycolytic metabolism under hypoxia by decreasing the nuclear translocation of hypoxia-inducible factor-1α, thereby reducing its protein levels [88]. Suppression of glycolytic metabolism in cancer cells is important for inhibiting tumor growth and progression as high glycolytic metabolism leads to increased cancer cell proliferation. Overall, the findings demonstrate that SFN plays several roles in suppressing malignant aggressiveness, such as by decreasing cancer cell proliferation, in BC cells.

2.3.3. In Vitro Studies: Inflammation, Epithelial-to-Mesenchymal Transition, Epigenesis, and Others

In addition to reducing BC cell survival, SFN inhibits malignant aggressiveness by suppressing inflammation, cancer cell invasion, and metastasis. Several studies have shown that SFN downregulates

COX-2 expression in BC cells via regulation of p38 mitogen-activated protein kinase (MAPK) and NF-κB [104–106]. Moreover, p38 MARK is positively associated with glutathione transferase and thioredoxin reductase-1—both antioxidant enzymes—following SFN treatment [105]. Furthermore, SFN can inhibit epithelial-to-mesenchymal transition (EMT)—an important mediator of cancer cell invasion and metastasis—via regulation of COX-2/matrix metalloproteinase (MMP)-2, -9/ZEB1, Snail, and miR-200c/ZEB1 in BC cells [106].

SFN was found to inhibit histone status in BC cells, which is associated with reduced levels of histone H1 phosphorylation via modification of histone acetyltransferase and histone deacetylase activity [26]. Changes in histone H1 status were previously reported to be associated with carcinogenesis and prognosis of BC [107]. Based on these findings, SFN is speculated to inhibit carcinogenesis and progression of BC via epigenetic modification [26].

Recently, the physiological and pathological roles of gut microbiota have garnered great interest. Research has shown how they affect systematic metabolism, inflammation, and the immune system, contributing to carcinogenesis, malignant potential, and cancer progression, of which similar findings have been reported in UC [108–110]. Interestingly, SFN was found to normalize gut microbiota dysbiosis by increasing the abundance of *Bacteroides fragilis* and *Clostridium* cluster I in a BBN-induced BC animal model [111], suppressing BBN-induced histological changes, including sub-mucosal capillary growth. While the detailed mechanisms of the anti-carcinogenic function of SFN in this model is not fully clear, normalization of intestinal flora has been shown to repair intestinal barrier dysfunction and injured mucosal epithelium via regulation of tight junction proteins, including ZO-1, claudin-1, occludin, and mucin-2 [111]. Moreover, SFN plays crucial roles in the inflammatory status of this model, as it decreases pro-inflammatory factors such as IL-6 and secretory immunoglobin A, which are increased by carcinogenesis [111]. The authors conclude that these gut microbiota-related beneficial effects of SFN led to its anti-carcinogenic effects in BC via complex mechanisms that involve inflammation and the immune system [111]. A summary of the molecular mechanisms of the anti-cancer effects of SFN is shown in Table 3.

Table 3. *In vitro* molecular mechanisms of the anti-cancer effects of sulforaphane.

Anti-Cancer Effect	Underlying Molecular Mechanisms	Reference
Cell growth ↓	Increased IGFBP-3 expression and decreased NF-κB expression	Dang et al., 2014 [96]
Cell growth ↓	Increased cyclin B1 and Cdk1 phosphorylation and their complex effects	Park et al., 2014 [91]
Cell growth ↓	Suppression of HIF-1α-mediated glycolytic metabolism under hypoxic conditions	Xia et al., 2019 [88]
Apoptosis ↑	Increased expression of the cyclin-dependent kinase inhibitor p27	Shan et al., 2006 [93]
Apoptosis ↑	Increased caspase-3/7 and PARP expression and decreased survivin, EGFR, and HER2/neu expression	Abboui et al., 2012 [99]
Apoptosis ↑	Increased IGFBP-3 expression and decreased NF-κB expression	Dang et al., 2014 [96]
Apoptosis ↑	Activation of ROS-mediated caspase-3/9 and PARP, ER stress, and Nrf2	Jo et al., 2014 [92]
Apoptosis ↑	Activation of caspase-3, 8, and 9 and PARP via ROS-dependent pathways	Park et al., 2014 [91]
Apoptosis ↑	Reversal of TRAIL activity via regulation of caspases, MMP, DR5, ROS, and Nrf2	Jin et al., 2018 [103]
Invasion ↓	Regulation of EMT and COX-2/MMP2,9/ZEB1, Snail, and miR-200c/ZEB1 pathways	Shan et al., 2013 [93]
Migration ↓	Regulation of autophagy activation	Bao et al., 2014 [112]

IGFBP, insulin-like growth-factor-binding protein; NF-κB, nuclear factor-kappa B; HIF, hypoxia-inducible factor; PARP, poly ADP-ribose polymerase; EGFR, epidermal growth factor receptor; HER, human EGFR-related; ROS, reactive oxygen species; ER, endoplasmic reticulum; Nrf2, nuclear factor erythroid 2-related factor; MMP, matrix metalloproteinase; DR5, death receptor 5; EMT, epithelial-to-mesenchymal transition; COX, cyclooxygenase.

2.3.4. In Vivo Studies

In vivo studies with the chemical-induced BC animal model have shown that SFN inhibits carcinogenesis, tumor growth, and progression via a complex mechanism that includes prevention of DNA damage [94]. In a murine UM-UC-3 xenograft model, tumor growth rates and tumor weights in the SFN group were found lower than in the control group (not significant and $p < 0.05$, respectively) [51]. Furthermore, this model showed decreases in tumor volumes in SFN-treated mice (12 mg/kg bodyweight for 5 weeks) with an inhibitory rate of 63% via increased caspase-3 and cytochrome *c* expression and decreased survivin expression [113]. In addition to the apoptosis-related pathways, several other molecules have been suggested to be associated with the anti-cancer effects of SFN, based on *in vivo* studies. Thus, further *in vivo* studies are essential for understanding the efficacy and limitations of an SFN-based treatment strategy against BC.

2.3.5. Combination Therapy of Sulforaphane and Other Therapeutic Agents

Although several clinical trials on the anti-cancer effects of SFN and broccoli sprout extracts have been performed, the results were unsatisfactory [114,115]; for example, no or minimum effects are detected on serum and tissue biomarkers of patients with prostate and breast cancer. Although a similar clinical trial has not been performed for patients with BC, the clinical effects of SFN monotherapy are also predicted to be unsatisfactory. Therefore, the efficacy of a combination therapy of SFN and other therapeutic agents was investigated in BC cells.

A combination therapy of acetazolamide (AZ; a carbonic anhydrase inhibitor) and SFN showed suppressed proliferative and clonogenic effects and stimulated apoptotic activity via caspase-3 and PARP activation [116]. In addition, the PI3K/Akt signaling pathway was found to play an important role in the anti-cancer effects of this combination therapy. The authors thus conclude that AZ + SFN is a potential therapeutic strategy for BC. Another study examined the effects of two ITCs (AITC + SFN) on the lung cancer cell line A549 [117]; their anti-carcinogenic effects showed higher inhibitory effects on tumor growth and cancer cell migration and greater stimulation of apoptosis compared with that of ATIC or SFN alone. Moreover, oxidative stress, including ROS, is associated with these activities. Although this study was not performed on BC cells, we believe that a combination of different ITCs may be effective for the prevention and treatment of BC. Indeed, in the BC cell line UM-UC-3, pro-apoptotic activity of BITC or PEITC alone is stronger than that of AITC or SFN alone [72]. Moreover, ≥20 µM SFN significantly suppresses cell proliferation in the BC cell line BIU87, whereas 10 µM SFN had no significant effect [96,112]. Therefore, more detailed studies on the combination of various ITC types, dosages, and durations are necessary to identify the most efficacious combination therapy of the ITC members.

Nevertheless, there are potential limitations of SFN-based therapies. Novel immunotherapy strategies, such as immune checkpoint inhibitors, have been recently established as standard therapy for patients with advanced/metastatic BC [118,119]. While we speculate that a combination of immunotherapy and SFN may be useful for the prevention and treatment of BC, a combination of SFN with T cell-mediated cancer immunotherapies is not recommended because SFN can function both as an anti- and pro-carcinogenic factor due to its effects on tumor and immune cells [120].

2.4. Phenethyl Isothiocyanate

Similar to other ITC members, PEITC can suppress carcinogenesis and malignant aggressiveness in various types of malignancies [121]. Suppression of various cancer-promoting characteristics, such as cancer cell proliferation, invasion, and angiogenesis, via regulation of the Bcl-2 protein family, caspases, and matrix metalloproteinases are reported as the potential molecular mechanisms underlying the tumor-suppressive activities of PEITC [121–123].

2.4.1. In Vitro Studies

PEITC was shown to have anti-cancer regulatory effects on cancer cell survival and apoptosis in BC cells [124]; PEITC inhibits cell viability in a dose-dependent manner and enhances apoptotic potential, as measured by caspases activities in T24 cells [124]. However, as shown in Table 4, the detailed molecular mechanisms underlying these anti-cancer effects in BC cells are not fully understood. It was reported that PEITC inhibits cell proliferation and stimulates apoptosis in the human adriamycin (ADM)-resistant bladder carcinoma cell line T24/ADM [123]. Interestingly, this study showed that PEITC increases intracellular drug accumulation potential and DNA topoisomerase II expression, and decreases multidrug resistance-related factors, such as multidrug resistance gene (MDR1), multidrug resistance-associated protein (MRP1), and glutathione S-transferase π [123]. In general, such changes by PEITC lead to increased chemosensitivity. Additionally, the authors clarified the detailed molecular mechanism underlying multidrug resistance reversal potential, which includes downregulation of NF-κB, survivin, Twist, and Akt and upregulation of PTEN and JNK by PEITC. As chemotherapeutic regimens including ADM are the standard therapy for patients with advanced UC [125,126], these findings highlight PEITC as a potential therapeutic agent for BC treatment, especially in patients with drug-resistant BC [123]. While we agree with their conclusion, clinical trials testing this hypothesis have yet to be performed.

Table 4. *In vitro* molecular mechanism of the anti-cancer effects of phenethyl isothiocyanate.

Anti-Cancer Effect	Underlying Molecular Mechanisms	Reference
Apoptosis ↑	Via caspase-9, a major regulator, and Bcl-2, Bax, Bak, and Bcl-xl	Tang & Zhang, 2005 [70]
Apoptosis ↑	Decreased NF-κB, survivin, Twist, and Akt expression and increased PTEN and JNK expression	Tang et al., 2013 [123]

Bcl, B-cell lymphoma-2; Bax, Bcl-2-associated X protein; Bak, BCL2-antagonist/killer; NF-κB, nuclear factor-kappa B; JNK, c-Jun N-terminal kinase.

Although BITC has been suggested to suppress cell growth by upregulating miR-99a expression via regulation of the c-Jun/AP-1 pathway in BC [79,80], this pathway plays no significant role in the anti-proliferative effects of PEITC in BC cells [127]. *In vitro* molecular mechanisms of the anti-cancer effects of PEITC are shown in Table 4.

2.4.2. In Vivo Studies

PEITC is suggested to play crucial roles in preventing the initiation step of carcinogenesis and inhibiting tumor progression in a variety of malignancies [121]. However, in a chemically BBN-induced BC animal model using male human c-Ha-ras proto-oncogene transgenic rats, microscopic BC is observed in the BBN alone (16 weeks) and BBN (8 weeks) → PEITC (8 weeks) groups; but not in the PEITC (8 weeks) → BBN (8 weeks) group [128]. This finding indicates that PEITC can inhibit the carcinogenic process after initiation. However, a conclusion cannot be drawn due to the limited information on *in vivo* SFN activities in BC.

2.4.3. Combination Therapy of Phenethyl Isothiocyanate and Other Therapeutic Agents

We previously introduced a novel treatment strategy that combines AITC and cisplatin for lung cancer cells (Section 2.1.4). Similarly, the efficacy of a combination therapy of PEITC and cisplatin was demonstrated in several studies. For instance, cervical cancer cells (HeLa) treated for 24 h with 5 μM PEITC and 10 μM cisplatin show typical features of apoptosis, such as cell shrinkage, membrane blebbing, and cell detachment, with a 4-fold increase in caspase-3 activity; these significant changes are not observed for either treatment alone [122]. The same study also showed that PEITC increases the pro-apoptotic activity of cisplatin in C33A cervical cancer and MCF-7 breast cancer cells; interestingly, this pro-apoptotic activity is not detected in normal human mammary epithelial MCF-10A cells [122]. Another study on non-small cell lung cancer cells (A549) showed that the percentage cell survival after treatment with AITC (15 μM) or cisplatin (5 μM) alone is 79.2 ± 3.8% and 55.9 ± 3.4%, respectively, whereas cell survival in the combination group is 46.2 ± 2.7% [129]. Notably, when PITC and cisplatin are co-encapsulated in liposomal nanoparticles, A549 cell survival further decreased to 33.3 ± 2.9% [129]. Similar results were obtained in another non-small cell lung cancer cells (H596), where the percentage cell survival after treatment with liposomal-PEITC-cisplatin or free PITC + cisplatin is 55.0 ± 9.5% and 28.6 ± 6.3%, respectively (p < 0.001) [129]. Moreover, the liposomal nanoparticles containing both PEITC and cisplatin have the advantage of increased circulation time in the bloodstream and accumulation in tumors [130]. Therefore, co-encapsulated PITC and cisplatin in liposomal nanoparticles may be a potential therapeutic strategy for advanced/metastatic UC.

3. Carcinogenic Potential of Isothiocyanates

There is general consensus that all ITC members possess anti-cancer effects in BC cells. However, several studies have also suggested the carcinogenic potential of ITCs in BC. In this section, we will discuss the relationships between BITC, SFN, and PEITC and carcinogenic changes in BC. To our knowledge, AITC has not been shown to promote tumorigenesis and carcinoma in BC; nevertheless, we cannot conclude that AITC has no carcinogenic potential as there is limited information on the biological and pathological effects of AITC in BC.

3.1. Carcinogenic Potential of Benzyl Isothiocyanate

In a two-stage carcinogenesis model, rats treated with BITC and with BBN initiation show neoplastic lesions, including papillary or nodular-hyperplasia (100%), papilloma (38%), and carcinoma (100%); these frequencies are higher than in rats under a basal diet (57%, 5%, and 24%, respectively) [131]. The frequencies of papilloma and carcinoma are also lower than those in rats with initiation + BITC (papilloma = 17% and carcinoma = 0%) and rats without initiation. Therefore, BITC may enhance the carcinogenic process in rats with initiation alone. However, in a BBN-induced BC rat model, oral administration of 10, 100, or 1,000 ppm BBN suppresses carcinogenic pathological changes [83]; moreover, epithelial hyperplasia of the urinary bladder is detected in rats treated with 100 or 1,000 ppm BITC, even without BBN [83]. Furthermore, the same research group showed that these neoplastic changes increase in rats with initiation treatment of 500 ppm BBN and subsequent low dose (25 ppm) BBN exposure, and their frequencies are further increased by additional treatment with 100 and 1000 ppm BITC in a dose-dependent manner [84]. In a similar experiment without initiation treatment, dysplasia, papilloma, and carcinoma were rare, although almost all rats had hyperplasia, except for the control and 100 ppm BITC groups [84]. Thus, BITC may stimulate carcinogenesis in a high-risk population of BBN-induced BC cases [83,84,132].

3.2. Carcinogenic Potential of Sulforaphane

As shown in a previous study, ≥20 µM SFN decreases cell viability and migration of T24 BC cells [112]. However, the study also showed that a low concentration of SFN promotes BC cell proliferation and migration [112], where 1–5 µM SFN or 2.5 and 3.75 SFN increase cell growth to approximately 120–130% and cell migration to 128 and 133% compared with those of control [112]. Thus, a biphasic effect of SFN on cell growth and migration of BC cells was suggested. Mechanistically, activation of autophagy by SFN is speculated to be associated with upregulated cell migration in an *in vivo* study using the autophagy inhibitor 3-methyladenine in T24 cells. The authors also found an enhanced protective effect in conjunction with selenium against free radical-induced cell death. Although this mechanism was confirmed in human hepatocyte cells (HHL-5) and breast cancer cells (MCF-7) rather than in BC cells, the benefits, and risks of SFN have been shown to be dependent on its doses and interactions with the microenvironment, including autophagy and selenium.

3.3. Carcinogenic Potential of Phenethyl Isothiocyanate

In an animal model of dimethylbenzanthracene-induced mammary carcinogenesis, continuous oral administration of 1200 ppm PEITC induces hyperplasia in the urinary bladder [133]. However, another study showed a high frequency of carcinoma (11 of 12 rats; 91.7%) with oral administration of 0.1% PEITC in rats for 48 weeks [134]; the authors thus conclude that PEITC has carcinogenic activities in the rat urinary bladder. By contrast, in a two-stage carcinogenesis model, rats treated with PEITC with BBN initiation exhibit papillary or nodular-hyperplasia (100%), papilloma (24%), and carcinoma (100%). Meanwhile, frequencies of papilloma (17%) and carcinoma (33%) are lower in rats without initiation than in those with initiation [131]. In studies showing the carcinogenic potential of PEITC according to initiation, specifically in a rat medium-term multi-organ carcinogenesis model, oral treatment with 0.1% PEITC after the initiation period leads to incidences of papillary or nodular-hyperplasia and tumors [135]. However, the authors showed that PEITC provided during the initiation period is not associated with carcinogenic activity [135]. These findings suggest that PEITC may stimulate carcinogenesis of UC during the post-initiation period. Another study, however, demonstrated that PEITC increases the incidences of papillary or nodular hyperplasia, dysplasia, and carcinoma in a dose-dependent manner; thus, > 0.01% PEITC enhances rat urinary bladder carcinogenesis and > 0.05% PEITC has tumorigenic potential. [136]. Collectively, these findings indicate that carcinogenic potential of PEITC administration may be modulated by complex mechanisms that involve timing and dosage.

When 0.1% BITC or 0.1% PEITC is administered in the diet to 6-week-old F344 rats for 1, 2, 3, and 7 days, a significant reduction of urinary pH levels compared to the normal control is detected, starting at day 1 [132]. Similarly, a reduction is detected in the urinary concentration of Na and Cl, whereas K is reduced. The same study also showed that thickness of the urinary bladder urothelium is significantly increased by administration of both BITC and PEITC and that inflammation, vacuolation, erosion, and apoptosis/single cell necrosis occur in the urinary bladder lesion; these morphological changes are not observed in normal control rats [132]. Furthermore, the cell proliferation potential, evaluated by the BrdU labeling index in male rats treated with BITC and female rats with BITC + PEITC, is significantly higher than that of control rats [132]. By contrast, when 0.1% BITC or 0.1% PEITC is administered for 14 days, histopathological simple hyperplasia and papillary/nodular hyperplasia are detected in 100% and 86% and 100% and 60% of the cases, respectively [132]. The authors thus suggest that continuous proliferation of bladder epithelial cells by BITC and PEITC plays important roles in pathological changes, including inflammation and the early stage of carcinogenesis [132]. Taken together, these findings are extremely important for the consideration of ITC treatment strategies, especially BITC and PEITC, for UC. However, we should note the difference in administered levels of ITCs in these studies. Although the mean daily consumption of BITC and PEITC in rats was approximately 80 mg/kg/day [132], these levels do not reflect human physiological conditions, i.e., 30 g of fresh watercress = 7.6 mg of PEITC per person and 0.8 mg from fresh (0.5 mg) and cooked (0.3 mg) Swede-turnips = 0.28 mg/person/day of PEITC [137,138].

4. Further Considerations

As previously mentioned, ITCs exhibit their anti- and pro-carcinogenic activities via complex mechanisms. In this review, we mainly introduced the findings of pre-clinical *in vivo* and *in vitro* studies for easier understanding across the field. However, we would be remiss if we do not mention that other cancer-related factors and signaling molecules affect the biological activities and anti-cancer effects of ITCs in malignancies. These include direct/indirect interactions with Nrf2 and NF-κB, the Nrf2-Kelch-like ECH-associated protein (Keap) 1-antioxidant response element (ARE) signaling pathway, and antioxidant enzymes, such as NAD(P)H quinone reductase (NQO1) and glutathione S transferases (GSTs), through the Nrf2-Keap1-ARE signaling pathway are closely associated with ITC-induced bioactivity [139–141]. We would like to emphasize that further basic research is essential for uncovering the utility and limitations of ITCs in cancer treatment, including BC.

Another important issue to consider is the carcinogenic risk factors of BC, which are affected by a variety of harmful chemical compounds (e.g., cigarette smoke) or physiologically active substances (e.g., sex hormones) [142–144]. With regards to cigarette smoke, cytochrome P450 and phase II detoxification enzymes, such as DOQ1, GSTs, and glucuronosyltransferase inhibit the formation of carcinogenic compounds from tobacco-specific carcinogens, and PEITC modulates such cancer preventive activities [145]. This finding supports the hypothesis that PEITC may suppress the tobacco-related cancer risk in smokers. Indeed, a clinical trial showed that metabolic activation of a tobacco-specific lung carcinogen is significantly suppressed by PEIT treatment [146]. We believe that the cancer risk of BC in smokers may be suppressed by ITCs though similar anti-carcinogenic mechanisms, and thus there is value in performing such clinical trials for BC. Furthermore, the frequency of BC is known to be remarkably higher in men than in women, which is perhaps due to the testosterone-androgen receptor pathways [147]. Interestingly, PEITC was reported to suppress testosterone-induced cancer cell proliferation by downregulating the testosterone-androgen receptor pathway in prostate cancer [148]. Meanwhile, other research has shown that estrogen-mediated pathways are associated with malignant potential and tumor growth of BC [143,144]. In addition, SFN was found to regulate tumor growth of breast cancer cells by modulating estrogen activities [149]. Unfortunately, there is little information on the influence of ITC-mediated sex hormone activity on the malignant potential of BC. Nevertheless, there is a possibility that ITCs affect carcinogenesis and malignant aggressiveness by regulating sex hormones in BC. This highlights the need for designing studies to identify the biological roles of ITCs according to patient background and environment, including occupation, diet, and health habits.

5. Conclusions

In this review, we discussed the anti-cancer effects of ITCs in BC. The research suggests that all ITC members can suppress carcinogenesis, tumor development, and progression *in vivo* and *in vitro*. Furthermore, regulation of cell proliferation, cell cycle, and apoptosis play crucial roles in the ITC-induced anti-cancer effects, and such phenomena are mainly regulated by complex mechanisms involving caspases, Bcl-2 family proteins, and mitochondrial activities. While changes in cancer-related molecules by ITCs may correspond to anti-cancer mechanisms in BC cells, some ITCs may have neoplastic and carcinogenic potential in BC. To clarify this issue, more detailed studies at the molecular level are essential. While there is a possibility that ITC-based treatment strategies can improve prognosis in patients with BC, further clinical trials with well-designed protocols are required to establish the optimal doses and types of ITCs for application in BC treatment [112]. In addition, it would be fruitful to investigate the anti-cancer effects and clinical utility of combination therapies of ITCs and new therapeutic strategies, including immunotherapy and gene therapy, for patients with BC.

Author Contributions: Conceptualization, Y.M.; supervision, H.S.; writing—original draft preparation, T.M., Y.M., T.Y., Y.M., A.O., K.M. and K.O. All authors have read and agreed to the published version of the manuscript. The authors declare that the content of this paper has not been published or submitted for publication elsewhere.

Funding: This research received no external funding.

Conflicts of Interest: The authors declare no conflict of interest.

References

1. Metts, M.C.; Metts, J.C.; Milito, S.J.; Thomas, C.R., Jr. Bladder cancer: A review of diagnosis and management. *J. Natl. Med. Assoc.* **2000**, *92*, 285–294. [PubMed]
2. Siegel, R.L.; Miller, K.D.; Jemal, A. Cancer statistics, 2019. *CA Cancer J. Clin.* **2019**, *69*, 7–34. [CrossRef] [PubMed]
3. Von der Maase, H.; Hansen, S.W.; Roberts, J.T.; Dogliotti, L.; Oliver, T.; Moore, M.J.; Bodrogi, I.; Albers, P.; Knuth, A. Gemcitabine and cisplatin versus methotrexate, vinblastine, doxorubicin, and cisplatin in advanced or metastatic bladder cancer: Results of a large, randomized, multinational, multicenter, phase III study. *J. Clin. Oncol.* **2000**, *18*, 3068–3077. [CrossRef] [PubMed]
4. Tripathi, A.; Plimack, E.R. Immunotherapy for Urothelial Carcinoma: Current Evidence and Future Directions. *Curr. Urol Rep.* **2018**, *19*, 109. [CrossRef]
5. Wang, H.; Liu, J.; Fang, K.; Ke, C.; Jiang, Y.; Wang, G.; Yang, T.; Chen, T.; Shi, X. Second-line treatment strategy for urothelial cancer patients who progress or are unfit for cisplatin therapy: A network meta-analysis. *BMC Urol.* **2019**, *19*, 125. [CrossRef]
6. Tan, W.P.; Tan, W.S.; Inman, B.A. PD-L1/PD-1 Biomarker for Metastatic Urothelial Cancer that Progress Post-platinum Therapy: A Systematic Review and Meta-analysis. *Bladder. Cancer* **2019**, *5*, 211–223. [CrossRef]
7. Hanna, K.S. Clinical Overview of Enfortumab Vedotin in the Management of Locally Advanced or Metastatic Urothelial Carcinoma. *Drugs* **2019**, in press. [CrossRef]

8. Sharma, P.; Sohn, J.; Shin, S.J.; Oh, D.Y.; Keam, B.; Lee, H.J.; Gizzi, M.; Kalinka, E.; de Vos, F.Y.F.L. Efficacy and Tolerability of Tremelimumab in Locally Advanced or Metastatic Urothelial Carcinoma Patients Who Have Failed First-Line Platinum-Based Chemotherapy. *Clin. Cancer Res* **2019**, in press.
9. Wan Mohd Tajuddin, W.N.B.; Lajis, N.H.; Abas, F.; Othman, I.; Naidu, R. Mechanistic Understanding of Curcumin's Therapeutic Effects in Lung Cancer. *Nutrients* **2019**, *11*, 989. [CrossRef]
10. Shu, P.; Tang, H.; Zhou, B.; Wang, R.; Xu, Y.; Shao, J.; Qi, M.; Xia, Y.; Huang, W.; Liu, S. Effect of Yiqi Huayu Jiedu decoction on stages II and III gastric cancer: A multicenter, prospective, cohort study. *Medicine* **2019**, *98*, e17875. [CrossRef]
11. Cullen, J.K.; Simmons, J.L.; Parsons, P.G.; Boyle, G.M. Topical treatments for skin cancer. Oral Intake of Royal Jelly Has Protective Effects Against Tyrosine Kinase Inhibitor-Induced Toxicity in Patients with Renal Cell Carcinoma: A Randomized, Double-Blinded, Placebo-Controlled Trial. *Adv. Drug Deliv. Rev.* **2019**, in press.
12. Emsen, B.; Ozdemir, O.; Engin, T.; Togar, B.; Cavusoglu, S.; Turkez, H. Inhibition of growth of U87MG human glioblastoma cells by Usnea longissima Ach. *An. Acad. Bras. Cienc.* **2019**, *91*, e20180994. [CrossRef] [PubMed]
13. Huang, Z.; Wei, P. Compound Kushen Injection for gastric cancer: A protocol of systematic review and meta-analysis. *Med. Baltimore* **2019**, *98*, e17927. [CrossRef] [PubMed]
14. Kim, K.I.; Kong, M.; Lee, S.H.; Lee, B.J. The efficacy and safety of Kyung-Ok-Ko on cancer-related fatigue in lung cancer patients: Study protocol for a randomized, patients-assessor blind, placebo-controlled, parallel-group, single-center trial. *Medicine* **2019**, *98*, e17717. [CrossRef]
15. Shi, C.S.; Li, J.M.; Chin, C.C.; Kuo, Y.H.; Lee, Y.R.; Huang, Y.C. Evodiamine Induces Cell Growth Arrest, Apoptosis and Suppresses Tumorigenesis in Human Urothelial Cell Carcinoma Cells. *Anticancer Res.* **2017**, *37*, 1149–1159.
16. Falke, J.; Parkkinen, J.; Vaahtera, L.; Hulsbergen-van de Kaa, C.A.; Oosterwijk, E.; Witjes, J.A. Curcumin as Treatment for Bladder Cancer: A Preclinical Study of Cyclodextrin-Curcumin Complex and BCG as Intravesical Treatment in an Orthotopic Bladder Cancer Rat Model. *Biomed. Res. Int.* **2018**, *2018*, 9634902. [CrossRef]
17. Yang, H.Y.; Chen, P.C.; Wang, J.D. Chinese herbs containing aristolochic acid associated with renal failure and urothelial carcinoma: A review from epidemiologic observations to causal inference. *Biomed. Res. Int.* **2014**, *2014*, 569325. [CrossRef]
18. Křížová, L.; Dadáková, K.; Kašparovská, J.; Kašparovský, T. Isoflavones. *Molecules* **2019**, *24*, 1076. [CrossRef]
19. Sagara, Y.; Miyata, Y.; Nomata, K.; Hayashi, T.; Kanetake, H. Green tea polyphenol suppresses tumor invasion and angiogenesis in N-butyl-(-4-hydroxybutyl) nitrosamine-induced bladder cancer. *Cancer Epidemiol.* **2010**, *34*, 350–354. [CrossRef]
20. Matsuo, T.; Miyata, Y.; Asai, A.; Sagara, Y.; Furusato, B.; Fukuoka, J.; Sakai, H. Green Tea Polyphenol Induces Changes in Cancer-Related Factors in an Animal Model of Bladder Cancer. *PLoS ONE* **2017**, *12*, e0171091. [CrossRef]
21. Araki, K.; Miyata, Y.; Ohba, K.; Nakamura, Y.; Matsuo, T.; Mochizuki, Y.; Sakai, H. *Medicines* **2018**, *6*, 2. [CrossRef] [PubMed]
22. Miyata, Y.; Matsuo, T.; Araki, K.; Nakamura, Y.; Sagara, Y.; Ohba, K.; Sakai, H. Anticancer Effects of Green Tea and the Underlying Molecular Mechanisms in Bladder Cancer. *Medicines* **2018**, *5*, 87. [CrossRef] [PubMed]
23. Miyata, Y.; Sakai, H. Anti-Cancer and Protective Effects of Royal Jelly for Therapy-Induced Toxicities in Malignancies. *Int. J. Mol. Sci.* **2018**, *19*, 3270. [CrossRef] [PubMed]
24. Yasuda, T.; Miyata, Y.; Nakamura, Y.; Sagara, Y.; Matsuo, T.; Ohba, K.; Sakai, H. High Consumption of Green Tea Suppresses Urinary Tract Recurrence of Urothelial Cancer via Down-regulation of Human Antigen-R Expression in Never Smokers. *In Vivo* **2018**, *32*, 721–729. [CrossRef] [PubMed]
25. Miyata, Y.; Shida, Y.; Hakariya, T.; Sakai, H. Anti-Cancer Effects of Green Tea Polyphenols Against Prostate Cancer. *Molecules* **2019**, *24*, 193. [CrossRef] [PubMed]
26. Abbaoui, B.; Telu, K.H.; Lucas, C.R.; Thomas-Ahner, J.M.; Schwartz, S.J.; Clinton, S.K.; Freitas, M.A.; Mortazavi, A. The impact of cruciferous vegetable isothiocyanates on histone acetylation and histone phosphorylation in bladder cancer. *J. Proteomics* **2017**, *156*, 94–103. [CrossRef] [PubMed]
27. Abbaoui, B.; Lucas, C.R.; Riedl, K.M.; Clinton, S.K.; Mortazavi, A. Cruciferous Vegetables, Isothiocyanates, and Bladder Cancer Prevention. *Mol. Nutr. Food Res.* **2018**, *62*, e1800079. [CrossRef]

28. Leone, A.; Diorio, G.; Sexton, W.; Schell, M.; Alexandrow, M.; Fahey, J.W.; Kumar, N.B. Sulforaphane for the chemoprevention of bladder cancer: Molecular mechanism targeted approach. *Oncotarget* **2017**, *8*, 35412–35424. [CrossRef]
29. Tang, L.; Zirpoli, G.R.; Guru, K.; Moysich, K.B.; Zhang, Y.; Ambrosone, C.B.; McCann, S.E. Consumption of raw cruciferous vegetables is inversely associated with bladder cancer risk. *Cancer Epidemiol. Biomarkers Prev.* **2008**, *17*, 938–944. [CrossRef]
30. Vieira, A.R.; Vingeliene, S.; Chan, D.S.; Aune, D.; Abar, L.; Navarro Rosenblatt, D.; Greenwood, D.C.; Norat, T. Fruits, vegetables, and bladder cancer risk: A systematic review and meta-analysis. *Cancer Med.* **2015**, *4*, 136–146. [CrossRef]
31. Xu, C.; Zeng, X.T.; Liu, T.Z.; Zhang, C.; Yang, Z.H.; Li, S.; Chen, X.Y. Fruits and vegetables intake and risk of bladder cancer: A PRISMA-compliant systematic review and dose-response meta-analysis of prospective cohort studies. *Med. Baltimore* **2015**, *94*, e759. [CrossRef] [PubMed]
32. Shapiro, T.A.; Fahey, J.W.; Wade, K.L.; Stephenson, K.K.; Talalay, P. Chemoprotective glucosinolates and isothiocyanates of broccoli sprouts: Metabolism and excretion in humans. *Cancer Epidemiol. Biomarkers Prev.* **2001**, *10*, 501–508. [PubMed]
33. Palliyaguru, D.L.; Yuan, J.M.; Kensler, T.W.; Fahey, J.W. Isothiocyanates: Translating the Power of Plants to People. *Mol. Nutr. Food Res.* **2018**, *62*, e1700965. [CrossRef] [PubMed]
34. Romeo, L.; Iori, R.; Rollin, P.; Bramanti, P.; Mazzon, E. Isothiocyanates: An Overview of Their Antimicrobial Activity against Human Infections. *Molecules* **2018**, *23*, 624. [CrossRef]
35. Novío, S.; Cartea, M.E.; Soengas, P.; Freire-Garabal, M.; Núñez-Iglesias, M.J. Effects of Brassicaceae Isothiocyanates on Prostate Cancer. *Molecules* **2016**, *21*, 626. [CrossRef]
36. Martin, S.L.; Royston, K.J.; Tollefsbol, T.O. The Role of Non-Coding RNAs and Isothiocyanates in Cancer. *Mol. Nutr. Food Res.* **2018**, *62*, e1700913. [CrossRef]
37. Mitsiogianni, M.; Koutsidis, G.; Mavroudis, N.; Trafalis, D.T.; Botaitis, S.; Franco, R.; Zoumpourlis, V.; Amery, T.; Galanis, A. The Role of Isothiocyanates as Cancer Chemo-Preventive, Chemo-Therapeutic and Anti-Melanoma Agents. *Antioxidants* **2019**, *8*, E106. [CrossRef]
38. Aytac, Z.; Dogan, S.Y.; Tekinay, T.; Uyar, T. Release and antibacterial activity of allyl isothiocyanate/β-cyclodextrin complex encapsulated in electrospun nanofibers. *Colloids Surf. B Biointerfaces* **2014**, *120*, 125–131. [CrossRef]
39. Subedi, L.; Venkatesan, R.; Kim, S.Y. Neuroprotective and Anti-Inflammatory Activities of Allyl Isothiocyanate through Attenuation of JNK/NF-κB/TNF-α Signaling. *Int. J. Mol. Sci.* **2017**, *18*, 1423. [CrossRef]
40. Chen, N.G.; Chen, K.T.; Lu, C.C.; Lan, Y.H.; Lai, C.H.; Chung, Y.T.; Yang, J.S.; Lin, Y.C. Allyl isothiocyanate triggers G2/M phase arrest and apoptosis in human brain malignant glioma GBM 8401 cells through a mitochondria-dependent pathway. *Oncol. Rep.* **2010**, *24*, 449–455.
41. Qin, G.; Li, P.; Xue, Z. Effect of allyl isothiocyanate on the viability and apoptosis of the human cervical cancer HeLa cell line *in vitro*. *Oncol. Lett.* **2018**, *15*, 8756–8760. [CrossRef] [PubMed]
42. Rajakumar, T.; Pugalendhi, P.; Thilagavathi, S.; Ananthakrishnan, D.; Gunasekaran, K. Allyl isothiocyanate, a potent chemopreventive agent targets AhR/Nrf2 signaling pathway in chemically induced mammary carcinogenesis. *Mol. Cell Biochem.* **2018**, *437*, 1–12. [CrossRef]
43. Sayeed, M.A.; Bracci, M.; Ciarapica, V.; Malavolta, M.; Provinciali, M.; Pieragostini, E.; Gaetani, S.; Monaco, F.; Lucarini, G. Allyl Isothiocyanate Exhibits No Anticancer Activity in MDA-MB-231 Breast Cancer Cells. *Int. J. Mol. Sci.* **2018**, *19*, 145. [CrossRef] [PubMed]
44. Savio, A.L.; da Silva, G.N.; de Camargo, E.A.; Salvadori, D.M. Cell cycle kinetics, apoptosis rates, DNA damage and TP53 gene expression in bladder cancer cells treated with allyl isothiocyanate (mustard essential oil). *Mutat. Res.* **2014**, *762*, 40–46. [CrossRef] [PubMed]
45. Kim, Y.J.; Lee, D.H.; Ahn, J.; Chung, W.J.; Jang, Y.J.; Seong, K.S.; Moon, J.H.; Ha, T.Y.; Jung, C.H. Pharmacokinetics, Tissue Distribution, and Anti-Lipogenic/Adipogenic Effects of Allyl-Isothiocyanate Metabolites. *PLoS ONE* **2015**, *10*, e0132151.
46. Sávio, A.L.; da Silva, G.N.; Salvadori, D.M. Inhibition of bladder cancer cell proliferation by allyl isothiocyanate (mustard essential oil). *Mutat. Res.* **2015**, *771*, 29–35. [CrossRef]
47. Blažević, I.; Đulović, A.; Maravić, A.; Čikeš Čulić, V.; Montaut, S.; Rollin, P. Antimicrobial and Cytotoxic Activities of Lepidium latifolium L.; Hydrodistillate, Extract and Its Major Sulfur Volatile Allyl Isothiocyanate. *Chem. Biodivers.* **2019**, *16*, e1800661. [CrossRef]

48. Geng, F.; Tang, L.; Li, Y.; Yang, L.; Choi, K.S.; Kazim, A.L.; Zhang, Y. Allyl isothiocyanate arrests cancer cells in mitosis, and mitotic arrest in turn leads to apoptosis via Bcl-2 protein phosphorylation. *J. Biol. Chem.* **2011**, *286*, 32259–32267. [CrossRef]
49. Hinata, N.; Shirakawa, T.; Zhang, Z.; Matsumoto, A.; Fujisawa, M.; Okada, H.; Kamidono, S.; Gotoh, A. Radiation induces p53-dependent cell apoptosis in bladder cancer cells with wild-type- p53 but not in p53-mutated bladder cancer cells. *Urol. Res.* **2003**, *31*, 387–396. [CrossRef]
50. Bhattacharya, A.; Li, Y.; Geng, F.; Munday, R.; Zhang, Y. The principal urinary metabolite of allyl isothiocyanate, N-acetyl-S-(N-allylthiocarbamoyl)cysteine, inhibits the growth and muscle invasion of bladder cancer. *Carcinogenesis* **2012**, *33*, 394–398. [CrossRef]
51. Munday, R.; Mhawech-Fauceglia, P.; Munday, C.M.; Paonessa, J.D.; Tang, L.; Munday, J.S.; Lister, C.; Wilson, P.; Fahey, J.W. Inhibition of urinary bladder carcinogenesis by broccoli sprouts. *Cancer Res.* **2008**, *68*, 1593–1600. [CrossRef] [PubMed]
52. Bhattacharya, A.; Li, Y.; Wade, K.L.; Paonessa, J.D.; Fahey, J.W.; Zhang, Y. Allyl isothiocyanate-rich mustard seed powder inhibits bladder cancer growth and muscle invasion. *Carcinogenesis* **2010**, *31*, 2105–2110. [CrossRef] [PubMed]
53. Miyata, Y.; Kanda, S.; Nomata, K.; Eguchi, J.; Kanetake, H. Expression of cyclooxygenase-2 and EP4 receptor in transitional cell carcinoma of the upper urinary tract. *J. Urol.* **2005**, *173*, 56–60. [CrossRef] [PubMed]
54. Miyata, Y.; Ohba, K.; Kanda, S.; Nomata, K.; Eguchi, J.; Hayashi, T.; Kanetake, H. Pathological function of prostaglandin E2 receptors in transitional cell carcinoma of the upper urinary tract. *Virchows Arch.* **2006**, *448*, 822–829. [CrossRef] [PubMed]
55. Van Kessel, K.E.; Zuiverloon, T.C.; Alberts, A.R.; Boormans, J.L.; Zwarthoff, E.C. Targeted therapies in bladder cancer: An overview of in vivo research. *Nat. Rev. Urol.* **2015**, *12*, 681–694. [CrossRef] [PubMed]
56. Benelli, R.; Venè, R.; Ferrari, N. Prostaglandin-endoperoxide synthase 2 (cyclooxygenase-2), a complex target for colorectal cancer prevention and therapy. *Transl. Res.* **2018**, *196*, 42–61. [CrossRef] [PubMed]
57. Ferreira, T.; Campos, S.; Silva, M.G.; Ribeiro, R.; Santos, S.; Almeida, J.; Pires, M.J.; Gil da Costa, R.M.; Córdova, C. The Cyclooxigenase-2 Inhibitor Parecoxib Prevents Epidermal Dysplasia in HPV16-Transgenic Mice: Efficacy and Safety Observations. *Int. J. Mol. Sci.* **2019**, *20*, 3902. [CrossRef]
58. Umezawa, S.; Higurashi, T.; Komiya, Y.; Arimoto, J.; Horita, N.; Kaneko, T.; Iwasaki, M.; Nakagama, H.; Nakajima, A. Chemoprevention of colorectal cancer: Past, present, and future. *Cancer Sci.* **2019**, *110*, 3018–3026. [CrossRef]
59. Mascan, B.; Marignol, L. Aspirin in the Management of Patients with Prostate Cancer Undergoing Radiotherapy: Friend or Foe? *Anticancer Res.* **2018**, *38*, 1897–1902.
60. Guo, Q.; Li, Q.; Wang, J.; Liu, M.; Wang, Y.; Chen, Z.; Ye, Y.; Guan, Q.; Zhou, Y. A comprehensive evaluation of clinical efficacy and safety of celecoxib in combination with chemotherapy in metastatic or postoperative recurrent gastric cancer patients: A preliminary, three-center, clinical trial study. *Medicine (Baltimore)* **2019**, *98*, e16234. [CrossRef]
61. Bhattacharya, A.; Li, Y.; Shi, Y.; Zhang, Y. Enhanced inhibition of urinary bladder cancer growth and muscle invasion by allyl isothiocyanate and celecoxib in combination. *Carcinogenesis* **2013**, *34*, 2593–2599. [CrossRef] [PubMed]
62. Ling, X.; Westover, D.; Cao, F.; Cao, S.; He, X.; Kim, H.R.; Zhang, Y.; Chan, D.C.; Li, F. Synergistic effect of allyl isothiocyanate (AITC) on cisplatin efficacy in vitro and in vivo. *Am. J. Cancer Res.* **2015**, *5*, 2516–2530. [PubMed]
63. Chang, W.J.; Chen, B.H.; Inbaraj, B.S.; Chien, J.T. Preparation of allyl isothiocyanate nanoparticles, their anti-inflammatory activity towards RAW 264.7 macrophage cells and anti-proliferative effect on HT1376 bladder cancer cells. *J. Sci Food Agric.* **2019**, *99*, 3106–3116. [CrossRef] [PubMed]
64. Liu, P.; Behray, M.; Wang, Q.; Wang, W.; Zhou, Z.; Chao, Y.; Bao, Y. Anti-cancer activities of allyl isothiocyanate and its conjugated silicon quantum dots. *Sci. Rep.* **2018**, *18*, 1084. [CrossRef]
65. Ibrahim, A.; Al-Hizab, F.A.; Abushouk, A.I.; Abdel-Daim, M.M. Nephroprotective Effects of Benzyl Isothiocyanate and Resveratrol Against Cisplatin-Induced Oxidative Stress and Inflammation. *Front. Pharmacol.* **2018**, *9*, 1268. [CrossRef]

66. Tang, Y.; Naito, S.; Abe-Kanoh, N.; Ogawa, S.; Yamaguchi, S.; Zhu, B.; Murata, Y.; Nakamura, Y. Benzyl isothiocyanate attenuates the hydrogen peroxide-induced interleukin-13 expression through glutathione S-transferase P induction in T lymphocytic leukemia cells. *J. Biochem. Mol. Toxicol.* **2018**, *32*, e22054. [CrossRef]
67. Huang, Y.P.; Jiang, Y.W.; Chen, H.Y.; Hsiao, Y.T.; Peng, S.F.; Chou, Y.C.; Yang, J.L.; Hsia, T.C.; Chung, J.G. Benzyl Isothiocyanate Induces Apoptotic Cell Death Through Mitochondria-dependent Pathway in Gefitinib-resistant NCI-H460 Human Lung Cancer Cells In Vitro. *Anticancer Res.* **2018**, *38*, 5165–5176. [CrossRef]
68. Ma, L.; Chen, Y.; Han, R.; Wang, S. Benzyl isothiocyanate inhibits invasion and induces apoptosis via reducing S100A4 expression and increases PUMA expression in oral squamous cell carcinoma cells. *Braz. J. Med. Biol. Res.* **2019**, *52*, e8409. [CrossRef]
69. Xie, B.; Zhao, L.; Guo, L.; Liu, H.; Fu, S.; Fan, W.; Lin, L.; Chen, J.; Wang, B.; Fan, L.; et al. Benzyl isothiocyanate suppresses development and metastasis of murine mammary carcinoma by regulating the Wnt/β-catenin pathway. *Mol. Med. Rep.* **2019**, *20*, 1808–1818. [CrossRef]
70. Tang, L.; Zhang, Y. Mitochondria are the primary target in isothiocyanate-induced apoptosis in human bladder cancer cells. *Mol. Cancer Ther.* **2005**, *4*, 1250–1259. [CrossRef]
71. Tang, L.; Li, G.; Song, L.; Zhang, Y. The principal urinary metabolites of dietary isothiocyanates, N-acetylcysteine conjugates, elicit the same anti-proliferative response as their parent compounds in human bladder cancer cells. *Anticancer Drugs* **2006**, *17*, 297–305. [CrossRef] [PubMed]
72. Tang, L.; Zhang, Y. Dietary isothiocyanates inhibit the growth of human bladder carcinoma cells. *J. Nutr.* **2004**, *134*, 2004–2010. [CrossRef] [PubMed]
73. Izquierdo, L.; Ingelmo-Torres, M.; Mallofré, C.; Lozano, J.J.; Verhasselt-Crinquette, M.; Leroy, X.; Colin, P.; Comperat, E.; Roupret, M.; Alcaraz, A.; et al. Prognostic value of microRNA expression pattern in upper tract urothelial carcinoma. *BJU Int.* **2014**, *113*, 813–821. [CrossRef]
74. Braicu, C.; Cojocneanu-Petric, R.; Chira, S.; Truta, A.; Floares, A.; Petrut, B.; Achimas-Cadariu, P.; Berindan-Neagoe, I. Clinical and pathological implications of miRNA in bladder cancer. *Int. J. Nanomed.* **2015**, *10*, 791–800. [CrossRef] [PubMed]
75. Nordentoft, I.; Birkenkamp-Demtroder, K.; Agerbæk, M.; Theodorescu, D.; Ostenfeld, M.S.; Hartmann, A.; Borre, M.; Ørntoft, T.F.; Dyrskjøt, L. miRNAs associated with chemo-sensitivity in cell lines and in advanced bladder cancer. *BMC Med. Genomics* **2012**, *5*, 40. [CrossRef] [PubMed]
76. Liu, Y.; Li, B.; Yang, X.; Zhang, C. MiR-99a-5p inhibits bladder cancer cell proliferation by directly targeting mammalian target of rapamycin and predicts patient survival. *J. Cell Biochem.* **2019**, *120*, 19330–19337. [CrossRef] [PubMed]
77. Inamoto, T.; Uehara, H.; Akao, Y.; Ibuki, N.; Komura, K.; Takahara, K.; Takai, T.; Uchimoto, T.; Saito, K. A Panel of MicroRNA Signature as a Tool for Predicting Survival of Patients with Urothelial Carcinoma of the Bladder. *Dis. Markers* **2018**, *2018*, 5468672. [CrossRef]
78. Tsai, T.F.; Lin, J.F.; Chou, K.Y.; Lin, Y.C.; Chen, H.E.; Hwang, T.I. miR-99a-5p acts as tumor suppressor via targeting to mTOR and enhances RAD001-induced apoptosis in human urinary bladder urothelial carcinoma cells. *Onco Targets Ther.* **2018**, *11*, 239–252. [CrossRef]
79. Tsai, T.F.; Chen, P.C.; Lin, Y.C.; Chou, K.Y.; Chen, H.E.; Ho, C.Y.; Lin, J.F.; Hwang, T.I. Benzyl isothiocyanate promotes miR-99a expression through ERK/AP-1-dependent pathway in bladder cancer cells. *Environ. Toxicol.* **2020**, *35*, 47–54. [CrossRef]
80. Feng, Y.; Kang, Y.; He, Y.; Liu, J.; Liang, B.; Yang, P.; Yu, Z. microRNA-99a acts as a tumor suppressor and is down-regulated in bladder cancer. *BMC Urol.* **2014**, *14*, 50. [CrossRef]
81. Tsai, T.F.; Lin, Y.C.; Chen, H.E.; Chou, K.Y.; Lin, J.F.; Hwang, T.I.S. Involvement of the insulin-like growth factor I receptor and its downstream antiapoptotic signaling pathway is revealed by dysregulated micro-RNA in bladder carcinoma. *Urol Sci.* **2014**, *25*, 58–64. [CrossRef]
82. Ganji, S.M.; Saidijam, M.; Amini, R.; Mousavi-Bahar, S.H.; Shabab, N.; Seyedabadi, S.; Mahdavinezhad, A. Evaluation of MicroRNA-99a and MicroRNA-205 Expression Levels in Bladder Cancer. *Int J. Mol. Cell Med.* **2017**, *6*, 87–95. [PubMed]

83. Okazaki, K.; Yamagishi, M.; Son, H.Y.; Imazawa, T.; Furukawa, F.; Nakamura, H.; Nishikawa, A.; Masegi, T.; Hirose, M. Simultaneous treatment with benzyl isothiocyanate, a strong bladder promoter, inhibits rat urinary bladder carcinogenesis by N-butyl-N-(4-hydroxybutyl)nitrosamine. *Nutr. Cancer* **2002**, *42*, 211–216. [CrossRef] [PubMed]
84. Okazaki, K.; Umemura, T.; Imazawa, T.; Nishikawa, A.; Masegi, T.; Hirose, M. Enhancement of urinary bladder carcinogenesis by combined treatment with benzyl isothiocyanate and N-butyl-N-(4-hydroxybutyl)nitrosamine in rats after initiation. *Cancer Sci.* **2003**, *94*, 948–952. [CrossRef]
85. Di Pasqua, A.J.; Hong, C.; Wu, M.Y.; McCracken, E.; Wang, X.; Mi, L.; Chung, F.L. Sensitization of non-small cell lung cancer cells to cisplatin by naturally occurring isothiocyanates. *Chem. Res. Toxicol.* **2010**, *23*, 1307–1309. [CrossRef]
86. Lee, Y.; Kim, Y.J.; Choi, Y.J.; Lee, J.W.; Lee, S.; Chung, H.W. Enhancement of cisplatin cytotoxicity by benzyl isothiocyanate in HL-60 cells. *Food Chem. Toxicol.* **2012**, *50*, 2397–2406. [CrossRef]
87. Wolf, M.A.; Claudio, P.P. Benzyl isothiocyanate inhibits HNSCC cell migration and invasion, and sensitizes HNSCC cells to cisplatin. *Nutr. Cancer* **2014**, *66*, 285–294. [CrossRef]
88. Xia, Y.; Kang, T.W.; Jung, Y.D.; Zhang, C.; Lian, S. Sulforaphane Inhibits Nonmuscle Invasive Bladder Cancer Cells Proliferation through Suppression of HIF-1α-Mediated Glycolysis in Hypoxia. *J. Agric. Food Chem.* **2019**, *67*, 7844–7854. [CrossRef]
89. Bernkopf, D.B.; Daum, G.; Brückner, M.; Behrens, J. Sulforaphane inhibits growth and blocks Wnt/β-catenin signaling of colorectal cancer cells. *Oncotarget* **2018**, *9*, 33982–33994. [CrossRef]
90. Kan, S.F.; Wang, J.; Sun, G.X. Sulforaphane regulates apoptosis- and proliferation-related signaling pathways and synergizes with cisplatin to suppress human ovarian cancer. *Int. J. Mol. Med.* **2018**, *42*, 2447–2458. [CrossRef]
91. Park, H.S.; Han, M.H.; Kim, G.Y.; Moon, S.K.; Kim, W.J.; Hwang, H.J.; Park, K.Y.; Choi, Y.H. Sulforaphane induces reactive oxygen species-mediated mitotic arrest and subsequent apoptosis in human bladder cancer 5637 cells. *Food Chem. Toxicol.* **2014**, *64*, 157–165. [CrossRef] [PubMed]
92. Jo, G.H.; Kim, G.Y.; Kim, W.J.; Park, K.Y.; Choi, Y.H. Sulforaphane induces apoptosis in T24 human urinary bladder cancer cells through a reactive oxygen species-mediated mitochondrial pathway: The involvement of endoplasmic reticulum stress and the Nrf2 signaling pathway. *Int. J. Oncol.* **2014**, *45*, 1497–1506. [CrossRef] [PubMed]
93. Shan, Y.; Sun, C.; Zhao, X.; Wu, K.; Cassidy, A.; Bao, Y. Effect of sulforaphane on cell growth, G(0)/G(1) phase cell progression and apoptosis in human bladder cancer T24 cells. *Int. J. Oncol.* **2006**, *29*, 883–888. [CrossRef] [PubMed]
94. Ding, Y.; Paonessa, J.D.; Randall, K.L.; Argoti, D.; Chen, L.; Vouros, P.; Zhang, Y. Sulforaphane inhibits 4-aminobiphenyl-induced DNA damage in bladder cells and tissues. *Carcinogenesis* **2010**, *31*, 1999–2003. [CrossRef] [PubMed]
95. Cullinan, S.B.; Diehl, J.A. Coordination of ER and oxidative stress signaling: The PERK/Nrf2 signaling pathway. *Int. J. Biochem. Cell Biol.* **2006**, *38*, 317–332. [CrossRef] [PubMed]
96. Dang, Y.M.; Huang, G.; Chen, Y.R.; Dang, Z.F.; Chen, C.; Liu, F.L.; Guo, Y.F.; Xie, X.D. Sulforaphane inhibits the proliferation of the BIU87 bladder cancer cell line via IGFBP-3 elevation. *Asian Pac. J. Cancer Prev.* **2014**, *15*, 1517–1520. [CrossRef] [PubMed]
97. Baxter, R.C. IGF binding proteins in cancer: Mechanistic and clinical insights. *Nat. Rev. Cancer.* **2014**, *14*, 329–341. [CrossRef]
98. Patel, M.; Horgan, P.G.; McMillan, D.C.; Edwards, J. NF-κB pathways in the development and progression of colorectal cancer. *Transl. Res.* **2018**, *197*, 43–56. [CrossRef]
99. Abbaoui, B.; Riedl, K.M.; Ralston, R.A.; Thomas-Ahner, J.M.; Schwartz, S.J.; Clinton, S.K.; Mortazavi, A. Inhibition of bladder cancer by broccoli isothiocyanates sulforaphane and erucin: Characterization, metabolism, and interconversion. *Mol. Nutr. Food Res.* **2012**, *56*, 1675–1687. [CrossRef]
100. Hao, L.; Zhao, Y.; Li, Z.G.; He, H.G.; Liang, Q.; Zhang, Z.G.; Shi, Z.D.; Zhang, P.Y.; Han, C.H. Tumor necrosis factor-related apoptosis-inducing ligand inhibits proliferation and induces apoptosis of prostate and bladder cancer cells. *Oncol. Lett.* **2017**, *13*, 3638–3640. [CrossRef]
101. Yuan, S.Y.; Shiau, M.Y.; Ou, Y.C.; Huang, Y.C.; Chen, C.C.; Cheng, C.L.; Chiu, K.Y.; Wang, S.S.; Tsai, K.J. Miconazole induces apoptosis via the death receptor 5-dependent and mitochondrial-mediated pathways in human bladder cancer cells. *Oncol. Rep.* **2017**, *37*, 3606–3616. [CrossRef] [PubMed]

102. Levidou, G.; Thymara, I.; Saetta, A.A.; Papanastasiou, P.; Pavlopoulos, P.; Sakellariou, S.; Fragkou, P.; Patsouris, E.; Korkolopoulou, P. TRAIL and osteoprotegerin (OPG) expression in bladder urothelial carcinoma: Correlation with clinicopathological parameters and prognosis. *Pathology* **2013**, *45*, 138–144. [CrossRef] [PubMed]
103. Jin, C.Y.; Molagoda, I.M.N.; Karunarathne, W.A.H.M.; Kang, S.H.; Park, C.; Kim, G.Y.; Choi, Y.H. TRAIL attenuates sulforaphane-mediated Nrf2 and sustains ROS generation, leading to apoptosis of TRAIL-resistant human bladder cancer cells. *Toxicol. Appl. Pharmacol.* **2018**, *352*, 132–141. [CrossRef] [PubMed]
104. Shan, Y.; Wu, K.; Wang, W.; Wang, S.; Lin, N.; Zhao, R.; Cassidy, A.; Bao, Y. Sulforaphane down-regulates COX-2 expression by activating p38 and inhibiting NF-kappaB-DNA-binding activity in human bladder T24 cells. *Int. J. Oncol.* **2009**, *34*, 1129–1134. [PubMed]
105. Shan, Y.; Wang, X.; Wang, W.; He, C.; Bao, Y. p38 MAPK plays a distinct role in sulforaphane-induced up-regulation of ARE-dependent enzymes and down-regulation of COX-2 in human bladder cancer cells. *Oncol. Rep.* **2010**, *23*, 1133–1138.
106. Shan, Y.; Zhang, L.; Bao, Y.; Li, B.; He, C.; Gao, M.; Feng, X.; Xu, W.; Zhang, X.; Wang, S. Epithelial-mesenchymal transition, a novel target of sulforaphane via COX-2/MMP2, 9/Snail, ZEB1 and miR-200c/ZEB1 pathways in human bladder cancer cells. *J. Nutr. Biochem.* **2013**, *24*, 1062–1069. [CrossRef]
107. Telu, K.H.; Abbaoui, B.; Thomas-Ahner, J.M.; Zynger, D.L.; Clinton, S.K.; Freitas, M.A.; Mortazavi, A. Alterations of histone H1 phosphorylation during bladder carcinogenesis. *J. Proteome Res.* **2013**, *12*, 3317–3326. [CrossRef]
108. Schwabe, R.F.; Jobin, C. The microbiome and cancer. *Nat. Rev. Cancer.* **2013**, *13*, 800–812. [CrossRef]
109. Markowski, M.C.; Boorjian, S.A.; Burton, J.P.; Hahn, N.M.; Ingersoll, M.A.; Maleki Vareki, S.; Pal, S.K.; Sfanos, K.S. The Microbiome and Genitourinary Cancer: A Collaborative Review. *Eur. Urol.* **2019**, *75*, 637–646. [CrossRef]
110. Nagano, T.; Otoshi, T.; Hazama, D.; Kiriu, T.; Umezawa, K.; Katsurada, N.; Nishimura, Y. Novel cancer therapy targeting microbiome. *Onco. Targets Ther.* **2019**, *12*, 3619–3624. [CrossRef]
111. He, C.; Huang, L.; Lei, P.; Liu, X.; Li, B.; Shan, Y. Sulforaphane Normalizes Intestinal Flora and Enhances Gut Barrier in Mice with BBN-Induced Bladder Cancer. *Mol. Nutr. Food Res.* **2018**, *62*, e1800427. [CrossRef] [PubMed]
112. Bao, Y.; Wang, W.; Zhou, Z.; Sun, C. Benefits and risks of the hormetic effects of dietary isothiocyanates on cancer prevention. *PLoS ONE* **2014**, *9*, e114764. [CrossRef]
113. Wang, F.; Shan, Y. Sulforaphane retards the growth of UM-UC-3 xenographs, induces apoptosis, and reduces survivin in athymic mice. *Nutr. Res.* **2012**, *32*, 374–380. [CrossRef]
114. Alumkal, J.J.; Slottke, R.; Schwartzman, J.; Cherala, G.; Munar, M.; Graff, J.N.; Beer, T.M.; Ryan, C.W.; Koop, D.R. A phase II study of sulforaphane-rich broccoli sprout extracts in men with recurrent prostate cancer. *Invest. N. Drugs* **2015**, *33*, 480–489. [CrossRef]
115. Atwell, L.L.; Hsu, A.; Wong, C.P.; Stevens, J.F.; Bella, D.; Yu, T.W.; Pereira, C.B.; Lohr, C.V.; Christensen, J.M.; Dashwood, R.H.; et al. Absorption and chemopreventive targets of sulforaphane in humans following consumption of broccoli sprouts or a myrosinase-treated broccoli sprout extract. *Mol. Nutr. Food Res.* **2015**, *59*, 424–433. [CrossRef]
116. Islam, S.S.; Mokhtari, R.B.; Akbari, P.; Hatina, J.; Yeger, H.; Farhat, W.A. Simultaneous Targeting of Bladder Tumor Growth, Survival, and Epithelial-to-Mesenchymal Transition with a Novel Therapeutic Combination of Acetazolamide (AZ) and Sulforaphane (SFN). *Target Oncol.* **2016**, *11*, 209–227. [CrossRef]
117. Rakariyatham, K.; Yang, X.; Gao, Z.; Song, M.; Han, Y.; Chen, X.; Xiao, H. Synergistic chemopreventive effect of allyl isothiocyanate and sulforaphane on non-small cell lung carcinoma cells. *Food Funct.* **2019**, *10*, 893–902. [CrossRef]
118. Jiang, D.M.; Sridhar, S.S. Prime time for immunotherapy in advanced urothelial cancer. *Asia Pac. J. Clin. Oncol.* **2018**, *14* (Suppl. S5), 24–32. [CrossRef]
119. Fan, Z.; Liang, Y.; Yang, X.; Li, B.; Cui, L.; Luo, L.; Jia, Y.; Wang, Y.; Niu, H. A meta-analysis of the efficacy and safety of PD-1/PD-L1 immune checkpoint inhibitors as treatments for metastatic bladder cancer. *Onco Targets Ther.* **2019**, *12*, 1791–1801. [CrossRef]
120. Liang, J.; Hänsch, G.M.; Hübner, K.; Samstag, Y. Sulforaphane as anticancer agent: A double-edged sword? Tricky balance between effects on tumor cells and immune cells. *Adv. Biol. Regul.* **2019**, *71*, 79–87. [CrossRef]

121. Gupta, P.; Wright, S.E.; Kim, S.H.; Srivastava, S.K. Phenethyl isothiocyanate: A comprehensive review of anti-cancer mechanisms. *Biochim. Biophys. Acta.* **2014**, *1846*, 405–424. [PubMed]
122. Wang, X.; Govind, S.; Sajankila, S.P.; Mi, L.; Roy, R.; Chung, F.L. Phenethyl isothiocyanate sensitizes human cervical cancer cells to apoptosis induced by cisplatin. *Mol. Nutr. Food Res.* **2011**, *55*, 1572–1581. [CrossRef] [PubMed]
123. Tang, K.; Lin, Y.; Li, L.M. The role of phenethyl isothiocyanate on bladder cancer ADM resistance reversal and its molecular mechanism. *Anat. Rec. Hoboken* **2013**, *296*, 899–906. [CrossRef] [PubMed]
124. Pullar, J.M.; Thomson, S.J.; King, M.J.; Turnbull, C.I.; Midwinter, R.G.; Hampton, M.B. The chemopreventive agent phenethyl isothiocyanate sensitizes cells to Fas-mediated apoptosis. *Carcinogenesis* **2004**, *25*, 765–772. [CrossRef]
125. Teply, B.A.; Kim, J.J. Systemic therapy for bladder cancer—A medical oncologist's perspective. *J. Solid Tumors* **2014**, *4*, 25–35. [CrossRef]
126. Zargar, H.; Shah, J.B.; van Rhijn, B.W.; Daneshmand, S.; Bivalacqua, T.J.; Spiess, P.E.; Black, P.C.; Kassouf, W.; Collaborators. Neoadjuvant Dose Dense MVAC versus Gemcitabine and Cisplatin in Patients with cT3-4aN0M0 Bladder Cancer Treated with Radical Cystectomy. *J. Urol.* **2018**, *199*, 1452–1458. [CrossRef]
127. Yao, S.; Zhang, Y.; Li, J. c-jun/AP-1 activation does not affect the antiproliferative activity of phenethyl isothiocyanate, a cruciferous vegetable-derived cancer chemopreventive agent. *Mol. Carcinog.* **2006**, *45*, 605–612. [CrossRef]
128. Tachibana, H.; Gi, M.; Kato, M.; Yamano, S.; Fujioka, M.; Kakehashi, A.; Hirayama, Y.; Koyama, Y.; Tamada, S.; Nakatani, T.; et al. Carbonic anhydrase 2 is a novel invasion-associated factor in urinary bladder cancers. *Cancer Sci.* **2017**, *108*, 331–337. [CrossRef]
129. Sun, M.; Shi, Y.; Dang, U.J.; Di Pasqua, A.J. Phenethyl Isothiocyanate and Cisplatin Co-Encapsulated in a Liposomal Nanoparticle for Treatment of Non-Small Cell Lung Cancer. *Molecules* **2019**, *24*, 801. [CrossRef]
130. Yang, Y.-T.; Shi, Y.; Jay, M.; Di Pasqua, A.J. Enhanced toxicity of cisplatin with chemosensitizer phenethyl isothiocyanate toward non-small cell lung cancer cells when delivered in liposomal nanoparticles. *Chem. Res. Toxicol.* **2014**, *27*, 946–948. [CrossRef]
131. Hirose, M.; Yamaguchi, T.; Kimoto, N.; Ogawa, K.; Futakuchi, M.; Sano, M.; Shirai, T. Strong promoting activity of phenylethyl isothiocyanate and benzyl isothiocyanate on urinary bladder carcinogenesis in F344 male rats. *Int. J. Cancer* **1998**, *77*, 773–777. [CrossRef]
132. Akagi, K.; Sano, M.; Ogawa, K.; Hirose, M.; Goshima, H.; Shirai, T. Involvement of toxicity as an early event in urinary bladder carcinogenesis induced by phenethyl isothiocyanate, benzyl isothiocyanate, and analogues in F344 rats. *Toxicol. Pathol.* **2003**, *31*, 388–396. [CrossRef] [PubMed]
133. Lubet, R.A.; Steele, V.E.; Eto, I.; Juliana, M.M.; Kelloff, G.J.; Grubbs, C.J. Chemopreventive efficacy of anethole trithione, N-acetyl-L-cysteine, miconazole and phenethylisothiocyanate in the DMBA-induced rat mammary cancer model. *Int. J. Cancer* **1997**, *72*, 95–101. [CrossRef]
134. Sugiura, S.; Ogawa, K.; Hirose, M.; Takeshita, F.; Asamoto, M.; Shirai, T. Reversibility of proliferative lesions and induction of non-papillary tumors in rat urinary bladder treated with phenylethyl isothiocyanate. *Carcinogenesis* **2003**, *24*, 547–553. [CrossRef]
135. Ogawa, K.; Futakuchi, M.; Hirose, M.; Boonyaphiphat, P.; Mizoguchi, Y.; Miki, T.; Shirai, T. Stage and organ dependent effects of 1-O-hexyl-2,3,5-trimethylhydroquinone, ascorbic acid derivatives, n-heptadecane-8,10-dione and phenylethyl isothiocyanate in a rat multiorgan carcinogenesis model. *Int. J. Cancer* **1998**, *76*, 851–856. [CrossRef]
136. Ogawa, K.; Hirose, M.; Sugiura, S.; Cui, L.; Imaida, K.; Ogiso, T.; Shirai, T. Dose dependent promotion by phenylethyl isothiocyanate, a known chemopreventer, of two-stage rat urinary bladder and liver carcinogenesis. *Nutr. Cancer* **2001**, *40*, 134–139. [CrossRef]
137. Sones, K.; Heaney, R.K.; Fenwick, G.R. An estimate of the mean daily Intake of glucosinolates from cruciferous vegetables in the UK. *J. Sci. Food Agric.* **1984**, *35*, 712–720. [CrossRef]
138. Chung, F.L.; Morse, M.A.; Eklind, K.I.; Lewis, J. Quatitation of human uptake of the anticarcinogen phenethyl isothiocyanate after a watercress meal. *Cancer Epidemiol. Biomark. Prev.* **1992**, *1*, 383–388.
139. Krajka-Kuźniak, V.; Paluszczak, J.; Szaefer, H.; Baer-Dubowska, W. The activation of the Nrf2/ARE pathway in HepG2 hepatoma cells by phytochemicals and subsequent modulation of phase II and antioxidant enzyme expression. *J. Physiol. Biochem.* **2015**, *71*, 227–738. [CrossRef]

140. Becker, T.M.; Juvik, J.A. The Role of Glucosinolate Hydrolysis Products from Brassica Vegetable Consumption in Inducing Antioxidant Activity and Reducing Cancer Incidence. *Diseases* **2016**, *4*, 22. [CrossRef]
141. Soundararajan, P.; Kim, J.S. Anti-Carcinogenic Glucosinolates in Cruciferous Vegetables and Their Antagonistic Effects on Prevention of Cancers. *Molecules* **2018**, *23*, 2983. [CrossRef] [PubMed]
142. Cumberbatch, M.G.K.; Jubber, I.; Black, P.C.; Esperto, F.; Figueroa, J.D.; Kamat, A.M.; Kiemeney, L.; Lotan, Y.; Pang, K.; Silverman, D.T. Epidemiology of Bladder Cancer: A Systematic Review and Contemporary Update of Risk Factors in 2018. *Eur. Urol.* **2018**, *74*, 784–795. [CrossRef] [PubMed]
143. Ou, Z.; Wang, Y.; Chen, J.; Tao, L.; Zuo, L.; Sahasrabudhe, D.; Joseph, J.; Wang, L.; Yeh, S. Estrogen receptor β promotes bladder cancer growth and invasion via alteration of miR-92a/DAB2IP signals. *Exp. Mol. Med.* **2018**, *50*, 152. [CrossRef] [PubMed]
144. Ye, X.; Guo, J.; Zhang, H.; Meng, Q.; Ma, Y.; Lin, R.; Yi, X.; Lu, H.; Bai, X.; Cheng, J. The enhanced expression of estrogen-related receptor α in human bladder cancer tissues and the effects of estrogen-related receptor α knockdown on bladder cancer cells. *J. Cell Biochem.* **2019**, *120*, 13841–13852. [CrossRef]
145. Ioannides, C.; Konsue, N. A principal mechanism for the cancer chemopreventive activity of phenethyl isothiocyanate is modulation of carcinogen metabolism. *Drug Metab. Rev.* **2015**, *47*, 356–373. [CrossRef]
146. Yuan, J.M.; Stepanov, I.; Murphy, S.E.; Wang, R.; Allen, S.; Jensen, J.; Strayer, L.; Adams-Haduch, J.; Upadhyaya, P.; Le, C. Clinical Trial of 2-Phenethyl Isothiocyanate as an Inhibitor of Metabolic Activation of a Tobacco-Specific Lung Carcinogen in Cigarette Smokers. *Cancer Prev. Res.* **2016**, *9*, 396–405. [CrossRef]
147. Sanguedolce, F.; Cormio, L.; Carrieri, G.; Calò, B.; Russo, D.; Menin, A.; Pastore, A.L.; Greco, F.; Bozzini, G.; Galfano, A. Role of androgen receptor expression in non-muscle-invasive bladder cancer: A systematic review and meta-analysis. *Histol. Histopathol.* **2019**, in press.
148. Beklemisheva, A.A.; Feng, J.; Yeh, Y.A.; Wang, L.G.; Chiao, J.W. Modulating testosterone stimulated prostate growth by phenethyl isothiocyanate via Sp1 and androgen receptor down-regulation. *Prostate* **2007**, *67*, 863–870. [CrossRef]
149. Gianfredi, V.; Vannini, S.; Moretti, M.; Villarini, M.; Bragazzi, N.L.; Izzotti, A.; Nucci, D. Sulforaphane and Epigallocatechin Gallate Restore Estrogen Receptor Expression by Modulating Epigenetic Events in the Breast Cancer Cell Line MDA-MB-231: A Systematic Review and Meta-Analysis. *J. Nutrigenet. Nutrigenomics* **2017**, *10*, 126–135. [CrossRef]

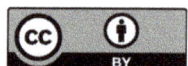

© 2020 by the authors. Licensee MDPI, Basel, Switzerland. This article is an open access article distributed under the terms and conditions of the Creative Commons Attribution (CC BY) license (http://creativecommons.org/licenses/by/4.0/).

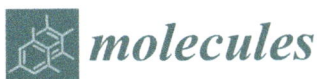

Review

Antiangiogenic Effects of Coumarins against Cancer: From Chemistry to Medicine

Mohammad Bagher Majnooni [1], Sajad Fakhri [2], Antonella Smeriglio [3], Domenico Trombetta [3], Courtney R. Croley [4], Piyali Bhattacharyya [5], Eduardo Sobarzo-Sánchez [6,7], Mohammad Hosein Farzaei [2,*] and Anupam Bishayee [4,*]

1. Student Research Committee, Kermanshah University of Medical Sciences, Kermanshah 6714415153, Iran; mb.majnooni64@yahoo.com
2. Pharmaceutical Sciences Research Center, Health Institute, Kermanshah University of Medical Sciences, Kermanshah 6734667149, Iran; pharmacy.sajad@yahoo.com
3. Department of Chemical, Biological, Pharmaceutical and Environmental Sciences, University of Messina, Viale Palatucci, 98168 Messina, Italy; asmeriglio@unime.it (A.S.); domenico.trombetta@unime.it (D.T.)
4. Lake Erie College of Osteopathic Medicine, Bradenton, FL 34211, USA; CCroley48578@med.lecom.edu
5. Escuela de Ciencias de la Salud, Universidad Ana G. Méndez, Recinto de Gurabo, Gurabo, PR 00778, USA; pbhattacharyya@suagm.edu
6. Laboratory of Pharmaceutical Chemistry, Department of Organic Chemistry, Faculty of Pharmacy, University of Santiago de Compostela, 15782 Santiago de Compostela, Spain; e.sobarzo@usc.es or eduardo.sobarzo@ucentral.cl
7. Instituto de Investigación e Innovación en Salud, Facultad de Ciencias de la Salud, Universidad Central de Chile, Santiago 8330507, Chile
* Correspondence: mh.farzaei@gmail.com (M.H.F.); abishayee@lecom.edu or abishayee@gmail.com (A.B.)

Academic Editor: Kyoko Nakagawa-Goto
Received: 27 October 2019; Accepted: 19 November 2019; Published: 24 November 2019

Abstract: Angiogenesis, the process of formation and recruitment of new blood vessels from pre-existing vessels, plays an important role in the development of cancer. Therefore, the use of antiangiogenic agents is one of the most critical strategies for the treatment of cancer. In addition, the complexity of cancer pathogenicity raises the need for multi-targeting agents. Coumarins are multi-targeting natural agents belonging to the class of benzopyrones. Coumarins have several biological and pharmacological effects, including antimicrobial, antioxidant, anti-inflammation, anticoagulant, anxiolytic, analgesic, and anticancer properties. Several reports have shown that the anticancer effect of coumarins and their derivatives are mediated through targeting angiogenesis by modulating the functions of vascular endothelial growth factor as well as vascular endothelial growth factor receptor 2, which are involved in cancer pathogenesis. In the present review, we focus on the antiangiogenic effects of coumarins and related structure-activity relationships with particular emphasis on cancer.

Keywords: coumarins; antiangiogenic; cancer; natural agents; chemistry; medicine

1. Introduction

Angiogenesis (also known as neovascularization), the growth of blood vessels from the existing vasculature, has been shown to play a critical role in the development of various diseases, including rheumatoid arthritis, diabetic retinopathy, asthma, endometriosis, psoriasis, obesity, and cancer [1–3]. Inflammation, tissue ischemia, and hypoxia which cause the release of the angiogenesis factors, such as vascular endothelial growth factor (VEGF), cytokines, cell adhesion molecules, and nitric oxide (NO), are among the most important triggers of angiogenesis [4]. In 1971, Folkman reported that tumor metastasis occurs as a consequence of angiogenesis [5]. This was the starting point for the design and use of bevacizumab, thalidomide, sunitinib, and axitinib as antiangiogenic drugs in the treatment of a variety of cancers [6–8]. Considering the crucial role of angiogenesis in the progression of cancer, investigating novel and potential antiangiogenic compounds is of great importance to combat cancer. Several naturally occurring compounds, including vinblastine, vincristine, paclitaxel, were reported as antiangiogenic and anticancer agents. Besides, other natural compounds with antiangiogenic activities, such as resveratrol, artemisinin, boswellic acid, and cannabidiol, have shown enormous potential for cancer prevention and therapy [9–13]. For instance, endocannabinoid 2-arachidonoyl-glycerol showed a promising anticancer effect in several cell lines [14]. Overall, cancer remains a clinical challenge, despite advancements in its treatment. This raises the need to investigate novel multi-target agents to attenuate multiple signaling pathways involved in tumor progression.

Growing evidence has introduced coumarins as potential multi-targeting agents with various pharmacological effects and medicinal uses [15]. Coumarins, with their 2H-1-benzopyran-2-one structure, are natural compounds that exist in various plant families, including Apiaceae, Asteraceae, Fabaceae, Rutaceae, Moraceae, Oleaceae, and Thymelaeaceae [16]. Apiaceae is the greatest family of plants containing coumarin compounds [16]. Also, due to the antioxidant [17], anti-inflammatory [18], anxiolytic [19], analgesic [20], neuroprotective [21], cardioprotective [22], antidiabetic [23], and anticancer [24] activities of coumarins [25], researchers have studied the synthesis of various coumarin derivatives, in addition to their purification from natural sources [26]. Both synthetic and natural coumarins have shown noticeable anticancer effects in vitro and in vivo through various mechanisms [27], including the inhibition of angiogenesis [28,29]. From a mechanistic point of view, some coumarins have shown promising antiangiogenic effects through the interaction with and repression of signaling mediators involved in angiogenesis [30,31].

In this review, we focus on the cellular signaling pathways of angiogenesis and recent pharmacological antiangiogenic agents, emphasizing natural and synthetic coumarins with antiangiogenic effects as well as their pharmacological mechanisms and structure-activity relationship in cancer.

2. Angiogenesis: Biology and Cellular Signaling

Angiogenesis could be controlled by achieving a balance among activating cytokines and growth factors on one hand and inhibiting agents on the other, which stimulate or inhibit endothelial cells (ECs), respectively. Proangiogenic agents include growth factors, namely, VEGF, fibroblast growth factors, epidermal growth factor (EGF), transforming growth factor-β (TGF-β), platelet-derived growth factor (PDGF), placental growth factor (PGF), hepatocyte growth factor/scatter factor (HGF/SF), and cytokines, such as tumor necrosis factor-α (TNF-α), colony-stimulating factor-1 (CSF-1), and interleukin-8 (IL-8) [32–35]. ECs, fibroblasts, platelets, smooth muscle cells, inflammatory cells, and cancer cells are involved in producing angiogenic growth factors and cytokines [4].

VEGF and FGF have been considered as promising antiangiogenic targets [35]. VEGF mainly acts through tyrosine kinase VEGF receptor 2 (VEGFR2) [36]. Furthermore, bioactive lipids, such as prostaglandin E_2 (PGE$_2$), and sphingosine-1-phosphate (S1P), matrix degenerating enzymes, namely, matrix metalloproteinases (MMP) and heparinases, small mediators (e.g., NO, peroxynitrite, serotonin, and histamine), angiopoietins (Ang), and erythropoietin are among other activators of angiogenesis [35]. In order to attract other angiogenesis-stimulating factors, cancer cells induce a situation of hypoxia by increasing the demand for nutrients and oxygen. In the hypoxic condition, hypoxia-inducible factor-1α (HIF-1α), together with released anti-apoptotic factors, growth factors, and cytokines, provokes angiogenesis [4,37].

On the other hand, angiogenesis could be suppressed by inhibiting proteins, which are classified into either direct or indirect angiogenesis inhibitors. The first class of inhibitors directly suppress ECs in the growing vasculature, while the second class indirectly suppress either tumor cells or other tumor-associated stromal cells [35,38]. This direct inhibitory effect could also be mediated by integrin receptors through several intracellular signaling pathways [39]. Angiostatin, endostatin, arrestin, canstatin, and tumstatin are released by the proteolysis of distinct endothelial cell-matrix molecules and prevent vascular ECs from proliferating and migrating in response to angiogenesis inducers [40]. Interferons, retinoic acid, IL-1, IL-12, tissue inhibitor of metalloproteinases, and multimerin 2 are other angiogenesis inhibitors [41,42].

As previously mentioned, angiogenesis is controlled by a balance between activators and inhibitors of angiogenesis. Hypoxia, as a critical determinant, causes an imbalance between activators and inhibitors by inducing the upregulation of HIF-1α, which elevates the expression of pro-angiogenesis agents as well as suppresses the expression of angiogenesis inhibitors [43]. Therefore, all the mediators in these pathways could be therapeutic targets to inhibit angiogenesis.

3. Recent Advancement in Pharmacological Antiangiogenic Agents

Several angiogenesis inhibitors have been found since Folkman first presented the concept of introducing angiogenesis inhibitors as anticancer drugs [5]. RNA interference (RNAi) therapy, chimeric antigen receptor T cell therapy, gene therapy, and pharmacological agents are auspicious antiangiogenic interventions [44]. According to the United States Food and Drug Administration (FDA), approved antiangiogenic agents are classified into two major groups, namely, monoclonal antibodies (mAbs) and small molecules [45].

VEGF receptors (VEGFRs) and related downstream signaling pathways are crucial targets of mAbs. Small molecules also target receptors, including PDGFR, VEGFR, Fms-like tyrosine kinase 3, and c-Kit receptor, and signaling proteins such as Raf, mitogen-activated protein kinase (MAPK), mammalian target of rapamycin (mTOR), and phosphoinositide 3-kinases (PI3K). Besides, the antiangiogenic/anticancer effects of FDA-approved herbal drugs, including vinca [46], taxan [47], camptothecins [48], podophyllotoxins [49], and homoharringtonine [50], related receptors, and downstream signaling pathways have now been confirmed [13].

VEGF (A–D), PDGF (A–D), HGF [51,52], and FGF [53,54] bind to VEGFR (1 and 2), PDGFR (α and β), MET [55,56], and FGFR (1-4) tyrosine kinase receptors, respectively, and activate downstream signaling pathways, thereby regulating cell growth, differentiation, and angiogenesis [54,57–59]. Their overactivation is attributed to several mutations promoting tumor vascularization in different types of cancers [60,61], while their inhibitors exert antitumor effects [62]. Bevacizumab, aflibercept, and ramucirumab have been developed as antiangiogenic agents to target the VEGF/VEGFR signaling pathway [63].

Angiopoietins (Ang1–4) bind to the Tie2 receptor. While Ang1 helps the vessels stabilize, Ang2 is secreted by ECs in response to proangiogenic factors, including hypoxia, cytokines, and inflammation [64]. Ang/Tie2-targeted therapy is challenging, since it could be either antitumor or protumor, depending on the context [65].

The rearranged during transfection (RET) protein binds receptor tyrosine kinases (RTKs) associated with normal development, maintenance, and maturation of cells and tissues [66]. However, its mutation is related to the growth and progression of tumors [66,67]. Therefore, RET inhibition could be of great importance in combating cancer.

Multi-targeting antiangiogenic drugs are shown in Figure 1. These drugs exert anticancer effects through simultaneously modulating several signaling pathways involved in angiogenesis.

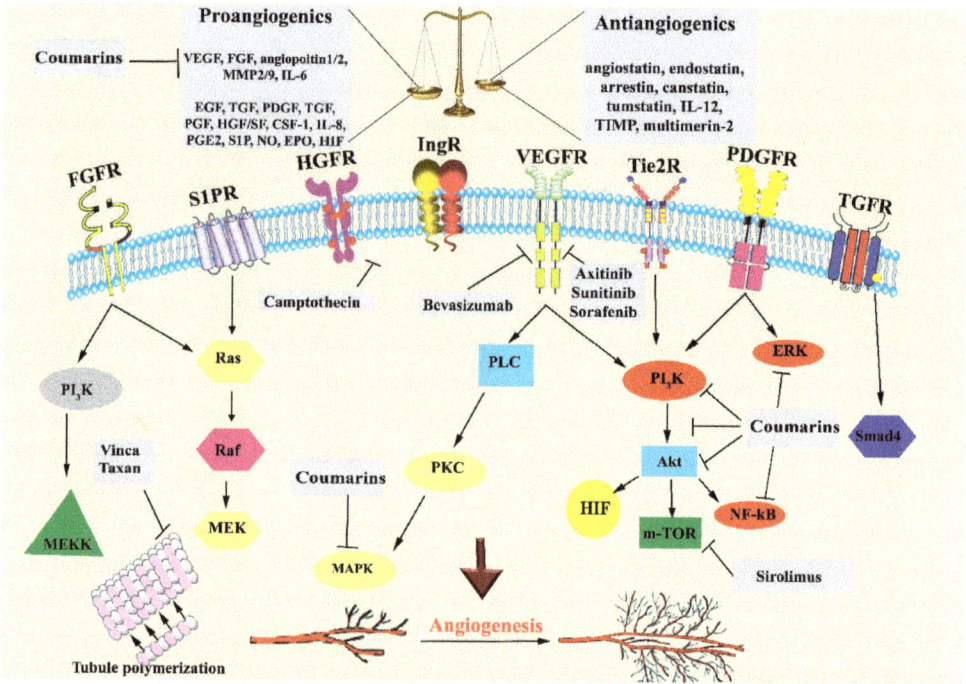

Figure 1. Signaling pathways and therapeutic targets of antiangiogenic and anticancer drugs and agents. VEGF, vascular endothelial growth factor; FGF, fibroblast growth factor; EGF, epidermal growth factor; TGF-β, transforming growth factor-β; PDGF, platelet-derived growth factor; PGF, placental growth factor; HGF/SF, hepatocyte growth factor/scatter factor; TNF-α, tumor necrosis factor-α; CSF-1, colony-stimulating factor-1; IL, interleukin; MMP, matrix metalloproteinase; TIMPs, tissue inhibitors of metalloproteinases; S1PR, sphingosine-1-phosphate receptor; NO, nitric oxide; PI3K:,phosphatidylinositol-3-kinase; PLC, phospholipase C; PKC, protein kinase C; HIF, hypoxia-inducible factor; and m-TOR: mammalian target of rapamycin.

4. Coumarins

4.1. Chemical Structure and Sources

Coumarin ($C_9H_6O_2$, 2H-1-benzopyran-2-one, 146.145 g/mol) and its derivatives (Figure 2) are a large class of natural compounds that are widely distributed in the plant kingdom and are biosynthesized from ortho-hydroxy-cinnamic acid in the shikimic acid pathways [68]. In terms of chemical structure, coumarins are subdivided into four main groups: (a) simple coumarins, such as heparin and scopoletin; (b) furanocoumarins (linear and angular), such as bergapten and imperatorin; (c) pyranocoumarins, such as grandivittin and agasyllin; (d) dicoumarins and pyrone-substituted coumarins, such as phenylcoumarins (Figure 2) [69–71].

Coumarins are isolated and purified from fruits, leaves, stems, roots, and flowers of more than 40 plant families. The Apiaceae represents a family of plants with the highest number of species producing coumarins, including *Anethum graveolens*, *Angelica dahurica*, *Apium graveolens*, *Petroselinum crispum* and *Heracleum mantegazzianum*. Other plant families producing coumarins are Rutaceae (*Citrus aurantium*, *Citrus sinensis*, and *Melicope glabra*), Asteraceae (*Matricaria recutita* and *Achillea millefolium*), Fabaceae (*Melilotus officinalis* and *Glycyrriza glabra*), and Moraceae (*Ficus carica*) [16,72–76].

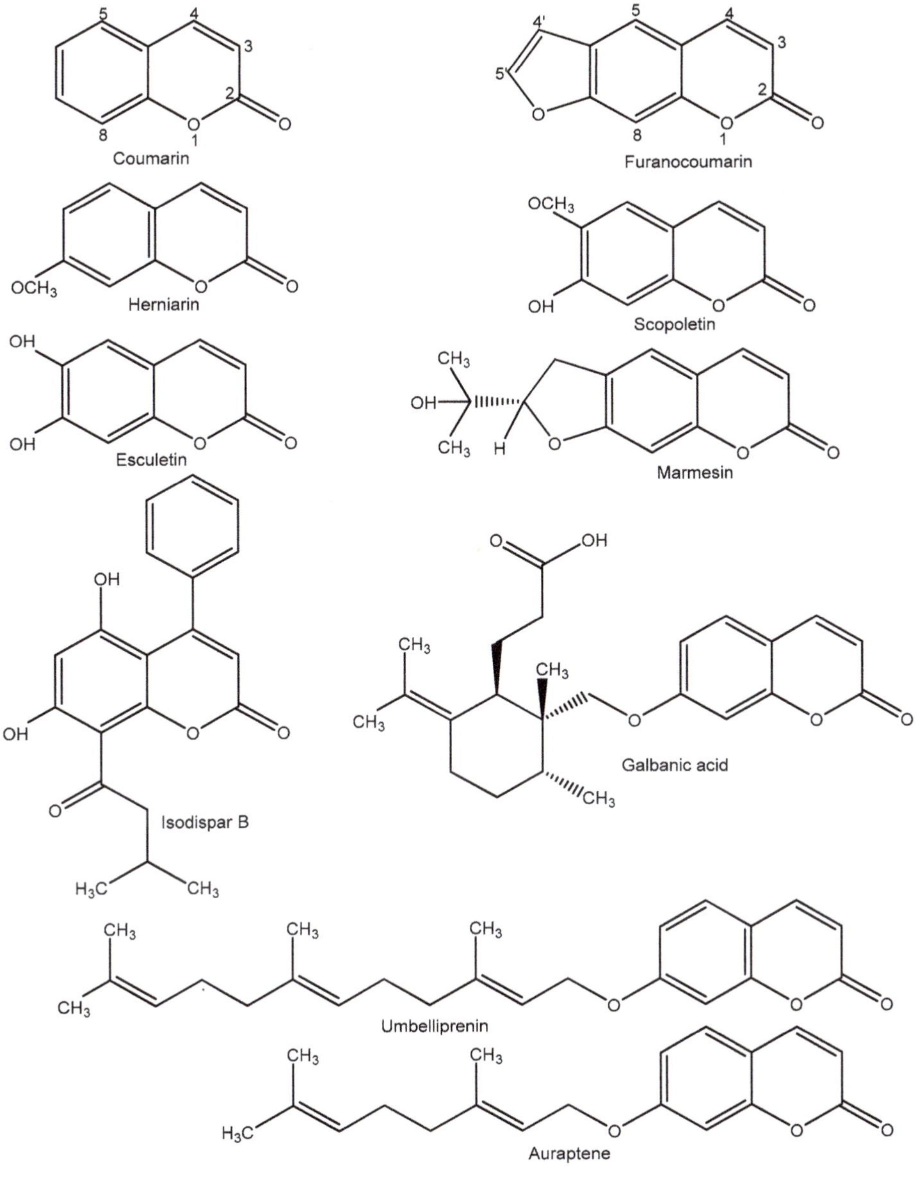

Figure 2. *Cont.*

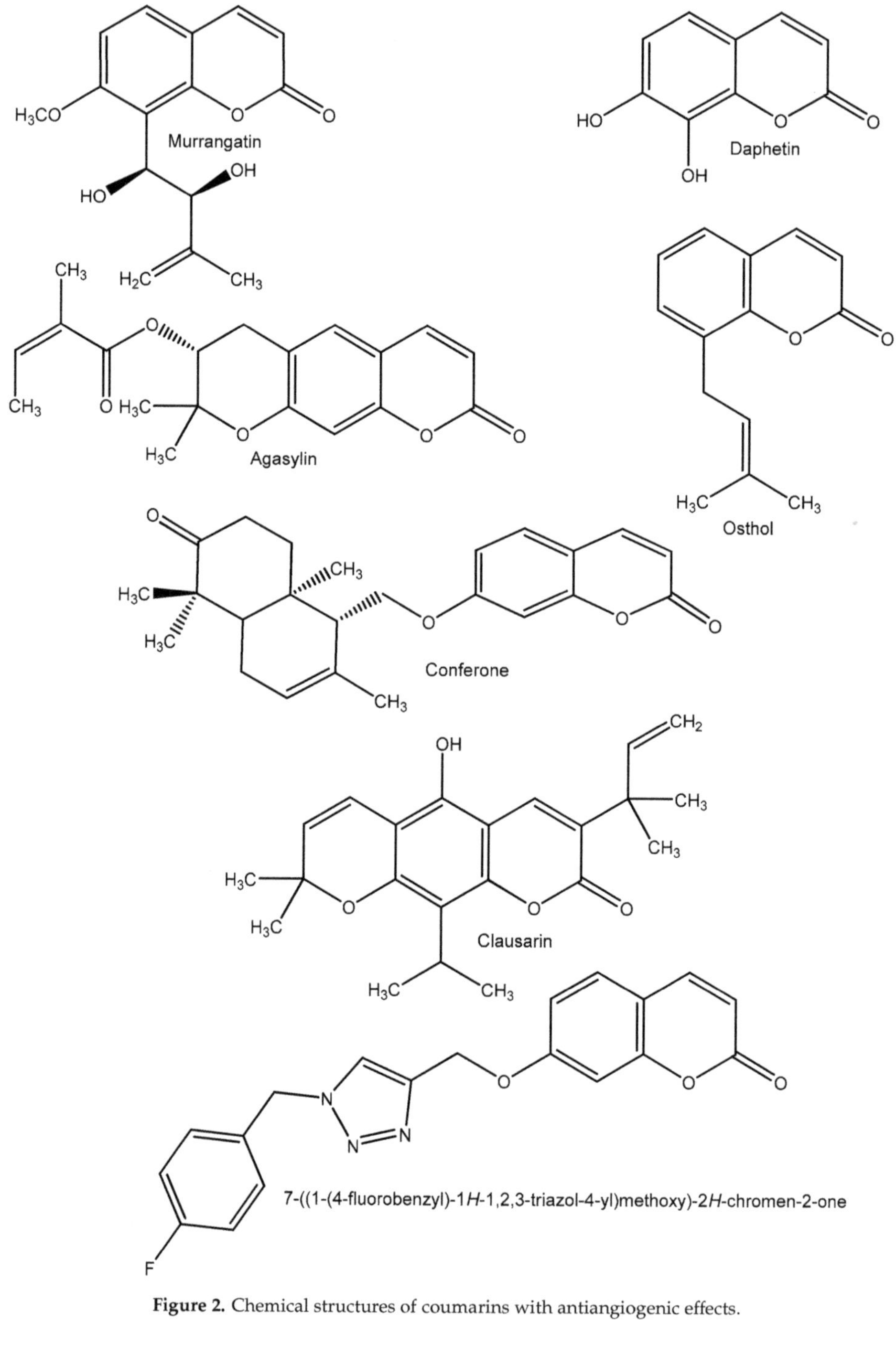

Figure 2. Chemical structures of coumarins with antiangiogenic effects.

4.2. Biological and Pharmacological Effects of Coumarins

Coumarins have several biological and pharmacological effects. For example, coumarins isolated from the bark of *M. glabra* showed antioxidant properties [73]. In this line, antimicrobial effects of coumarins from the fruits of *H. mantegazzianum* Sommier & Levier as well as *Peucedanum luxurians* Tamamsch were reported [76,77]. Antiviral effects of coumarins isolated from *Prangos ferulacea* L. have been shown by Shokoohinia et al. [78]. In addition, anxiolytic effects of coumarin derivatives, purified from the root of *Biebersteinia multifida* DC, have been demonstrated [79]. Other coumarins, such as umbelliferone and pimpinellin, were isolated from the root of *Zosima absinthifolia* and these compounds showed anti-Alzheimer effects [80]. Kontogiorgis and co-workers [81] designed and synthesized coumarin derivatives based on azomethine, with anti-inflammatory activities. Synthesized coumarins based on 3,4-dihydro-2H-benzothiazines showed analgesic effects in formalin- and acetic acid-induced writhing tests [82]. Additionally, various coumarins have shown antiulcerogenic [83], spasmolytic [84], anticoagulant [85], vasorelaxant [86], cytotoxic, and anticancer activities [87].

On the other hand, hepatotoxicity, nausea, and diarrhea were reported as the side effects of coumarin derivatives [88,89].

4.3. Coumarins as Anticancer Agents

As the second leading cause of death worldwide, cancer is one of the most critical diseases that threaten public health and imposes a high cost on countries' health systems each year. Because of the resistance of cancer cells to conventional drugs used in chemotherapy as well as the side effects of these drugs, it is necessary to find new anticancer agents. Undoubtedly, medicinal plants are one of the richest sources of biologically active compounds and potential novel anticancer drugs. Coumarins are natural compounds with low to moderate side effects, which have been introduced by researchers as promising anticancer compounds [29,90–92]. Several coumarins also inhibit cytochrome P450, thereby affecting the blood concentration of various anticancer drugs. In this line, bergamottin inhibits cytochrome P450 and reduces the effects of various carcinogenic agents [93].

The anticancer and cytotoxic activities of synthetic and natural coumarins with different functional groups on their basic structure (Figure 2) have been reported by several investigators. These studies showed the anticancer activity of coumarins against breast cancer [89], colon cancer [94], lung cancer [24], ovarian cancer [95], hepatocellular carcinoma [96], bladder carcinoma [97], leukemia [98], and other types of cancer in vitro and in vivo, via different mechanisms, including free-radical scavenging, antioxidant activity [99], induction of cell cycle arrest [100], interaction with various signaling pathways with important role in cell differentiation and proliferation [101], telomerase and carbonic anhydrase inhibition [102,103], and antiangiogenic activity [104]. For example, Taniguchi and co-workers [105] isolated eight coumarins from the leaves of *Rhizophora mucronata* and reported the anticancer effects of methoxyinophyllum P, calocoumarin B, and calophyllolide against HeLa cells (cervical cancer), with IC_{50} equal to 3.8, 29.9, and 36.4 µM, respectively, and HL-60 cells (promyelocytic leukemia cells) with IC_{50} of 12.9, 2.6, and 2.2 µM, respectively. Also, three hemiterpene ether coumarins, isolated from *Artemisia armeniaca* Lam, showed cytotoxic effects in HL-60 and K562 cells (chronic myelogenous leukemia cells). In their study, armenin showed the highest cytotoxic effect through cycle arrest, with IC_{50} equal to 22.5 and 71.1 µM for K562 and HL-60 cells, respectively [106].

Among coumarins, clausarin, nordentatin, dentatin, and xanthoxyletin, isolated from dichloromethane extraction of root bark of *Clausena harmandiana*, showed high cytotoxic activities [107]. In this study, clausarin (Figure 2) showed the highest cytotoxic activity, which was superior to that of cisplatin used as a positive control, against hepatocellular carcinoma (HepG2, $IC_{50} = 17.6 \pm 2.1$ µM), colorectal carcinoma (HCT116, $IC_{50} = 44.9 \pm 1.4$ µM), and lung adenocarcinoma (SK-LU-1, $IC_{50} = 6.9 \pm 1.6$ µM) cell lines. Clausarin also showed the highest antioxidant activity in the 2,2-diphenyl-1-picryl-hydrazyl-hydrate scavenging assay. From a mechanistic point of view, apoptosis induction was reported as an anticancer mechanism of coumarins [107].

On the other hand, several studies have been carried out on the synthesis of coumarins to produce coumarin derivatives with improved anticancer effects. Among them, synthetic scopoletin derivatives have shown promising antitumor activities. In their study, out of 20 synthesized derivatives of scopoletin, 5 compounds showed the greatest effects (IC$_{50}$ < 2 µM) in MCF-7 and MDA-MB 231 cells (human breast adenocarcinoma cell line) as well as in HT29 cells (human colorectal adenocarcinoma cell line). The relationship between the increase in Log P value and the increase in cytotoxic activity was established in this investigation. Cell cycle arrest was also suggested as the anticancer mechanism of these compounds [108].

Besides, Zang et al. [105] synthesized novel anticancer analogs of geiparvarin using a bioisosteric transformation method. In their study, it was also shown that adding electron-withdrawing substituents to the benzene rings, such as 7-((1-(4-fluorobenzyl)-1H-1,2,3-triazol-4-yl)methoxy)-4Hchromen-4-one (Figure 2), increased their cytotoxic effects in a human hepatoma cell line (QGY-7701, IC$_{50}$ = 14.37 ± 9.93) and a colon carcinoma cell line (SW480, IC$_{50}$ = 11.18 ± 2.16) compared with geiparvarin (IC$_{50}$ = 17.68 ± 0.40 and 20.34 ± 0.75, respectively) [109]. Additionally, Cui and co-workers [110] showed the anticancer effects of three synthesized coumarins derived from triphenylethylene, occurring through the inhibition of angiogenesis.

Considering the above investigations on the anticancer effects of coumarin derivatives, these compounds could be developed as anticancer drugs.

5. Coumarin and Angiogenesis Inhibition

Inhibition of angiogenesis is one of the most critical anticancer mechanisms of secondary plant metabolites, including coumarins. Natural and synthetic coumarins with different structures can inhibit the factors involved in angiogenesis, migration, proliferation, and differentiation of endothelial cells in vitro and in vivo. Coumarins act by blocking various molecular signaling pathways, involving growth factors (e.g., VEGFs, TNF-α, and FGF-2), cytokines (e.g., IL-1 and IL-6), angiogenic enzymes (e.g., MMP), endothelial-specific receptor tyrosine kinases (e.g., Tie2), and adhesion molecules (e.g., intercellular adhesion molecule-1) [30,111,112].

5.1. Natural Coumarins with Antiangiogenic Effects

The antiangiogenic effects of coumarins from natural sources, especially isolated and purified from plants, are reported in several studies. Scopoletin [113,114], esculetin [104], herniarin [115], decursin, and decursinol [116] with coumarin structure, as well as imperatorin [117] and psoralidine [118] with furanocoumarin structure (Figure 2), are among the natural antiangiogenic coumarins.

Pan and co-workers [119] showed the antiangiogenic effects of scopoletin, isolated from *Erycibe obtusifolia* Benth stem, in vitro and in vivo. In their study, scopoletin markedly reduced the number of blood vessel branch points after a 48-h treatment with the dose of 100 nmol/egg in the chick chorioallantoic membrane (CAM) model. Additionally, the inhibitory effects of scopoletin on migration, proliferation, and tube formation of human umbilical vein endothelial cells (HUVECs) induced by VEGF (10 ng/mL) were observed. These investigators showed that the proliferation of HUVECs was significantly inhibited by 100 µM scopoletin after 72 h, and tube formation and migration of HUVECs were inhibited following treatment with 100 µM scopoletin by 52.4% and 38.1%, respectively [119].

Decursin and decursinol angelate, isolated from *Angelica gigas* root, showed substantial antiangiogenic effects in vitro and in vivo [120]. These natural coumarins significantly decreased the development of blood vessels in transgenic zebrafish embryos at 20 µM concentration as well as in the CAM model at 6 µM/egg. In their study, the inhibition of VEGFR2 (one of the most important receptors of VEGF) and other angiogenesis signaling pathway related to VGEF, such as phosphorylated extracellular signal-regulated kinase (p-ERK) and MAPK as well as phosphorylated-c-Jun N-terminal kinase (JNK) in ECs were observed [116].

The antiangiogenic effect of marmesin (Figure 2), a furanocoumarin isolated from ethanolic extract of the twigs of *Broussonetia kazinoki*, was reported by Kim et al. [121]. They showed that marmesin at 10 μM significantly inhibited the expression and activity of MMP-2 in response to VEGF-A (10 ng/mL) in HUVECs. Besides, marmesin reduced EC proliferation, migration, invasion, tube formation and also induced cell cycle arrest in a concentration-dependent manner. Marmesin at 10 μM also inhibited the development of angiogenesis in the rat aortic ring model. VEGF-A stimulated various critical molecules of angiogenesis signaling pathways, such as focal adhesion kinase (FAK), Src kinase, MEK, ERK, Akt, and p70S6K. These pathways were inhibited by 10 μM marmesin [121]. In another study, osthol, columbianadin and columbianetin acetate, three coumarins isolated from *Angelicae Pubescentis* Radix, showed inhibitory effects on the secretion of monocyte chemoattractant protein-1, a pro-inflammation factor and one of the most important migration-regulating chemokines [122]. On the other hand, conferone, a sesquiterpene coumarin isolated from *Ferula szwitziana*, showed antiangiogenic and cytotoxic effects on a human colorectal adenocarcinoma cell line (HT-29) through reducing proangiogenic factors, including angiopoietin 1 and 2 [123]. Besides, daphnetin (7,8-hydroxy coumarin), another natural coumarin, inhibited the expression of MAPK, VEGFR2, ERK1/2, AKT, FAK, and cSrc, which are involved in angiogenesis [124] (Table 1). Also, inhibiting PI3K/AKT activity, another angiogenesis inducer pathway, is one of the antiangiogenic mechanisms of murrangatin purified from *Micromelum falcatum* [125]. Moreover, reducing and blocking VEGF and MMPs are among the most important antiangiogenic mechanisms of coumarins such as galbanic acid [126], umbelliprenin [127], imperatorin [117], auraptene [128], esculetin [31], osthole [129], and scopolin [130] (Table 1).

Table 1. Natural coumarins with antiangiogenic effects and their mechanisms.

Coumarin	Sources	Mechanism of Action	Concentrations	Reference
Galbanic acid	*Ferula assafoetida*	Decreases molecular angiogenesis pathways including VEGF, MAPK, JNK, and AKT	5, 10, 20, 40 μM for in vitro study and 0.1, 1 mg/Kg for Lewis lung cancer (LLC) mouse model, intraperitoneally (i.p.) injected once daily for 18 days	[126]
Umbelliprenin	*Ferula* species	Reduces and blocks angiogenesis marker activity including Ki-67, CD31, VEGF, MMP2, MMP9, and E-cadherin	3, 6.25, 12.5, 25, 50, 100, and 200 μg/mL	[127]
Murrangatin	*Micromelum falcatum*	Inhibition of phosphoinositol 3-kinase (PI3K)/AKT activity as angiogenic inducer	10, 50, 100 μM	[125]
Imperatorin	*Angelica dahurica* and *Angelica archangelica*	Blocks the expression of nuclear factor (NF-κB) target genes, such as MMP-9, VEGF, IL-6 that are induced by TNF-α	50, 100, 150 μM	[117]
Auraptene	*Citrus sinensis*	Inhibition of angiogenesis via suppression of MMP-2,9	12.5, 25, 50, 100 μM	[128]
Esculetin	*Artemisia scoparia*	Inhibition of angiogenesis via decreasing MMP expression and blocking phosphorylation of VEGFR-2, ERK1/2, Akt, and endothelial nitric oxide synthase (eNOS) induced by VEGF (20 ng/mL)	12.5, 25, 50 μg/ml	[31]
Osthol	*Cnidium monnieri*	Reduction of microvessel density (MVD) with blocked expression of VEGF and NF-κB	61, 122, and 244 mg/kg, i.p, once daily for two weeks in a mouse model of hepatocellular carcinoma (HCC)	[129]
Conferone	*Ferula szwitsiana*	Reduction of the production of the pro-angiogenic factors VEGF, Angiopoietin-1, and Angiopoietin -2	20 μM	[123]
Daphnetin	*Changbai daphne*	Inhibition of the expression of proteins involved in angiogenesis induced by VEGF such as MAPK, VEGFR2, ERK1/2, AKT, focal adhesion kinase (FAK), cSrc, and MMP and inhibition of NF-κB induced by TNF-α	37.5, 75, 150 μM	[124]
Scopolin	*Erycibe obtusifolia* Benth	Decreases VEGF, FGF-2 and IL-6 expressions	25, 50, 100 mg/kg, i.p, once daily for 10 days	[130]

5.2. Synthetic Coumarins with Antiangiogenic Effects

Angiogenesis is a critical process in the development and progression of cancer, as demonstrated by various pre-clinical and clinical evidence. Among natural-based entities, coumarins present little cytotoxicity, while demonstrating more powerful antiangiogenic effects than conventional cytotoxic drugs [131,132]. Semi-synthesized and synthesized products from natural coumarins, used as lead compounds, led to the discovery of interesting antiangiogenic and non-cytotoxic molecules. Coumarins with interesting antiangiogenic and non-cytotoxic properties almost entirely mimic the behavior of the physiological ligands of the main therapeutic targets [132]. Recently, several sulfonyl derivatives of coumarins have been studied as cytotoxic and antiangiogenic agents against HepG2 hepatocellular carcinoma cells in vitro. All synthesized coumarins showed no cytotoxic effect but exhibited a high antimigration activity through the inhibition of MMP-2. CD105 was over-expressed in all cases and, therefore, was not involved in the antimigration activity [132]. In other cases, no statistically significant difference in gene expression of CD44 was found. A synthesized coumarin, 2-oxo-2H-chromene-6-sulfonyl derivative, was found to be the most promising antiangiogenic agent, since it was able to inhibit the migratory activity mediated by MMP-2 and down-regulate CD105; however, it did not show any effect on CD44.

On the other hand, the antiangiogenic capacity of several sulfonyl derivatives of coumarins was evaluated using molecular docking studies. In these studies, it was also observed that the compounds showed better docking scores with respect to the I52 ligand, with the nitro derivatives being the best, due to the ability of the nitro group to better coordinate the Zn^{++} ion within the binding site. However, the in vitro antiangiogenic activity of sulfonyl derivatives of coumarins was not statistically significant. Only the 2-oxo-2H-chromene-6-sulfonyl derivative with N-acetylpyrazolone substitution at the 6-position showed a promising antiangiogenic activity, exhibiting better binding interactions with the active site and a docking score comparable to that of the inhibitor I52 (−16.22 vs. 18.18 kJmol-1, respectively) [132].

NF-κB is another protein factor, which plays a pivotal role in gene expression and, therefore, is involved in proliferation, angiogenesis, and metastasis, as well as in drug resistance in cancer. In light of this, the development of angiogenesis inhibitors is of significant importance in the treatment of many cancers. Recently, the effects of 26 new synthetic coumarins were tested against hepatocellular carcinoma cells [133]. The investigators identified (7-carbethoxyamino-2-oxo-2H-chromen-4-yl)-methylpyrrolidine-1-carbodithioate as the most promising one, because it was cytotoxic in a time- and concentration-dependent manner and it was able to hinder the binding of NF-κB to DNA, therefore inhibiting the expression of several genes, such as *cyclin D1, Bcl-2, survivin, MMP12,* and *c-Myc.* Furthermore, it was able to reduce cell migration and invasion induced by CXCL12, a cytokine that plays a pivotal role in angiogenesis by recruiting endothelial progenitor cells from the bone marrow [133].

Analysis of data present in the existing literature shows that it is possible to identify, through structure-activity analysis, coumarin derivatives more suitable for a given type of tumor. The coumarin derivatives that possess an N-aryl carboxamide, a phenyl substitution at the C-3 position, and 1, 2, 3-triazolyl, trihydroxystilbene, and amino substitutions at the C-4 position were the most effective in targeting lung cancer [24].

Preliminary in vitro results revealed that some coumarin-tethered isoxazolines exhibited significant antiproliferative effect against a human melanoma cancer cell line (UACC 903). Only one derivative with a 3,4-dimethoxy substitution did not show any cytotoxicity against a normal fibroblast cell line (FF2441) in the same concentration range. These results were corroborated in the Ehrlich ascites carcinoma animal model, highlighting significantly lowered cell viability, body weight, ascites volume as well as a down-regulation of angiogenesis and tumor growth [134].

Histone deacetylase 1 (HDAC1), a key element in the control of cell proliferation and differentiation as well as in angiogenesis, represents an attractive therapeutic target for new inhibitors of angiogenesis. In this regard, the benzamidic derivatives of coumarins were found to be the most promising candidates. Four compounds of N-(4-((2-aminophenyl)carbamoyl) benzyl)-2-oxo-2H-chromene-3-carboxamide derivatives showed the most promising cytotoxic effect, calculated as IC_{50} in the range of 0.53–57.59 µM, on several cancer cells, including HCT116, A2780, MCF7, PC-3, HL60, and A549, without any effects on a human normal cell line (HUVEC, IC_{50} > 100 µM). Moreover, they showed a strong HDAC1-inhibitory activity (IC_{50} 0.47–0.87 µM) with N-(4-((2-aminophenyl) carbamoyl) benzyl)-7-((3,4-dichlorobenzyl)oxy)-2-oxo-2H-chromene-3-carboxamide, showing an IC_{50} value similar to that of the reference drug entinostat (0.47 ± 0.02 µM vs. 0.41 ± 0.06 µM) [135].

Another interesting coumarin derivative investigated is (E)-2-(4-methoxybenzyloxy)-3-prenyl-4-methoxy-N-hydroxycinamide (BMX), a semisynthetic derivative of osthole and a coumarin found in several plant species, such as Cnidium monnieri L, Angelica archangelica L, and Angelica pubescens Maxim. BMX was found to inhibit VEGF-induced proliferation, migration, and endothelial tube formation in HUVECs. These activities were also corroborated by ex vivo and in vivo studies decreasing VEGF-induced microvessel sprouting from aortic rings and HCT116 colorectal cancer cells. Moreover, BMX inhibited HCT116 cell proliferation and the growth of xenografts of HCT116 cells in vivo [136].

Scopoletin is a well-known natural coumarin with antiangiogenic properties. To develop new and robust angiogenesis inhibitors, several scopoletin derivatives were designed and synthesized. According to the study of Tabana et al. [137], scopoletin inhibited VEGF-A, ERK1, and FGF-2, and is thereby considered a strong antiangiogenic agent. In another study, among several scopoletin analogs, three compounds, including 4-bromo-phenyl and 4-chloro-phenyl scopoletin derivatives and 2-hydroxy-3-(piperidin-1-yl)-propoxy)-6-methoxy-2H-chromen-2-one, were able to inhibit VEGF-stimulated proliferation, migration, and tube formation of HUVECs. These results showed a significant decrease in the VEGF-triggered phosphorylated forms of ERK1/2 and Akt, which was corroborated by in vivo observations on chick chorioallantoic membrane [138]. Luo and co-workers also showed that 3-aryl-4-anilino/aryloxy-2H-chromen-2-one analogues significantly affected breast cancer through the inhibition of estrogen receptor-α and VEGFR-2 [139]. In another study, coumarin-conjugated benzophenone analogs showed promising antitumor activity against Ehrlich ascites carcinoma and Dalton's lymphoma ascites cell lines. In this study, a compound with a bromo group in the benzophenone structure markedly showed antiangiogenic effects through the inhibition of VEGF [28]. In a more recent study by Makowska et al. [140], a series of 2-imino-2H-chromen-3-yl-1,3,5-triazine compounds were synthesized. Among them, 4-[7-(diethylamino)-2-imino-2H-chromen-3-yl]-6-(4-phenylpiperazin-1-yl)-1,3,5-triazin-2-amine showed the greatest cytotoxic effects against several human cancer cell lines, which underscores the promising role of synthetic coumarins in combating cancer. Figure 1 illustrates how coumarins inhibit various angiogenic signaling pathways.

6. Conclusions

Considering the crucial role of angiogenesis in cancer development, antiangiogenic agents have significant potential to fight cancer. Thus, investigating novel drugs to attenuate or prevent angiogenesis-associated complications in cancer is of great importance. The several clinical limitations and side effects related to the administration of current antiangiogenic agents for cancer treatment raise the need to find alternative treatments. Natural and synthetic coumarins have shown a variety of pharmacological properties. They have demonstrated prominent anticancer effects by targeting multiple signaling pathways involved in several types of cancer.

Recently, studies have focused on the antiangiogenic effects of coumarins according to their structure-activity relationships. The present review reports the currently available literature data on the signaling and regulatory pathways of angiogenesis, as well as on antiangiogenic and anticancer mechanisms of natural and synthetic coumarins, critically analyzing and highlighting their use as possible therapeutic strategies. These studies are essential to identify novel and effective anticancer agents with fewer side effects than conventional drugs. It is also critical to identify potential synergies that may allow reducing the side effects of cytotoxic medicines and increasing the quality of life of patients. Additional studies should focus on additional in vitro and in vivo experiments followed by well-controlled clinical trials to reveal the exact signaling pathways involved in cancer angiogenesis as well as the precise pharmacological mechanisms of coumarins. In addition, there is a need to investigate and adjust novel antiangiogenic coumarin lead compounds to develop more potent and efficient anticancer drugs with lower toxicity. In addition, an appropriate drug delivery system should be introduced to overcome the existing pharmacokinetic challenges of coumarin administration. Such research will unveil the potential of coumarins in the prevention, attenuation, and treatment of angiogenesis in cancer.

Author Contributions: Conceptualization, M.B.M., and M.H.F.; drafting the manuscript, M.B.M., S.F., A.S., D.T., and M.H.F.; review and editing the paper: M.B.M., S.F., E.S.-S., M.H.F., C.R.C., P.B., and A.B.; revising, M.B.M., S.F., M.H.F., and A.B.

Funding: This research did not receive any specific grant from funding agencies in the public, commercial, or not-for-profit sectors.

Acknowledgments: The authors thank Yalda Shokoohinia for her excellent and helpful suggestions.

Conflicts of Interest: The authors declared no conflict of interest.

References

1. Carmeliet, P.; Jain, R.K. Angiogenesis in cancer and other diseases. *Nature* **2000**, *407*, 249. [CrossRef] [PubMed]
2. Ribatti, D.; Puxeddu, I.; Crivellato, E.; Nico, B.; Vacca, A.; Levi-Schaffer, F. Angiogenesis in asthma. *Clin. Exp. Allergy* **2009**, *39*, 1815–1821. [CrossRef] [PubMed]
3. Rodríguez-Caso, L.; Reyes-Palomares, A.; Sánchez-Jiménez, F.; Quesada, A.R.; Medina, M.Á. What is known on angiogenesis-related rare diseases? A systematic review of literature. *J. Cell. Mol. Med.* **2012**, *16*, 2872–2893. [CrossRef] [PubMed]
4. Ucuzian, A.A.; Gassman, A.A.; East, A.T.; Greisler, H.P. Molecular mediators of angiogenesis. *J. Burn. Care. Res.* **2010**, *31*, 158–175. [CrossRef]
5. Folkman, J. Tumor angiogenesis: Therapeutic implications. *N. Engl. J. Med.* **1971**, *285*, 1182–1186.
6. Al-Abd, A.M.; Alamoudi, A.J.; Abdel-Naim, A.B.; Neamatallah, T.A.; Ashour, O.M. Anti-angiogenic agents for the treatment of solid tumors: Potential pathways, therapy and current strategies–a review. *J. Adv. Res.* **2017**, *8*, 591–605. [CrossRef]
7. EL-Meghawry, E.; Rahman, H.; Abdelkarim, G.; Najda, A. Natural products against cancer angiogenesis. *Tumor. Biol.* **2016**, *37*, 14513–14536.
8. Quesada, A.R.; Muñoz-Chápuli, R.; Medina, M.A. Anti-angiogenic drugs: From bench to clinical trials. *Med. Res. Rev.* **2006**, *26*, 483–530. [CrossRef]
9. Aviello, G.; Romano, B.; Borrelli, F.; Capasso, R.; Gallo, L.; Piscitelli, F.; Di Marzo, V.; Izzo, A.A. Chemopreventive effect of the non-psychotropic phytocannabinoid cannabidiol on experimental colon cancer. *J. Mol. Med.* **2012**, *90*, 925–934. [CrossRef]
10. Wang, Z.; Dabrosin, C.; Yin, X.; Fuster, M.M.; Arreola, A.; Rathmell, W.K.; Generali, D.; Nagaraju, G.P.; El-Rayes, B.; Ribatti, D.; et al. Broad targeting of angiogenesis for cancer prevention and therapy. *Sem. Can. Biol.* **2015**, *35*, S224–S243. [CrossRef]
11. Bishayee, A.; Darvesh, A.S. Angiogenesis in hepatocellular carcinoma: A potential target for chemoprevention and therapy. *Curr. Cancer Drug Targets* **2012**, *12*, 1095–1118.
12. Rajasekar, J.; Perumal, M.K.; Vallikannan, B. A critical review on anti-angiogenic property of phytochemicals. *J. Nutr. Biochem.* **2019**, *71*, 1–15. [CrossRef] [PubMed]
13. Fakhri, s.; Abbaszadeh, F.; Jorjani, M.; Pourgholami, M.H. The effects of anticancer medicinal herbs on vascular endothelial growth factor based on pharmacological aspects: A review study. *Nutr. Cancer* **2019**, *25*, 1–15. [CrossRef] [PubMed]

14. Pagano, E.; Borrelli, F.; Orlando, P.; Romano, B.; Monti, M.; Morbidelli, L.; Aviello, G.; Imperatore, R.; Capasso, R.; Piscitelli, F. Pharmacological inhibition of MAGL attenuates experimental colon carcinogenesis. *Pharmacol. Res.* **2017**, *119*, 227–236. [CrossRef]
15. Kumar, S.; Kumari, R.; Mishra, S. Pharmacological properties and their medicinal uses of Cinnamomum: A review. *J. Pharm. Pharmacol.* **2019**, *71*, 1735–1761. [CrossRef]
16. Ribeiro, C.V.C.; Kaplan, M.A.C. Tendências evolutivas de famílias produtoras de cumarinas em Angiospermae. *Química Nova* **2002**, *25*, 533–538. [CrossRef]
17. Borges Bubols, G.; da Rocha Vianna, D.; Medina-Remon, A.; von Poser, G.; Maria Lamuela-Raventos, R.; Lucia Eifler-Lima, V.; Cristina Garcia, S. The antioxidant activity of coumarins and flavonoids. *Mini. Rev. Med. Chem.* **2013**, *13*, 318–334.
18. Gagliotti Vigil de Mello, S.V.; Frode, T.S. In Vitro and In Vivo Experimental Model-based Approaches for Investigating Anti-inflammatory Properties of Coumarins. *Curr. Med. Chem.* **2018**, *25*, 1446–1476. [CrossRef]
19. Orhan, I.E. Potential of Natural Products of Herbal Origin as Monoamine Oxidase Inhibitors. *Curr. Pharm. Des.* **2016**, *22*, 268–276. [CrossRef]
20. Ghate, M.; Kusanur, R.A.; Kulkarni, M.V. Synthesis and in vivo analgesic and anti-inflammatory activity of some bi heterocyclic coumarin derivatives. *Eur. J. Med. Chem.* **2005**, *40*, 882–887. [CrossRef]
21. Jameel, E.; Umar, T.; Kumar, J.; Hoda, N. Coumarin: A privileged scaffold for the design and development of antineurodegenerative agents. *Chem. Biol. Drug. Des.* **2016**, *87*, 21–38. [CrossRef]
22. Najmanova, I.; Dosedel, M.; Hrdina, R.; Anzenbacher, P.; Filipsky, T.; Riha, M.; Mladenka, P. Cardiovascular effects of coumarins besides their antioxidant activity. *Curr. Top. Med. Chem.* **2015**, *15*, 830–849. [CrossRef] [PubMed]
23. Li, H.; Yao, Y.; Li, L. Coumarins as potential antidiabetic agents. *J. Pharm. Pharmacol.* **2017**, *69*, 1253–1264. [CrossRef] [PubMed]
24. Kumar, M.; Singla, R.; Dandriyal, J.; Jaitak, V. Coumarin derivatives as anticancer agents for lung cancer therapy: A review. *Anti-Cancer Agents Med. Chem.* **2018**, *18*, 964–984. [CrossRef] [PubMed]
25. Ren, Q.-C.; Gao, C.; Xu, Z.; Feng, L.-S.; Liu, M.-L.; Wu, X.; Zhao, F. Bis-coumarin derivatives and their biological activities. *Curr. Top. Med. Chem.* **2018**, *18*, 101–113. [CrossRef] [PubMed]
26. Pereira, T.M.; Franco, D.P.; Vitorio, F.; Kummerle, A.E. Coumarin Compounds in Medicinal Chemistry: Some Important Examples from the Last Years. *Curr. Top. Med. Chem.* **2018**, *18*, 124–148. [CrossRef]
27. Kaur, M.; Kohli, S.; Sandhu, S.; Bansal, Y.; Bansal, G. Coumarin: A promising scaffold for anticancer agents. *Anti-Cancer Agents Med. Chem.* **2015**, *15*, 1032–1048. [CrossRef]
28. Vijay Avin, B.R.; Thirusangu, P.; Lakshmi Ranganatha, V.; Firdouse, A.; Prabhakar, B.T.; Khanum, S.A. Synthesis and tumor inhibitory activity of novel coumarin analogs targeting angiogenesis and apoptosis. *Eur. J. Med. Chem.* **2014**, *75*, 211–221. [CrossRef]
29. Thakur, A.; Singla, R.; Jaitak, V. Coumarins as anticancer agents: A review on synthetic strategies, mechanism of action and SAR studies. *Eur. J. Med. Chem.* **2015**, *101*, 476–495. [CrossRef]
30. Pan, R.; Gao, X.; Lu, D.; Xu, X.; Xia, Y.; Dai, Y. Prevention of FGF-2-induced angiogenesis by scopoletin, a coumarin compound isolated from Erycibe obtusifolia Benth, and its mechanism of action. *Int. Immunopharmacol.* **2011**, *11*, 2007–2016. [CrossRef]
31. Park, S.L.; Won, S.Y.; Song, J.-H.; Lee, S.-Y.; Kim, W.-J.; Moon, S.-K. Esculetin inhibits VEGF-induced angiogenesis both in vitro and in vivo. *Am. J. Chin. Med.* **2016**, *44*, 61–76. [CrossRef] [PubMed]
32. Amini, A.; Masoumi, M.S.; Morris, L.D.; Pourgholami, H.M. The critical role of vascular endothelial growth factor in tumor angiogenesis. *Curr. Cancer Drug Targets.* **2012**, *12*, 23–43. [CrossRef] [PubMed]
33. Simons, M.; Gordon, E.; Claesson-Welsh, L. Mechanisms and regulation of endothelial VEGF receptor signalling. *Nat. Rev. Mol. Cell Biol.* **2016**, *17*, 611. [CrossRef] [PubMed]
34. Bergers, G.; Benjamin, L.E. Angiogenesis: Tumorigenesis and the angiogenic switch. *Nat. Rev. Can.* **2003**, *3*, 401. [CrossRef]
35. El-Kenawi, A.E.; El-Remessy, A.B. Angiogenesis inhibitors in cancer therapy: Mechanistic perspective on classification and treatment rationales. *Brit. J. Pharmacol.* **2013**, *170*, 712–729. [CrossRef]

36. Pourgholami, M.H.; Khachigian, L.M.; Fahmy, R.G.; Badar, S.; Wang, L.; Chu, S.W.L.; Morris, D.L. Albendazole inhibits endothelial cell migration, tube formation, vasopermeability, VEGF receptor-2 expression and suppresses retinal neovascularization in ROP model of angiogenesis. *Bioch. Bioph. Res. Commun.* **2010**, *397*, 729–734. [CrossRef]
37. Folkman, J. Angiogenesis and Apoptosis, Seminars in cancer biology, Semin. *Cancer Biol.* **2003**, *13*, 159–167. [CrossRef]
38. Folkman, J. Opinion: Angiogenesis: An organizing principle for drug discovery? *Nat. Rev. Drug Discov.* **2007**, *6*, 273. [CrossRef]
39. Mundel, T.M.; Kalluri, R. Type IV collagen-derived angiogenesis inhibitors. *Microvasc. Res.* **2007**, *74*, 85–89. [CrossRef]
40. Ribatti, D. Endogenous inhibitors of angiogenesis: A historical review. *Leuk. Res.* **2009**, *33*, 638–644. [CrossRef]
41. Rajabi, M.; Mousa, S. The role of angiogenesis in cancer treatment. *Biomedicines* **2017**, *5*, 34. [CrossRef] [PubMed]
42. Kerbel, R.S. Tumor angiogenesis. *N. Engl. J. Med.* **2008**, *358*, 2039–2049. [CrossRef] [PubMed]
43. Pugh, C.W.; Ratcliffe, P.J. Regulation of angiogenesis by hypoxia: Role of the HIF system. *Nat. Med.* **2003**, *9*, 677. [CrossRef] [PubMed]
44. Ohlfest, J.R.; Demorest, Z.L.; Motooka, Y.; Vengco, I.; Oh, S.; Chen, E.; Scappaticci, F.A.; Saplis, R.J.; Ekker, S.C.; Low, W.C. Combinatorial antiangiogenic gene therapy by nonviral gene transfer using the sleeping beauty transposon causes tumor regression and improves survival in mice bearing intracranial human glioblastoma. *Mol. Ther.* **2005**, *12*, 778–788. [CrossRef]
45. Abdalla, A.M.; Xiao, L.; Ullah, M.W.; Yu, M.; Ouyang, C.; Yang, G. Current challenges of cancer anti-angiogenic therapy and the promise of nanotherapeutics. *Theranostics* **2018**, *8*, 533. [CrossRef]
46. Marimpietri, D.; Brignole, C.; Nico, B.; Pastorino, F.; Pezzolo, A.; Piccardi, F.; Cilli, M.; Di Paolo, D.; Pagnan, G.; Longo, L. Combined therapeutic effects of vinblastine and rapamycin on human neuroblastoma growth, apoptosis, and angiogenesis. *Clin. Can. Res.* **2007**, *13*, 3977–3988. [CrossRef]
47. Li, W.; Tang, Y.-X.; Wan, L.; Cai, J.-H.; Zhang, J. Effects of combining Taxol and cyclooxygenase inhibitors on the angiogenesis and apoptosis in human ovarian cancer xenografts. *Oncol. Lett.* **2013**, *5*, 923–928. [CrossRef]
48. Nakashio, A.; Fujita, N.; Tsuruo, T. Topotecan inhibits VEGF-and bFGF-induced vascular endothelial cell migration via downregulation of the PI3K-Akt signaling pathway. *Int. J. Cancer* **2002**, *98*, 36–41. [CrossRef]
49. Sang, C.-Y.; Xu, X.-H.; Qin, W.-W.; Liu, J.-F.; Hui, L.; Chen, S.-W. DPMA, a deoxypodophyllotoxin derivative, induces apoptosis and anti-angiogenesis in non-small cell lung cancer A549 cells. *Bioorg. Med. Chem. Lett.* **2013**, *23*, 6650–6655. [CrossRef]
50. Xiu-jin, Y.; Mao-fang, L. Homoharringtonine induces apoptosis of endothelium and down-regulates VEGF expression of K562 cells. *J. Zhejiang. Univ. Sci. A* **2004**, *5*, 230–234.
51. Graveel, C.R.; Tolbert, D.; Woude, G.F.V. MET: A critical player in tumorigenesis and therapeutic target. *Cold. Spring. Harb. Perspect. Biol.* **2013**, *5*, a009209. [CrossRef]
52. You, W.-K.; McDonald, D.M. The hepatocyte growth factor/c-Met signaling pathway as a therapeutic target to inhibit angiogenesis. *BMB. Rep.* **2008**, *41*, 833. [CrossRef] [PubMed]
53. Beenken, A.; Mohammadi, M. The FGF family: Biology, pathophysiology and therapy. *Nat. Rev. Drug Discov.* **2009**, *8*, 235. [CrossRef] [PubMed]
54. Turner, N.; Pearson, A.; Sharpe, R.; Lambros, M.; Geyer, F.; Lopez-Garcia, M.A.; Natrajan, R.; Marchio, C.; Iorns, E.; Mackay, A. FGFR1 amplification drives endocrine therapy resistance and is a therapeutic target in breast cancer. *Cancer Res.* **2010**, *70*, 2085–2094. [CrossRef] [PubMed]
55. Lu, K.V.; Chang, J.P.; Parachoniak, C.A.; Pandika, M.M.; Aghi, M.K.; Meyronet, D.; Isachenko, N.; Fouse, S.D.; Phillips, J.J.; Cheresh, D.A. VEGF inhibits tumor cell invasion and mesenchymal transition through a MET/VEGFR2 complex. *Cancer Cell* **2012**, *22*, 21–35. [CrossRef] [PubMed]
56. Jahangiri, A.; De Lay, M.; Miller, L.M.; Carbonell, W.S.; Hu, Y.-L.; Lu, K.; Tom, M.W.; Paquette, J.; Tokuyasu, T.A.; Tsao, S. Gene expression profile identifies tyrosine kinase c-Met as a targetable mediator of antiangiogenic therapy resistance. *Clin. Cancer Res.* **2013**, *19*, 1773–1783. [CrossRef]

57. Cao, Y.; Cao, R.; Hedlund, E.-M. R Regulation of tumor angiogenesis and metastasis by FGF and PDGF signaling pathways. *J. Mol. Med.* **2008**, *86*, 785–789. [CrossRef]
58. Heldin, C.-H. Targeting the PDGF signaling pathway in tumor treatment. *Cell Commun. Signal.* **2013**, *11*, 97. [CrossRef]
59. Wu, E.; Palmer, N.; Tian, Z.; Moseman, A.P.; Galdzicki, M.; Wang, X.; Berger, B.; Zhang, H.; Kohane, I.S. Comprehensive dissection of PDGF-PDGFR signaling pathways in PDGFR genetically defined cells. *PLoS ONE* **2008**, *3*, e3794. [CrossRef]
60. Cao, Y. Multifarious functions of PDGFs and PDGFRs in tumor growth and metastasis. *Trend. Mol. Med.* **2013**, *19*, 460–473. [CrossRef]
61. Levitzki, A. PDGF receptor kinase inhibitors for the treatment of PDGF driven diseases. *Cytokine Growth Factor Rev.* **2004**, *15*, 229–235. [CrossRef] [PubMed]
62. Lu, C.; Shahzad, M.M.; Moreno-Smith, M.; Lin, Y.; Jennings, N.B.; Allen, J.K.; Landen, C.N.; Mangala, L.S.; Armaiz-Pena, G.N.; Schmandt, R. Targeting pericytes with a PDGF-B aptamer in human ovarian carcinoma models. *Cancer Biol. Ther.* **2010**, *9*, 176–182. [CrossRef] [PubMed]
63. Zhao, Y.; Adjei, A.A. Targeting angiogenesis in cancer therapy: Moving beyond vascular endothelial growth factor. *Oncologist* **2015**, *20*, 660–673. [CrossRef] [PubMed]
64. Cascone, T.; Heymach, J.V. Targeting the angiopoietin/Tie2 pathway: Cutting tumor vessels with a double-edged sword? *J. Clin. Oncol.* **2011**, *30*, 441–444. [CrossRef] [PubMed]
65. Gerald, D.; Chintharlapalli, S.; Augustin, H.G.; Benjamin, L.E. Angiopoietin-2: An attractive target for improved antiangiogenic tumor therapy. *Cancer Res.* **2013**, *73*, 1649–1657. [CrossRef] [PubMed]
66. Mulligan, L.M. RET revisited: Expanding the oncogenic portfolio. *Nat. Rev. Cancer* **2014**, *14*, 173. [CrossRef] [PubMed]
67. Ibáñez, C.F. Structure and physiology of the RET receptor tyrosine kinase. *Cold Spring Harb. Perspect. Biol.* **2013**, *5*, a009134. [CrossRef]
68. Santos-Sánchez, N.F.; Salas-Coronado, R.; Hernández-Carlos, B.; Villanueva-Cañongo, C. Shikimic Acid Pathway in Biosynthesis of Phenolic Compounds. In *Plant Physiological Aspects of Phenolic Compounds*; IntechOpen: London, UK, 2019.
69. Jain, P.; Joshi, H. Coumarin: Chemical and pharmacological profile. *JAPS* **2012**, *2*, 236–240.
70. Stefanachi, A.; Leonetti, F.; Pisani, L.; Catto, M.; Carotti, A. Coumarin: A natural, privileged and versatile scaffold for bioactive compounds. *Molecules* **2018**, *23*, 250. [CrossRef]
71. Venugopala, K.N.; Rashmi, V.; Odhav, B. Review on natural coumarin lead compounds for their pharmacological activity. *BioMed. Res. Int.* **2013**, *2013*, 963248. [CrossRef]
72. Hroboňová, K.; Machyňáková, A.; Čižmárik, J. Determination of dicoumarol in Melilotus officinalis L. by using molecularly imprinted polymer solid-phase extraction coupled with high performance liquid chromatography. *J. Chromatogr. A* **2018**, *1539*, 93–102. [CrossRef] [PubMed]
73. Kassim, N.K.; Rahmani, M.; Ismail, A.; Sukari, M.A.; Ee, G.C.L.; Nasir, N.M.; Awang, K. Antioxidant activity-guided separation of coumarins and lignan from Melicope glabra (Rutaceae). *Food Chem.* **2013**, *139*, 87–92. [CrossRef] [PubMed]
74. Pfeifer, I.; Murauer, A.; Ganzera, M. Determination of coumarins in the roots of Angelica dahurica by supercritical fluid chromatography. *J. Pharm. Biomed. Anal.* **2016**, *129*, 246–251. [CrossRef] [PubMed]
75. Teixeira, D.M.; Patão, R.F.; Coelho, A.V.; da Costa, C.T. Comparison between sample disruption methods and solid–liquid extraction (SLE) to extract phenolic compounds from Ficus carica leaves. *J. Chromatogr. A* **2006**, *1103*, 22–28. [CrossRef]
76. Walasek, M.; Grzegorczyk, A.; Malm, A.; Skalicka-Woźniak, K. Bioactivity-guided isolation of antimicrobial coumarins from Heracleum mantegazzianum Sommier & Levier (Apiaceae) fruits by high-performance counter-current chromatography. *Food Chem.* **2015**, *186*, 133–138.
77. Widelski, J.; Luca, S.V.; Skiba, A.; Chinou, I.; Marcourt, L.; Wolfender, J.-L.; Skalicka-Wozniak, K. Isolation and Antimicrobial Activity of Coumarin Derivatives from Fruits of Peucedanum luxurians Tamamsch. *Molecules* **2018**, *23*, 1222. [CrossRef]
78. Shokoohinia, Y.; Sajjadi, S.-E.; Gholamzadeh, S.; Fattahi, A.; Behbahani, M. Antiviral and cytotoxic evaluation of coumarins from Prangos ferulacea. *Pharm. Biol.* **2014**, *52*, 1543–1549. [CrossRef]

79. Monsef-Esfahani, H.R.; Amini, M.; Goodarzi, N.; Saiedmohammadi, F.; Hajiaghaee, R.; Faramarzi, M.A.; Tofighi, Z.; Ghahremani, M.H. Coumarin compounds of Biebersteinia multifida roots show potential anxiolytic effects in mice. *DARU* **2013**, *21*, 51. [CrossRef]
80. Karakaya, S.; Koca, M.; Yılmaz, S.V.; Yıldırım, K.; Pınar, N.M.; Demirci, B.; Brestic, M.; Sytar, O. Molecular docking studies of coumarins isolated from extracts and essential oils of Zosima absinthifolia Link as potential inhibitors for Alzheimer's disease. *Molecules* **2019**, *24*, 722. [CrossRef]
81. Kontogiorgis, C.A.; Savvoglou, K.; Hadjipavlou-Litina, D.J. Antiinflammatory and antioxidant evaluation of novel coumarin derivatives. *J. Enzym. Inhib. Med. Chem.* **2006**, *21*, 21–29. [CrossRef]
82. Alipour, M.; Khoobi, M.; Emami, S.; Fallah-Benakohal, S.; Ghasemi-Niri, S.F.; Abdollahi, M.; Foroumadi, A.; Shafiee, A. Antinociceptive properties of new coumarin derivatives bearing substituted 3, 4-dihydro-2 H-benzothiazines. *DARU* **2014**, *22*, 9. [CrossRef] [PubMed]
83. Bighetti, A.; Antonio, M.; Kohn, L.; Rehder, V.; Foglio, M.; Possenti, A.; Vilela, L.; Carvalho, J. Antiulcerogenic activity of a crude hydroalcoholic extract and coumarin isolated from Mikania laevigata Schultz Bip. *Phytomedicine* **2005**, *12*, 72–77. [CrossRef] [PubMed]
84. Sadraei, H.; Shokoohinia, Y.; Sajjadi, S.; Ghadirian, B. Antispasmodic effect of osthole and Prangos ferulacea extract on rat uterus smooth muscle motility. *Res. Pharm. Sci.* **2012**, *7*, 141. [PubMed]
85. Chen, I.-S.; Chang, C.-T.; Sheen, W.-S.; Teng, C.-M.; Tsai, I.-L.; Duh, C.-Y.; Ko, F.-N. Coumarins and antiplatelet aggregation constituents from Formosan Peucedanum japonicum. *Phytochemistry* **1996**, *41*, 525–530. [CrossRef]
86. Dongmo, A.; Azebaze, A.; Nguelefack, T.; Ouahouo, B.; Sontia, B.; Meyer, M.; Nkengfack, A.; Kamanyi, A.; Vierling, W. Vasodilator effect of the extracts and some coumarins from the stem bark of Mammea africana (Guttiferae). *J. Ethnopharmacol.* **2007**, *111*, 329–334. [CrossRef]
87. Sakunpak, A.; Matsunami, K.; Otsuka, H.; Panichayupakaranant, P. Isolation of new monoterpene coumarins from Micromelum minutum leaves and their cytotoxic activity against Leishmania major and cancer cells. *Food Chem.* **2013**, *139*, 458–463. [CrossRef]
88. Lake, B.G.; Grasso, P. Comparison of the hepatotoxicity of coumarin in the rat, mouse, and Syrian hamster: A dose and time response study. *Fundam. Appl. Toxicol.* **1996**, *34*, 105–117. [CrossRef]
89. Musa, M.A.; Cooperwood, J.S.; Khan, M.O.F. A review of coumarin derivatives in pharmacotherapy of breast cancer. *Curr. Med. Chem.* **2008**, *15*, 2664–2679. [CrossRef]
90. Amaral, R.; dos Santos, S.; Andrade, L.; Severino, P.; Carvalho, A. Natural Products as Treatment against Cancer: A Historical and Current Vision. *Clin. Oncol.* **2019**, *4*, 1562.
91. Devji, T.; Reddy, C.; Woo, C.; Awale, S.; Kadota, S.; Carrico-Moniz, D. Pancreatic anticancer activity of a novel geranylgeranylated coumarin derivative. *Bioorganic Med. Chem. Lett.* **2011**, *21*, 5770–5773. [CrossRef]
92. Siegel, R.L.; Miller, K.D.; Jemal, A. Cancer statistics, 2019. *CA. Cancer J. Clin.* **2019**, *69*, 7–34. [CrossRef] [PubMed]
93. Foroozesh, M.; Sridhar, J.; Goyal, N.; Liu, J. Coumarins and P450s, Studies Reported to-Date. *Molecules* **2019**, *24*, 1620. [CrossRef]
94. Saidu, N.E.B.; Valente, S.; Bana, E.; Kirsch, G.; Bagrel, D.; Montenarh, M. Coumarin polysulfides inhibit cell growth and induce apoptosis in HCT116 colon cancer cells. *Bioorganic Med. Chem.* **2012**, *20*, 1584–1593. [CrossRef] [PubMed]
95. Nordin, N.; Fadaeinasab, M.; Mohan, S.; Hashim, N.M.; Othman, R.; Karimian, H.; Iman, V.; Ramli, N.; Ali, H.M.; Majid, N.A. Pulchrin A, a new natural coumarin derivative of Enicosanthellum pulchrum, induces apoptosis in ovarian cancer cells via intrinsic pathway. *PLoS ONE* **2016**, *11*, e0154023. [CrossRef] [PubMed]
96. Wang, J.; Lu, M.; Dai, H.; Zhang, S.; Wang, H.; Wei, N. Esculetin, a coumarin derivative, exerts in vitro and in vivo antiproliferative activity against hepatocellular carcinoma by initiating a mitochondrial-dependent apoptosis pathway. *Braz. J. Med. Biol. Res.* **2015**, *48*, 245–253. [CrossRef] [PubMed]
97. Haghighitalab, A.; Matin, M.M.; Bahrami, A.R.; Iranshahi, M.; Saeinasab, M.; Haghighi, F. In vitro investigation of anticancer, cell-cycle-inhibitory, and apoptosis-inducing effects of diversin, a natural prenylated coumarin, on bladder carcinoma cells. *Z. Nat. C J. Biosci.* **2014**, *69*, 99–109. [CrossRef] [PubMed]
98. Hejchman, E.; Taciak, P.; Kowalski, S.; Maciejewska, D.; Czajkowska, A.; Borowska, J.; Śladowski, D.; Młynarczuk-Biały, I. Synthesis and anticancer activity of 7-hydroxycoumarinyl gallates. *Pharm. Rep.* **2015**, *67*, 236–244. [CrossRef]

99. Zahri, S.; Razavi, S.M.; Moatamed, Z. Antioxidant activity and cytotoxic effect of aviprin and aviprin-3″-O-d-glucopyranoside on LNCaP and HeLa cell lines. *Nat. Prod. Res.* **2012**, *26*, 540–547. [CrossRef]
100. Chuang, J.-Y.; Huang, Y.-F.; Lu, H.-F.; Ho, H.-C.; Yang, J.-S.; Li, T.-M.; Chang, N.-W.; Chung, J.-G. Coumarin induces cell cycle arrest and apoptosis in human cervical cancer HeLa cells through a mitochondria-and caspase-3 dependent mechanism and NF-κB down-regulation. *In Vivo* **2007**, *21*, 1003–1009.
101. Aas, Z.; Babaei, E.; Feizi, M.A.H.; Dehghan, G. Anti-proliferative and apoptotic effects of dendrosomal farnesiferol C on gastric cancer cells. *Asian. Pac. J. Cancer Prev.* **2015**, *16*, 5325–5329. [CrossRef]
102. Lv, N.; Sun, M.; Liu, C.; Li, J. Design and synthesis of 2-phenylpyrimidine coumarin derivatives as anticancer agents. *Bioorg. Med. Chem. Lett.* **2017**, *27*, 4578–4581. [CrossRef] [PubMed]
103. Maresca, A.; Temperini, C.; Pochet, L.; Masereel, B.; Scozzafava, A.; Supuran, C.T. Deciphering the mechanism of carbonic anhydrase inhibition with coumarins and thiocoumarins. *J. Med. Chem.* **2009**, *53*, 335–344. [CrossRef] [PubMed]
104. Mokdad-Bzeouich, I.; Kovacic, H.; Ghedira, K.; Chebil, L.; Ghoul, M.; Chekir-Ghedira, L.; Luis, J. Esculin and its oligomer fractions inhibit adhesion and migration of U87 glioblastoma cells and in vitro angiogenesis. *Tumor. Biol.* **2016**, *37*, 3657–3664. [CrossRef] [PubMed]
105. Taniguchi, K.; Funasaki, M.; Kishida, A.; Sadhu, S.K.; Ahmed, F.; Ishibashi, M.; Ohsaki, A. Two new coumarins and a new xanthone from the leaves of Rhizophora mucronata. *Bioorg. Med. Chem. Lett.* **2018**, *28*, 1063–1066. [CrossRef] [PubMed]
106. Mojarrab, M.; Emami, S.A.; Delazar, A.; Tayarani-Najaran, Z. Cytotoxic Properties of Three Isolated Coumarin-hemiterpene Ether Derivatives from Artemisia armeniaca Lam. *IJPR* **2017**, *16*, 221. [PubMed]
107. Jantamat, P.; Weerapreeyakul, N.; Puthongking, P. Cytotoxicity and Apoptosis Induction of Coumarins and Carbazole Alkaloids from Clausena Harmandiana. *Molecules* **2019**, *24*, 3385. [CrossRef]
108. Liu, W.; Hua, J.; Zhou, J.; Zhang, H.; Zhu, H.; Cheng, Y.; Gust, R. Synthesis and in vitro antitumor activity of novel scopoletin derivatives. *Bioorg. Med. Chem. Lett.* **2012**, *22*, 5008–5012. [CrossRef]
109. Zhang, Y.; Lv, Z.; Zhong, H.; Geng, D.; Zhang, M.; Zhang, T.; Li, Y.; Li, K. Convenient synthesis of novel geiparvarin analogs with potential anti-cancer activity via click chemistry. *Eur. J. Med. Chem.* **2012**, *53*, 356–363. [CrossRef]
110. Cui, N.; Lin, D.-D.; Shen, Y.; Shi, J.-G.; Wang, B.; Zhao, M.-Z.; Zheng, L.; Chen, H.; Shi, J.-H. Triphenylethylene-Coumarin Hybrid TCH-5c Suppresses Tumorigenic Progression in Breast Cancer Mainly Through the Inhibition of Angiogenesis. *Anti-Cancer Agents. Med. Chem.* **2019**, *19*, 1253–1261. [CrossRef]
111. Nishida, N.; Yano, H.; Nishida, T.; Kamura, T.; Kojiro, M. Angiogenesis in cancer. *Vasc. Health. Risk Manag.* **2006**, *2*, 213. [CrossRef]
112. Sandhiutami, N.M.D.; Moordiani, M.; Laksmitawati, D.R.; Fauziah, N.; Maesaroh, M.; Widowati, W. In vitro assesment of anti-inflammatory activities of coumarin and Indonesian cassia extract in RAW264.7 murine macrophage cell line. *Iran. J. Basic. Med. Sci.* **2017**, *20*, 99. [PubMed]
113. Pan, R.; Dai, Y.; Yang, J.; Li, Y.; Yao, X.; Xia, Y. Anti-angiogenic potential of scopoletin is associated with the inhibition of ERK1/2 activation. *Drug. Dev. Res.* **2009**, *70*, 214–219. [CrossRef]
114. Pan, R.; Gao, X.H.; Li, Y.; Xia, Y.F.; Dai, Y. Anti-arthritic effect of scopoletin, a coumarin compound occurring in Erycibe obtusifolia Benth stems, is associated with decreased angiogenesis in synovium. *Fundam. Clin. Pharm.* **2010**, *24*, 477–490. [CrossRef] [PubMed]
115. Anegundi, N.; Pancharatna, K. 7-Hydroxycoumarin Elicit Anti-Angiogenic Effects Through Cellular Apoptosis in Developing Embryos of Zebrafish (Danio Rerio). *Eur. Sci. J.* **2017**, *13*, 53. [CrossRef]
116. Jung, M.H.; Lee, S.H.; Ahn, E.-M.; Lee, Y.M. Decursin and decursinol angelate inhibit VEGF-induced angiogenesis via suppression of the VEGFR-2-signaling pathway. *Carcinogenesis* **2009**, *30*, 655–661. [CrossRef]
117. Wang, K.S.; Lv, Y.; Wang, Z.; Ma, J.; Mi, C.; Li, X.; Xu, G.H.; Piao, L.X.; Zheng, S.Z.; Jin, X. Imperatorin efficiently blocks TNF-α-mediated activation of ROS/PI3K/Akt/NF-κB pathway. *Oncol. Rep.* **2017**, *37*, 3397–3404. [CrossRef]
118. Bronikowska, J.; Szliszka, E.; Jaworska, D.; Czuba, Z.P.; Krol, W. The coumarin psoralidin enhances anticancer effect of tumor necrosis factor-related apoptosis-inducing ligand (TRAIL). *Molecules* **2012**, *17*, 6449–6464. [CrossRef]

119. Pan, R.; Dai, Y.; Gao, X.-H.; Lu, D.; Xia, Y.-F. Inhibition of vascular endothelial growth factor-induced angiogenesis by scopoletin through interrupting the autophosphorylation of VEGF receptor 2 and its downstream signaling pathways. *Vascul. Pharm.* **2011**, *54*, 18–28. [CrossRef]
120. Zhang, J.; Li, L.; Jiang, C.; Xing, C.; Kim, S.-H.; Lu, J. Anti-cancer and other bioactivities of Korean *Angelica gigas* Nakai (AGN) and its major pyranocoumarin compounds. *Anticancer. Agents. Med. Chem.* **2012**, *12*, 1239–1254. [CrossRef]
121. Kim, J.H.; Kim, J.K.; Ahn, E.K.; Ko, H.J.; Cho, Y.R.; Lee, C.H.; Kim, Y.K.; Bae, G.U.; Oh, J.S.; Seo, D.W. Marmesin is a novel angiogenesis inhibitor: Regulatory effect and molecular mechanism on endothelial cell fate and angiogenesis. *Cancer Lett.* **2015**, *369*, 323–330. [CrossRef]
122. Yang, Y.; Zhu, R.; Li, J.; Yang, X.; He, J.; Wang, H.; Chang, Y. Separation and Enrichment of Three Coumarins from Angelicae Pubescentis Radix by Macroporous Resin with Preparative HPLC and Evaluation of Their Anti-Inflammatory Activity. *Molecules* **2019**, *24*, 2664. [CrossRef] [PubMed]
123. Cheraghi, O.; Dehghan, G.; Mahdavi, M.; Rahbarghazi, R.; Rezabakhsh, A.; Charoudeh, H.N.; Iranshahi, M.; Montazersaheb, S. Potent anti-angiogenic and cytotoxic effect of conferone on human colorectal adenocarcinoma HT-29 cells. *Phytomedicine* **2016**, *23*, 398–405. [CrossRef] [PubMed]
124. Kumar, A.; Sunita, P.; Jha, S.; Pattanayak, S.P. Daphnetin inhibits TNF-α and VEGF-induced angiogenesis through inhibition of the IKK s/IκBα/NF-κB, Src/FAK/ERK 1/2 and Akt signalling pathways. *Clin. Exp. Pharm. Physiol.* **2016**, *43*, 939–950. [CrossRef] [PubMed]
125. Long, W.; Wang, M.; Luo, X.; Huang, G.; Chen, J. Murrangatin suppresses angiogenesis induced by tumor cell-derived media and inhibits AKT activation in zebrafish and endothelial cells. *Drug Des. Devel. Ther.* **2018**, *12*, 3107–3115. [CrossRef]
126. Kim, K.H.; Lee, H.J.; Jeong, S.J.; Lee, H.J.; Lee, E.O.; Kim, H.S.; Zhang, Y.; Ryu, S.Y.; Lee, M.H.; Lü, J.; et al. Galbanic acid isolated from Ferula assafoetida exerts in vivo anti-tumor activity in association with anti-angiogenesis and anti-proliferation. *Pharm. Res.* **2011**, *28*, 597–609. [CrossRef]
127. Alizadeh, M.N.; Rashidi, M.; Muhammadnejad, A.; Zanjani, T.M.; Ziai, S.A. Antitumor effects of umbelliprenin in a mouse model of colorectal cancer. *Iran. J. Pharm. Res.* **2018**, *17*, 976–985.
128. Jamialahmadi, K.; Salari, S.; Alamolhodaei, N.S.; Avan, A.; Gholami, L.; Karimi, G. Auraptene Inhibits Migration and Invasion of Cervical and Ovarian Cancer Cells by Repression of Matrix Metalloproteinasas 2 and 9 Activity. *J. Pharm.* **2018**, *21*, 177.
129. Yao, F.; Zhang, L.; Jiang, G.; Liu, M.; Liang, G.; Yuan, Q. Osthole attenuates angiogenesis in an orthotopic mouse model of hepatocellular carcinoma via the downregulation of nuclear factor-κB and vascular endothelial growth factor. *Oncol. Lett.* **2018**, *16*, 4471–4479. [CrossRef]
130. Pan, R.; Dai, Y.; Gao, X.; Xia, Y. Scopolin isolated from Erycibe obtusifolia Benth stems suppresses adjuvant-induced rat arthritis by inhibiting inflammation and angiogenesis. *Int. Immunopharmacol.* **2009**, *9*, 859–869. [CrossRef]
131. Lee, S.; Sivakumar, K.; Shin, W.-S.; Xie, F.; Wang, Q. Synthesis and anti-angiogenesis activity of coumarin derivatives. *Bioorg. Med. Chem. Lett.* **2006**, *16*, 4596–4599. [CrossRef]
132. El-Sawy, E.R.; Ebaid, M.S.; Rady, H.M.; Shalby, A.B.; Ahmed, K.M.; Abo-Salem, H.M. Synthesis and molecular docking of novel non-cytotoxic anti-angiogenic sulfonyl coumarin derivatives against hepatocellular carcinoma cells in vitro. *J. App. Pharm. Sci.* **2017**, *7*, 049–066.
133. Neelgundmath, M.; Dinesh, K.R.; Mohan, C.D.; Li, F.; Dai, X.; Siveen, K.S.; Paricharak, S.; Mason, D.J.; Fuchs, J.E.; Sethi, G. Novel synthetic coumarins that targets NF-κB in hepatocellular carcinoma. *Bioorganic Med. Chem. Lett.* **2015**, *25*, 893–897. [CrossRef] [PubMed]
134. Lingaraju, G.S.; Balaji, K.S.; Jayarama, S.; Anil, S.M.; Kiran, K.R.; Sadashiva, M.P. Synthesis of new coumarin tethered isoxazolines as potential anticancer agents. *Bioorganic Med. Chem. Lett.* **2018**, *28*, 3606–3612. [CrossRef] [PubMed]
135. Abdizadeh, T.; Kalani, M.R.; Abnous, K.; Tayarani-Najaran, Z.; Khashyarmanesh, B.Z.; Abdizadeh, R.; Ghodsi, R.; Hadizadeh, F. Design, synthesis and biological evaluation of novel coumarin-based benzamides as potent histone deacetylase inhibitors and anticancer agents. *Eur. J. Med. Chem.* **2017**, *132*, 42–62. [CrossRef]
136. Yang, H.Y.; Hsu, Y.F.; Chiu, P.T.; Ho, S.J.; Wang, C.H.; Chi, C.C.; Huang, Y.H.; Lee, C.F.; Li, Y.S.; Ou, G.; et al. Anti-Cancer Activity of an Osthole Derivative, NBM-T-BMX-OS01: Targeting Vascular Endothelial Growth Factor Receptor Signaling and Angiogenesis. *PLoS ONE* **2013**, *8*, e81592. [CrossRef]

137. Tabana, Y.M.; Hassan, L.E.A.; Ahamed, M.B.K.; Dahham, S.S.; Iqbal, M.A.; Saeed, M.A.; Khan, M.S.S.; Sandai, D.; Majid, A.S.A.; Oon, C.E. Scopoletin, an active principle of tree tobacco (Nicotiana glauca) inhibits human tumor vascularization in xenograft models and modulates ERK1, VEGF-A, and FGF-2 in computer model. *Microvasc. Res.* **2016**, *107*, 17–33. [CrossRef]
138. Cai, X.; Yang, J.; Zhou, J.; Lu, W.; Hu, C.; Gu, Z.; Huo, J.; Wang, X.; Cao, P. Synthesis and biological evaluation of scopoletin derivatives. *Bioorganic Med. Chem.* **2013**, *21*, 84–92. [CrossRef]
139. Luo, G.; Li, X.; Zhang, G.; Wu, C.; Tang, Z.; Liu, L.; You, Q.; Xiang, H. Novel SERMs based on 3-aryl-4-aryloxy-2H-chromen-2-one skeleton-A possible way to dual ERα/VEGFR-2 ligands for treatment of breast cancer. *Eur. J. Med. Chem.* **2017**, *140*, 252–273. [CrossRef]
140. Makowska, A.; Sączewski, F.; Bednarski, P.; Sączewski, J.; Balewski, Ł. Hybrid Molecules Composed of 2, 4-Diamino-1, 3, 5-triazines and 2-Imino-Coumarins and Coumarins. Synthesis and Cytotoxic Properties. *Molecules* **2018**, *23*, 1616. [CrossRef]

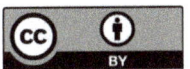

© 2019 by the authors. Licensee MDPI, Basel, Switzerland. This article is an open access article distributed under the terms and conditions of the Creative Commons Attribution (CC BY) license (http://creativecommons.org/licenses/by/4.0/).

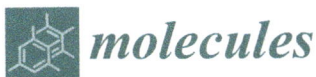

Review

Novel Antiretroviral Structures from Marine Organisms

Karlo Wittine, Lara Saftić, Željka Peršurić and Sandra Kraljević Pavelić *

University of Rijeka, Department of Biotechnology, Centre for high-throughput technologies, Radmile Matejčić 2, 51000 Rijeka, Croatia

* Correspondence: sandrakp@biotech.uniri.hr; Tel.: +385-51-584-550

Academic Editor: Kyoko Nakagawa-Goto
Received: 2 September 2019; Accepted: 19 September 2019; Published: 26 September 2019

Abstract: In spite of significant advancements and success in antiretroviral therapies directed against HIV infection, there is no cure for HIV, which scan persist in a human body in its latent form and become reactivated under favorable conditions. Therefore, novel antiretroviral drugs with different modes of actions are still a major focus for researchers. In particular, novel lead structures are being sought from natural sources. So far, a number of compounds from marine organisms have been identified as promising therapeutics for HIV infection. Therefore, in this paper, we provide an overview of marine natural products that were first identified in the period between 2013 and 2018 that could be potentially used, or further optimized, as novel antiretroviral agents. This pipeline includes the systematization of antiretroviral activities for several categories of marine structures including chitosan and its derivatives, sulfated polysaccharides, lectins, bromotyrosine derivatives, peptides, alkaloids, diterpenes, phlorotannins, and xanthones as well as adjuvants to the HAART therapy such as fish oil. We critically discuss the structures and activities of the most promising new marine anti-HIV compounds.

Keywords: antiretroviral agents; anti-HIV; marine metabolites; natural products; drug development

1. Introduction

Human immunodeficiency virus (HIV) infections pose a global challenge given that in 2017, according to the World Health Organization data, 36.9 million people were living with HIV and additional 1.8 million people were becoming newly infected globally (Table 1). HIV targets immune cells and impairs the human defense against pneumonia, tuberculosis, and shingles as well as certain types of cancer [1]. The most advanced stage of HIV infection is the Acquired Immunodeficiency Syndrome (AIDS), which can take from two to 15 years to develop, depending on the individual [2].

Table 1. Summary of the global human immunodeficiency virus (HIV) epidemic (2017) according to World Health Organization (WHO) data.

	People Living with HIV in 2017	People Newly Infected with HIV in 2017	HIV-Related Deaths in 2017
total	36.9 million (31.3–43.9 million)	1.8 million (1.4–2.4 million)	940,000 (670,000–1.3 million)
adults	35 million (29.6–41.7 million)	1.6 million (1.3–2.1 million)	830 000 (590,000–1.2 million)
women	18.2 million (15.6–21.4 million)		
men	16.8 million (13.9–20.4 million)		
children (<15 years)	1.8 million (1.3–2.4 million)	180,000 (110,000–260,000)	110,000 (63,000–160,000)

HIV has two viral forms: HIV-1 (the most common form that accounts for around 95% of all infections worldwide) and HIV-2 (relatively uncommon and less infectious). HIV-1 consists of groups M, N, O, and P with at least nine genetically distinct subtypes of HIV-1 within group M (A, B, C, D, F, G, H, J, and K). Additionally, different subtypes can combine genetic material to form a hybrid virus known as the 'circulating recombinant form' (CRFs) (Figure 1). HIV-2 consists of eight known groups (A to H). Of these, only groups A and B are pandemic. The HIV-2 mechanism is not clearly defined and neither is its difference from HIV-1. However, the transmission rate is much lower in HIV-2 than in HIV-1. HIV-2 is estimated to be more than 55% genetically distinct from HIV-1.

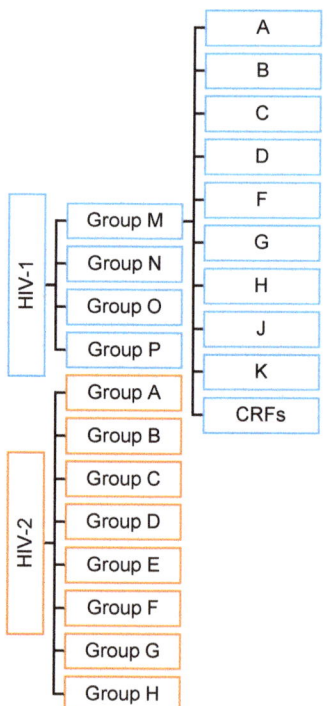

Figure 1. HIV types and strains classification.

The HIV-1 genome has reading frames coding for structural and regulatory proteins. The *gag* gene encodes the Pr55Gag precursor of inner structural proteins p24 (capsid protein, CA), p17 (matrix protein, MA), p7 (nucleoprotein, NC), and p6 involved in the virus particle release. The *pol* gene encodes the Pr160GagPol precursor of the viral enzymes p10 (protease, PR), p51 (reverse transcriptase, RT), p15 (RNase H), and p32 (integrase, IN). The *env* gene encodes the PrGp160 precursor of the gp120 (surface glycoprotein, SU) and gp41 (transmembrane protein, TM). Other genes include *tat*, encoding p14 (transactivator protein), *rev*, encoding p19 (RNA splicing regulator), *nef*, encoding p27 (negative regulating factor), *vif*, encoding p23 (viral infectivity protein), *vpr*, encoding p15 (virus protein r), *vpu*, encoding p16 (virus protein unique), *vpx* in HIV2, encoding p15 (virus protein x), and *tev*, encoding p26 (tat/rev protein) [3].

The HIV infections are extremely problematic as the virus targets the CD4+ memory T-cells population, which is essential for organism immunity. HIV can attach itself to the host cell through 1) a relatively nonspecific interaction with negatively charged cell-surface heparan sulfate proteoglycans [4], 2) specific interactions between the Env and $\alpha 4\beta 7$ integrin [5,6], and/or 3) the interaction with pattern-recognition receptors, such as the dendritic cell-specific intercellular adhesion molecular 3-grabbing non-integrin (DC-SIGN) [7]. The attachment of HIV in any of the abovementioned ways can increase the efficacy of infection because it brings Env, a heavily glycosylated trimer of gp120 and gp41 heterodimers, into close proximity with the viral receptor CD4 and co-receptor [8]. Finally, in order for the viral entry to occur, Env needs to bind itself to the host protein CD4 [9,10].

The binding of the HIV glycoprotein gp120 to the host cell CD4 receptor causes conformational changes of the gp120 glycoprotein, which uncover additional binding sites that interact with distinct proteins on the host cell membrane, known as β-chemokine co-receptors (mainly CCR5 and CXCR4), which facilitate the virus entry into the cell [11].

After the infection, a progressive decline of CD4 + cells consequently leads to the failure of the immune system function and the development of opportunistic infections that usually lead to death [1]. In HIV-infected patients, immunodeficiency develops both as a result of the viral replication and the failure of the patients' homeostatic mechanisms. The continuous viral presence in the patients after the application of therapy is attributed to the CD4 + T-cell homeostasis owing to a pool of latently infected and resting CD4 + T-cells, macrophages, and follicular dendritic cells that remain in the organism. Indeed, the complex interactions of the patient's immune system with the virus, and vice versa after the viral suppression, are thought to be crucial for the control of disease progression [12,13].

Current therapeutic approaches mainly target proteins that are vital for the viral cycle. One of the prominent examples is the linear 36-amino acid synthetic peptide enfuviritide (T20, Fuzeon), developed by Hoffmann-La Roche, and the first FDA approved fusion inhibitor for the treatment of HIV-1/AIDS acting through the binding to the gp41 subunit of the HIV-1 envelope glycoprotein. This induces a conformational change that brings the viral and cellular membranes into close enough proximity for the fusion and the subsequent viral entry into the host-cell to occur. Nevertheless, several restrictions, such as a low genetic barrier for drug resistance and a short in vivo half-life, limit its clinical use [14–17].

Other various FDA-approved antiretroviral drugs from seven mechanistic classes of inhibitors of the HIV replication are also available for the treatment of infected patients, namely, the nucleoside reverse-transcriptase inhibitors NRTIs, non-nucleoside reverse-transcriptase (RT) inhibitors NNRTIs, protein inhibitors PIs, fusion inhibitors, entry inhibitors—CCR5 co-receptor antagonists, HIV integrase strand transfer inhibitors, and multi-class combinations. None of the mentioned drug classes alone or in combination, the latter being known as the highly active antiretroviral therapy (HAART), can eradicate the HIV infection, and effective vaccines remain unavailable.

The difficulties of HIV-1 vaccine research are, in part, a result of 1) the unavailability of a model for natural immunity related to HIV; 2) the existence of genetically distinct subtypes of HIV and frequent mutations; 3) unidentified correlates of specific immune response to HIV; 4) lack of a reliable, non-human animal model for HIV infection (SIV in monkeys vs. HIV in humans).

The established latent pro-viral reservoirs in the patient's body can stochastically begin to reproduce viral particles, which makes the HIV disease practically incurable. From over 160 compounds identified so far as latency-reversing agents (LRAs), none have led to a promising cure [18].

Several rare and long-term remissions of HIV cases are described in the literature. For example, Berlin, London, and Düsseldorf's patients underwent bone marrow transplantation with stem cells from a donor with a rare genetic mutation of the CCR5. The Mississippi baby received a very early antiretroviral therapy that extended the time of the viral rebound for more than 27 months. There undoubtedly remains a lot to be learned from these cases, and further investigation of stem-cell transplantation in people living with HIV is required [19–21].

The currently used antiretroviral treatment, alone or in combination, extends the quality and life expectancy of HIV-infected individuals but does not cure them. Drug resistance, along with the emergence of drug-resistant virus strains, a high-cost of the lifetime treatment regimen, cell toxicity, and serious side effects of currently used anti-HIV drugs [2] underlie the need for a synthetic development of new drugs or the search for active anti-HIV molecules in natural sources. Mother Nature has been perfecting its chemistry for three billion years, and most of it has been done in water. Intense competition and feeding pressure as well as non-static marine environmental conditions yield compounds with chemical and structural features generally not found in terrestrial natural products.

New efficient molecules directed against HIV should demonstrate better performance in comparison with the currently approved drugs and suppress the HIV virus and/or eliminate the latent HIV reservoirs present in the human body.

Around 60% of drugs currently available on the market are derived or inspired by nature [22]. Turning to nature for drug development holds great potential, especially when it comes to marine organisms. Only few marine-derived drugs have been approved on the market so far but many are in the preclinical or clinical stage of development [23]. Marine organisms make up to two-thirds of Earth's species and produce, as a consequence of living in a highly competitive environment, unique and structurally diverse metabolites. Over the last 40 years, bioprospecting efforts have resulted in over 20,000 compounds of marine origin. The highest share of marine metabolites (up to 70%) are obtained from marine sponges, corals, and microorganisms, while mollusks, ascidians, and algae metabolites form only a minor part [24]. Oceans are, indeed, still a rather underexploited habitat, and biodiversity appears to be higher in the oceans than on land, which might be relevant when focusing on the marine environment as an untapped reservoir of novel antiretroviral candidates. In the discovery of new antiviral marine-derived drugs, researchers usually implement two strategies. They either screen the extracts from different strains (e.g., cyanobacteria, microalgae) or search directly for bioactive molecules in organisms—extract and purify them for evaluation within the drug development pipeline. It is thought that the marine environment might yield more potent anti-HIV candidates characterized by a higher efficiency (lower effective dose) and a better selectivity and which do not induce resistance development. This could, of course, only be speculation based on some of the previous success stories in the discovery of drugs from natural sources such as, e.g., lovastatin and paclitaxel. However, nature generally does create more sophisticated and perfected systems with a complex mode of action.

An excellent example is protein lectin, derived from marine red algae *Griffithsia* sp. named Griffithsin with mid-picomolar activities, which groups it among the most potent HIV entry inhibitors reported so far [25]. It inhibits the HIV infection by binding itself to high mannose glycan structures on the surface of gp120, altering the gp120 structure or its oligomeric state [26]. This interaction relies on the specific trimeric "sugar tower," including N295 and N448 [27]. Griffithsin can also prevent infections caused by other glycoprotein-enveloped viruses such as the Ebola virus, hepatitis C virus, and the severe acute respiratory syndrome coronavirus. It has been shown that the dimerization of Griffithsin is necessary for a high potency inhibition of HIV-1 [28]. However, the discrepancy between the HIV gp120 binding activity and the HIV inhibitory activity points to the presence of mechanism unrelated to a merely simple HIV gp120 binding [26]. The most promising application of Griffithsin would be its incorporation into vaginal and rectal gels, creams, or suppositories acting as an antiviral microbicide to prevent the transmission of HIV.

Despite the vast number of structurally diverse and unique bioactive molecules from the marine environment, the global marine pharmaceutical pipeline includes only eight approved drugs: Adcetris®, Cytosar-U®, Halaven®, Yondelis®, Carragelose®, Vira-A®, Lovaza®, and Prialt® [29]. Overall, it has taken 20 to 30 years from their discovery to their entry into the market. A sustainable supply, structural complexity, optimization of formulation, and ADMET properties, and a scale-up issue have prevented further development of several highly promising marine compounds. It is by no means an easy task to identify a marine candidate that may be considered as a potential drug. Initial high costs of developing a natural product into a drug could be balanced out with careful long-term considerations (biodiversity, supply, and technical, market) [30].

This paper provides an overview of natural marine metabolites that were first identified in the period between 2013 and 2018 or the previously identified marine constituents with a recently confirmed anti-HIV activity that could be potentially used or further optimized as novel ant-HIV agents. We also comprehensively summarize anti-HIV activities for several categories of marine structures including chitosan and its derivatives, sulfated polysaccharides, lectins, bromotyrosine derivatives, peptides, alkaloids, diterpenes, phlorotannins, and xanthones as well as fish oil as an auxiliary to HAART therapy.

2. Marine Compounds in the Treatment of HIV/AIDS

2.1. Chitosan and Its Derivatives

Chitosan (**2**, Figure 2), a natural marine byproduct, is a poly-cationic linear polysaccharide derived from chitin (**1**, Figure 2) after partial deacetylation. Chitin is a structural element in the exoskeleton of mainly shrimps and crabs and is mainly composed of the randomly distributed β-(1-4)-linked D-glucosamine and N-acetyl-D-glucosamine. It has been previously shown that this compound can exhibit a large scale of different bioactivities and can also be used as a carrier for anti-HIV drugs [31]. Chitosan is loaded with saquinavir, an anti-HIV drug with a protease inhibitory activity, which showed better cell targeting efficiency than saquinavir alone [32]. Furthermore, trimethyl chitosan has improved Atripla, an anti-HIV drug consisting of efavirenz, emtricitabine, and tenofovir disoproxil fumarate, anti-HIV 1 activity, and has allowed it to be used in lower concentrations [33]. The antiretroviral activity is manifested in the chitosan-specific cationic nature that allows the formation of electrostatic complexes or multilayer structures with other negatively charged polymers [34]. Karagozlu et al. reported about new QMW-COS and WMQ-COS oligomers with anti-HIV activities. These oligomers are conjugates of chitosan and the Gln-Met-Trp peptide, which were constructed as a continuation of the authors' previous research, in which a high potency of synthetically constructed chitosan oligomers was confirmed in anti-HIV therapy. More specifically, it was shown that these oligomers suppress syncytium formation, which occurs as a fusion of infected cells with neighboring cells, induced by HIV in a dose-dependent manner. However, the authors also noticed that after a certain period, the number of syncytia once again increased, suggesting that the cells should be re-treated with QMW-COS and WMQ-COS oligomers to maintain the primary therapeutically-relevant effect. The inhibition of the HIV-1 induced lytic effect, determined by the cell viability assay, showed that IC_{50} for QMW-COS was 48.14 µg/mL and was almost identical for WMQ-COS, 48.01 µg/mL. These oligomers effectively reduced the HIV load but showed no effects on HIV-1 RT and protease in vitro. Higher dosages were also required for the reduction in the HIV-1IIIB p24 antigen production assessed by the ELISA assay and the HIV-1$_{RTMDR}$ p24 antigen production. The highest difference between the compounds was reflected in IC_{50} values obtained from studies on the virus-induced luciferase activity in infected cells, where QMW-COS had a higher potency in comparison with WMQ-COS. Lastly, the authors determined the effects of oligomers on the interaction between gp41 and CD4 by using the CD4-gp41 ELISA assay, whereby both oligomers showed high potency. The effect of these oligomers was highest when they were applied immediately upon the HIV-1 infection of cells, indicating that they should be used as a potential treatment in the early stages of HIV infection, probably at the entry stage [31].

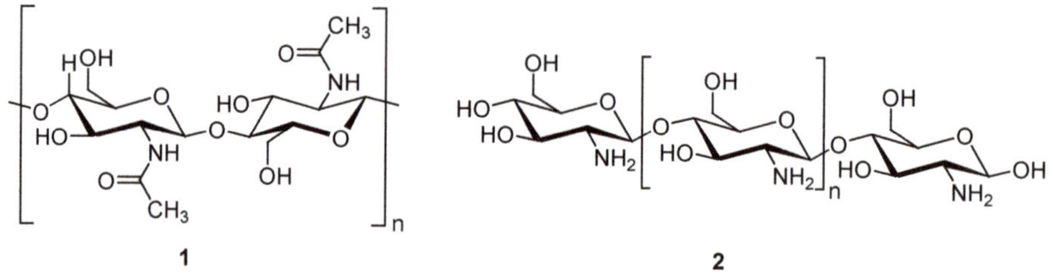

Figure 2. Chemical structures of chitin (1) and chitosan (2).

2.2. Sulfated Polysaccharides

Sulfated polysaccharides (SP) are the most studied class of antiviral polysaccharides that are structural components of the alga cell wall where they play both the storage and structural role. They are an important source of galactans, commercially known as agar and carrageenan in red alga (Rhodophyta), fucans (fucoidan, sargassan, ascophyllan, and glucuronoxylofucan) in brown alga (Phaeophyta), and ulvans-sulfated heteropolysaccharides that contain galactose, xylose, arabinose, mannose, glucuronic acid, or glucose [35–37]. Many studies indicate that, in marine algae, sulfated polysaccharides facilitate water and ion retention in extracellular matrices, which is an important mechanism for coping with desiccation and osmotic stress in a highly salted environment [38–40]. The antiviral activity of this group of compounds is mainly connected to the degree of sulfation, constituent sugars, molecular weight, conformation, and dynamic stereochemistry [41,42]. The effect of counter cation should also be considered as an important factor in observed biological activity.

The antagonizing effect of the negatively charged sulfated polysaccharides on the HIV-1 entry into cells may be due to 1) their binding onto the positively charged V3 domain of gp120, thereby preventing the virus attachment to the cell surface [43–45] or 2) the masking of the docking sites of gp120 for sCD4 on the surface of T lymphocytes, thereby disrupting the CD4-gp120 interaction [46–48] and subsequently inhibiting the expression of the viral antigen and the activity of the viral reverse transcriptase [49,50].

2.2.1. Heparan Sulfate

Heparinoid polysaccharides can interact with the positive-charge regions of cell-surface glycoproteins, leading to a shielding effect on these regions, which prevents the binding of viruses to the cell surface [51]. The sulfated polysaccharides content in marine mollusks is high in comparison with the bovine mucosal heparin (73.5%) and the porcine mucosal heparin (72.8%) [52]. The acidic sulfate groups on heparin (3, Figure 3), or heparin-like compounds, can inhibit HIV through electrostatic interactions with basic amino-acid residues of the transcriptional activator Tat protein [53].

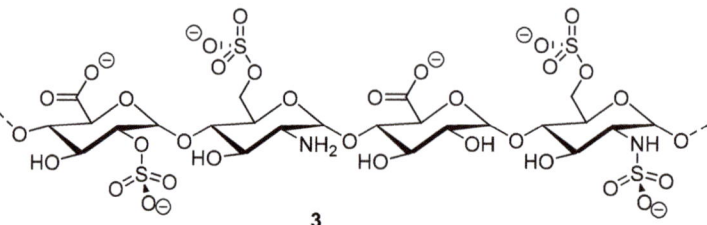

Figure 3. Structure of heparan sulfate (3).

2.2.2. Fucose Containing SP

So far, the main anti-infectious activities documented for the fucose-containing SP are those against viruses [54]. More importantly, these polysaccharides are selective inhibitors of various enveloped viruses, including HIV [54–56]. FCSP acts during the early phase of infection by blocking the virus attachment and entry into the host cells, but may also inhibit subsequent replication stages in vitro [57].

2.2.3. Fucoidans

Three fucoidans extracted from three brown seaweeds (*Sargassum mcclurei*, *Sargassum polycystum*, *Turbinara ornata*) inhibit the early stages of HIV-1 entry into target cells, with IC_{50} ranging from 0.33 to 0.7 µM. Neither the sulfate content nor the position of sulfate groups are related to the anti-HIV activity of fucoidans, suggesting the involvement of other structural parameters such as the molecular weight, the type of glycosidic linkage, or even a unique fucoidan sequence [56]. Although the presence of sulfo-groups seems to be necessary for anti-HIV activity [58], these data do not support random sulfation as the main antiviral factor.

Sulfated fucan polysaccharides, ascophyllan (**4**, Figure 4), and two fucoidans (S and A) (**5** and **6**, Table 2), derived from different sources, significantly inhibit (IC_{50} 1.3; 0.3; 0.6 µg/mL) the early step of HIV-1 (R9 and JR-Fl) infection. They also inhibit the VSV-G-pseudotype HIV-1 infection in HeLa cells [59].

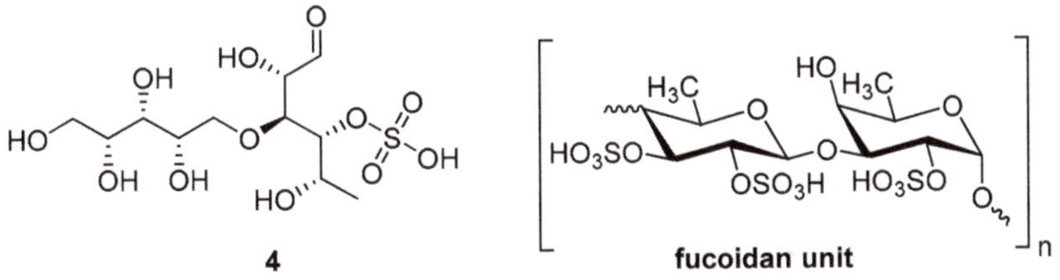

Figure 4. Structure of ascophyllan (**4**) and fucoidan unit.

Table 2. Chemical composition of polyscharides (Fuc, Fucose; Xyl, Xylose; Glu, Glucose; Man, Mannose; Gal, Galactose) in ascophyllan, S- and A-fucoidan.

	Neutral Sugars					Uronic Acid	SO_3^-
	Fuc	Xyl	Glu	Man	Gal		
ascophyllan (**4**)	15.5	13.4	0.3	3.4	0.6	21.4	9.6
S-fucoidan (**5**)	24.8	1.9	0.8	1	3.1	9.6	22.6
A-fucoidan (**6**)	28.4	4.3	2.0	0.8	5.1	5.8	19.4

Chondroitin sulfate with fucosylated branches (FuCS) (**7**, Figure 5) has also attracted attention as an HIV antiviral compound. Depolymerized fucosylated CS, extracted from the sea cucumber, has shown in vitro activity against a range of viral strains, including the resistant ones [60]. FuCS is effective in blocking the laboratory strain HIV-1IIIB entry and replication by inhibiting the p24 antigen production (4.26 and 0.73 µg/mL, respectively) and the infection of the clinic isolate HIV-1KM018 and HIV-1TC-2 (23.75 and 31.86 µg/mL, respectively) as well as suppressing the HIV-1 drug-resistant virus. Additionally, FuCS is also effective in T-20-resistant strains (EC50 values ranging from 0.76 to 1.13 µg/mL). The depolymerized fragments seem to maintain a similar anti-HIV action at the early stages of infection, apparently through interaction with an HIV envelope glycoprotein gp120. The sulfated fucose branches appear necessary for antiviral activity, which is also affected by molecular weight and carboxylation [61]. While the in vitro results of the fucosylated CS against HIV are promising, it is questionable whether the antiviral activity would be maintained in vivo. Other polyanionic HIV entry inhibitors, which advanced into clinical trials, failed to prove effective against the heterosexual HIV-1 transmission. This was related to factors not considered in previous development stages, such as the presence of seminal plasma and the concentration and retention of polyanionic inhibitors [62].

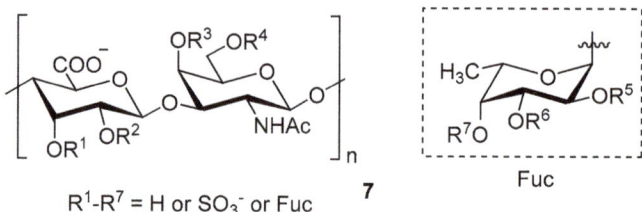

Figure 5. General chemical structure of fucosylated chondroitin sulfate (7).

The complex chemical architecture and the sulfate patterning of marine polysaccharides depends on numerous factors (species, tidal cycles, environmental variations (e.g., salinity), harvesting season, plant age, geographical location etc.) [39,63–69], making isolation, purification, and comprehensive chemical characterization a highly challenging task [70]. The development of many polysaccharides into clinical application is hindered by the still limited view of their sophisticated and diverse nature. Despite having good antiviral effects, the use of carbohydrate drugs is still in its infancy, and intensive structure-activity and in vivo studies are needed in the future.

A relatively new strategy in inducing immunity and developing an HIV vaccine is to use carbohydrates. The major difficulty of such an approach lies in mimicking the specific glycan protective epitope. Gp120 of HIV is a highly glycosylated envelope surface glycoprotein responsible for the receptor and co-receptor binding, which, together with gp41, comprises the heterodimeric envelope trimer spikes of HIV. N-linked glycans, mainly mannose and complex-type, cover much of the gp120 surface-accessible face of the HIV envelope spike forming the glycan shield. Inadequate mimicry of the glycan shield, tolerance mechanisms, and/or the inability to induce a domain-exchange are reflecting difficulties in creating the proper specificity of Abs [71]. Most of the vaccines for HIV-1 in preclinical trials are based on a Manα1-2Man oligomannosyl epitope (various conjugates, engineered yeast strains, and modified glycoproteins) [72–79]. Better specificity could potentially be gained using carbohydrates of marine origin.

2.3. Lectins

Lectins are a group of proteins that specifically, but reversibly, bind glycosylated molecules on the cell surface. Precisely, this group of molecules can affect cell-cell interactions, protect cells from pathogens, influence cell adhesion, and affect the intracellular glycoprotein translocation [80]. Recently, lectins have become promising agents for antiretroviral therapy, and different researches have confirmed their anti-HIV properties. Their antiretroviral activity is manifested through an alteration of the interaction between HIV gp120 or gp41 and the corresponding receptors [81], which, in the end, inhibit the HIV cell function, HIV infectivity, and the formation of the syncytium, multi-nucleated cells [82–84].

Several published review papers describe the previously found marine lectins with antiretroviral action [85,86]. For example, Gogineni et al. reported about some new, unusual lectins, such as the β-galactose specific lectin (CVL), CGL, DTL, DTL-A, SVL-1, and SVL-2 [86]. Additionally, Akkouh et al. reported about some new algal lectins, such as *Boodlea Coacta* Lectin, Griffithsin and *Oscillatoria Agardhii* Agglutinin (OAA), and some cyanobacterial lectins, such as Cyanovirin-N, Scytovirin, Microcystis Viridis Lectin, and Microvirin.

However, in the last few years, there has not been as much research focused on anti-HIV lectins from marine sources. Only Hirayama et al. (2016) reported about the new high-mannose specific lectin and its recombinants that possess anti-HIV activity [87]. In their research performed on the red alga *Kappaphycus alvarezii*, authors confirmed KAA-1 and KAA-2, two KAA mannose-binding lectin isomers, as potent anti-HIV agents. The anti-HIV role of action of these two compounds includes a strong binding to the virus envelope glycoprotein gp120 and, consequently, the inhibition of HIV entry into the host cells. These KAA recombinants, as well as the native one, inhibited the HIV-1 entry at IC_{50}s (neutralization assay in Jurkat cells) of 7.3–12.9 nM. Authors concluded in the end that KAAs, besides their strong inhibitory effect on HIV entry into the cells, have a potential as agents in treatments against other viruses possessing high mannose glycans on their envelope as well.

2.4. Peptides

It has been shown that the majority of marine peptides have strong anti-HIV activity. They are usually isolated from marine organisms through the process of enzymatic hydrolysis [88]. The most common source of such constituents is marine sponges that are known for their unique metabolome [89] and are a source of more than 36% of all marine bioactive compounds [90]. Their bioactive peptides can be found in cyclic or linear forms and contain unusual amino acids that form unique structures rarely found in other species. Antiretroviral activity of such structures works on several different levels: blocking of virus entry, inhibition of the cytopathic viral activity, neutralization of viral particles, or inhibition of viral fusion and entry [89,91].

Recently, Shin et al. discovered two new depsipeptides from marine sponges *Stelletta sp.*, stellettapeptin A (**8**, Figure 6), and stellettapeptin B (**9**, Figure 6), with the inhibition of the cytopathic effect of HIV-1 infection [92]. Confirming the mentioned theory about the unique metabolome of marine sponges, the authors revealed that these two compounds have previously undescribed nonproteinogenic amino-acid parts on peptides that are rarely found in nature. Namely, stellettapeptin A and stellettapeptin B have an unexpected polyketide subunit, 3-hydroxy-6,8-dimethylnon-4-enoic acid, 3-OHGln, and 3-OHAsn residues. Their high potency is witnessed through low EC_{50} values (inhibition of the cytotoxic effect upon HIV infection)—values of 23 nM for stellettapeptin A and 27 nM for stellettapeptin B.

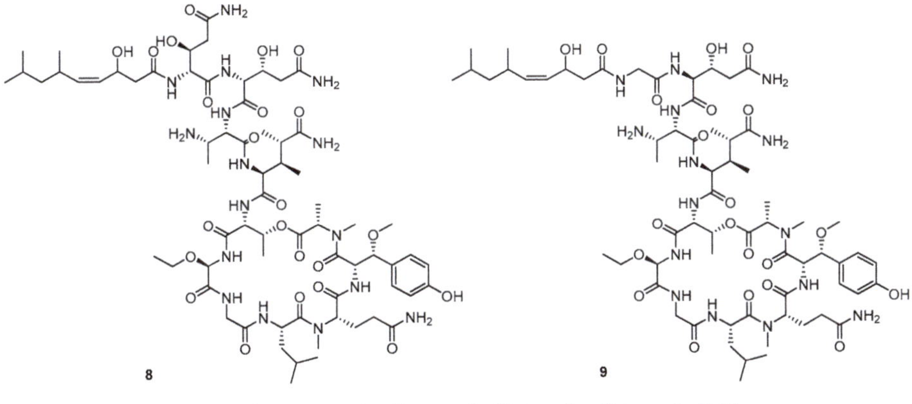

Figure 6. Structures of stelletapeptin (**8**) A and stelletapeptin B (**9**).

Furthermore, newly discovered anti-HIV constituents derived from marine sponges *Verongula rigida* and *Aiolochoria crassa* with amino-acid structure were published by Gomez-Archila et al. (2014) [93]. In their paper, they evaluated and confirmed the anti-HIV effect of 11 bromotyrosine derivatives (Table 3), whereby aeroplysinin-1 (**10**), 19-deoxyfistularin 3 (**15**), purealidin B (**16**), fistularin 3 (**17**) and 3-bromo-5-hydroxy-O-methyltyrosine (**18**, Figure 7) were the most potent in their anti-HIV activity. Aeroplysinin 1 (**15**) and purealidin B (**16**), compounds found in *V. rigida* species inhibited the HIV-1 replication in a dose-dependent manner by more than 50%. Specifically, for aeroplysinin 1, HIV-a replication was inhibited by 74% at a concentration of 20 µM, whereas purealidin was less potent with inhibitory power of 57% at a concentration of 80 µM. These two compounds had been previously isolated; however, their anti-HIV activity was proven in this research. The same was with 3-bromo-5-hydroxy-O-methyltyrosine (**18**) that has a relatively high percentage of inhibition of HIV activity (47%) in a dose-dependent manner. However, the exact mechanism of action remains unclear. In the same study, additional tests with these compounds on the HIV RT inhibition (qPCR of the early and late transcripts), nuclear import (qPCR analysis of 2-LTR transcript), and HIV entry inhibition (viral infectivity assay) were performed. The results showed that aeroplysinin-1 (**10**), 19-deoxyfistularin 3 (**15**), purealidin B (**16**), fistularin 3 (**17**), and 3-bromo-5-hydroxy-O-methyltyrosine (**18**) influenced the nuclear import of the HIV virus with around or more than 50% of inhibition: aeroplysinin-1 (**10**) showed 67% of inhibition at 10 µM, 19-deoxyfistularin 3 62% inhibition at 20 µM, purealidin B 66% of inhibition at 20 µM, fistularin 3 47% of inhibition at 10 µM, and 3-bromo-5-hydroxy-O-methyltyrosine 73% of inhibition at 80 µM. Viral RT inhibition was not high for all compounds, whereby the highest results were around 50% of inhibition. For example, purealidin B had 58% of inhibition at 20 µM in the qPCR analysis of early transcripts. As for the HIV entry inhibition, all compounds were active in a dose-depended manner, with the highest results of inhibition obtained for 3,5-dibromo-N,N,N,O-tetramethyltyraminium (**13**), from 14% to 30%. Finally, the authors stressed the structural similarity of these compounds with the HIV integrase and protease inhibitors, suggesting that these compounds can have a broader mode of antiviral action.

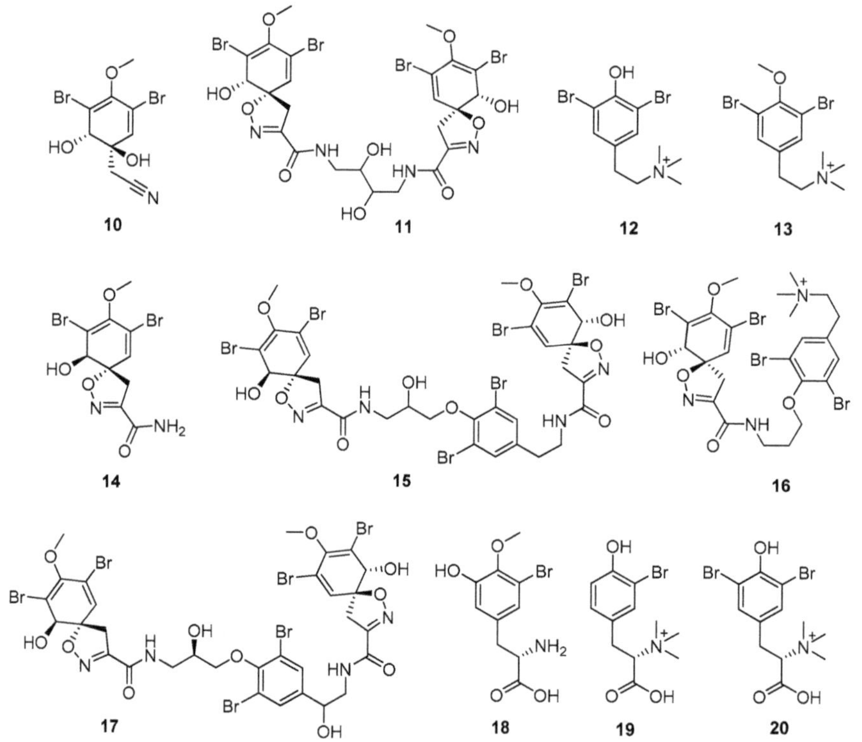

Figure 7. Structures of aeroplysinin-1 (**10**), dihydroxyaerothionin (**11**), 3,4-dibromo-N,N,N-trimethyltyraminium (**12**), 3,5-dibromo-N,N,N,O-tetramethyltyraminium (**13**), purealidin R (**14**), 19-deohxyfistularin 3 (**15**), purealidin B (**16**), fistularin-3 (**17**), 3-bromo-5-hydroxy-O-methyltyrosine (**18**), 3-bromo-N,N,N-trimethyltyrosinium (**19**), and 3,5-dibromo-N,N,N-trimethyltyrosinium (**20**).

Table 3. Summary of anti-HIV compounds from marine organisms.

Group	Compound	Location	Organism	Assay	Dose	Activity	Structure	Reference
Peptide + chitosan oligomer	QMW-COS	not disclosed [a]	marine byproduct	IC$_{50}$—inhibition of HIV-1 induced lytic effects (cell viability assay); IC$_{50}$—inhibition of HIV-1$_{IIIB}$ p24 antigen production (ELISA); IC$_{50}$—inhibition of HIV-1$_{KTMDR}$ p24 antigen production (ELISA); IC$_{50}$—inhibition of virus-induced luciferase activity in infected TZM-bl cells; IC$_{50}$—inhibition of the interaction between gp41 and CD4 (CD4-gp41 ELISA)	48.14 µg/mL; 67.35 µg/mL; 81.03 µg/mL; 68.13 µg/mL; 39.13 µg/mL	**anti-HIV-1**; inhibition of the HIV entry at an early stage, blocking the fusion of HIV-1 infected cells, interference of gp41-CD4 binding	glutamine (Q), methionine (M), tryptophan (W)	[31]
	WMQ-COS	not disclosed [a]	marine byproduct	IC$_{50}$—Inhibition of HIV-1 induced lytic effects (cell viability assay); IC$_{50}$—inhibition of HIV-IIIB p24 antigen production (ELISA); IC$_{50}$—inhibition of HIV-1$_{KTMDR}$ p24 antigen production (ELISA); IC$_{50}$—inhibition of virus-induced luciferase activity in infected TZM-bl cells; IC$_{50}$—inhibition of interaction between gp41 and CD4 (CD4-gp41 ELISA)	48.01 µg/mL; 98.73 µg/mL; 144.02 µg/mL; 250 µg/mL; 51.48 µg/mL	**anti-HIV-1**; inhibition of the HIV entry at an early stage	tryptophan (W), methionine (M), glutamine (Q)	[31]
Sulfated polysaccharides	heparan sulfate (3)	not disclosed	-	EC$_{50}$—inhibition of HIV-1$_{IIIB}$ strain (syncytia assay); EC$_{50}$—inhibition of HIV-1$_{IIIB}$ strain (p24 assay); EC$_{50}$—inhibition of HIV-1$_{IIIB}$/H9 strain (co-cultivation assay); EC$_{50}$—inhibition of HIV-1$_{RF}$ strain (p24 assay); EC$_{50}$—inhibition of HIV-1$_{KM018}$ strain (p24 assay); EC$_{50}$—inhibition of HIV-1$_{TC-2}$ strain (p24 assay); EC$_{50}$—inhibition of HIV-1$_{A17}$ strain (p24 assay); EC$_{50}$—inhibition of HIV-1$_{RF/V82F/I84V}$ strain (p24 assay); EC$_{50}$—inhibition of HIV-1$_{L10R/M46I/L63P/V82T/I84V}$ strain (p24 assay); EC$_{50}$—inhibition of HIV-1$_{CBL-20}$ strain (syncytia assay); EC$_{50}$—inhibition of HIV-1$_{ROD}$ strain (syncytia assay)	0.24 µg/mL; 0.73 µg/mL; 4.26 µg/mL; 1.14 µg/mL; 23.75 µg/mL; 31.86 µg/mL; 1.09 µg/mL; 0.95 µg/mL; 1.12 µg/mL; 71.76 µg/mL; 97.63 µg/ml	**anti-HIV-1**; electrostatic interactions with basic amino acid residues of Tat		[53]

Table 3. *Cont.*

Group	Compound	Location	Organism	Assay	Dose	Activity	Structure	Reference
	fucose containing	Nha Trang bay, Vietnam	*Sargassum mcclurei*, *Sargassum polycystum*, and *Turbinara Ornate* brown seaweeds	U373-CD4-CXCR4 cells 211 infected with pseudotype viral IC$_{50}$—inhibition (F$_{SP}$ crude extract)-(p24 ELISA) IC$_{50}$—inhibition (F$_{TO}$ crude extract)-(p24 ELISA) IC$_{50}$—inhibition (F$_{SM}$ crude extract)-(p24 ELISA)	0.34 µg/mL 0.39 µg/mL 0.96 µg/mL	**anti-HIV-1**; inhibition of the early phase of infection, by blocking the virus attachment and entry into the host cells		[56]
	ascophyllan (4)	not disclosed	different sources	IC$_{50}$—inhibition of HIV-1$_{89}$-real-time PCR	1.3 µg/mL	**anti-HIV-1**; early step of HIV-1 (R9 and JR-FI) infection; inhibition of VSV-G-pseudotyped HIV-1 infection in HeLa cells		[59]
	fucoidan S (5) fucoidan A (6)	not disclosed	different sources	IC$_{50}$—inhibition of HIV-1$_{89}$-real-time PCR (fucoidan S) IC$_{50}$—inhibition of HIV-1$_{89}$-real-time PCR (fucoidan A)	0.3 µg/mL 0.6 µg/ml	**anti-HIV-1**; early step of HIV-1 (R9 and JR-FI) infection; inhibition of VSV-G-pseudotyped HIV-1 infection in HeLa cells		[59]
	chondroitin sulfate (7)	not disclosed		EC$_{50}$—HIV-1 p24 detection-PBMC assay-inhibition of HIV-1$_{IIIB}$, HIV-1$_{L10R/M46I/L63P/V82T/I84V}$, HIV-1$_{A17}$, HIV-1$_{RF}$, and HIV-1$_{RF/V82F/I84V}$ strains	0.01–0.08 µM	**anti-HIV-1**; inhibition of HIV-1 replication; inhibition of the HIV-1 entry		[61]
Lectins	KAA-1	not disclosed	red alga *Kappaphycus alvarezii*	IC$_{50}$—neutralization assay in Jurkat cells (median tissue culture infectious dose (TCID50) method using Jurkat cells)	9.2 nM	**anti-HIV-1**; inhibition of the HIV-1 entry		[87]
	KAA-2	not disclosed	red alga *Kappaphycus alvarezii*	IC$_{50}$—neutralization assay in Jurkat cells (median tissue culture infectious dose (TCID50) method using Jurkat cells)	7.3 nM	**anti-HIV-1**; inhibition of the HIV-1 entry		[87]

Table 3. Cont.

Group	Compound	Location	Organism	Assay	Dose	Activity	Structure	Reference
Peptides	stellettapeptin A (8)	north-western Australia	marine sponge *Stelletta sp.*	EC$_{50}$—inhibition of the cytotoxic effect upon HIV-1 infection	23 nm	**anti-HIV-1**; cytopathic effect of HIV-1 infection		[92]
	stellettapeptin B (9)	north-western Australia	marine sponge *Stelletta sp.*	EC$_{50}$—inhibition of the cytotoxic effect upon HIV-1 infection	27 nm	**anti-HIV-1**; cytopathic effect of HIV-1 infection		[92]
Bromotyrosine derivatives	aeroplysinin-1 (10)	Colombia	marine sponge *Verongula rigida*	% of inhibition of HIV-1 replication by flow cytometry % of reverse transcription inhibition (qPCR analysis of late transcripts) % of nuclear import inhibition (qPCR analysis of 2-LTR transcript) % of HIV entry inhibition (viral infectivity assay)	74% of inhibition at 20 µM 48% of inhibition at 10 µM 67% of inhibition at 10 µM dose dependent manner 2–20%	**anti-HIV-1**; inhibition of HIV-1 replication, RT, nuclear import and entry		[93]
	3,5-dibromo-*N,N,N,O*-tetramethyl Tyraminium (13)	Colombia	marine sponge *Verongula rigida*	% of HIV entry inhibition (viral infectivity assay)	dose depended manner 14–30%	**anti-HIV-1**; inhibition of HIV-1 entry		[93]
	19-deoxy fistularin 3 (15)	Colombia	marine sponge *Verongula rigida*	% of reverse transcription inhibition (qPCR analysis of early transcripts) % of reverse transcription inhibition (qPCR analysis of late transcripts) % of nuclear import inhibition (qPCR analysis of 2-LTR transcript)	35% inhibition at 20 µM 11% inhibition at 20 µM 62% inhibition at 20 µM	**anti-HIV-1**; inhibition of HIV-1 replication, RT, nuclear import		[93]

Table 3. *Cont.*

Group	Compound	Location	Organism	Assay	Dose	Activity	Structure	Reference
	purealidin B (16)	Colombia	marine sponge *Verongula rigida*	% of inhibition of HIV-1 replication by flow cytometry % of reverse transcription inhibition (qPCR analysis of early transcripts) % of reverse transcription inhibition (qPCR analysis of late transcripts) % of nuclear import inhibition (qPCR analysis of 2-LTR transcript) % of HIV entry inhibition (viral infectivity assay)	57% of inhibition at 80 µM 58% of inhibition at 20 µM 34% of inhibition at 20 µM 66% of inhibition at 20 µM dose depended manner 2–11%	**anti-HIV-1**; inhibition of HIV-1 replication, RT, nuclear import and entry		[93]
	fistularin 3 (17)	Colombia	marine sponge *Verongula rigida*	% of reverse transcription inhibition (qPCR analysis of late transcripts) % of nuclear import inhibition (qPCR analysis of 2-LTR transcript) % of HIV entry inhibition (viral infectivity assay)	24% of inhibition at 5 µM, 47% of inhibition at 10 µM, dose depended manner 11–13%	**anti-HIV-1**; inhibition of, HIV-1 RT, nuclear import and HIV-1 entry		[93]
	3-bromo-5-hydroxy-O-methyltyrosine (18)	Colombia	marine sponge *Aiolochroia crassa*	% of inhibition of HIV-1 replication by flow cytometry % of reverse transcription inhibition (qPCR analysis of early transcripts) % of reverse transcription inhibition (qPCR analysis of late transcripts) % of nuclear import inhibition (qPCR analysis of 2-LTR transcript) % of HIV entry inhibition (viral infectivity assay)	47% of inhibition at 80 µM, 54% of inhibition at 160 µM, 50% of inhibition at 40 µM, 73% of inhibition at 80 µM, dose depended manner 2–12%	**anti-HIV-1**; inhibition of HIV-1 replication, RT, nuclear import and entry		[93]

Table 3. Cont.

Group	Compound	Location	Organism	Assay	Dose	Activity	Structure	Reference
Peptides	APCHP (21)	not disclosed	Alaska pollack	EC_{50}—against anti-HIV-1 induced cell lysis (MTT assay) EC_{50}—HIV-1-induced RT activation in MT-4 cells EC_{50}—against p24 production (western blot)	459 µM (0.403 mg/mL) 374 µM (0.327 mg/mL) 405 µM (0.356 mg/mL)	anti-HIV-1; inhibition of induced syncytia formation by interference of HIV fusion inhibition of cell lysis, RT activity and production of p24 antigen		[94]
	SM-peptide	not disclosed	*Spirulina maxima*	IC_{50}—protective activity on HIV-1-induced cell lysis-MTT assay % of RT Inhibition in HIV-1-infected cells (reverse transcriptase assay kit) % of HIV-1 p24 antigen production (p24 antigen production assay)	0.691 mM (0.475 mg/mL) 90% inhibition at 1.093 mM (0.75 mg/mL) 95% of inhibition at 1.093 mM (0.75 mg/mL)	anti-HIV-1; inhibition of the HIV-1 RT activity and p24 antigen production	Leu-Asp-Ala-Val-Asn-Arg	[95]
Alkaloids	aspernigrin C (22)	Yongxing Island, South China Sea	marine fungus *Aspergillus niger* SCSIO Jcw6F30 isolated from marine alga *Sargassum sp.*	IC_{50}—inhibitory effects on infection by CCR5-tropic HIV-1 SF162 in TZM-bl cells	4.7 µM	anti-HIV-1		[96]
	malformin C (23)	Yongxing Island, South China Sea	marine fungus *Aspergillus niger* SCSIO Jcw6F30 isolated from marine alga *Sargassum sp.*	IC_{50}—inhibitory effects on infection by CCR5-tropic HIV-1 SF162 in TZM-bl cells	1.4 µM	anti-HIV-1		[96]

Table 3. Cont.

Group	Compound	Location	Organism	Assay	Dose	Activity	Structure	Reference
	eutypellazine E (24)	South Atlantic Ocean	deep-sea sediment fungus *Eutypella sp.* MCCC 3A00281	IC$_{50}$—anti-HIV bioassay-pNL4.3.Env.-Luc co-transfected 293T cells	3.2 µM	**anti-HIV-1;** inhibitory effects against HIV-1 replication		[97]
	eutypellazine J (25)	South Atlantic Ocean	deep-sea sediment fungus *Eutypella sp.* MCCC 3A00281	IC$_{50}$—anti-HIV bioassay-pNL4.3.Env.-Luc co-transfected 293T cells reactivation activity-In vitro latent HIV reactivating assay-flow cytometry-based screening	4.9 µM 80 µM	**anti-HIV-1;** inhibitory effects against HIV-1 replication, latency reactivating agent		[97]
	debromo-hymenialdisine (26)	Coral reefs in the Red Sea	*S. carteri* sponge extract	% of reduction of HIV-1 replication-cell-based assay	30% of inhibition at 13 µM	**anti-HIV 1;** decrease the transcription of the HIV-1, abrogate the G2-checkpoint of the cell cycle		[98]
	Hymenialdisine (27)	Coral reefs in the Red Sea	*S. carteri* sponge extract	% of reduction of HIV-1 replication-cell-based assay	<40% of inhibition at 3.1 µM	**anti-HIV 1;** decrease the transcription of the HIV-1, abrogate the G2-checkpoint of the cell cycle		[98]

Table 3. Cont.

Group	Compound	Location	Organism	Assay	Dose	Activity	Structure	Reference
	Oroidin (28)	Coral reefs in the Red Sea	*S. carteri* sponge extract	% of inhibition - HIV-1 RT biochemical assay % of reduction of HIV-1 replication-cell-based assay	90% of inhibition at >25 µM 50% of inhibition at 50 µM	anti-HIV-1; inhibition of HIV-1 RT, reduction of HIV-1 replication		[98]
	3-(phenetyl amino) demethyl(oxy) aaptamine (29)	Woody Island (Yongxing, Hainan, China) and Seven Connected Islets in the South China Sea	*A. aptos* sponge extract	% of inhibition against HIV-1 replication-anti-HIV-1 activity assay-cell-based VSVG/HIV-1 pseudotyping system	88% of inhibition at 10 µM	anti-HIV-1; inhibitory effects against HIV-1 replication		[99]
	3-(isopentyl amino) demethyl(oxy) aaptamine (30)	Woody Island (Yongxing, Hainan, China) and Seven Connected Islets in the South China Sea	*A. aptos* sponge extract	% of inhibition against HIV-1 replication-anti-HIV-1 activity assay-cell-based VSVG/HIV-1 pseudotyping system	72.3% of inhibition at 10 µM	anti-HIV-1; inhibitory effects against HIV-1 replication		[99]
	bengamide A (31)	not disclosed	screening of previously isolated compounds (originally isolated from the sponge *Jaspis cf. coriacea*)	EC$_{50}$—multi-cycle viral replication assay % inhibition of p24^{Gag} production-of PBMC assay-p24^{Gag} was quantified by ELISA EC$_{50}$—inhibition of LTR promoter-driven gene expression-LTR-based reporter assays	0.015 µM >90% of inhibition at 0.3 µM 0.17 µM	anti-HIV-1; inhibition of NF-κB-mediated retroviral gene expression		[100]
	haliclony-cyclamine A + B (32)	not disclosed	screening of previously isolated compounds	EC$_{50}$—multi-cycle viral replication assay	3.8 µM	anti-HIV-1; inhibitory effects against HIV-1 replication		[100]

Table 3. *Cont.*

Group	Compound	Location	Organism	Assay	Dose	Activity	Structure	Reference
	keramamine C (33)	not disclosed	screening of previously isolated compounds	EC$_5$—multi-cycle viral replication assay	3.4 µM	**anti-HIV-1**; inhibitory effects against HIV-1 replication		[100]
	stachybotrin D (34)	Xisha Island, China	sponge *Xestospongia testudinaris*	EC$_{50}$—inhibitory Effects on Wild-Type and NNRTI-Resistant HIV-1 Replication: EC$_{50}$—inhibition of VSVG/HIV-1$_{wt}$ EC$_{50}$—inhibition of VSVG/HIV-1$_{RT-K103N}$ EC$_{50}$—inhibition of VSVG/HIV-1$_{RT-L100I,K103N}$ EC$_{50}$—inhibition of VSVG/HIV-1$_{RT-K103N,V108I}$ EC$_{50}$—inhibition of VSVG/HIV-1$_{RT-K103N,G190A}$ EC$_{50}$—inhibition of VSVG/HIV-1$_{RT-K103N,P225H}$	8.4 µM 7.0 µM 23.8 µM 13.3 µM 14.2 µM 6.2 µM	**anti-HIV-1**; HIV-1 RT inhibition (inhibitory effects on wild type and five NNRTI-resistant HIV-1 strains)		[101]
Diterpenes	dolabelladienetriol A (35)	Atol das Rocas, in Northeast Brazil	brown alga *Dictyota pfaffii*	EC$_{50}$—inhibition of the cytopathic effect of HIV-1-MT-2 cells—MTT method	2.9 µM	**anti-HIV-1**;- inhibition of the cytopathic effect of HIV-1		[102]
	dolabelladienetriol B (36)	Atol das Rocas, in Northeast Brazil	brown alga *Dictyota pfaffii*	EC$_{50}$—inhibition of the cytopathic effect of HIV-1-MT-2 cells—MTT method	4.1 µM	**anti-HIV-1**;- inhibition of the cytopathic effect of HIV-1		[102]
	dolastane (38)	Praia do Velho, Angra dos Reis, in the south of Rio de Janeiro State, Brazil	brown alga *Canistrocarpus cervicornis*	EC$_{50}$—inhibition of HIV-1 replication-CXCR4-tropic HIV-1-MTT method	0.35 µM	**anti-HIV-1**; inhibition of HIV-1 replication, potent effect on HIV-1 infectivity		[103]

Table 3. *Cont.*

Group	Compound	Location	Organism	Assay	Dose	Activity	Structure	Reference
	dolastane (39)	Praia do Velho, Angra dos Reis, in the south of Rio de Janeiro State, Brazil	brown alga *Canistrocarpus cervicornis*	EC$_{50}$—inhibition of HIV-1 replication-CXCR4-tropic HIV-1–MTT method	0.794 µM	**anti-HIV-1;** inhibition of HIV-1 replication, potent effect on HIV-1 infectivity		[103]
	secodolastane diterpene (40)	Praia do Velho, Angra dos Reis, in the south of Rio de Janeiro State, Brazil	brown alga *Canistrocarpus cervicornis*	EC$_{50}$—inhibition of HIV-1 replication-CXCR4-tropic HIV-1–MTT method	3.67 µM	**anti-HIV-1;** inhibition of HIV-1 replication		[103]
	8,10,18-trihydroxy-2,6-dolabelladiene (41)	Atol das Rocas reef, Brazil	brown alga *Dictyota friabilis*	EC$_{50}$—inhibition of the cytopathic effect of HIV-1-MT-2 cells—MTT method	6.16 µM	**anti-HIV-1;** inhibition of the cytopathic effect of HIV-1		[104,105]
	oxygenated dolabellane (42)	Santa Marta Bay (Colombian Caribbean Sea	octocoral *Eunicea laciniata*	EC$_{50}$—inhibition of HIV-1-Inhibition of the cytopathic effect of HIV-1-MT-2 cells—MTT method	3.9 µM	**anti-HIV-1;** inhibition of the cytopathic effect of HIV-1		[106]
	oxygenated dolabellane (43)	Santa Marta Bay (Colombian Caribbean Sea	octocoral *Eunicea laciniata*	EC$_{50}$—inhibition of the cytopathic effect of HIV-1-MT-2 cells—MTT method	0.73 µM	**anti-HIV-1;** inhibition of the cytopathic effect of HIV-1		[106]
	oxygenated dolabellane (44)	Santa Marta Bay (Colombian Caribbean Sea	octocoral *Eunicea laciniata*	EC$_{50}$—inhibition of HIV-1-Inhibition of the cytopathic effect of HIV-1-MT-2 cells—MTT method	0.69 µM	**anti-HIV-1;** inhibition of the cytopathic effect of HIV-1		[106]

Table 3. *Cont.*

Group	Compound	Location	Organism	Assay	Dose	Activity	Structure	Reference
	8,4‴-dieckol (45)	not disclosed	brown alga, *Ecklonia cava*	Inhibition of syncytia formation on C8166 cells (HIV-1_IIIB, HIV-1_RF and HIV-1_A1)-inverted microscope Inhibition of the cytopathic effect of HIV-1-C8166 cells—MTT method Effect on p24 antigen production-p24 antigen capture ELISA and immunoblast analysis RT activity assay—commercial fluorescence RT assay kit Inhibition of HIV-1 replication-Luciferase gene reporter assay	Inhibition in dose-depended manner * Cell viability was more than 90% dose-dependent inhibition Inhibited 91% activity of HIV-1_IIIB RT and approximately 80% for rest of the HIV-1 strains tested, HIV-1_KMDR1 strain was inhibited at a ratio of 76.1% At the highest concentration, inhibition was more than 80% for all viral strains except for RTMDR1 (76.33%)	**anti-HIV-1**; inhibition of the cytopathic effects of HIV-1: inhibition of syncytia formation, lytic effects, inhibition of viral p24 antigen production, HIV-1 entry inhibition and RT inhibition		[107]
	penicillixanthone A (46)	not disclosed	from the jellyfish-derived fungus *Aspergillus fumigates*	IC$_{50}$—inhibition of PXA on infection by CCR5-tropic HIV-1 in TZM-bl cells IC$_{50}$—inhibition of PXA on infection by CXCR4-tropic HIV-1 in TZM-bl cells	0.36 µM 0.26 µM	**anti-HIV-1**; inhibition of infection against CCR5-tropic HIV-1 SF162 and CXCR4-tropic HIV-1 NL4-3		[108]
	docosahexanoic acid (48)	not disclosed		In vivo study on male rat models-Male F344 (control) and HIV-1Tg rats		**anti-HIV-1**; neuroprotective effect on neuroinflammations induced by ethanol (in the presence of HIV viral proteins)		[109]

Table 3. *Cont.*

Group	Compound	Location	Organism	Assay	Dose	Activity	Structure	Reference
Phlorotannins and xanthones	radicicol (49)	Tutuila, American Samoa	H. fuscoatra	EC$_{50}$—In Vitro Model of HIV-1 Latency-high-throughput primary cell-based HIV-1 latency assay	9.1 µM	anti-HIV-1; reactivation of latent viral loads in CD4+ T-cells		[110]
	pochonin B (50)	Tutuila, American Samoa	H. fuscoatra	EC$_{50}$—In Vitro Model of HIV-1 Latency-high-throughput primary cell-based HIV-1 latency assay	39.6 µM	anti-HIV-1; reactivation of latent viral loads in CD4+ T-cells		[110]
Auxiliary therapy to HAART therapy—fish oil	pochonin C (51)	Tutuila, American Samoa	H. fuscoatra	EC$_{50}$—In Vitro Model of HIV-1 Latency-high-throughput primary cell-based HIV-1 latency assay	6.3 µM	anti-HIV-1; reactivation of latent viral loads in CD4+ T-cells		[110]
Others	truncateol O (52)	Yongxing Island, Hainan Province of China	sponge-associated fungus *Truncatella angustata*	IC$_{50}$—Anti-HIV bioassays-VSV-G pseudotyped HIV-1-Luciferase assay system	39 µM	anti-HIV-1; inhibition of the HIV replication		[111]
	truncateol P (53)	Yongxing Island, Hainan Province of China	sponge-associated fungus *Truncatella angustata*	IC$_{50}$—Anti-HIV bioassays-VSV-G pseudotyped HIV-1-Luciferase assay system	16.1 µM	anti-HIV-1; inhibition of the HIV replication		[111]

[a] Tripeptide conjugates of chitosan (a natural marine byproduct), prepared in the laboratory.

Marine sponges are not the sole source of bioactive proteins. For example, Jang et al. reported about a new small hydroxyproline-rich peptide from Alaska Pollack collagen (APHCP, **21**, Figure 8) that exhibits a unique antiviral activity [94]. This peptide is a Gly-Pro-Hyp-Gly-Pro-Hyp-Gly-Pro-Hyp-Gly peptide, and the authors showed that the most important part of a peptide for anti-HIV activity is the hydroxyl group at hydroxyproline, whereas a peptide with only prolines does not exhibit antiviral activity. Its anti-HIV 1 mode of action is manifested through the inhibition of the induced syncytia formation by the interference of an HIV fusion, inhibition of cell lysis, RT activity, and the production of the p24 antigen. It was shown that APHCP can decrease the HIV-1 induced cell lysis at a potency around EC_{50} of 459 μM (EC_{50} against anti-HIV-1 induced cell lysis—MTT assay). Additionally, through the inhibition of the viral RT at EC_{50} at 374 μM, this peptide's crucial role in the inhibition of the conversion of viral RNA to DNA was also confirmed. With EC_{50} of 405 μM, this compound effectively suppressed the p24 production in viral cells, as determined by the Western blot analysis.

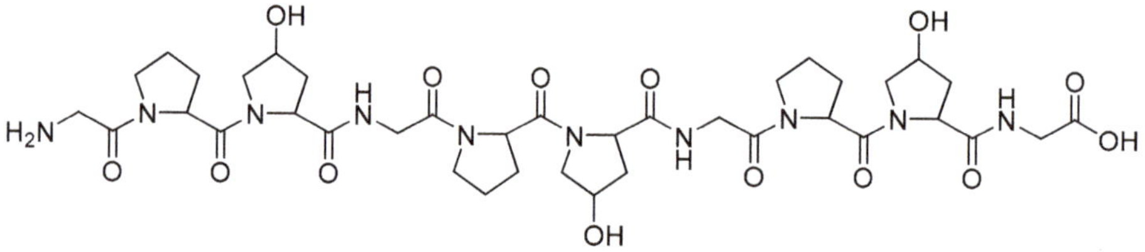

Figure 8. Structure of the Alaska Pollack collagen hydroxyl proline (APCHP) peptide (**21**).

Similarly, one new anti-HIV peptide was isolated from *Spirulina maxima* (SM-peptide) [95]–the Leu-Asp-Ala-Val-Asn-Arg peptide, and the authors showed its HIV-1 infection inhibition in a human T cell line MT4. The peptide inhibited cell lysis, p24 antigen production, and HIV-1 RT. Specifically, IC_{50} (obtained by a cell viability assay) against an anti-HIV 1 infection was determined as 0.691 mM, the inhibition of the HIV-1-induced RT activation (RT assay kit) in MT4 cells was at a high 90% at a concentration of 1.093 mM, and the p24 production (p24 antigen production assay) was inhibited at 95% at a concentration of 1.093 mM.

2.5. Alkaloids

Marine organisms are well-established sources of natural alkaloids. Although the term 'alkaloid' seems puzzling and is prone to scientific controversy, alkaloids are generally defined as nitrogen-containing compounds derived from plants and animals. Relatively few alkaloids from marine sources have been found to possess antiretroviral properties and, so far, none have found their clinical use.

Aspernigrin C (**22**, Figure 9) and malformin C (**23**, Figure 9) have been isolated from marine-derived black aspergili, *Aspergillus niger* SCSIO Jcw6F30, and their inhibitory activity against the chemokine receptor subtype 5 (CCR5) tropic HIV-1 SF162 has been evaluated. They show potent inhibition of infection with IC_{50} values 4.7 ± 0.4 μM and 1.4 ± 0.06 μM, which is comparable to the nucleoside reverse transcriptase inhibitor—abacavir (IC_{50} = 0.8 ± 0.1 μM) and the HIV-1 entry inhibitor ADS-J1 (IC_{50} = 0.8 ± 0.1 μM). In comparison to other aspernigrins, it has been suggested that the 2-methylsuccinic moiety is responsible for the potency of aspernigrin C [96].

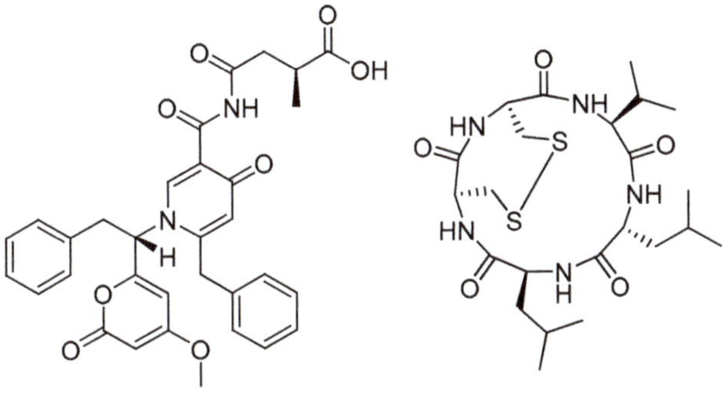

Figure 9. Structures of aspernigrin C (**22**) and malformin C (**23**).

Thiodiketopiperazine-type alkaloids, eutypellazines A-M, isolated from the EtOAc extract of the fermentation broth of deep-sea sediment fungus *Eutypella sp.* shows potent inhibitory effects against pNL4.3.Env-.Luc co-transfected 293T HIV model cells. Eutypellazine E (**24**, Figure 10) exerts activity in a low micromolar range (IC$_{50}$ = 3.2 ± 0.4 µM), while eutypellazine J (**25**, Figure 10) shows a reactivating effect toward latent HIV-1 in J-Lat A2 cells. This could be used as a promising strategy to expunge the HIV-1 infection by activating latent virus cellular reservoirs in combination with HAART [97].

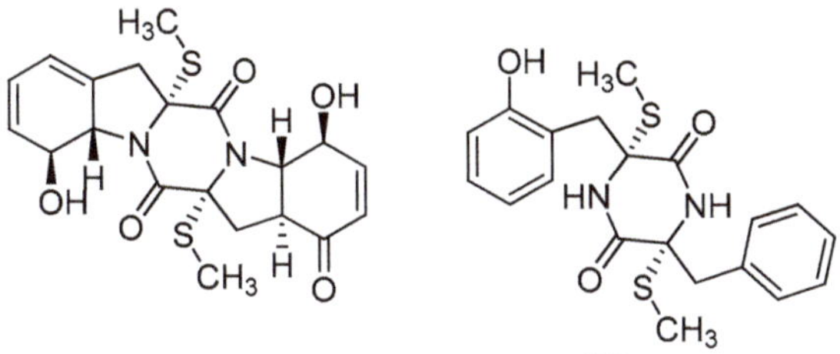

Figure 10. Structures of eutypellazine E (**24**) and eutypellazine J (**25**).

The *S. carteri* Red Sea sponge extract yields three previously characterized compounds: debromohymenialdisine (DBH) (**26**, Figure 11), hymenialdisine (HD) (**27**, Figure 11), and oroidin (**28**, Figure 11). DBH and HD exhibited a 30–40% inhibition of HIV-1 at 3.1 µM and 13 µM but with associated cytotoxicity. Conversely, oroidin displayed a 50% inhibition of viral replication at 50 µM without observed cytotoxicity. Also, it showed inhibition of HIV-1 reverse transcriptase up to 90% at 25 µMc [98].

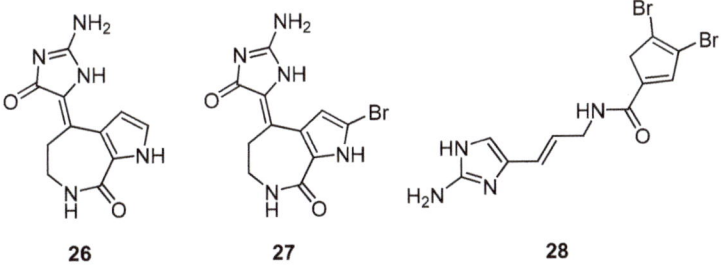

Figure 11. Structures of debromohymenialdisine (**26**), 10Z-hymenialdisine (**27**), and oroidin (**28**).

The two known alkaloids of the aaptamine family containing 1*H*-benz[*de*]-1,6-naphthyridine skeleton, namely 3-(phenetylamino)demethyl(oxy)aaptamine (**29**, Figure 12) and 3-(isopentylamino)demethyl(oxy)aaptamine (**30**, Figure 11), were isolated from the sponge *A. aptos*. They exhibited anti-HIV activity, with inhibitory rates of 88.0% and 72.3%, respectively, at a concentration of 10 µM [99].

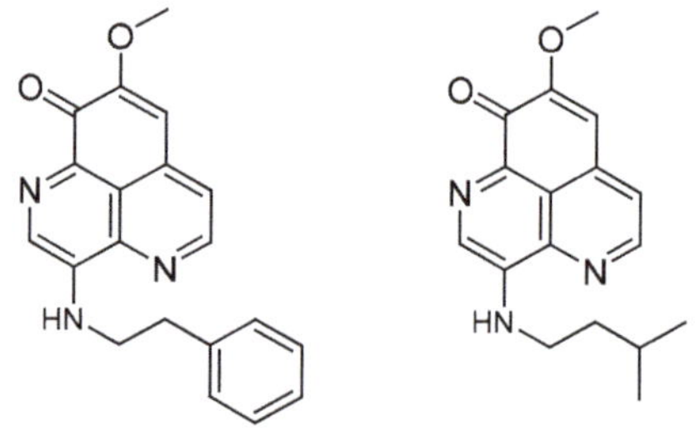

Figure 12. Structures of 3-(phenetylamino)dimethyl(oxo)aaptamine (**29**) and 3-(isopentylamino)dimethyl (oxo)aaptamine (**30**).

Bengamide A (**31**, Figure 13), haliclonycyclamine A+B (**32**, Figure 13) and keramamine C (**33**, Figure 13) inhibit HIV-1 with a 50% effective concentration of 3.8 µM or less. The most potent among them, bengamide A, blocked HIV-1 in a T cell line with an EC_{50} of 0.015 µM (which was comparable to control antiretrovirals indinavir 0.029 µM, efavirenz 0.0024 µM, and raltegravir 0.011 µM) and in peripheral blood mononuclear cells with EC_{50} of 0.032 µM. It was concluded that HIV-1 LTR NF-κB response elements are required for a bengamide A-mediated inhibition of LTR-dependent gene expression [100].

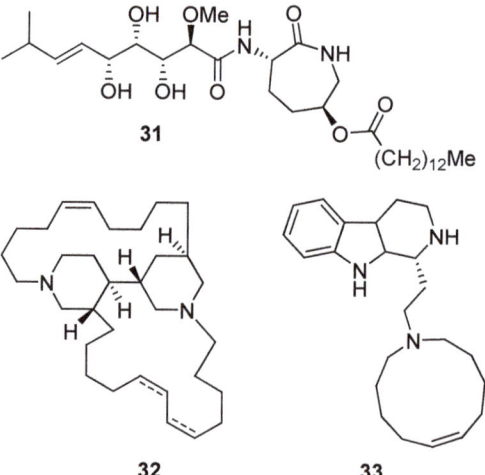

Figure 13. Structures of bengamide A (**31**), haliclonacyclamines A + B (**32**), keramamine C (**33**).

Phenylspirodrimane, stachybotrin D (**34**, Figure 14) isolated from the sponge-derived fungus *Stachybotrys chartarum* MXH-X73, was discovered to be a HIV-1 *RT* inhibitor, which showed inhibitory effects on the wild type (EC_{50} 8.4 µM) and five NNRTI-resistant HIV-1 strains (EC_{50} 7.0; 23.8; 13.3; 14.2; 6.2 µM) [101].

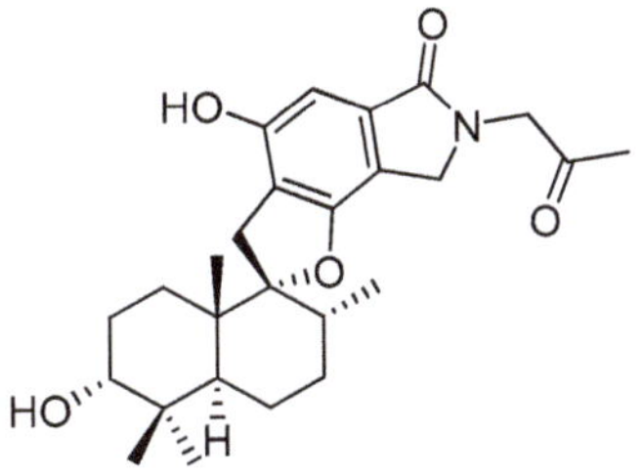

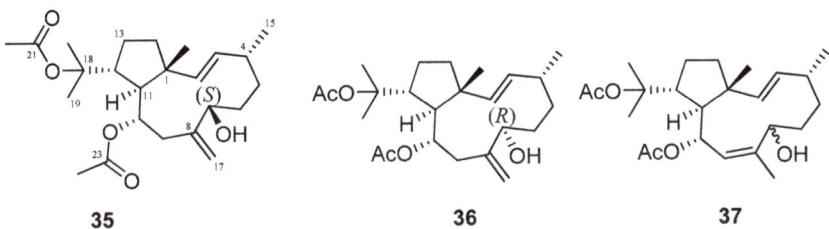

Figure 14. Structure of stachybotrin D (**34**).

2.6. Diterpenes

Many terpenes from marine natural products demonstrated anti-HIV properties. Mechanisms of action involve blocking of different steps of the HIV-1 replicative cycle as reverse transcriptase inhibitors, protease inhibitors, or entry inhibitors. Among them, diterpenes from marine algae are nowadays in the spotlight due to their promising anti-HIV activities [102]. Dolabellane diterpenes are compounds from the diterpene group that have recently been extensively studied for their anti-HIV activity. Pardo-Vargas et al. characterized three new dolabellane diterpenes isolated from the marine brown alga *Dictyota pfaffii* from Northeast Brazil: (1R*,2E,4R*,7S,10S*,11S*,12R*)10,18-diacetoxy-7-hydroxy-2,8(17)-dolabelladiene, (1R*,2E,4R*,7R*,10S*,11S*,12R*)10,18-diacetoxy-7-hydroxy-2,8(17)-dolabelladiene, (1R*,2E,4R*,8E,10S*,11S,12R*)10,18-diacetoxy-7-hydroxy-2,8-dolabelladiene, named dolabelladienols A–C (**35–37**, Figure 15), respectively [102]. In particular, the new compounds, dolabelladienols A and B, showed potent anti-HIV-1 activities that can be confirmed with their low IC_{50} values of 2.9 and 4.1 µM and low cytotoxic activity against MT-2 lymphocyte tumor cells. These promising anti-HIV-1 agents were even more active than previously known 2,6-dolabelladienes series.

Figure 15. Structures of the new dolabellane diterpenoids dolabelladienols A–C (**35–37**).

De Souza Barros et al. tested marine dolastanes (**38, 40**, Figure 16) and secodolastane diterpenes (**39**, Figure 16) isolated from the brown alga *Canistrocarpus cervicornis* for anti-HIV-1 activity [103]. They observed that the marine diterpenes **38–40** inhibit the HIV-1 replication in a dose-dependent manner (EC_{50} values of 0.35, 3.67, and 0.794 µM) without a cytotoxic effect (CC_{50} values ranging from 935 to 1910 µM). Additionally, they investigated the virucidal effect of these diterpenes and their potential use as microbicides. Dolastane-diterpenes **38** and **40** showed a potent effect on HIV-1 infectivity, whereas no virucidal effect was observed for secodolastane diterpene **39**, demonstrating another mechanism of antiretroviral activity. Therefore, the authors suggested a potential use of marine dolastanes **38** and **40** as microbicides that could directly inhibit virus infectivity and possibly act before the virus penetrates the target cells [103].

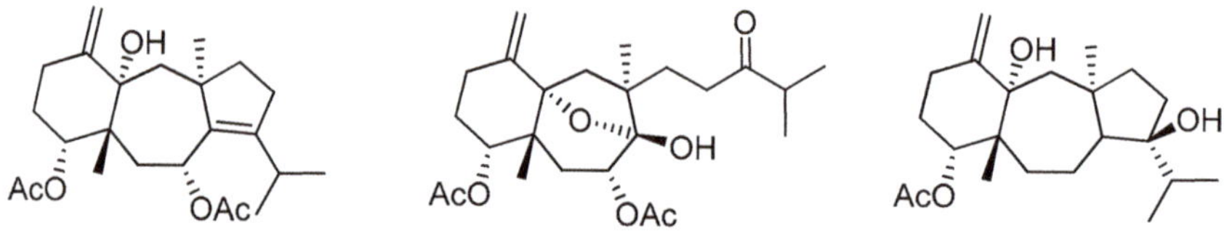

Figure 16. Structures of marine dolastanes (**38** and **40**) and secodolastane diterpene (**39**) derived from *Canistrocarpus cervicornis*.

Dolabelladienetriol from brown alga *Dictyota* spp has also been evaluated as a potential microbicide against HIV-1 in tissue explants. Namely, Stephens et al. examined the 8,10,18-trihydroxy-2,6-dolabelladiene (**41**, Figure 17) in pretreated peripheral blood cells (PBMC) and macrophages along with their protective effect in the ex vivo explant model of the uterine cervix [104]. Pre-treatment of peripheral PBMC and macrophages with dolabelladienotriol showed inhibitory effects on HIV-1 replication. Furthermore, in the explant model dolabelladienetriol inhibited viral replication in a dose-dependent manner from 20 to 99% in concentrations of 0.15 and 14.4 µM without a loss in the viability of the tissue. The authors concluded that this compound has great potential as a possible microbicide. The same compound was also theoretically analyzed as an inhibitor of the wild-type and mutants' HIV-1 reverse transcriptase [105]. Firstly, the structure-activity relationship studies revealed that a low dipole moment and high HOMO (highest occupied molecular orbital)-LUMO (lowest unoccupied molecular orbital) gap values are related to the antiviral activity. Secondly, molecular docking studies with RT wild-type and mutants showed a seahorse-like conformation of 8,10,18-trihydroxy-2,6-dolabelladiene, hydrophobic interactions, and hydrogen bonds with important residues of the binding pocket. Finally, the authors suggested a new derivative of the 8,10,18-trihydroxy-2,6-dolabelladiene with an aromatic moiety in the double bond to improve its biological activity.

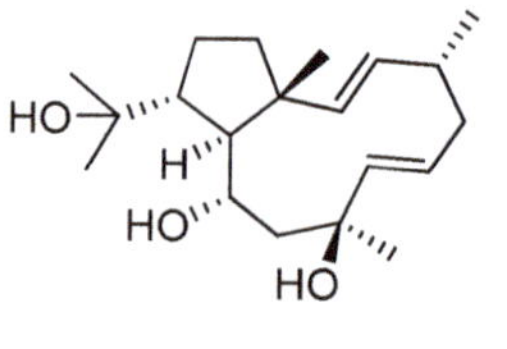

Figure 17. Structure of (1*R*,2*E*,4*R*,6*E*,8*S*,10*S*,11*S*,12*R*)-8,10,18-trihydroxy-2,6-dolabelladiene (**41**).

Although dolabellane diterpenes of brown alga *Dictyota* spp showed a strong anti-HIV-1 activity, this was not confirmed for dolabellane diterpenes isolated from octocorals. Therefore, some chemical transformations have been conducted to improve the anti-HIV-1 potency of the main dolabellane 13-keto-1(*R*),11(*S*)-dolabella-3(*E*),7(*E*),12(18)-triene from Caribbean octocoral *Eunicea laciniata* [106]. Oxygenated dolabellanes derivatives (**42–44**, Figure 18), obtained by epoxidation, epoxide opening, and allylic oxidation of ketodolbellatriene have shown significantly improved antiviral activities and a low cytotoxicity to MT-2 cells, which makes them promising antiviral compounds.

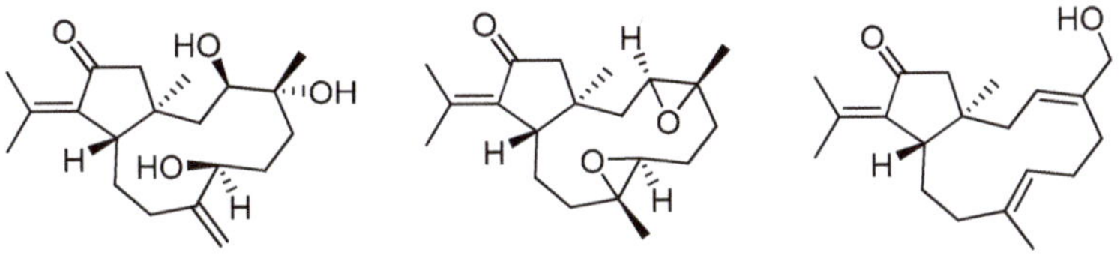

Figure 18. Structures of semi-synthesized oxygenated dolabellanes (**42**–**44**) originally isolated from the Caribbean octocoral *Eunicea laciniata*.

2.7. Phlorotannins and Xanthones

Phlorotannins are tannin derivatives made from several phloroglucinol units linked to each other in different ways. Phlorotannins contain phenyl linkage (fucols), ether linkage (fuhalols and phlorethols), phenyl and ether linkage (fucophloroethols), and dibenzodioxin linkage (eckols) [86,107]. So far, a series of phlorotannins have been identified with potent anti-HIV activity. For example, 8,8′-bieckol and 6,6′-bieckol from marine brown alga *Ecklonia cava* has shown an enhanced HIV-1 inhibitory effect [112,113]. Karadeniz et al. reported that 8,4‴-dieckol (**45**, Figure 19) is another phlorotannin derivative isolated from the same brown alga that could be used as a drug candidate for the development of new generation anti-HIV therapeutic agents [107]. The compound showed HIV-1 inhibitory activity at noncytotoxic concentrations. More precisely, the results indicated that 8,4‴-dieckol inhibited the cytopathic effects of HIV-1, including HIV-1 induced syncytia formation, lytic effects, and viral p24 antigen production. Furthermore, 8,4‴-dieckol inhibited an HIV-1 entry and RT enzyme with the inhibition ratio of 91% at a concentration of 50 µM.

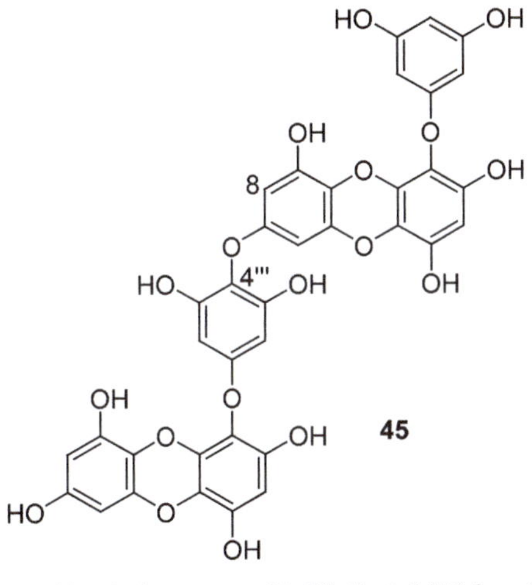

Figure 19. Chemical structure of 8,4‴-dieckol (**45**) from *E. cava*.

Recently, for the first time, xanthone dimer was identified as a potential anti-HIV-1 agent [108]. Xanthones are secondary metabolites from higher plant families, fungi, and lichen [114,115]. Although structurally related to flavonoids, xanthones are not as frequently encountered in nature [9]. Penicillixanthone A (PXA) (**46**, Figure 20), a natural xanthone dimer, has been isolated from the jellyfish-derived fungus *Aspergillus fumigates* with fourteen other natural products [108]. However, only penicillixanthone A showed inhibitory activities in an HIV infection. Marine-derived PXA displayed potent anti-HIV-1 activity against CCR5-tropic HIV-1 SF162 and CXCR4-tropic HIV-1 NL4-3, with IC_{50} of 0.36 and 0.26 µM, respectively. A molecular docking study confirmed that PXA might bind to either CCR5 or CXCR4 to prevent HIV entry into target cells. Therefore, PXA, as a CCR5/CXCR4 dual-coreceptor antagonist, may be seen as a new potential lead product type for the development of anti-HIV therapeutics.

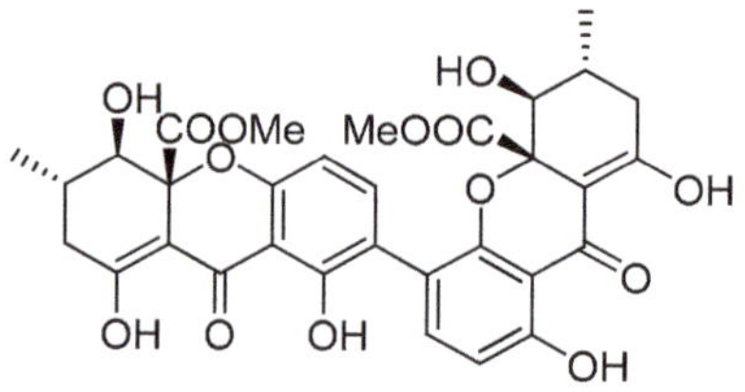

Figure 20. Structure of penicillixanthone A (**46**).

2.8. Fish Oil as an Adjuvant to HAART Therapy

HAART therapy can cause severe side effects, e.g., insulin resistance, lipoatrophy, dyslipidemia, and abnormalities of fat distribution. Therefore, finding an adequate diet and supplementation to lower the negative effects of the HAART combination therapy is desirable [116]. Fish oil contains omega-3 polyunsaturated fatty acids (PUFA), eicosapentaenoic (EPA, 20:5n-3) (**47**, Figure 21) and docosahexaenoic (DHA, 22:6n-3) (**48**, Figure 21) acids, which may have beneficial effects for HIV-infected patients. It has been shown that the addition of fish oil to the diet of HIV-infected individuals receiving usual antiretroviral therapy can significantly lower serum triglycerides levels [117], which is highly relevant knowing that HIV dyslipidemia is a serious problem related to an increased frequency of cardiovascular disease.

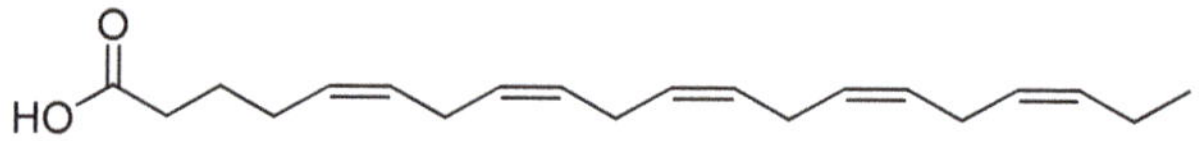

Figure 21. Structures of eicosapentanoic (**47**) and docosahexanoic acid (**48**).

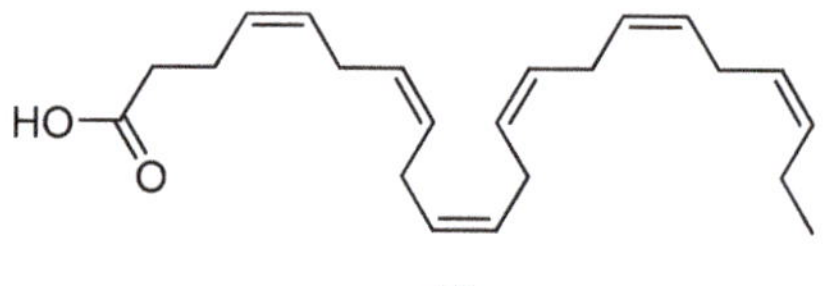

Recently, He et al. analyzed the influence of DHA on the locomotor activity in ethanol-treated HIV-1 transgenic rats [109]. The prevalence of alcohol use and alcohol abuse in infected individuals is much higher, and numerous ethanol and HIV-1 viral proteins have synergistic effects on inflammation in the central nervous system [118–120]. HIV remains in the body in its latent form after HAART therapy and, as such, can induce neuroinflammation. DHA depletion has been found to be associated with various neurological abnormalities, and its administration can have a neuroprotective effect. DHA taken daily could reverse the effects of the ethanol negative effect on the locomotor activity in the presence of HIV viral proteins. An in vivo study, using real-time quantitative PCR, showed that the addition of DHA can reduce elevated levels of IL-6, IL-18, and increase the expression of NF-κB in the striatum. This proved the potential of this fish oil constituent as an adjuvant in HIV patients' treatment that can help in lowering the interactive effects of ethanol consumption during HIV infection.

2.9. Others

Resorcyclic acid lactones, namely radicicol (**49**, Figure 22) pochonin B (**50**, Figure 22) and C (**51**, Figure 22) isolated from *H. fuscoatra* exhibited a 92–98% reactivation efficiency of the latent HIV-1 relative to SAHA (subeoylanilide hydroxamic acid, vorinostat, HDAC inhibitor) and EC_{50} of 9.1, 39.6 and 6.3 µM [110]. The reactivation strategy is, indeed, a promising strategy to expunge the HIV-1 infection by reactivating latent viral loads, mainly in CD4 + T-cells, which quickly rebound when antiviral treatment is interrupted. It was noted that all active compounds contain Michael acceptor functionality. The PKC-independent mechanism of reactivation of the latent HIV-1 remains to be elucidated.

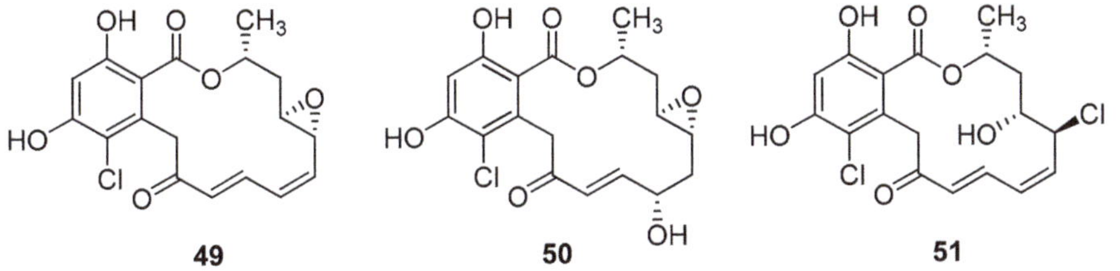

Figure 22. Structures of radicicol (**49**), pochonin B (**50**), pochonin C (**51**).

A team of researchers led by Zhao isolated new isoprenylated cyclohexanols from the sponge-associated fungus *Truncatella angustata* named truncateols O-V [111]. In vitro testing showed that truncateols O and P (**52** and **53**, Figure 23), analogues bearing the alkynyl group in the side chain, exhibit a significant inhibition toward the HIV-1 virus with IC_{50} values of 39.0 µM and 16.1 µM, respectively. These compounds could be considered as new anti-HIV lead compounds due to lower cytotoxicity (CC_{50} > 100 µM) in comparison with the positive control efavirenz (CC_{50} = 40.6 µM).

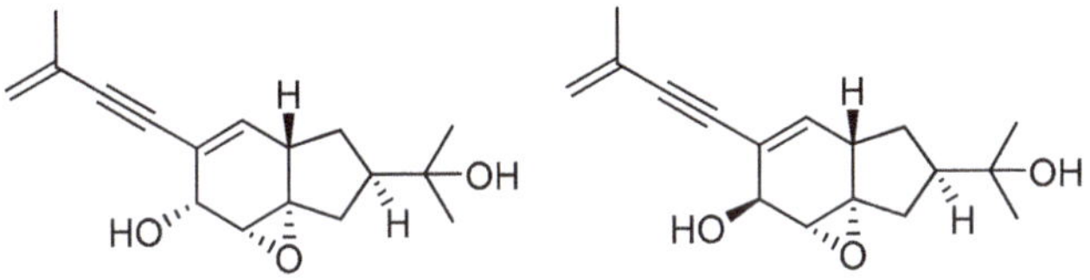

Figure 23. Structures of truncateols O (**52**) and P (**53**).

3. Future Directions in the Anti-HIV Marine Drug Development

Marine organisms have been acknowledged as a precious source of bioactive compounds that may provide novel anti-HIV structures or lead structures for structural optimization. A large amount of evidence from scientific research confirmed a high biological potential of these compounds to treat serious diseases, including infective ones. Some of the marine-derived bioactive compounds discovered much earlier have emerged with novel properties and potential applications after a decade or two. Isolation and structural elucidation of compounds from marine organisms is not an easy task and still carries challenges. Identification of all the compounds is a daunting task, especially with regards to complex structural motifs that may be present in a single marine extract. Taxonomic knowledge is still insufficient to enable unambiguous species classification that can result in the false prediction of chemical constituents and hamper structural analysis. Furthermore, a temporal lag between the discovery, chemical characterization, and associated pharmacological activities is quite common, and the majority of marine metabolites are usually tested for anticancer activity, whereas anti-HIV and other possible biological effects are neglected or mostly not performed due to a lack of funding. Targeted assays and in vivo analyses are similarly performed only for some of the potential candidates, while the translation into clinical trials remains very limited. Thus, the financial gap is certainly a relevant factor contributing to the slow drug development process in this area. In particular, the development of anti-HIV compounds, which act by mechanisms that differ from existing antivirals, requires a well-designed and focused approach to studying the mode of action. Libraries should be created for specifically defined crude extracts, their corresponding simplified fractions as well as for pure compounds for a well-balanced natural product discovery program. Additionally, there exist but few publications in which scientists have tried to modify known compounds of marine origin to improve their bioactivity. We are, however, continuously witnessing advancements in the deep-sea exploration technology, sampling strategies, genome sequencing, genome mining, genetic engineering, chemo-enzymatic synthesis, nanoscale NMR structure determination, and development and optimization of suitable fermentation strategies to ensure a continued supply of unique bioactive compounds from the oceans. Therefore, the grounds have been met for a broad, international effort based on scientific collaboration that would rely on well-equipped infrastructure and human resources as a prerequisite for a full advancement in the field and development of new drug candidates for the pharmaceutical market in the future.

Author Contributions: K.W. devised the main conceptual idea and, together with L.S. and Ž.P., wrote the manuscript parts related to medicinal chemistry. K.W. and Ž.P. performed literature searches and L.S. prepared the table. S.K.P. participated in the manuscript writing and wrote and discussed parts relevant for clinical applications, shaped the paper concept, and performed the final revision.

Funding: We want to thank the Croatian Government and the European Union (European Regional Development Fund—the Competitiveness and Cohesion Operational Programme—KK.01.1.1.01) for funding this research through project Bioprospecting of the Adriatic Sea (KK.01.1.1.01.0002) granted to The Scientific Centre of Excellence for Marine Bioprospecting—BioProCro. We also acknowledge the project "Research Infrastructure for Campus-based Laboratories at the University of Rijeka," co-financed by European Regional Development Fund (ERDF) and the University of Rijeka research grant uniri-biomed-18-133 (1277).

Conflicts of Interest: The authors declare no conflict of interests.

References

1. AVERT. Symptoms and Stages of HIV Infection. Available online: https://www.avert.org/about-hiv-aids/symptoms-stages (accessed on 12 April 2019).
2. HIV/AIDS. Available online: https://www.who.int/news-room/fact-sheets/detail/hiv-aids (accessed on 12 April 2019).
3. Li, G.; Piampongsant, S.; Faria, N.R.; Voet, A.; Pineda-Peña, A.-C.; Khouri, R.; Lemey, P.; Vandamme, A.-M.; Theys, K. An integrated map of HIV genome-wide variation from a population perspective. *Retrovirology* **2015**, *12*, 18. [CrossRef] [PubMed]
4. Saphire, A.C.S.; Bobardt, M.D.; Zhang, Z.; David, G.; Gallay, P.A. Syndecans Serve as Attachment Receptors for Human Immunodeficiency Virus Type 1 on Macrophages. *J. Virol.* **2001**, *75*, 9187–9200. [CrossRef] [PubMed]
5. Arthos, J.; Cicala, C.; Martinelli, E.; Macleod, K.; Van Ryk, D.; Wei, D.; Xiao, Z.; Veenstra, T.D.; Conrad, T.P.; Lempicki, R.A.; et al. HIV-1 envelope protein binds to and signals through integrin $\alpha_4\beta_7$, the gut mucosal homing receptor for peripheral T cells. *Nat. Immunol.* **2008**, *9*, 301–309. [CrossRef] [PubMed]
6. Cicala, C.; Martinelli, E.; McNally, J.P.; Goode, D.J.; Gopaul, R.; Hiatt, J.; Jelicic, K.; Kottilil, S.; Macleod, K.; O'Shea, A.; et al. The integrin $\alpha_4\beta_7$ forms a complex with cell-surface CD4 and defines a T-cell subset that is highly susceptible to infection by HIV-1. *PNAS* **2009**, *106*, 20877–20882. [CrossRef] [PubMed]
7. Geijtenbeek, T.B.; Kwon, D.S.; Torensma, R.; van Vliet, S.J.; van Duijnhoven, G.C.; Middel, J.; Cornelissen, I.L.; Nottet, H.S.; KewalRamani, V.N.; Littman, D.R.; et al. DC-SIGN, a dendritic cell-specific HIV-1-binding protein that enhances trans-infection of T cells. *Cell* **2000**, *100*, 587–597. [CrossRef]
8. Orloff, G.M.; Orloff, S.L.; Kennedy, M.S.; Maddon, P.J.; McDougal, J.S. Penetration of CD4 T cells by HIV-1. The CD4 receptor does not internalize with HIV, and CD4-related signal transduction events are not required for entry. *J. Immunol.* **1991**, *146*, 2578–2587. [PubMed]

9. Maddon, P.J.; Dalgleish, A.G.; McDougal, J.S.; Clapham, P.R.; Weiss, R.A.; Axel, R. The T4 gene encodes the AIDS virus receptor and is expressed in the immune system and the brain. *Cell* **1986**, *47*, 333–348. [CrossRef]
10. McDougal, J.; Kennedy, M.; Sligh, J.; Cort, S.; Mawle, A.; Nicholson, J. Binding of HTLV-III/LAV to T4+ T cells by a complex of the 110K viral protein and the T4 molecule. *Science* **1986**, *231*, 382–385. [CrossRef]
11. Alkhatib, G. The biology of CCR5 and CXCR4. *Curr. Opin. HIV AIDS* **2009**, *4*, 96–103. [CrossRef]
12. Okoye, A.A.; Picker, L.J. CD4(+) T-cell depletion in HIV infection: Mechanisms of immunological failure. *Immunol. Rev.* **2013**, *254*, 54–64. [CrossRef]
13. Schrager, L.K.; D'Souza, M.P. Cellular and anatomical reservoirs of HIV-1 in patients receiving potent antiretroviral combination therapy. *JAMA* **1998**, *280*, 67–71. [CrossRef] [PubMed]
14. Berkhout, B.; Eggink, D.; Sanders, R.W. Is there a future for antiviral fusion inhibitors? *Curr. Opin. Virol.* **2012**, *2*, 50–59. [CrossRef] [PubMed]
15. Greenberg, M.L.; Cammack, N. Resistance to enfuvirtide, the first HIV fusion inhibitor. *J. Antimicrob. Chemother.* **2004**, *54*, 333–340. [CrossRef] [PubMed]
16. Baldwin, C.E.; Sanders, R.W.; Deng, Y.; Jurriaans, S.; Lange, J.M.; Lu, M.; Berkhout, B. Emergence of a drug-dependent human immunodeficiency virus type 1 variant during therapy with the T20 fusion inhibitor. *J. Virol.* **2004**, *78*, 12428–12437. [CrossRef] [PubMed]
17. Rimsky, L.T.; Shugars, D.C.; Matthews, T.J. Determinants of human immunodeficiency virus type 1 resistance to gp41-derived inhibitory peptides. *J. Virol.* **1998**, *72*, 986–993. [PubMed]
18. Abner, E.; Jordan, A. HIV "shock and kill" therapy: In need of revision. *Antiviral Res.* **2019**, *166*, 19–34. [CrossRef]
19. Hütter, G.; Nowak, D.; Mossner, M.; Ganepola, S.; Müßig, A.; Allers, K.; Schneider, T.; Hofmann, J.; Kücherer, C.; Blau, O.; et al. Long-Term Control of HIV by CCR5 Delta32/Delta32 Stem-Cell Transplantation. *N. Engl. J. Med.* **2009**, *360*, 692–698. [CrossRef] [PubMed]
20. Ananworanich, J.; Robb, M.L. The transient HIV remission in the Mississippi baby: Why is this good news? *J. Int. AIDS Soc.* **2014**, *17*, 19859. [CrossRef]
21. The Lancet HIV. Like London buses, two putative cure cases arrive at once. *Lancet HIV* **2019**, *6*, e205. [CrossRef]
22. Newman, D.J.; Cragg, G.M. Natural Products as Sources of New Drugs from 1981 to 2014. *J. Nat. Prod.* **2016**, *79*, 629–661. [CrossRef]
23. Erakovic Haber, V.; Spaventi, R. Discovery and Development of Novel Drugs. In *Progress in Molecular and Subcellular Biology*; Springer: Cham, Switzerland, 2017; Volume 55, pp. 91–104.
24. Blunt, J.W.; Copp, B.R.; Hu, W.-P.; Munro, M.H.G.; Northcote, P.T.; Prinsep, M.R. Marine natural products. *Nat. Prod. Rep.* **2009**, *26*, 170. [CrossRef] [PubMed]
25. Mori, T.; O'Keefe, B.R.; Sowder, R.C.; Bringans, S.; Gardella, R.; Berg, S.; Cochran, P.; Turpin, J.A.; Buckheit, R.W.; McMahon, J.B.; et al. Isolation and Characterization of Griffithsin, a Novel HIV-inactivating Protein, from the Red Alga *Griffithsia* sp. *J. Biol. Chem.* **2005**, *280*, 9345–9353. [CrossRef] [PubMed]
26. Xue, J.; Gao, Y.; Hoorelbeke, B.; Kagiampakis, I.; Zhao, B.; Demeler, B.; Balzarini, J.; Liwang, P.J. The role of individual carbohydrate-binding sites in the function of the potent anti-HIV lectin griffithsin. *Mol. Pharm.* **2012**, *9*, 2613–2625. [CrossRef] [PubMed]
27. Huang, X.; Jin, W.; Griffin, G.E.; Shattock, R.J.; Hu, Q. Removal of two high-mannose N-linked glycans on gp120 renders human immunodeficiency virus 1 largely resistant to the carbohydrate-binding agent griffithsin. *J. Gen. Virol.* **2011**, *92*, 2367–2373. [CrossRef] [PubMed]
28. Xue, J.; Hoorelbeke, B.; Kagiampakis, I.; Demeler, B.; Balzarini, J.; Liwang, P.J. The griffithsin dimer is required for high-potency inhibition of HIV-1: Evidence for manipulation of the structure of gp120 as part of the griffithsin dimer mechanism. *Antimicrob. Agents Chemother.* **2013**, *57*, 3976–3989. [CrossRef] [PubMed]
29. Gerwick, W.H.; Moore, B.S. Lessons from the Past and Charting the Future of Marine Natural Products Drug Discovery and Chemical Biology. *Chem. Biol.* **2012**, *19*, 85–98. [CrossRef] [PubMed]
30. Martins, A.; Vieira, H.; Gaspar, H.; Santos, S.; Martins, A.; Vieira, H.; Gaspar, H.; Santos, S. Marketed Marine Natural Products in the Pharmaceutical and Cosmeceutical Industries: Tips for Success. *Mar. Drugs* **2014**, *12*, 1066–1101. [CrossRef] [PubMed]
31. Karagozlu, M.Z.; Karadeniz, F.; Kim, S.-K. Anti-HIV activities of novel synthetic peptide conjugated chitosan oligomers. *Int. J. Biol. Macromol.* **2014**, *66*, 260–266. [CrossRef] [PubMed]

32. Ramana, L.N.; Sharma, S.; Sethuraman, S.; Ranga, U.; Krishnan, U.M. Evaluation of chitosan nanoformulations as potent anti-HIV therapeutic systems. *Biochim. Biophys. Acta* **2014**, *1840*, 476–484. [CrossRef]
33. Shohani, S.; Mondanizadeh, M.; Abdoli, A.; Khansarinejad, B.; Salimi-Asl, M.; Ardestani, M.; Ghanbari, M.; Haj, M.; Zabihollahi, R. Trimethyl Chitosan Improves Anti-HIV Effects of Atripla as a New Nanoformulated Drug. *Curr. HIV Res.* **2017**, *15*, 56–65. [CrossRef]
34. Cheung, R.C.F.; Ng, T.B.; Wong, J.H.; Chan, W.Y. Chitosan: An Update on Potential Biomedical and Pharmaceutical Applications. *Mar. Drugs* **2015**, *13*, 5156–5186. [CrossRef] [PubMed]
35. Wijesekara, I.; Pangestuti, R.; Kim, S.-K. Biological activities and potential health benefits of sulfated polysaccharides derived from marine algae. *Carbohydr. Polym.* **2011**, *84*, 14–21. [CrossRef]
36. Jiao, G.; Yu, G.; Zhang, J.; Ewart, H.S. Chemical structures and bioactivities of sulfated polysaccharides from marine algae. *Mar. Drugs* **2011**, *9*, 196–223. [CrossRef] [PubMed]
37. Gupta, S.; Abu-Ghannam, N. Recent developments in the application of seaweeds or seaweed extracts as a means for enhancing the safety and quality attributes of foods. *Innov. Food Sci. Emerg. Technol.* **2011**, *12*, 600–609. [CrossRef]
38. Aquino, R.S.; Grativol, C.; Mourão, P.A.S. Rising from the Sea: Correlations between Sulfated Polysaccharides and Salinity in Plants. *PLoS ONE* **2011**, *6*, e18862. [CrossRef]
39. Torode, T.A.; Marcus, S.E.; Jam, M.; Tonon, T.; Blackburn, R.S.; Hervé, C.; Knox, J.P. Monoclonal Antibodies Directed to Fucoidan Preparations from Brown Algae. *PLoS One* **2015**, *10*, e0118366. [CrossRef] [PubMed]
40. Deniaud-Bouët, E.; Kervarec, N.; Michel, G.; Tonon, T.; Kloareg, B.; Hervé, C. Chemical and enzymatic fractionation of cell walls from Fucales: Insights into the structure of the extracellular matrix of brown algae. *Ann. Bot.* **2014**, *114*, 1203–1216. [CrossRef]
41. Adhikari, U.; Mateu, C.G.; Chattopadhyay, K.; Pujol, C.A.; Damonte, E.B.; Ray, B. Structure and antiviral activity of sulfated fucans from Stoechospermum marginatum. *Phytochemistry* **2006**, *67*, 2474–2482. [CrossRef]
42. Zhang, H.; Wang, J.-Q.; Nie, S.-P.; Wang, Y.-X.; Cui, S.W.; Xie, M.-Y. Sulfated modification, characterization and property of a water-insoluble polysaccharide from Ganoderma atrum. *Int. J. Biol. Macromol.* **2015**, *79*, 248–255. [CrossRef]
43. Witvrouw, M.; De Clercq, E. Sulfated polysaccharides extracted from sea algae as potential antiviral drugs. *Gen. Pharmacol.* **1997**, *29*, 497–511. [CrossRef]
44. Meiyu, G.; Fuchuan, L.; Xianliang, X.; Jing, L.; Zuowei, Y.; Huashi, G. The potential molecular targets of marine sulfated polymannuroguluronate interfering with HIV-1 entry. Interaction between SPMG and HIV-1 rgp120 and CD4 molecule. *Antiviral Res.* **2003**, *59*, 127–135. [CrossRef]
45. Damonte, E.B.; Matulewicz, M.C.; Cerezo, A.S. Sulfated seaweed polysaccharides as antiviral agents. *Curr. Med. Chem.* **2004**, *11*, 2399–2419. [CrossRef] [PubMed]
46. Witvrouw, M.; Schols, D.; Andrei, G.; Snoeck, R.; Ikeda, S.; Pauwels, R.; Van Schepdael, A.; Arnout, J.; Claes, P.; Desmyter, J.; et al. New Polyacetal Polysulphate Active against Human Immunodeficiency Virus and other Enveloped Viruses. *Antivir. Chem. Chemother.* **1992**, *3*, 351–360. [CrossRef]
47. Parish, C.R.; Jakobsen, K.B.; Coombe, D.R.; Bacic, A. Isolation and characterization of cell adhesion molecules from the marine sponge, Ophlitaspongia tenuis. *Biochim. Biophys. Acta* **1991**, *1073*, 56–64. [CrossRef]
48. Lynch, G.; Low, L.; Li, S.; Sloane, A.; Adams, S.; Parish, C.; Kemp, B.; Cunningham, A.L. Sulfated polyanions prevent HIV infection of lymphocytes by disruption of the CD4-gp120 interaction, but do not inhibit monocyte infection. *J. Leukoc. Biol.* **1994**, *56*, 266–272. [CrossRef] [PubMed]
49. Talyshinsky, M.M.; Souprun, Y.Y.; Huleihel, M.M. Anti-viral activity of red microalgal polysaccharides against retroviruses. *Cancer Cell Int.* **2002**, *2*, 8. [CrossRef] [PubMed]
50. Gerenčer, M.; Turecek, P.L.; Kistner, O.; Mitterer, A.; Savidis-Dacho, H.; Barrett, N.P. In vitro and in vivo anti-retroviral activity of the substance purified from the aqueous extract of Chelidonium majus L. *Antiviral Res.* **2006**, *72*, 153–156. [CrossRef]
51. Neyts, J.; Snoeck, R.; Schols, D.; Balzarini, J.; Esko, J.D.; Van Schepdael, A.; De Clercq, E. Sulfated polymers inhibit the interaction of human cytomegalovirus with cell surface heparan sulfate. *Virology* **1992**, *189*, 48–58. [CrossRef]
52. Vidhyanandhini, R.; Saravanan, R.; Vairamani, S.; Shanmugam, A. The anticoagulant activity and structural characterization of fractionated and purified glycosaminoglycans from venerid clam Meretrix casta (Chemnitz). *J. Liq. Chromatogr. Relat. Technol.* **2014**, *37*, 917–929. [CrossRef]

53. Li, P.; Sheng, J.; Liu, Y.; Li, J.; Liu, J.; Wang, F. Heparosan-Derived Heparan Sulfate/Heparin-Like Compounds: One Kind of Potential Therapeutic Agents. *Med. Res. Rev.* **2013**, *33*, 665–692. [CrossRef]
54. Ahmadi, A.; Zorofchian Moghadamtousi, S.; Abubakar, S.; Zandi, K. Antiviral Potential of Algae Polysaccharides Isolated from Marine Sources: A Review. *Biomed. Res. Int.* **2015**, *2015*, 1–10. [CrossRef] [PubMed]
55. Rabanal, M.; Ponce, N.M.A.; Navarro, D.A.; Gómez, R.M.; Stortz, C.A. The system of fucoidans from the brown seaweed Dictyota dichotoma: Chemical analysis and antiviral activity. *Carbohydr. Polym.* **2014**, *101*, 804–811. [CrossRef] [PubMed]
56. Thuy, T.T.T.; Ly, B.M.; Van, T.T.T.; Van Quang, N.; Tu, H.C.; Zheng, Y.; Seguin-Devaux, C.; Mi, B.; Ai, U. Anti-HIV activity of fucoidans from three brown seaweed species. *Carbohydr. Polym.* **2015**, *115*, 122–128. [CrossRef] [PubMed]
57. Hoshino, T.; Hayashi, T.; Hayashi, K.; Hamada, J.; Lee, J.B.; Sankawa, U. An antivirally active sulfated polysaccharide from Sargassum horneri (TURNER) C. AGARDH. *Biol. Pharm. Bull.* **1998**, *21*, 730–734. [CrossRef] [PubMed]
58. Schaeffer, D.J.; Krylov, V.S. Anti-HIV Activity of Extracts and Compounds from Algae and Cyanobacteria. *Ecotoxicol. Environ. Saf.* **2000**, *45*, 208–227. [CrossRef] [PubMed]
59. Ueno, M.; Nogawa, M.; Siddiqui, R.; Watashi, K.; Wakita, T.; Kato, N.; Ikeda, M.; Okimura, T.; Isaka, S.; Oda, T.; et al. Acidic polysaccharides isolated from marine algae inhibit the early step of viral infection. *Int. J. Biol. Macromol.* **2019**, *124*, 282–290. [CrossRef]
60. Huang, N.; Wu, M.-Y.; Zheng, C.-B.; Zhu, L.; Zhao, J.-H.; Zheng, Y.-T. The depolymerized fucosylated chondroitin sulfate from sea cucumber potently inhibits HIV replication via interfering with virus entry. *Carbohydr. Res.* **2013**, *380*, 64–69. [CrossRef] [PubMed]
61. Lian, W.; Wu, M.; Huang, N.; Gao, N.; Xiao, C.; Li, Z.; Zhang, Z.; Zheng, Y.; Peng, W.; Zhao, J. Anti-HIV-1 activity and structure–activity-relationship study of a fucosylated glycosaminoglycan from an echinoderm by targeting the conserved CD4 induced epitope. *Biochim. Biophys. Acta* **2013**, *1830*, 4681–4691. [CrossRef]
62. Pirrone, V.; Wigdahl, B.; Krebs, F.C. The rise and fall of polyanionic inhibitors of the human immunodeficiency virus type 1. *Antiviral Res.* **2011**, *90*, 168–182. [CrossRef]
63. Torode, T.A.; Siméon, A.; Marcus, S.E.; Jam, M.; Le Moigne, M.-A.; Duffieux, D.; Knox, J.P.; Hervé, C. Dynamics of cell wall assembly during early embryogenesis in the brown alga Fucus. *J. Exp. Bot.* **2016**, *67*, 6089–6100. [CrossRef]
64. Raimundo, S.C.; Avci, U.; Hopper, C.; Pattathil, S.; Hahn, M.G.; Popper, Z.A. Immunolocalization of cell wall carbohydrate epitopes in seaweeds: Presence of land plant epitopes in Fucus vesiculosus L. (Phaeophyceae). *Planta* **2016**, *243*, 337–354. [CrossRef] [PubMed]
65. Andrade, L.R.; Leal, R.N.; Noseda, M.; Duarte, M.E.R.; Pereira, M.S.; Mourão, P.A.S.; Farina, M.; Amado Filho, G.M. Brown algae overproduce cell wall polysaccharides as a protection mechanism against the heavy metal toxicity. *Mar. Pollut. Bull.* **2010**, *60*, 1482–1488. [CrossRef]
66. Zvyagintseva, T.N.; Shevchenko, N.M.; Chizhov, A.O.; Krupnova, T.N.; Sundukova, E.V.; Isakov, V.V. Water-soluble polysaccharides of some far-eastern brown seaweeds. Distribution, structure, and their dependence on the developmental conditions. *J. Exp. Mar. Bio. Ecol.* **2003**, *294*, 1–13. [CrossRef]
67. Mak, W.; Hamid, N.; Liu, T.; Lu, J.; White, W.L. Fucoidan from New Zealand Undaria pinnatifida: Monthly variations and determination of antioxidant activities. *Carbohydr. Polym.* **2013**, *95*, 606–614. [CrossRef] [PubMed]
68. Fletcher, H.R.; Biller, P.; Ross, A.B.; Adams, J.M.M. The seasonal variation of fucoidan within three species of brown macroalgae. *Algal Res.* **2017**, *22*, 79–86. [CrossRef]
69. Stengel, D.B.; Connan, S.; Popper, Z.A. Algal chemodiversity and bioactivity: Sources of natural variability and implications for commercial application. *Biotechnol. Adv.* **2011**, *29*, 483–501. [CrossRef]
70. Fitton, J.H.; Stringer, D.N.; Karpiniec, S.S. Therapies from Fucoidan: An Update. *Mar. Drugs* **2015**, *13*, 5920–5946. [CrossRef]
71. Astronomo, R.D.; Burton, D.R. Carbohydrate vaccines: Developing sweet solutions to sticky situations? *Nat. Rev. Drug Discov.* **2010**, *9*, 308–324. [CrossRef]
72. Wang, Y.; Ye, X.-S.; Zhang, L.-H. Oligosaccharide assembly by one-pot multi-step strategy. *Org. Biomol. Chem.* **2007**, *5*, 2189. [CrossRef]

73. Astronomo, R.D.; Lee, H.-K.; Scanlan, C.N.; Pantophlet, R.; Huang, C.-Y.; Wilson, I.A.; Blixt, O.; Dwek, R.A.; Wong, C.-H.; Burton, D.R. A Glycoconjugate Antigen Based on the Recognition Motif of a Broadly Neutralizing Human Immunodeficiency Virus Antibody, 2G12, Is Immunogenic but Elicits Antibodies Unable To Bind to the Self Glycans of gp120. *J. Virol.* **2008**, *82*, 6359–6368. [CrossRef]
74. Luallen, R.J.; Lin, J.; Fu, H.; Cai, K.K.; Agrawal, C.; Mboudjeka, I.; Lee, F.-H.; Montefiori, D.; Smith, D.F.; Doms, R.W.; et al. An Engineered Saccharomyces cerevisiae Strain Binds the Broadly Neutralizing Human Immunodeficiency Virus Type 1 Antibody 2G12 and Elicits Mannose-Specific gp120-Binding Antibodies. *J. Virol.* **2008**, *82*, 6447–6457. [CrossRef] [PubMed]
75. Dunlop, D.C.; Ulrich, A.; Appelmelk, B.J.; Burton, D.R.; Dwek, R.A.; Zitzmann, N.; Scanlan, C.N. Antigenic mimicry of the HIV envelope by AIDS-associated pathogens. *AIDS* **2008**, *22*, 2214–2217. [CrossRef] [PubMed]
76. Joyce, J.G.; Krauss, I.J.; Song, H.C.; Opalka, D.W.; Grimm, K.M.; Nahas, D.D.; Esser, M.T.; Hrin, R.; Feng, M.; Dudkin, V.Y.; et al. An oligosaccharide-based HIV-1 2G12 mimotope vaccine induces carbohydrate-specific antibodies that fail to neutralize HIV-1 virions. *PNAS* **2008**, *105*, 15684–15689. [CrossRef] [PubMed]
77. Astronomo, R.D.; Kaltgrad, E.; Udit, A.K.; Wang, S.-K.; Doores, K.J.; Huang, C.-Y.; Pantophlet, R.; Paulson, J.C.; Wong, C.-H.; Finn, M.G.; et al. Defining Criteria for Oligomannose Immunogens for HIV Using Icosahedral Virus Capsid Scaffolds. *Chem. Biol.* **2010**, *17*, 357–370. [CrossRef] [PubMed]
78. Wang, S.-K.; Liang, P.-H.; Astronomo, R.D.; Hsu, T.-L.; Hsieh, S.-L.; Burton, D.R.; Wong, C.-H. Targeting the carbohydrates on HIV-1: Interaction of oligomannose dendrons with human monoclonal antibody 2G12 and DC-SIGN. *PNAS* **2008**, *105*, 3690–3695. [CrossRef] [PubMed]
79. Wang, L.-X. Toward oligosaccharide- and glycopeptide-based HIV vaccines. *Curr. Opin. Drug Discov. Devel.* **2006**, *9*, 194–206. [PubMed]
80. Kumar, K.K.; Reddy, G.S.; Reddy, B.; Shekar, P.C.; Sumanthi, J.; Chandra, K.I.P. Biological role of lectins: A review. *J. Orofac. Sci.* **2012**, *4*, 20. [CrossRef]
81. Balzarini, J. Inhibition of HIV entry by carbohydrate-binding proteins. *Antiviral Res.* **2006**, *71*, 237–247. [CrossRef]
82. Balzarini, J.; Neyts, J.; Schols, D.; Hosoya, M.; Van Damme, E.; Peumans, W.; De Clercq, E. The mannose-specific plant lectins from Cymbidium hybrid and Epipactis helleborine and the (N-acetylglucosamine)n-specific plant lectin from Urtica dioica are potent and selective inhibitors of human immunodeficiency virus and cytomegalovirus replication. *Antiviral Res.* **1992**, *18*, 191–207. [CrossRef]
83. Hansen, J.E.; Nielsen, C.M.; Nielsen, C.; Heegaard, P.; Mathiesen, L.R.; Nielsen, J.O. Correlation between carbohydrate structures on the envelope glycoprotein gp120 of HIV-1 and HIV-2 and syncytium inhibition with lectins. *AIDS* **1989**, *3*, 635–641. [CrossRef]
84. Sato, T.; Hori, K. Cloning, expression, and characterization of a novel anti-HIV lectin from the cultured cyanobacterium, Oscillatoria agardhii. *Fish. Sci.* **2009**, *75*, 743–753. [CrossRef]
85. Akkouh, O.; Ng, T.B.; Singh, S.S.; Yin, C.; Dan, X.; Chan, Y.S.; Pan, W.; Cheung, R.C.F. Lectins with anti-HIV activity: A review. *Molecules* **2015**, *20*, 648–668. [CrossRef] [PubMed]
86. Gogineni, V.; Schinazi, R.F.; Hamann, M.T. Role of Marine Natural Products in the Genesis of Antiviral Agents. *Chem. Rev.* **2015**, *115*, 9655–9706. [CrossRef] [PubMed]
87. Hirayama, M.; Shibata, H.; Imamura, K.; Sakaguchi, T.; Hori, K. High-Mannose Specific Lectin and Its Recombinants from a Carrageenophyta Kappaphycus alvarezii Represent a Potent Anti-HIV Activity Through High-Affinity Binding to the Viral Envelope Glycoprotein gp120. *Mar. Biotechnol.* **2016**, *18*, 144–160. [CrossRef] [PubMed]
88. Vo, T.-S.; Kim, S.-K. Potential Anti-HIV Agents from Marine Resources: An Overview. *Mar. Drugs* **2010**, *8*, 2871–2892. [CrossRef] [PubMed]
89. Cheung, R.C.F.; Ng, T.B.; Wong, J.H. Marine Peptides: Bioactivities and Applications. *Mar. Drugs* **2015**, *13*, 4006–4043. [CrossRef] [PubMed]
90. Qaralleh, H. Chemical and bioactive diversities of marine sponge Neopetrosia. *Bangladesh J. Pharmacol.* **2016**, *11*, 433. [CrossRef]
91. ANEIROS, A.; GARATEIX, A. Bioactive peptides from marine sources: Pharmacological properties and isolation procedures. *J. Chromatogr. B* **2004**, *803*, 41–53. [CrossRef]
92. Shin, H.J.; Rashid, M.A.; Cartner, L.K.; Bokesch, H.R.; Wilson, J.A.; McMahon, J.B.; Gustafson, K.R. Stellettapeptins A and B, HIV-inhibitory cyclic depsipeptides from the marine sponge *Stelletta* sp. *Tetrahedron Lett.* **2015**, *56*, 4215–4219. [CrossRef]

93. Wildeman;Gomez-Archila, L.G.; Galeano, E.; Martínez, A.; Castrillón, F.J.D.; Rugeles, M.T. Bromotyrosine Derivatives from Marine Sponges Inhibit the HIV-1 Replication in Vitro. *Vitae* **2014**, *21*, 114–125.
94. Jang, I.S.; Park, S.J. Hydroxyproline-containing collagen peptide derived from the skin of the Alaska pollack inhibits HIV-1 infection. *Mol. Med. Rep.* **2016**, *14*, 5489–5494. [CrossRef] [PubMed]
95. Jang, I.-S.; Park, S.J. A Spirulina maxima-derived peptide inhibits HIV-1 infection in a human T cell line MT4. *Fish. Aquat. Sci.* **2016**, *19*, 37. [CrossRef]
96. Zhou, X.; Fang, W.; Tan, S.; Lin, X.; Xun, T.; Yang, B.; Liu, S.; Liu, Y. Aspernigrins with anti-HIV-1 activities from the marine-derived fungus Aspergillus niger SCSIO Jcsw6F30. *Bioorg. Med. Chem. Lett.* **2016**, *26*, 361–365. [CrossRef] [PubMed]
97. Niu, S.; Liu, D.; Shao, Z.; Proksch, P.; Lin, W. Eutypellazines A–M, thiodiketopiperazine-type alkaloids from deep sea derived fungus Eutypella sp. MCCC 3A00281. *RSC Adv.* **2017**, *7*, 33580–33590. [CrossRef]
98. O'Rourke, A.; Kremb, S.; Bader, T.; Helfer, M.; Schmitt-Kopplin, P.; Gerwick, W.; Brack-Werner, R.; Voolstra, C. Alkaloids from the Sponge Stylissa carteri Present Prospective Scaffolds for the Inhibition of Human Immunodeficiency Virus 1 (HIV-1). *Mar. Drugs* **2016**, *14*, 28. [CrossRef] [PubMed]
99. Yu, H.-B.; Yang, F.; Sun, F.; Li, J.; Jiao, W.-H.; Gan, J.-H.; Hu, W.-Z.; Lin, H.-W. Aaptamine derivatives with antifungal and anti-HIV-1 activities from the South China Sea sponge Aaptos aaptos. *Mar. Drugs* **2014**, *12*, 6003–6013. [CrossRef] [PubMed]
100. Tietjen, I.; Williams, D.E.; Read, S.; Kuang, X.T.; Mwimanzi, P.; Wilhelm, E.; Markle, T.; Kinloch, N.N.; Naphen, C.N.; Tenney, K.; et al. Inhibition of NF-κB-dependent HIV-1 replication by the marine natural product bengamide A. *Antiviral Res.* **2018**, *152*, 94–103. [CrossRef] [PubMed]
101. Ma, X.; Li, L.; Zhu, T.; Ba, M.; Li, G.; Gu, Q.; Guo, Y.; Li, D. Phenylspirodrimanes with Anti-HIV Activity from the Sponge-Derived Fungus Stachybotrys chartarum MXH-X73. *J. Nat. Prod.* **2013**, *76*, 2298–2306. [CrossRef] [PubMed]
102. Pardo-Vargas, A.; de Barcelos Oliveira, I.; Stephens, P.; Cirne-Santos, C.; de Palmer Paixão, I.; Ramos, F.; Jiménez, C.; Rodríguez, J.; Resende, J.; Teixeira, V.; et al. Dolabelladienols A–C, New Diterpenes Isolated from Brazilian Brown Alga Dictyota pfaffii. *Mar. Drugs* **2014**, *12*, 4247–4259. [CrossRef]
103. de Souza Barros, C.; Cirne-Santos, C.C.; Garrido, V.; Barcelos, I.; Stephens, P.R.S.; Giongo, V.; Teixeira, V.L.; de Palmer Paixão, I.C.N. Anti-HIV-1 activity of compounds derived from marine alga Canistrocarpus cervicornis. *J. Appl. Phycol.* **2016**, *28*, 2523–2527. [CrossRef]
104. Stephens, P.R.S.; Cirne-Santos, C.C.; de Souza Barros, C.; Teixeira, V.L.; Carneiro, L.A.D.; Amorim, L.; dos, S.C.; Ocampo, J.S.P.; Castello-Branco, L.R.R.; de Palmer Paixão, I.C.N. Diterpene from marine brown alga Dictyota friabilis as a potential microbicide against HIV-1 in tissue explants. *J. Appl. Phycol.* **2017**, *29*, 775–780. [CrossRef]
105. Miceli, L.; Teixeira, V.; Castro, H.; Rodrigues, C.; Mello, J.; Albuquerque, M.; Cabral, L.; de Brito, M.; de Souza, A.; Miceli, L.A.; et al. Molecular Docking Studies of Marine Diterpenes as Inhibitors of Wild-Type and Mutants HIV-1 Reverse Transcriptase. *Mar. Drugs* **2013**, *11*, 4127–4143. [CrossRef] [PubMed]
106. Pardo-Vargas, A.; Ramos, F.A.; Cirne-Santos, C.C.; Stephens, P.R.; Paixão, I.C.P.; Teixeira, V.L.; Castellanos, L. Semi-synthesis of oxygenated dolabellane diterpenes with highly in vitro anti-HIV-1 activity. *Bioorg. Med. Chem. Lett.* **2014**, *24*, 4381–4383. [CrossRef] [PubMed]
107. Karadeniz, F.; Kang, K.-H.; Park, J.W.; Park, S.-J.; Kim, S.-K. Anti-HIV-1 activity of phlorotannin derivative 8,4'''-dieckol from Korean brown alga Ecklonia cava. *Biosci. Biotechnol. Biochem.* **2014**, *78*, 1151–1158. [CrossRef] [PubMed]
108. Tan, S.; Yang, B.; Liu, J.; Xun, T.; Liu, Y.; Zhou, X. Penicillixanthone A, a marine-derived dual-coreceptor antagonist as anti-HIV-1 agent. *Nat. Prod. Res.* **2017**, 1–5. [CrossRef] [PubMed]
109. He, J.; Huang, W.; Zheng, S.; Vigorito, M.; Chang, S.L. Effects of docosahexaenoic acid on locomotor activity in ethanol-treated HIV-1 transgenic rats. *J. Neurovirol.* **2018**, *24*, 88–97. [CrossRef] [PubMed]
110. Mejia, E.J.; Loveridge, S.T.; Stepan, G.; Tsai, A.; Jones, G.S.; Barnes, T.; White, K.N.; Drašković, M.; Tenney, K.; Tsiang, M.; et al. Study of Marine Natural Products Including Resorcyclic Acid Lactones from Humicola fuscoatra That Reactivate Latent HIV-1 Expression in an in Vitro Model of Central Memory CD4+ T Cells. *J. Nat. Prod.* **2014**, *77*, 618–624. [CrossRef] [PubMed]
111. Zhao, Y.; Liu, D.; Proksch, P.; Zhou, D.; Lin, W. Truncateols O–V, further isoprenylated cyclohexanols from the sponge-associated fungus Truncatella angustata with antiviral activities. *Phytochemistry* **2018**, *155*, 61–68. [CrossRef]

112. Ahn, M.-J.; Yoon, K.-D.; Min, S.-Y.; Lee, J.S.; Kim, J.H.; Kim, T.G.; Kim, S.H.; Kim, N.-G.; Huh, H.; Kim, J. Inhibition of HIV-1 reverse transcriptase and protease by phlorotannins from the brown alga Ecklonia cava. *Biol. Pharm. Bull.* **2004**, *27*, 544–547. [CrossRef]
113. Artan, M.; Li, Y.; Karadeniz, F.; Lee, S.-H.; Kim, M.-M.; Kim, S.-K. Anti-HIV-1 activity of phloroglucinol derivative, 6,6′-bieckol, from Ecklonia cava. *Bioorg. Med. Chem.* **2008**, *16*, 7921–7926. [CrossRef]
114. Cardona, M.L.; Fernández, I.; Pedro, J.R.; Serrano, A. Xanthones from Hypericum reflexum. *Phytochemistry* **1990**, *29*, 3003–3006. [CrossRef]
115. Negi, J.S.; Bisht, V.K.; Singh, P.; Rawat, M.S.M.; Joshi, G.P. Naturally Occurring Xanthones: Chemistry and Biology. *J. Appl. Chem.* **2013**, *2013*, 1–9. [CrossRef]
116. Ahmed, M.; Husain, N.E. Managing dyslipidemia in HIV/AIDS patients: Challenges and solutions. *HIV/AIDS* **2014**, *7*, 1. [CrossRef] [PubMed]
117. Vieira, A.D.S.; Silveira, G.R.M. da Effectiveness of n-3 fatty acids in the treatment of hypertriglyceridemia in HIV/AIDS patients: A meta-analysis. *Cien. Saude Colet.* **2017**, *22*, 2659–2669. [CrossRef] [PubMed]
118. Maria Jose MB, M.N.; MB, M.J.; Agudelo, M.; Yndart, A.; Vargas-Rivera, M.E. Platelets Contribute to BBB Disruption Induced by HIV and Alcohol. *J. Alcohol. Drug Depend.* **2015**, *3*, 1–6. [CrossRef]
119. Flora, G.; Pu, H.; Lee, Y.W.; Ravikumar, R.; Nath, A.; Hennig, B.; Toborek, M. Proinflammatory synergism of ethanol and HIV-1 Tat protein in brain tissue. *Exp. Neurol.* **2005**, *191*, 2–12. [CrossRef] [PubMed]
120. Acheampong, E.; Mukhtar, M.; Parveen, Z.; Ngoubilly, N.; Ahmad, N.; Patel, C.; Pomerantz, R.J. Ethanol strongly potentiates apoptosis induced by HIV-1 proteins in primary human brain microvascular endothelial cells. *Virology* **2002**, *304*, 222–234. [CrossRef]

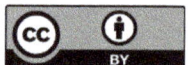

© 2019 by the authors. Licensee MDPI, Basel, Switzerland. This article is an open access article distributed under the terms and conditions of the Creative Commons Attribution (CC BY) license (http://creativecommons.org/licenses/by/4.0/).

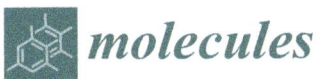

Review

Cytotoxic Effects of Diterpenoid Alkaloids Against Human Cancer Cells

Koji Wada * and Hiroshi Yamashita

Department of Medicinal Chemistry, Faculty of Pharmaceutical Sciences, Hokkaido University of Science, 4-1, Maeda 7-jo 15-choume, Teine-ku, Sapporo 006-8590, Japan; yama@hus.ac.jp
* Correspondence: kowada@hus.ac.jp; Tel.: +81-11-681-2161

Academic Editor: Kyoko Nakagawa-Goto
Received: 23 May 2019; Accepted: 21 June 2019; Published: 22 June 2019

Abstract: Diterpenoid alkaloids are isolated from plants of the genera *Aconitum*, *Delphinium*, and *Garrya* (Ranunculaceae) and classified according to their chemical structures as C_{18}-, C_{19}- or C_{20}-diterpenoid alkaloids. The extreme toxicity of certain compounds, e.g., aconitine, has prompted a thorough investigation of how structural features affect their bioactivities. Therefore, natural diterpenoid alkaloids and semi-synthetic alkaloid derivatives were evaluated for cytotoxic effects against human tumor cells [A549 (lung carcinoma), DU145 (prostate carcinoma), MDA-MB-231 (triple-negative breast cancer), MCF-7 (estrogen receptor-positive, HER2-negative breast cancer), KB (identical to cervical carcinoma HeLa derived AV-3 cell line), and multidrug-resistant (MDR) subline KB-VIN]. Among the tested alkaloids, C_{19}-diterpenoid (e.g., lipojesaconitine, delcosine and delpheline derivatives) and C_{20}-diterpenoid (e.g., kobusine and pseudokobusine derivatives) alkaloids exhibited significant cytotoxic activity and, thus, provide promising new leads for further development as antitumor agents. Notably, several diterpenoid alkaloids were more potent against MDR subline KB-VIN cells than the parental drug-sensitive KB cells.

Keywords: diterpenoid alkaloids; cytotoxicity; human tumor cells; lipojesaconitine; delcosine; delpheline; kobusine; pseudokobusine

---

1. Introduction

Cancer therapy mainly involves surgery, chemotherapy, radiation therapy, immunotherapy, monoclonal antibody therapy, and hormone therapy. Chemotherapy generally refers to the use of cytotoxic drugs to treat cancer. Plant alkaloids are one major class of chemotherapeutic drugs [1–9]. Chemotherapeutic drugs that affect cell division by preventing the normal functioning of micro-tubules include the vinca alkaloids.

Numerous diterpenoid alkaloids have been isolated from various *Aconitum*, *Delphinium*, and *Garrya* (Family Ranunculaceae) species and are classified according to their chemical structures as C_{18}-, C_{19}- or C_{20}-diterpenoid alkaloids (Figure 1) [10,11]. The C_{19}-diterpenoid alkaloids may be divided into six types: aconitine, lycoctonine, pyro (C_8=C_{15} or C_{15}=O), lactone (δ-valerolactone rather than cyclopentyl C-ring), 7,17-*seco*, and rearranged ones [10,11]. Most of the isolated C_{19}-diterpenoid alkaloids are aconitine- and lycoctonine-types and include aconitine, mesaconitine, hypaconitine and jesaconitine, all of which are extremely toxic. The C_{20}-diterpenoid alkaloids may be divided into ten types: atisine, denudatine, hetidine, hetisine, vakognavine, napelline, kusnezoline, racemulosine, arcutine, and tricalysiamide [10,11]. Most of the isolated C_{20}-diterpenoid alkaloids are atisine-, hetisine-, and napelline-types and include atisine, kobusine, pseudokobusine and lucidusculine, which are far less toxic [12].

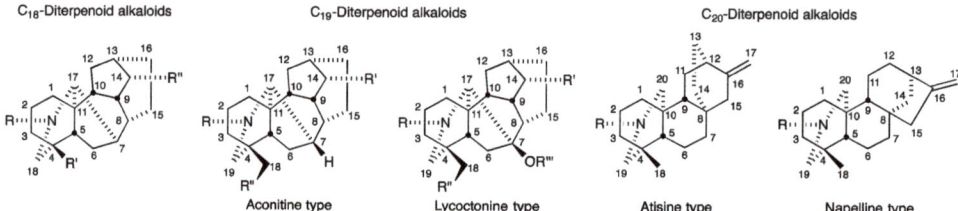

Figure 1. Classifications, general structures and numbering systems for C_{18}-, C_{19}-, and C_{20}-diterpenoid alkaloids.

The pharmacological properties of the C_{19}-diterpenoid alkaloids have been studied extensively and reviewed [12]. Aconitine is a toxin that exhibits activity both centrally and peripherally, acting predominantly on the cardiovascular and respiratory systems by preventing the normal closing of sodium channels [12]. This extreme toxicity resulted in the use of *Aconitum* extracts as poisons in hunting and warfare [13], although extracts were also used as traditional medicines by oral and topical routes. For example, the roots of *Aconitum* plants have been used as "bushi", an herbal drug in some prescriptions of traditional Japanese medicine for the treatment of hypometabolism, dysuria, cardiac weakness, chills, neuralgia, gout, and certain rheumatic diseases [14]. However, proper processing is essential to reduce the content of toxic alkaloids and avoid inadvertent poisoning [15–17]. Such obstacles encourage a good understanding of the relationships between structure and cytotoxic activity of aconitine and related compounds before they can be considered for modification and development as chemotherapeutic agents.

Our previous study demonstrated the effects of various naturally occurring and semi-synthetic C_{19}- and C_{20}-diterpenoid alkaloids on the growth of the A172 human malignant glioma cell line [18]. Antitumor properties and radiation-sensitizing effects of various types of novel derivatives prepared from C_{19}- and C_{20}-diterpenoid alkaloids were also investigated [19]. Two novel hetisine-type C_{20}-diterpenoid derivatives showed significant suppressive effects against the Raji non-Hodgkin's lymphoma cell line [20]. In addition, the effects of various semi-synthetic novel hetisine-type C_{20}-diterpenoid alkaloids on the growth of the A549 human lung cancer cell line were examined and subsequent structure-activity relationships for the antiproliferative effects against A549 cells were considered [21]. Since 2012, several diterpenoid alkaloid components and their derivatives exhibited antiproliferative activity against human tumor cell lines, including A549 (lung carcinoma), DU145 (prostate carcinoma), MDA-MB-231 (estrogen and progesterone receptor-negative & HER2-negative triple-negative breast cancer), MCF-7 (estrogen receptor-positive, HER2-negative breast cancer), KB (identical to cervical carcinoma HeLa derived AV-3 cell line), and multidrug-resistant (MDR) subline KB-VIN [P-glycoprotein (P-gp) overexpressing vincristine-resistant KB subline]. Among such alkaloids, C_{19}-diterpenoid (e.g., lipojesaconitine, delpheline, and delcosine derivative) and C_{20}-diterpenoid (e.g., kobusine and pseudokobusine derivatives) alkaloids have shown significant antiproliferative activity, as well as provided promising new leads for further development as antitumor agents.

2. Antiproliferative Activity of C_{19}-Diterpenoid Alkaloid Derivatives

2.1. Aconitine-Type C_{19}-Diterpenoid Alkaloids

The tested aconitine-type C_{19}-diterpenoid alkaloids included 21 natural alkaloids, aconitine (**1**), deoxyaconitine (**2**), jesaconitine (**3**), deoxyjesaconitine (**4**), aljesaconitine A (**5**), secojesaconitine (**6**), mesaconitine (**8**), hypaconitine (**9**), hokbusine A (**10**), 14-anisoyllasianine (**12**), *N*-deethylaljesaconitine A (**13**), aconine (**14**), lipomesaconitine (**15**), lipoaconitine (**16**), lipojesaconitine (**17**), neolinine (**18**), neoline (**19**), 14-benzoylneoline (**20**), isotalatizidine (**21**), karacoline (**22**), and 3-hydroxykaracoline (**23**), isolated from the rhizoma of *Aconitum japonicum* THUNB. subsp. *subcuneatum* (NAKAI) KADOTA [22–28] (Figure 2). Two synthetic aconitine-type C_{19}-diterpenoid alkaloids, 3,15-diacetyljesaconitine (**7**) [26] and 3-acetylmesaconitine (**11**) [29] prepared from secojesaconitine (**6**) and mesaconitine (**8**), respectively (Figure 2), were also tested.

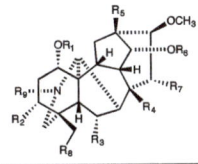

		R_1	R_2	R_3	R_4	R_5	R_6	R_7	R_8	R_9
1 *	aconitine	CH_3	OH	OCH_3	$OCOCH_3$	OH	Bz	OH	OCH_3	CH_2CH_3
2 *	deoxyaconitine	CH_3	H	OCH_3	$OCOCH_3$	OH	Bz	OH	OCH_3	CH_2CH_3
3 *	jesaconitine	CH_3	OH	OCH_3	$OCOCH_3$	OH	As	OH	OCH_3	CH_2CH_3
4 *	deoxyjesaconitine	CH_3	H	OCH_3	$OCOCH_3$	OH	As	OH	OCH_3	CH_2CH_3
5 *	aljesaconitine A	CH_3	OH	OCH_3	OCH_2CH_3	OH	As	OH	OCH_3	CH_2CH_3
6 *	see structure below									
7	3,15-diacetyljesaconitine	CH_3	$OCOCH_3$	OCH_3	$OCOCH_3$	OH	As	$OCOCH_3$	OCH_3	CH_2CH_3
8 *	mesaconitine	CH_3	OH	OCH_3	$OCOCH_3$	OH	Bz	OH	OCH_3	CH_3
9 *	hypaconitine	CH_3	H	OCH_3	$OCOCH_3$	OH	Bz	OH	OCH_3	CH_3
10 *	hokbusine A	CH_3	OH	OCH_3	OCH_3	OH	Bz	OH	OCH_3	CH_3
11	3-acetylmesaconitine	CH_3	$OCOCH_3$	OCH_3	$OCOCH_3$	OH	Bz	OH	OCH_3	CH_3
12 *	14-anisoyllasianine	CH_3	OH	OCH_3	NH_2	OH	As	OH	OCH_3	CH_2CH_3
13 *	N-deethylaljesaconitine A	CH_3	OH	OCH_3	OCH_2CH_3	OH	As	OH	OCH_3	H
14 *	aconine	CH_3	OH	OCH_3	OH	OH	H	OH	OCH_3	CH_2CH_3
15 *	lipomesaconitine	CH_3	OH	OCH_3	Olipo	OH	Bz	OH	OCH_3	CH_3
16 *	lipoaconitine	CH_3	OH	OCH_3	Olipo	OH	Bz	OH	OCH_3	CH_2CH_3
17 *	lipojesaconitine	CH_3	OH	OCH_3	Olipo	OH	As	OH	OCH_3	CH_2CH_3
18 *	neolinine	H	H	OCH_3	OH	H	H	H	OH	CH_2CH_3
19 *	neoline	H	H	OCH_3	OH	H	H	H	OCH_3	CH_2CH_3
20 *	14-benzoylneoline	H	H	OCH_3	OH	H	Bz	H	OCH_3	CH_2CH_3
21 *	isotalatizidine	H	H	H	OH	H	H	H	OCH_3	CH_2CH_3
22 *	karacoline	H	H	H	OH	H	H	H	H	CH_2CH_3
23 *	3-hydroxykaracoline	H	OH	H	OH	H	H	H	H	CH_2CH_3

Bz = COC_6H_5
As = $COC_6H_4OCH_3$ (p)
lipo = linoleoyl, palmitoyl, oleoyl, stearoyl, linolenoyl

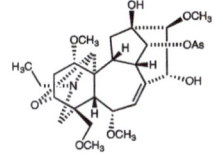

6 *   secojesaconitine

*: Natural alkaloid

Figure 2. Chemical structures of aconitine-type C_{19}-diterpenoid alkaloids **1–23**.

Eighteen of the 23 tested aconitine-type C_{19}-diterpenoid alkaloids, both natural alkaloids (**1~6, 8~10, 12~14, 18~23**) and synthetic analogs (**7** and **11**), were inactive (IC_{50} > 20 or 40 µM) [27,28,30] (Table 1). Three natural diterpenoid alkaloids (**15~17**) exhibited cytotoxic activity against five human tumor cell lines (A549, MDA-MB-231, MCF-7, KB, and MDR KB subline KB-VIN) (Table 1). Lipojesaconitine (**17**) showed significant cytotoxicity against four tested cell lines with IC_{50} values of 6.0 to 7.3 µM, but weak cytotoxicity against KB-VIN (IC_{50} = 18.6 µM) [28]. Lipomesaconitine (**15**) showed moderate cytotoxicity against the KB cell line (IC_{50} = 9.9 µM), but weak cytotoxicity against the other four human tumor cell lines (IC_{50} =17.2 ~ 21.5 µM) [27]. Lipoaconitine (**16**) was weakly cytotoxic (IC_{50} = 13.7 ~ 20.3 µM) against all five human tumor cell lines [28]. Based on the results, the fatty acid ester at C-8 and the anisoyl group at C-14 found in **17** may be important to the cytotoxic activity of aconitine-type C_{19}-diterpenoid alkaloids.

Table 1. Cytotoxic activity data for aconitine-type C_{19}-diterpenoid alkaloids and derivatives **1–23**.

Alkaloids	Cell Line/IC$_{50}$ (μM) [1]					
	A549	DU145	MDA-MB-231	MCF-7	KB	KB-VIN
Aconitine (**1**)	>20	>20	-	-	>20	>20
Deoxyaconitine (**2**)	>20	>20	-	-	>20	>20
Jesaconitine (**3**)	>20	>20	-	-	>20	>20
Deoxyjesaconitine (**4**)	>20	>20	-	-	>20	>20
Aljesaconitine A (**5**)	>20	>20	-	-	>20	>20
Secojesaconitine (**6**)	>20	>20	-	-	>20	>20
7	>20	>20	-	-	>20	>20
Mesaconitine (**8**)	>20	>20	-	-	>20	>20
Hypaconitine (**9**)	>20	>20	-	-	>20	>20
Hokbusine A (**10**)	>20	>20	-	-	>20	>20
11	>20	>20	-	-	>20	>20
14-Anisoyllasianine (**12**)	>40	-	>40	>40	>40	>40
N-Deethylaljesaconitine A (**13**)	>40	-	>40	>40	>40	>40
Aconine (**14**)	>40	-	>40	>40	>40	>40
Lipomesaconitine (**15**)	17.2 ± 2.3	-	20.0 ± 0.2	19.0 ± 1.0	10.0 ± 3.3	21.5 ± 0.9
Lipoaconitine (**16**)	17.4 ± 1.1	-	15.5 ± 0.5	16.0 ± 0.3	13.7 ± 1.3	20.3 ± 1.1
Lipojesaconitine (**17**)	7.3 ± 0.3	-	6.0 ± 0.2	6.7 ± 0.2	6.0 ± 0.2	18.6 ± 0.9
Neolinine (**18**)	>40	-	>40	>40	>40	>40
Neoline (**19**)	>20	>20	-	-	>20	>20
14-benzoylneoline (**20**)	>20	>20	-	-	>20	>20
Isotalatizidine (**21**)	>40	-	>40	>40	>40	>40
Karacoline (**22**)	>20	>20	-	-	>20	>20
3-Hydroxykaracoline (**23**)	>40	-	>40	>40	>40	>40
PXL [2] (nM)	4.8 ± 0.6	5.9 ± 1.9	8.4 ± 0.8	10.2 ± 0.9	5.8 ± 0.2	2405.4 ± 44.8

[1] Values are means ± standard deviation; [2] Paclitaxel (PXL; nM) was used as an experimental control.

2.2. Lycoctonine-Type (7,8-diol) C_{19}-Diterpenoid Alkaloids

The tested lycoctonine-type (7,8-diol) C_{19}-diterpenoid alkaloid group included 12 natural alkaloids, namely nevadensine (**24**), N-deethylnevadensine (**25**), and virescenine (**27**), purified from rhizoma of *Aconitum japonicum* subsp. *subcuneatum* [27], and 18-methoxygadesine (**26**), delphinifoline (**28**), delcosine (**34**), 14-acetyldelcosine (**34-43**), and 14-acetylbrowniine (**35**), purified from root of *Aconitum yesoense* var. *macroyesoense* (NAKAI) TAMURA [31–34], and andersonidine (**30**), pacifiline (**31**), pacifinine (**32**), and pacifidine (**33**), purified from seeds of *Delphinium elatum* cv. Pacific Giant [35] (Figure 3). The remaining tested C_{19}-diterpenoid alkaloids from this subtype were synthetic alkaloids, N-deethyldelsoline (**29**) [18], 1-acetyldelcosine (**34-1**) [36], 1,14-diacetyldelcosine (**34-2**) [37], 1-(4-trifluoromethylbenzoyl)delcosine (**34-24**) [30], delsoline (**34-42**) [37], 1,14-di-(4-nitrobenzoyl)-delcosine (**34-45**) [30], 14-acetyl-1-(4-nitrobenzoyl)delcosine (**34-46**) [30], and 1-acyl or 1,14-diacyldelcosine derivatives (**34-3~34-23**, **34-25~34-41**, **34-44**, and **34-47**) [38], prepared from delcosine (**34**) or delsoline (**34-42**) (Figure 3). These 42 C_{19}-diterpenoid alkaloids were evaluated for antiproliferative activity against four to five human tumor cell lines (A549, DU145, MDA-MB-231, MCF-7, KB, and KB-VIN) [30,38] (Table 2). Several tested lycoctonine-type (7,8-diol) C_{19}-diterpenoid alkaloids, both natural alkaloids (**24–28**, **30~33**) and a synthetic alkaloid (**29**), were inactive (IC$_{50}$ > 20 or 40 μM). All tested delcosine derivatives that contain an acetyl or methoxy group, both natural alkaloids (**34**, **34-43**, **35**) and synthetic analogs (**34-1**, **34-2**, **34-42**), were inactive (IC$_{50}$ > 20 μM). However, acylation, except with an acetyl group, of the C-1 and/or C-14 hydroxy group of **34** led to various degrees of antiproliferative activity. Among the C-1 esterified alkaloids, the synthetic derivatives **34-6**, **34-8**, **34-10**, and **34-18** exhibited significant potency against all cell lines (average IC$_{50}$ 9.3, 5.3, 5.0, and 6.9 μM, respectively). Also, alkaloids **34-3**, **34-16**, **34-17**, **34-21**, **34-25**, **34-27**, **34-31**, **34-32**, **34-38**, and **34-40** showed moderate potency toward all cell lines (average IC$_{50}$ 12.7–20.7 μM). While alkaloid **34-32** displayed good antiproliferative activity (IC$_{50}$ 8.7 μM) against KB cells, it was much less potent against A549, MDA-MB-231, and KB-VIN cells. Alkaloids **34-5**, **34-13**, **34-15**, **34-29**, **34-35**, **34-37**, and **34-41** exhibited only weak potency against all cell lines (average IC$_{50}$ 22.0–26.5 μM). Finally, alkaloids **34-24**, **34-30**, and **34-34** were inactive against all five human tumor cell lines, while **34-12**, **34-33**, and **34-39** showed limited potency.

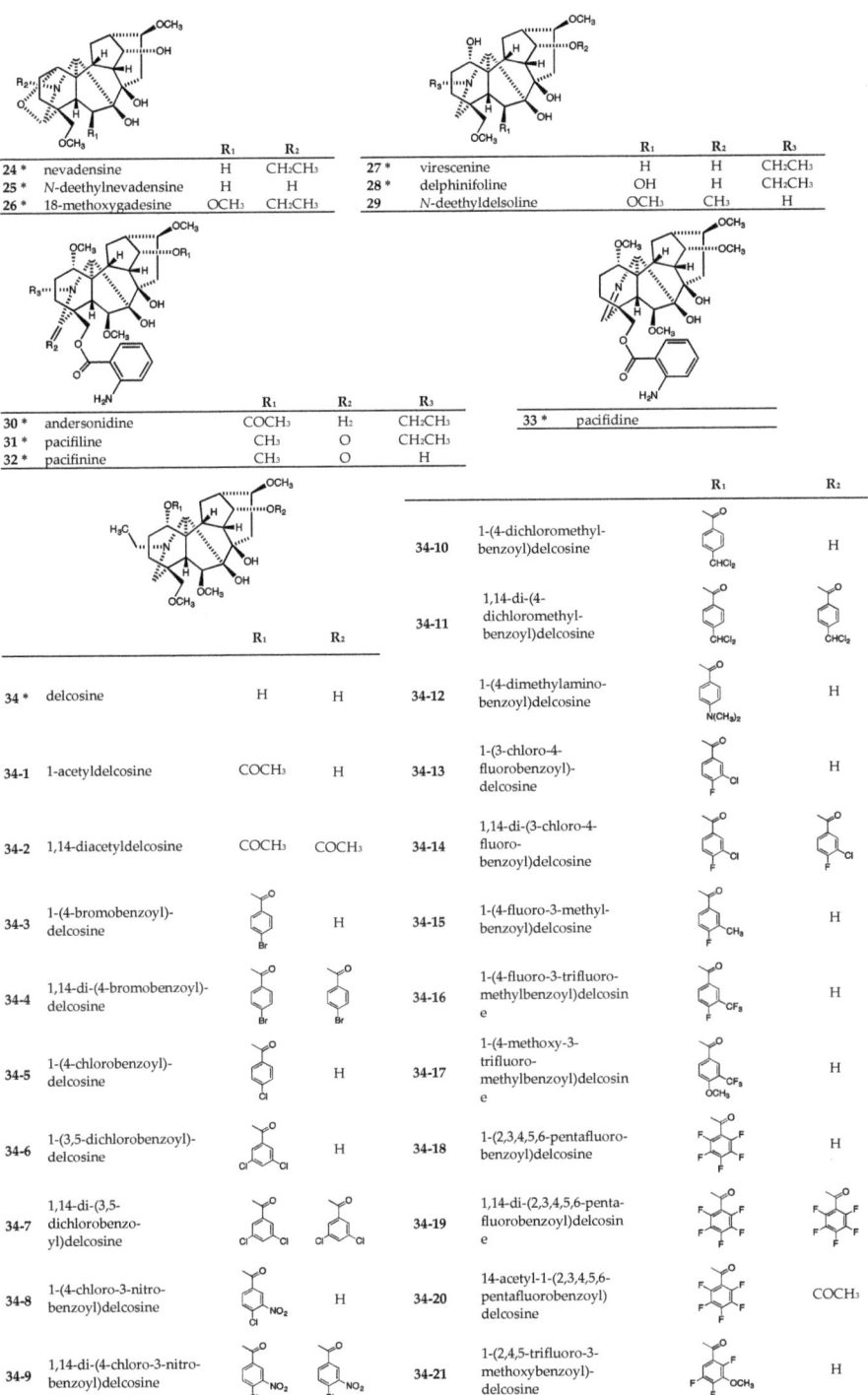

Figure 3. *Cont.*

		R₁	R₂			R₁	R₂
34-22	1,14-di-(2,4,5-trifluoro-3-methoxybenzoyl)delcosine	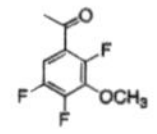	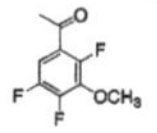	34-36	1,14-di-(2,2-difluoro-1,3-benzodioxole-4-carbonyl)delcosine	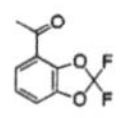	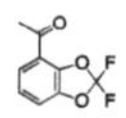
34-23	14-acetyl-1-(2,4,5-trifluoro-3-methoxybenzoyl)delcosine	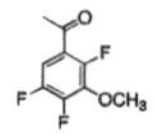	COCH₃	34-37	1-(phenylacethyl)delcosine	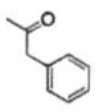	H
34-24	1-(4-trifluoromethylbenzoyl)delcosine	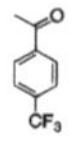	H	34-38	1-(3-trifluoromethylcinnamoyl)delcosine	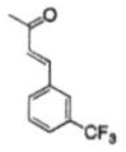	H
34-25	1-(3,5-bis-trifluoromethylbenzoyl)delcosine	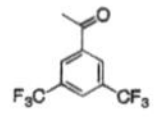	H	34-39	1-(4-nitrocinnamoyl)delcosine	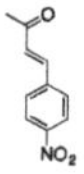	H
34-26	1,14-di-(3,5-bis-trifluoromethylbenzoyl)delcosine	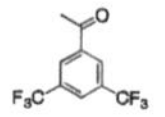	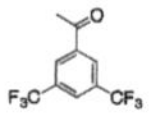	34-40	1-(naphthoyl)delcosine	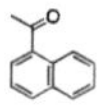	H
34-27	1-(4-trifluoromethylthiobenzoyl)delcosine	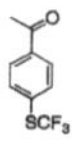	H	34-41	1-(anthraquinone-2-carbonyl)delcosine	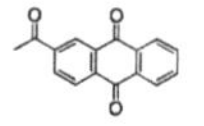	H
34-28	1,14-di-(4-trifluoromethylthiobenzoyl)delcosine	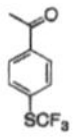	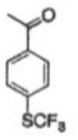	34-42	delsoline	H	CH₃
34-29	1-(3,5-dimethoxybenzoyl)delcosine	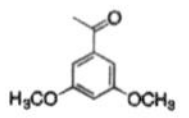	H		14-acetyldelcosine	H	COCH₃
34-30	1-(3,4,5-trimethoxybenzoyl)delcosine	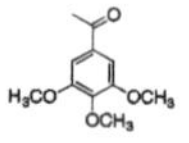	H	34-44	14-benzyldelcosine	H	CH₂C₆H₅
34-31	1-(3,5-diethoxybenzoyl)delcosine	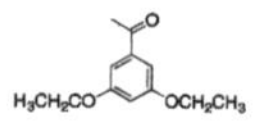	H	34-45	1,14-di-(4-nitrobenzoyl)delcosine	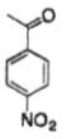	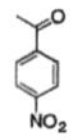
34-32	1-(4-benzyloxybenzoyl)delcosine	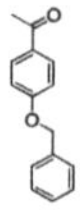	H	34-46	14-acetyl-1-(4-nitrobenzoyl)delcosine		COCH₃
34-33	1-(4-cyanobenzoyl)delcosine	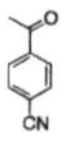	H	34-47	1,14-di-(4-ethoxybenzoyl)delcosine	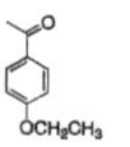	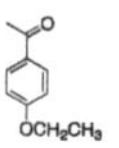
34-34	1-piperonyloyldelcosine	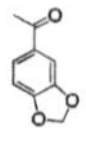	H	35*	14-acetylbrowniine	CH₃	COCH₃
34-35	1-(2,2-difluoro-1,3-benzodioxole-4-carbonyl)delcosine	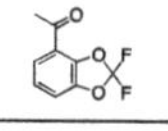	H				

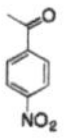

*: Natural alkaloid.

Figure 3. Chemical structures of lycoctonine-type (7,8-diol) C_{19}-diterpenoid alkaloids **24–35**.

Among the derivatives esterified at both C-1 and -14, alkaloids **34-19** and **34-20** exhibited significant potency against all five tested cell lines (average IC_{50} 4.9 and 5.0 µM, respectively). Alkaloid **34-9** (average IC_{50} 11.9 µM) showed significant antiproliferative activity against MDA-MB-231 and KB cells (IC_{50} 4.7 and 5.8 µM, respectively) comparable with **34-19** and **34-20**, but was less potent against MCF-7 and A549 (IC_{50} 12.2 and 24.8 µM, respectively) and inactive against KB-VIN. Alkaloid **34-23** exhibited only weak potency toward all cell lines (average IC_{50} 23.7 µM). Alkaloids **34-4**, **34-7**, **34-11**, **34-14**, **34-26**, **34-36**, **34-45**, **34-46**, and **34-47** were inactive against all five human tumor cell lines, while **34-22** and **34-28** showed limited potency.

Table 2. Cytotoxic activity data for lycoctonine-type (7,8-diol) C_{19}-diterpenoid alkaloids and synthetic analogs of delcosine 24~35.

Alkaloids	Cell Line/IC$_{50}$ (μM) [1]					
	A549	DU145	MDA-MB-231	MCF-7	KB	KB-VIN
Nevadensine (24)	>40	-	>40	>40	>40	>40
N-Deethylnevadensine (25)	>40	-	>40	>40	>40	>40
18-Methoxygadesine (26)	>20	>20	-	-	>20	>20
Virescenine (27)	>40	-	>40	>40	>40	>40
Delphinifoline (28)	>20	>20	-	-	>20	>20
N-Deethyldelsoline (29)	>20	>20	-	-	>20	>20
Andersonidine (30)	>20	>20	-	-	>20	>20
Pacifiline (31)	>20	>20	-	-	>20	>20
Pacifinine (32)	>20	>20	-	-	>20	>20
Pacifidine (33)	>20	>20	-	-	>20	>20
Delcosine (34)	>20	>20	-	-	>20	>20
34-1	>20	>20	-	-	>20	>20
34-2	>20	>20	-	-	>20	>20
34-3	20.6 ± 0.3	-	19.4 ± 1.0	17.9 ± 0.3	14.6 ± 0.6	17.1 ± 0.8
34-4	>40	-	>40	>40	>40	>40
34-5	18.7 ± 0.1	-	29.1 ± 1.6	25.8 ± 1.4	19.6 ± 0.3	21.1 ± 1.5
34-6	7.7 ± 0.9	-	8.6 ± 6.0	15.8 ± 4.2	5.6 ± 1.2	8.6 ± 1.9
34-7	>40	-	>40	>40	>40	>40
34-8	4.5 ± 0.5	-	5.0 ± 0.1	5.9 ± 0.3	5.4 ± 0.3	5.6 ± 0.4
34-9	24.8 ± 0.1	-	4.7 ± 0.1	12.2 ± 0.3	5.8 ± 0.4	>40
34-10	4.8 ± 0.3	-	4.8 ± 0.7	5.7 ± 0.4	4.3 ± 0.5	5.3 ± 0.4
34-11	>40	-	>40	>40	>40	>40
34-12	26.5 ± 0.3	-	>40	40.6 ± 2.5	27.8 ± 1.7	28.1 ± 3.0
34-13	20.8 ± 1.7	-	32.4 ± 1.8	25.9 ± 2.4	23.0 ± 2.4	21.5 ± 1.3
34-14	>40	-	>40	>40	>40	>40
34-15	21.7 ± 1.6	-	30.2 ± 2.7	26.9 ± 1.4	20.7 ± 1.2	21.5 ± 3.6
34-16	14.4 ± 2.1	-	20.1 ± 0.7	16.4 ± 2.1	13.6 ± 1.1	15.7 ± 0.8
34-17	11.4 ± 1.4	-	10.4 ± 1.7	22.5 ± 1.5	10.8 ± 1.9	11.8 ± 3.2
34-18	4.7 ± 0.1	-	5.3 ± 0.2	9.2 ± 0.4	5.8 ± 0.6	9.5 ± 0.5
34-19	4.9 ± 0.1	-	4.9 ± 0.1	5.3 ± 0.3	4.7 ± 0.1	4.9 ± 0.1
34-20	4.8 ± 0.1	-	4.6 ± 0.3	6.0 ± 0.1	4.8 ± 0.4	4.9 ± 0.4
34-21	20.8 ± 2.1	-	21.5 ± 0.6	21.4 ± 0.3	18.6 ± 1.7	15.0 ± 0.1
34-22	>40	-	>40	>40	>40	39.1 ± 2.0
34-23	23.8 ± 2.0	-	25.2 ± 1.0	23.3 ± 1.1	23.7 ± 1.1	22.6 ± 0.3
34-24	>20	>20	-	-	>20	>20
34-25	20.6 ± 1.2	-	21.3 ± 1.3	22.4 ± 1.2	20.8 ± 2.1	18.0 ± 1.0
34-26	>40	-	>40	>40	>40	>40
34-27	18.6 ± 2.6	-	19.7 ± 2.0	20.6 ± 1.2	22.2 ± 1.8	19.8 ± 1.9
34-28	33.0 ± 2.1	-	32.4 ± 1.7	31.1 ± 0.8	23.2 ± 1.1	40.0 ± 1.0
34-29	23.8 ± 2.6	-	33.4 ± 1.7	29.8 ± 1.2	22.8 ± 1.7	22.6 ± 2.4
34-30	>40	-	>40	>40	>40	>40
34-31	17.3 ± 2.2	-	23.1 ± 0.5	20.0 ± 0.7	16.2 ± 1.8	17.4 ± 1.9
34-32	16.5 ± 1.3	-	22.5 ± 0.8	-	8.71 ± 0.7	15.8 ± 0.8
34-33	40.9 ± 5.3	-	>40	>40	36.3 ± 1.0	29.3 ± 0.6
34-34	>40	-	>40	>40	>40	>40
34-35	21.2 ± 0.1	-	24.8 ± 1.6	24.6 ± 1.0	18.7 ± 1.2	21.7 ± 0.6
34-36	>40	-	>40	>40	>40	>40
34-37	23.8 ± 0.5	-	32.9 ± 1.0	22.6 ± 1.5	21.2 ± 0.1	19.2 ± 0.1
34-38	11.2 ± 0.7	>20	-	-	21.1 ± 3.9	19.5 ± 8.2
34-39	29.7 ± 0.7	-	43.2 ± 1.8	32.0 ± 0.6	36.0 ± 0.4	45.1 ± 3.4
34-40	18.5 ± 0.5	-	17.9 ± 0.5	15.5 ± 0.6	13.7 ± 0.1	14.2 ± 0.5
34-41	22.9 ± 0.5	-	20.7 ± 2.1	20.5 ± 1.0	21.6 ± 0.1	24.4 ± 0.5
34-42	>20	>20	-	-	>20	>20
14-Acetyldelcosine (34-43)	>20	>20	-	-	>20	>20
34-44	>20	>20	-	-	>20	>20
34-45	>20	>20	-	-	>20	>20
34-46	>20	>20	-	-	>20	>20
34-47	>20	>20	-	>20	>20	>20
14-Acetylbrowniine (35)	>20	>20	-	-	>20	>20
PXL[2] (nM)	4.8 ± 0.6	5.9 ± 1.9	8.4 ± 0.8	10.2 ± 0.9	5.8 ± 0.2	2405.4 ± 44.8

[1] Values are means ± standard deviation; [2] Paclitaxel (PXL; nM) was used as an experimental control.

Particularly, C-1 monoacylated delcosine derivatives (**34-3**, **34-6**, **34-8**, **34-10**, **34-13**, **34-21**, **34-25**, **34-27**, and **34-35**) were significantly more potent compared with corresponding C-1,14 diacylated delcosine derivatives (**34-4**, **34-7**, **34-9**, **34-11**, **34-14**, **34-22**, **34-23**, **34-26**, **34-28** and **34-36**). Thus, a C-1 acyloxy group and C-14 hydroxy group are crucial for enhanced antiproliferative activity of **1**-derivatives. Regarding alkaloids **34-18** (pentafluorobenzoate at C-1, hydroxy at C-14), **34-19** (pentafluorobenzoate at C-1 and C-14), and **34-20** (pentafluorobenzoate at C-1, acetate at C-14), all three alkaloids were essentially equipotent against three of the five tumor cell lines, while **34-18** was somewhat less potent than the diacylated alkaloids against MCF-7 and KB-VIN cells.

Striking observations from the data in Table 2 were the consistent identities of the most potent alkaloids. Alkaloids **34-8**, **34-10**, **34-19**, and **34-20** exhibited the highest potency against all five tested tumor cell lines with IC$_{50}$ values ranging from 4.3 to 6.0 µM. The same range of potency was found with alkaloid **34-18** against A549 cells, with alkaloids **34-9** and **34-18** against MDA-MB-231 cells, and with **34-6**, **34-9**, and **34-18** against KB cells. The potencies of **34-6** and **34-17** (IC$_{50}$ 5.6–11.8 µM) generally ranked somewhat below those of the most potent alkaloids, except against the MCF-7 cell line, where they were even less active.

The identity of the substituent(s) on the acyl group affected the antiproliferative potency. Notably, among the 1,14-diacyl and 1-acyl-14-acetyl derivatives, only alkaloids **34-19** and **34-20** with one or two pentafluorinated benzoyl esters, respectively, showed significant potency against all five tested cell lines. Alkaloid **34-9** with two 3-nitro-4-chlorobenzoyl groups showed good potency against certain cell lines. Similarly, the 1-monoacylated alkaloids with the highest potency against the five tumor cell lines contained 3-nitro-4-chloro- (**34-8**) and pentafluoro- (**34-18**) as well as 4-dichloro-methyl- (**34-10**) benzoyl esters. The chlorinated alkaloids **34-8** and **34-10** as well as **34-6**, which has 3,5-dichloro substitution on the benzoate ester, were more potent than **34-5** with only a single chloro group or **34-13** with chloro and fluoro groups. Similarly, alkaloid **34-18** showed increased antiproliferative activity against the five tumor cell lines compared with other fluorinated alkaloids **34-13**~**34-17**, **34-21**~**34-27**. Moreover, with some exceptions against certain cell lines, alkaloids with bromo (**34-3** and **34-4**), dimethylamino (**34-12**), dimethoxy (**34-29**), trimethoxy (**34-30**), diethoxy (**34-31**), benzyloxy (**34-32**), cyano (**34-33**), methylenedioxy (**34-34** and **34-35**), nitro (**34-45** and **34-46**), and ethoxy (**34-47**) substituted benzoate esters or phenylacetyl (**34-37**), cinnamoyl (**34-38** and **34-39**), 1-naphthoyl (**34-40**), and anthraquinone-2-carbonyl (**34-41**) esters were less potent or inactive.

Interestingly, the active alkaloids were generally effective against P-gp overexpressing MDR subline KB-VIN, while alkaloids such as vincristine and paclitaxel are ineffective due to excretion from the MDR cells by P-gp. These results suggest that these diterpenoids are not substrates for P-gp.

2.3. Lycoctonine-Type (7,8-methylenedioxy) C$_{19}$-Diterpenoid Alkaloids

The tested lycoctonine-type (7,8-methylenedioxy) C$_{19}$-diterpenoid alkaloids included 19 natural alkaloids, delcorine (**36**), delpheline (**37**), pacinine (**38**), yunnadelphinine (**39**), melpheline (**40**), bonvalotidine C (**41**), N-deethyl-N-formylpaciline (**42**), N-deethyl-N-formylpacinine (**43**), isodel-pheline (**44**), pacidine (**45**), eladine (**46**), N-formyl-4,19-secopacinine (**47**), N-formyl-4,19-secoyunna-delphinine (**48**), iminoisodelpheline (**49**), iminodelpheline (**50**), laxicyminine (**51**), N-deethyl-19-oxo-isodelpheline (**52**), N-deethyl-19-oxodelpheline (**53**), and 19-oxoisodelpheline (**54**), purified from seeds of *Delphinium elatum* cv. Pacific Giant [35,39–42] (Figure 4). The remaining 22 tested C$_{19}$-diterpenoids were synthetic derivatives (**37-1**~**37-22**) [43] prepared from **37** (Figure 4).

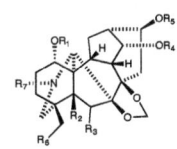

		R₁	R₂	R₃	R₄	R₅	R₆	R₇
36 *	delcorine	CH₃	H	β-OH	CH₃	CH₃	OCH₃	CH₂CH₃
37 *	delpheline	CH₃	H	β-OH	CH₃	CH₃	H	CH₂CH₃
38 *	pacinine	CH₃	H	=O	CH₃	CH₃	H	CH₂CH₃
39 *	yunnadelphinine	CH₃	H	=O	H	CH₃	H	CH₂CH₃
40 *	melpheline	CH₃	H	β-OH	CH₃	CH₃	H	CH₃
41 *	bonvalotidine C	CH₃	OH	=O	CH₃	CH₃	H	CH₂CH₃
42 *	N-deethyl-N-formylpaciline	CH₃	H	β-OCH₃	CH₃	CH₃	H	CHO
43*	N-deethyl-N-formylpacinine	CH₃	H	=O	CH₃	CH₃	H	CHO
44 *	isodelpheline	CH₃	H	β-OCH₃	H	CH₃	H	CH₂CH₃
45 *	pacidine	H	H	β-OH	CH₃	CH₃	H	CH₂CH₃
46 *	eladine	CH₃	H	β-OH	CH₃	H	H	CH₂CH₃

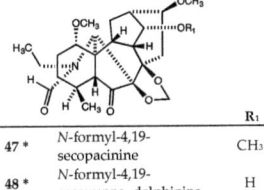

		R₁			R₁	R₂			
47 *	N-formyl-4,19-secopacinine	CH₃		49 *	iminoisodelpheline	CH₃	H	51 *	laxicyminine
48 *	N-formyl-4,19-secoyunna-delphinine	H		50 *	iminodelpheline	H	CH₃		

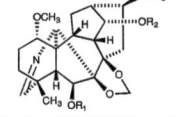

		R₁	R₂	R₃			R₁
52*	N-deethyl-19-oxoisodelpheline	CH₃	H	H	37-20	7,8-demethylenedelpheline	H
53*	N-deethyl-19-oxodelpheline	H	CH₃	H	37-21	7,8-demethylene-6-(3-trifluoro-methylbenzoyl)delpheline	
54 *	19-oxoisodelpheline	CH₃	H	CH₂CH₃			
37-22	19-oxodelpheline	H	CH₃	CH₂CH₃			

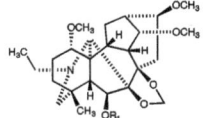

		R₁			R₁
37-1	6-(4-chlorobenzoyl)delpheline		37-6	6-(4-trifluoromethoxybenzoyl)delpheline	
37-2	6-(4-fluorobenzoyl)delpheline		37-7	6-(4-trifluoromethylthiobenzoyl)delpheline	
37-3	6-(4-nitrobenzoyl)delpheline		37-8	6-(methyl terephthaloyl)delpheline	
37-4	6-(4-anisoyl)delpheline		37-9	6-(3-trifluoromethylbenzoyl)delpheline	
37-5	6-(4-phenylbenzoyl)delpheline		37-10	6-(3,5-dinitrobenzoyl)delpheline	

Figure 4. *Cont.*

37-11	6-(3,4,5-trimethoxybenzoyl)delpheline			37-16	6-(4-ethoxybenzoyl)delpheline	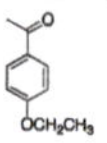
37-12	6-(3,4,5-trifluorobenzoyl)delpheline			37-17	6-(4-benzyloxybenzoyl)delpheline	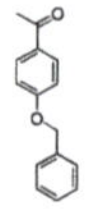
37-13	6-(3-trifluoromethylcinnamoyl)delpheline			37-18	6-(3-fluoro-4-trifluoromethyl-benzoyl)delpheline	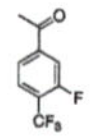
37-14	6-(4-fluorocinnamoyl)delpheline			37-19	6-(4-fluoro-3-methylbenzoyl)delpheline	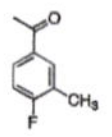
37-15	6-(6-trifluoromethylnicotinoyl)delpheline					

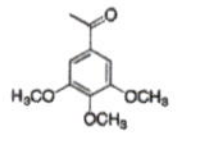

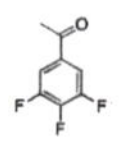

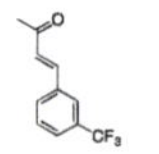

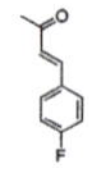

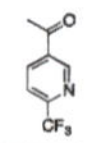

*: Natural alkaloid

Figure 4. Chemical structures of lycoctonine-type (7,8-methylenedioxy) C_{19}-diterpenoid alkaloids **36–54**.

All tested lycoctonine-type (7,8-methylenedioxy) C_{19}-diterpenoid alkaloids were evaluated for antiproliferative activity against human tumor cell lines [30,40–43] (Table 3). The lycoctonine-type (7,8-methylenedioxy) C_{19}-diterpenoid alkaloids, both the natural alkaloids (**36~54**) and synthetic analogs that did not contain a C-6 ester group (**37-20** and **37-22**), were inactive (IC_{50} > 20 or 40 μM). Among the C-6 esterified alkaloids, **37-1**, **37-17**, and **37-18** exhibited the highest average potency toward four tested cell lines (A549, DU145, KB and KB-VIN; average IC_{50} 9.83, 9.57, and 9.41 μM, respectively). Alkaloids **37-3**, **37-5~37-7**, **37-9**, **37-10**, **37-12**, **37-13**, **37-16**, and **37-19** showed moderate potency against all tested cell lines (average IC_{50} 13.9–20.8 μM). However, alkaloid **37-13** showed significantly increased cytotoxic activity (IC_{50} 10.2 μM) against A549 cells compared with **37-1**, **37-17**, and **37-18**, but was generally less potent against DU145 and KB cells. While alkaloids **37-12**, **37-13**, **37-16**, and **37-19** displayed good antiproliferative activity (IC_{50} 6.8, 9.1, 6.5, and 4.7 μM, respectively) against KB-VIN cells, they were much less potent against A549, DU145, and KB cells. Alkaloids **37-4** and **37-21** were inactive against all tested cancer cell lines, while **37-2**, **37-8**, **37-11**, and **37-14** exhibited only weak potency toward all cell lines (average IC_{50} 23.0–29.2 μM).

The most noticeable observations from the data in Table 3 were the degree and relative ratio of KB/KB-VIN potency. Among the four cancer cell lines tested, the highest potency was found against the KB-VIN cell line by alkaloids **37-17~37-19** (IC_{50} 4.22, 4.40, and 4.71 μM, respectively), followed by alkaloids **37-16**, **37-12**, **37-1**, **37-13**, and **37-9** (IC_{50} 6.50, 6.80, 8.27, 9.10, and 11.9 μM, respectively). Generally, all active alkaloids showed the highest potency against the KB-VIN cell line compared with the other three tested cancer cell lines. Moreover, alkaloids **37-12**, **37-16**, **37-13**, and **37-19** showed over two-fold selectivity between the two cell lines (ratio of IC_{50} KB/IC_{50} KB-VIN: 2.15, 2.28, 2.31, and 2.57, respectively). Alkaloids **37-2**, **37-5**, and **37-17** displayed weak selectivity between the KB and KB-VIN cell lines (ratio of IC_{50} KB/IC_{50} KB-VIN: 1.55, 1.36, and 1.62, respectively). Finally, alkaloids **37-1**, **37-3**, **37-6~37-9**, **37-11**, **37-14**, **37-15**, and **37-18** displayed similar potency against the KB and KB-VIN cell lines (ratio of IC_{50} KB/IC_{50} KB-VIN: 1.07, 1.17, 1.06, 1.21, 1.04, 1.25, 1.07, 1.07, 1.17, and 1.23, respectively).

The identity of the substituent on the C-6 acyl group affected the cytotoxic potency. For instance, the alkaloids with the highest potency against the KB-VIN cell line contained chloro (**37-1**), fluoro (**37-12**, **37-18**, and **37-19**), trifluoromethyl (**37-9**, **37-13**, and **37-18**), ethoxy (**37-16**), or benzyloxy (**37-17**) substituents on the acyl group. Against the KB-VIN cell line, alkaloids **37-18** and **37-19** with both fluoro and trifluoromethyl/methyl groups were more potent than **37-9** with only a single trifluoromethyl group and even more potent than **37-2** with a single fluoro group. Similarly, alkaloid **37-13** showed increased cytotoxic activity against most cell lines compared with the related fluorinated alkaloids **37-14** and **37-15**. Moreover, alkaloids with nitro, methoxy, phenyl, trifluoromethoxy, trifluoromethythio, and methyl carboxylate groups on a C-6 benzoate ester were generally less potent.

Table 3. Cytotoxic activity data for lycoctonine-type (7,8-methylenedioxy) C_{19}-diterpenoid alkaloids and synthetic analogs of delpheline **36~54**.

Alkaloids	Cell Line/IC$_{50}$ (µM) [1]					KB/KB-VIN Ratio
	A549	DU145	MDA-MB-231	KB	KB-VIN	
Delcorine (**36**)	>40	-	>40	>40	>40	-
Delpheline (**37**)	>20	>20	-	>20	>20	-
Pacinine (**38**)	>20	>20	-	>20	>20	-
Yunnadelphinine (**39**)	>20	>20	-	>20	>20	-
Melpheline (**40**)	>40	-	>40	>40	>40	-
Bonvalotidine C (**41**)	>40	-	>40	>40	>40	-
N-Deethyl-N-formylpaciline (**42**)	>40	-	>40	>40	>40	-
N-Deethyl-N-formylpacinine (**43**)	>40	-	>40	>40	>40	-
Isodelpheline (**44**)	>40	-	>40	>40	>40	-
Pacidine (**45**)	>40	-	>40	>40	>40	-
Eladine (**46**)	>40	-	>40	>40	>40	-
N-Formyl-4,19-secopacinine (**47**)	>40	-	>40	>40	>40	-
N-Formyl-4,19-secoyunnadelphinine (**48**)	>40	-	>40	>40	>40	-
Iminoisodelpheline (**49**)	>40	-	>40	>40	>40	-
Iminodelpheline (**50**)	>40	-	>40	>40	>40	-
Laxicyminine (**51**)	>40	-	>40	>40	>40	-
N-Deethyl-19-oxoisodelpheline (**52**)	>40	-	>40	>40	>40	-
N-Deethyl-19-oxo-delpheline (**53**)	>40	-	>40	>40	>40	-
19-Oxoisodelpheline (**54**)	>40	-	>40	>40	>40	-
37-1	14.8 ± 3.8	7.4 ± 1.2	-	8.9 ± 2.0	8.3 ± 1.6	1.07
37-2	38.1 ± 11.8	15.6 ± 5.4	-	23.3 ± 3.9	15.0 ± 6.5	1.55
37-3	22.7 ± 0.3	17.2 ± 3.3	-	20.7 ± 0.9	17.7 ± 3.5	1.17
37-4	>20	>20	-	>20	>20	-
37-5	24.1 ± 2.7	17.1 ± 11.4	-	23.6 ± 0.4	17.4 ± 7.4	1.36
37-6	18.7 ± 6.6	20.3 ± 7.1	-	20.1 ± 7.6	18.9 ± 5.0	1.06
37-7	21.1 ± 9.2	16.6 ± 12.7	-	21.7 ± 11.6	17.9 ± 4.2	1.21
37-8	28.7 ± 13.6	28.7 ± 7.2	-	24.3 ± 5.7	23.3 ± 3.7	1.04
37-9	21.2 ± 4.7	12.6 ± 3.0	-	14.9 ± 4.9	11.9 ± 3.3	1.25
37-10	20.9 ± 4.3	22.7 ± 6.0	-	19.1 ± 4.8	20.3 ± 2.7	0.94
37-11	30.8 ± 13.3	28.9 ± 4.7	-	29.5 ± 3.5	27.5 ± 3.1	1.07
37-12	19.9 ± 10.1	16.9 ± 6.7	-	14.6 ± 7.1	6.80 ± 5.0	2.15
37-13	10.2 ± 2.6	15.1 ± 6.0	-	21.0 ± 9.4	9.10 ± 1.5	2.31
37-14	22.4 ± 7.1	22.8 ± 8.5	-	25.9 ± 9.3	24.2 ± 4.4	1.07
37-15	29.7 ± 11.6	29.0 ± 5.4	-	21.8 ± 1.4	18.7 ± 5.2	1.17
37-16	20.0 ± 0.9	15.6 ± 2.6	-	14.8 ± 3.3	6.5 ± 2.2	2.28
37-17	14.1 ± 2.9	13.2 ± 5.7	-	6.8 ± 1.7	4.2 ± 1.1	1.62
37-18	16.5 ± 2.2	11.3 ± 7.9	-	5.4 ± 1.8	4.4 ± 0.8	1.23
37-19	25.6 ± 1.2	19.8 ± 4.6	-	12.1 ± 7.8	4.7 ± 1.4	2.57
37-20	>20	>20	-	>20	>20	-
37-21	>20	>20	-	>20	>20	-
37-22	>20	>20	-	>20	>20	-
PXL [2] (nM)	4.8 ± 0.6	5.9 ± 1.9	8.4 ± 0.8	5.8 ± 0.2	2405.4 ± 44.8	-

[1] Values are means ± standard deviation; [2] Paclitaxel (PXL; nM) was used as an experimental control.

3. Antiproliferative Activity of C_{20}-Diterpenoid Alkaloid Derivatives

3.1. Actaline and Napelline-Type C_{20}-Diterpenoid Alkaloids

One natural actaline-type C_{20}-diterpenoid alkaloid [44], aconicarchamine A (**55**), isolated from rhizoma of *Aconitum japonicum* subsp. *subcuneatum* [30], (Figure 5) and seven natural napelline-type C_{20}-diterpenoid alkaloids, lucidusculine (**57**), flavadine (**58**), 12-acetyllucidusculine (**59**), 1-acetyl-luciculine (**60**), dehydrolucidusculine (**61**), dehydroluciculine (**62**), and 12-acetyldehydroluciduscu-line (**63**), purified from roots of *Aconitum yesoense* var. *macroyesoense* [31–33], (Figure 5) were tested. Seven synthetic napelline-type C_{20}-diterpenoid alkaloid derivatives (**56-1**~**56-7**) [18,32,45] were prepared from luciculine (**56**) (Figure 5) and tested also. All tested actaline- and napelline-type C_{20}-diterpenoid alkaloids were evaluated for antiproliferative activity against four to five human tumor cell lines [28,30] (Table 4). Tested actaline- and napelline-type C_{20}-diterpenoid alkaloids, both the natural alkaloids (**55** and **57–63**) and synthetic analogs (**56-1**~**56-4**, **56-6**, and **56-7**), were inactive (IC$_{50}$ > 20 or 40 µM). Among the synthetic alkaloids, alkaloid **56-5** exhibited only weak potency toward the tested cell lines (A549, DU145, KB and KB-VIN; average IC_{50} 27.8 µM). Because the related alkaloids **57**, **60**, **56-2~56-4**, **56-6**, and **56-7** were inactive against all tested cancer cell lines, a C-1 hydroxy group, C-12 acyloxy group, and C-15 acetoxy group found in **56-5** could be needed for antiproliferative activity of luciculine derivatives.

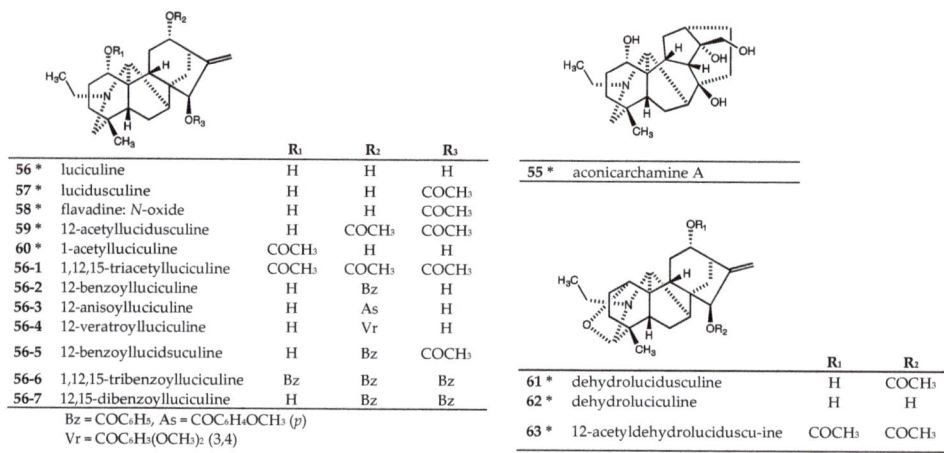

		R₁	R₂	R₃
56 *	luciculine	H	H	H
57 *	lucidusculine	H	H	COCH₃
58 *	flavadine: N-oxide	H	H	COCH₃
59 *	12-acetyllucidusculine	H	COCH₃	COCH₃
60 *	1-acetylluciculine	COCH₃	H	H
56-1	1,12,15-triacetylluciculine	COCH₃	COCH₃	COCH₃
56-2	12-benzoylluciculine	H	Bz	H
56-3	12-anisoylluciculine	H	As	H
56-4	12-veratroylluciculine	H	Vr	H
56-5	12-benzoyllucidsuculine	H	Bz	COCH₃
56-6	1,12,15-tribenzoylluciculine	Bz	Bz	Bz
56-7	12,15-dibenzoylluciculine	H	Bz	Bz

Bz = COC₆H₅, As = COC₆H₄OCH₃ (p)
Vr = COC₆H₃(OCH₃)₂ (3,4)

		R₁	R₂
55 *	aconicarchamine A		
61 *	dehydrolucidusculine	H	COCH₃
62 *	dehydroluciculine	H	H
63 *	12-acetyldehydroluciduscu-ine	COCH₃	COCH₃

*: Natural alkaloid

Figure 5. Chemical structures of actaline and napelline-type C_{20}-diterpenoid alkaloids **55~63**.

Table 4. Cytotoxic activity data for actaline and napelline-type C_{20}-diterpenoid alkaloids **55~63** and synthetic analogs **56-1~56-7** of luciculine.

Alkaloids	Cell Line/IC_{50} (µM) [1]					
	A549	DU145	MDA-MB-231	MCF-7	KB	KB-VIN
Aconicarchamine A (**55**)	>40	-	>40	>40	>40	>40
Lucidusculine (**57**)	>20	>20	-	-	>20	>20
Flavadine (**58**)	>20	>20	-	-	>20	>20
12-Acetyllucidusculine (**59**)	>20	>20	-	-	>20	>20
1-Acetylluciculine (**60**)	>20	>20	-	-	>20	>20
Dehydrolucidusculine (**61**)	>20	>20	-	-	>20	>20
Dehydroluciculine (**62**)	>20	>20	-	-	>20	>20
12-Acetyldehydrolucidusculine (**63**)	>20	>20	-	-	>20	>20
56-1	>20	>20	-	-	>20	>20
56-2	>20	>20	-	-	>20	>20
56-3	>20	>20	-	-	>20	>20
56-4	>20	>20	-	-	>20	>20
56-5	23.3 ± 6.1	28.1 ± 11.1	-	-	31.8 ± 10.5	27.8 ± 1.9
56-6	>20	>20	-	-	>20	>20
56-7	>20	>20	-	-	>20	>20
PXL [2] (nM)	4.8 ± 0.6	5.9 ± 1.9	8.4 ± 0.8	10.2 ± 0.9	5.8 ± 0.2	2405.4 ± 44.8

[1] Values are means ± standard deviation; [2] Paclitaxel (PXL; nM) was used as an experimental control.

3.2. Hetisine-Type (Analogs of Kobusine) C_{20}-Diterpenoid Alkaloids

Tested hetisine-type (analogs of kobusine) C_{20}-diterpenoid alkaloids included four natural alkaloids, ryosenamine (**64**), 9-hydroxynominine (**65**), and torokonine (**66**), isolated from rhizoma of *Aconitum japonicum* subsp. *subcuneatum* [27,28] (Figure 6) and kobusine (**67**), purified from roots of *Aconitum yesoense* var. *macroyesoense* [31] (Figure 6). Nineteen synthetic derivatives (**67-1~67-19**) [18,21,30,46,47] (Figure 6) prepared from **67** were tested also.

All tested hetisine-type (kobusine analogs) C_{20}-diterpenoid alkaloids were evaluated for antiproliferative activity against four human tumor cell lines [27,28,30] (Table 5). Fifteen of the 23 alkaloids, both natural (**64~67**) and synthetic (**67-1~67-4**, **67-6**, **67-9**, **67-11**, **67-12**, **67-15~67-17**), were inactive (IC$_{50}$ > 20 or 40 µM). Kobusine derivatives **67-5**, **67-7**, **67-10**, **67-18**, and **67-19** exhibited the highest average potency over the four tested cell lines (A549, DU145, KB and KB-VIN; average IC$_{50}$ 7.8, 6.1, 6.2, 6.8, and 4.7 µM, respectively), and alkaloids **67-8**, **67-13**, and **67-14** showed moderate potency (average IC$_{50}$ 16.6, 14.3, and 11.6 µM, respectively). However, while alkaloid **67-14** showed good cytotoxic activity (IC$_{50}$ 9.6 µM) against DU145 cells, it was much less potent against A549, KB, and KB-VIN cells.

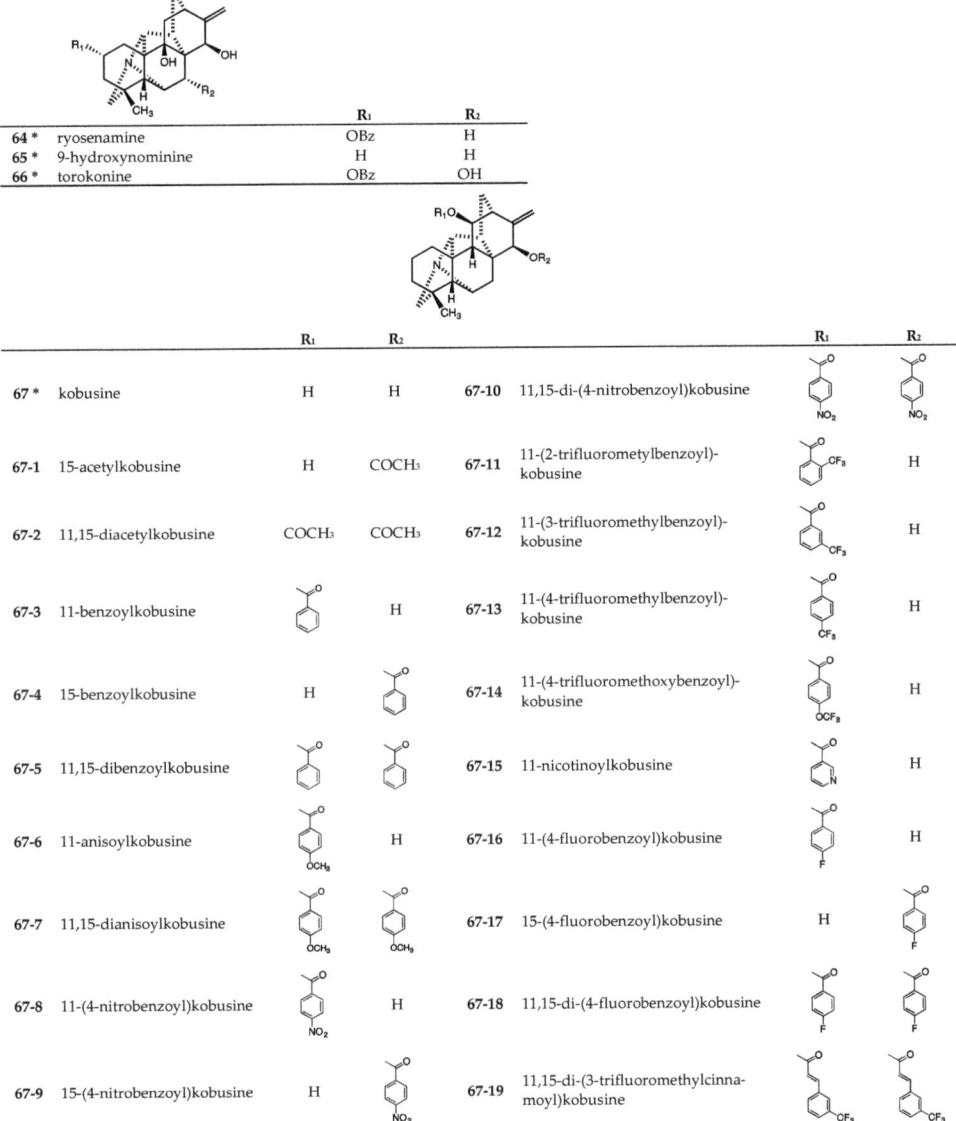

*: Natural alkaloid

Figure 6. Chemical structures of hetisine-type (analogs of kobusine) C$_{20}$-diterpenoid alkaloids **64~67-19**.

Table 5. Cytotoxic activity data for hetisine-type C_{20}-diterpenoid alkaloids 64~67 and synthetic derivatives 67-1~67-19 of kobusine.

Alkaloids	Cell Line/IC$_{50}$ (μM) [1]						KB/KB-VIN Ratio
	A549	DU145	MDA-MB-231	MCF-7	KB	KB-VIN	
Ryosenamine (64)	>40	-	>40	>40	>40	>40	
9-Hydroxynominine (65)	>40	-	>40	>40	>40	>40	
Torokonine (66)	>40	-	>40	>40	>40	>40	
Kobusine (67)	>20	>20	-	-	>20	>20	
67-1	>20	>20	-	-	>20	>20	
67-2	>20	>20	-	-	>20	>20	
67-3	>20	>20	-	-	>20	>20	
67-4	>20	>20	-	-	>20	>20	
67-5	8.4 ± 1.4	9.3 ± 3.0	-	-	6.0 ± 0.8	7.5 ± 3.7	0.80
67-6	>20	>20	-	-	>20	>20	
67-7	6.7 ± 2.4	7.1 ± 2.0	-	-	5.3 ± 0.3	5.2 ± 1.2	1.02
67-8	19.5 ± 3.3	15.3 ± 5.6	-	-	13.9 ± 2.8	17.9 ± 1.8	0.78
67-9	>20	>20	-	-	>20	>20	
67-10	6.9 ± 1.7	7.0 ± 2.2	-	-	5.3 ± 0.6	5.5 ± 0.7	0.96
67-11	>20	>20	-	-	>20	>20	
67-12	>20	>20	-	-	>20	>20	
67-13	17.2 ± 0.9	13.2 ± 2.8	-	-	12.7 ± 1.1	14.1 ± 1.0	0.90
67-14	14.1 ± 0.7	9.6 ± 2.4	-	-	11.7 ± 0.6	10.9 ± 0.7	1.07
67-15	>20	>20	-	-	>20	>20	
67-16	>20	>20	-	-	>20	>20	
67-17	>20	>20	-	-	>20	>20	
67-18	8.1 ± 4.7	6.8 ± 2.0	-	-	5.2 ± 0.6	7.1 ± 2.6	0.73
67-19	5.5 ± 1.9	6.2 ± 3.1	-	-	4.1 ± 0.7	3.1 ± 1.6	1.32
PXL [2] (nM)	4.8 ± 0.6	5.9 ± 1.9	8.4 ± 0.8	10.2 ± 0.9	5.8 ± 0.2	2405.4 ± 44.8	0.0067

[1] Values are means ± standard deviation; [2] Paclitaxel (PXL; nM) was used as an experimental control.

Among these analogs of **67**, esterification of C-15 in addition to C-11 increased potency significantly (compare **67-8** to **67-10**) or even converted an inactive to an active alkaloid (compare **67-3** to **67-5**, **67-6** to **67-7**, **67-16** to **67-18**). Consequently, all of the most potent analogs (**67-5**, **67-7**, **67-10**, **67-18**, and **67-19**) of **67** were esterified at both C-11 and C-15.

Striking observations from the data in Table 5 were the degree and comparative ratio of KB/KB-VIN potency. Five alkaloids (**67-5**, **67-7**, **67-10**, **67-18**, and **67-19**) were quite potent (IC$_{50}$ < 10 μM) against KB-VIN. Indeed, alkaloid **67-19** exhibited a significantly low IC$_{50}$ value of 3.1 μM. The ratios of KB to KB-VIN (IC$_{50}$ KB/IC$_{50}$ KB-VIN) were greater than 0.73 for all active alkaloids, with many alkaloids displaying comparable potency against the two cell lines, in contrast with paclitaxel (ratio of 0.0067). Alkaloid **67-19** showed over 1.3-fold selectivity with the greatest cytotoxic activity against KB-VIN (IC$_{50}$ KB/IC$_{50}$ KB-VIN: 1.32).

3.3. Hetisine-Type (Analogs of Pseudokobusine) C_{20}-Diterpenoid Alkaloids

The two tested natural hetisine-type (analogs of pseudokobusine) C_{20}-diterpenoid alkaloids pseudokobusine (**68**) and 15-veratroylpseudokobusine (**68-11**) were purified from the roots of *Aconitum yesoense* var. *macroyesoense* [31,32] (Figure 7). The 36 tested synthetic derivatives (**68-1~68-10**, **68-12~68-37**) [18,21,30,32,46–49] (Figure 7) were prepared from **68**.

All tested hetisine-type (**68** analogs) C_{20}-diterpenoid alkaloids were evaluated for antiproliferative activity against four human tumor cell lines [30] (Table 6). Many alkaloids, both natural alkaloids (**68** and **68-11**) and synthetic analogs (**68-1~68-3**, **68-6**, **68-8**, **68-9**, **68-14**, **68-16~68-18**, **68-21**, **68-23**, **68-25~68-31**, **68-33~68-37**), were inactive (IC$_{50}$ > 20 μM). The pseudokobusine derivatives **68-5**, **68-15**, **68-19**, **68-20**, **68-24**, and **68-32** exhibited the highest average potency over the tested cell lines (A549, DU145, KB and KB-VIN; average IC$_{50}$ 7.0, 5.2, 5.3, 7.4, 7.1, and 6.1 μM, respectively). Alkaloids **68-7**, **68-10**, **68-12**, **68-13**, and **68-22** showed moderate potency over all tested cell lines (average IC$_{50}$ 13.5-16.8 μM). However, although alkaloid **68-10** showed good cytotoxic activity (IC$_{50}$ 8.0 μM) against A549 cells, it was much less potent against DU145, KB, and KB-VIN cells.

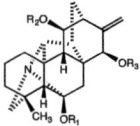

		R₁	R₂	R₃
68*	pseudokobusine	H	H	H
68-1	15-acetylpseudokobusine	H	H	COCH₃
68-2	11,15-diacetylpseudokobusine	H	COCH₃	COCH₃
68-3	6-benzoylpseudokobusine	COC₆H₅	H	H
68-4	6,11-dibenzoylpseudokobusine	COC₆H₅	COC₆H₅	H
68-5	11,15-dibenzoylpseudokobusine	H	COC₆H₅	COC₆H₅
68-6	6-anisoylpseudokobusine	CO-C₆H₄-OCH₃	H	H
68-7	11-anisoylpseudokobusine	H	CO-C₆H₄-OCH₃	H
68-8	6,11-dianisoylpseudokobusine	CO-C₆H₄-OCH₃	CO-C₆H₄-OCH₃	H
68-9	6,15-dianisoylpseudokobusine	CO-C₆H₄-OCH₃	H	CO-C₆H₄-OCH₃
68-10	11-veratroylpseudokobusine	H	CO-C₆H₃(OCH₃)₂	H
68-11*	15-veratroylpseudokobusine	H	H	CO-C₆H₃(OCH₃)₂
68-12	6,11-diveratroylpseudokobusine	CO-C₆H₃(OCH₃)₂	CO-C₆H₃(OCH₃)₂	H
68-13	6,15-diveratroylpseudokobusine	CO-C₆H₃(OCH₃)₂	H	CO-C₆H₃(OCH₃)₂
68-14	6-(4-nitrobenzoyl)pseudokobusine	CO-C₆H₄-NO₂	H	H
68-15	11-(4-nitrobenzoyl)pseudokobusine	H	CO-C₆H₄-NO₂	H
68-16	15-(4-nitrobenzoyl)pseudokobusine	H	H	CO-C₆H₄-NO₂
68-17	6,15-di-(4-nitrobenzoyl)pseudokobusine	CO-C₆H₄-NO₂	H	CO-C₆H₄-NO₂
68-18	6,11,15-tri-(4-nitrobenzoyl)pseudokobusine	CO-C₆H₄-NO₂	CO-C₆H₄-NO₂	CO-C₆H₄-NO₂

Figure 7. *Cont.*

		R₁	R₂	R₃
68-19	11,15-di-(3-nitrobenzoyl)pseudokobusine	H	3-nitrobenzoyl	3-nitrobenzoyl
68-20	11-(3-trifluoromethylbenzoyl)pseudokobusine	H	3-CF₃-benzoyl	H
68-21	6,11-di-(3-trifluoromethylbenzoyl)pseudokobusine	3-CF₃-benzoyl	3-CF₃-benzoyl	H
68-22	11-(4-trifluoromethylbenzoyl)pseudokobusine	H	4-CF₃-benzoyl	H
68-23	6-cinnamoylpseudokobusine	cinnamoyl	H	H
68-24	11-cinnamoylpseudokobusine	H	cinnamoyl	H
68-25	15-cinnamoylpseudokobusine	H	H	cinnamoyl
68-26	11-pivaloylpseudokobusine	H	pivaloyl	H
68-27	11-nicotinoylpseudokobusine	H	nicotinoyl	H
68-28	15-nicotinoylpseudokobusine	H	H	nicotinoyl
68-29	11,15-dinicotinoylpseudokobusine	H	nicotinoyl	nicotinoyl
68-30	15-propionylpseudokobusine	H	H	COCH₂CH₃
68-31	11,15-dipropionylpseudokobusine	H	COCH₂CH₃	COCH₂CH₃
68-32	11-tritylpseudokobusine	H	trityl	H

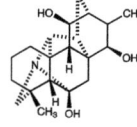

| 68-33 | dihydropseudokobusine | | | |

		R₁	R₂	R₃
68-34	N-benzyl-N,6-seco-6-dehydropseudokobusine	CH₂C₆H₅	H	H
68-35	N,11,15-triacetyl-N,6-seco-6-dehydropseudokobusine	COCH₃	COCH₃	COCH₃
68-36	N-acetyl-N,6-seco-6-dehydropseudokobusine	COCH₃	H	H
68-37	N-cinnamoyl-N,6-seco-6-dehydropseudokobusine	cinnamoyl	H	H

*: Natural alkaloid

Figure 7. Chemical structures of hetisine-type (analogs of pseudokobusine) C₂₀-diterpenoid alkaloids **68~68-37**.

Table 6. Cytotoxic activity data for hetisine-type C_{20}-diterpenoid alkaloids pseudokobusine (**68**) and its synthetic analogs **68-1**~**68-37**.

Alkaloids	Cell Line/IC$_{50}$ (μM) [1]				KB/KB-VIN Ratio
	A549	DU145	KB	KB-VIN	
Pseudokobusine (**68**)	>20	>20	>20	>20	
68-1	>20	>20	>20	>20	
68-2	>20	>20	>20	>20	
68-3	>20	>20	>20	>20	
68-4	19.3 ± 4.5	15.3 ± 4.3	12.8 ± 1.7	10.2 ± 0.9	1.25
68-5	8.8 ± 4.5	7.6 ± 2.5	5.2 ± 1.3	6.3 ± 0.6	0.83
68-6	>20	>20	>20	>20	
68-7	15.4 ± 3.7	13.2 ± 2.0	11.1 ± 5.5	15.7 ± 1.5	0.70
68-8	>20	>20	>20	>20	
68-9	>20	>20	>20	>20	
68-10	8.0 ± 5.1	15.3 ± 2.9	14.9 ± 3.6	20.1 ± 13.5	0.74
15-Veratroylpseudokobusine (**68-11**)	>20	>20	>20	>20	
68-12	16.0 ± 5.5	16.9 ± 7.8	19.7 ± 3.1	14.7 ± 7.0	1.34
68-13	15.2 ± 6.4	16.6 ± 7.9	18.1 ± 4.3	12.2 ± 5.6	1.48
68-14	>20	>20	>20	>20	
68-15	5.8 ± 0.7	7.2 ± 1.9	6.4 ± 0.8	6.4 ± 1.8	1.00
68-16	>20	>20	>20	>20	
68-17	>20	>20	>20	>20	
68-18	>20	>20	>20	>20	
68-19	5.0 ± 1.1	5.2 ± 1.8	5.6 ± 1.2	5.6 ± 2.9	1.00
68-20	6.8 ± 0.7	7.7 ± 3.8	8.9 ± 3.7	6.2 ± 1.3	1.44
68-21	>20	>20	>20	>20	
68-22	17.9 ± 7.2	14.5 ± 7.2	15.7 ± 4.1	13.9 ± 3.3	1.13
68-23	>20	>20	>20	>20	
68-24	8.4 ± 1.7	6.5 ± 0.5	7.0 ± 1.3	6.4 ± 0.9	1.09
68-25	>20	>20	>20	>20	
68-26	>20	>20	>20	>20	
68-27	>20	>20	>20	>20	
68-28	>20	>20	>20	>20	
68-29	>20	>20	>20	>20	
68-30	>20	>20	>20	>20	
68-31	>20	>20	>20	>20	
68-32	6.4 ± 1.2	6.0 ± 3.3	6.6 ± 3.1	5.2 ± 1.0	1.27
68-33	>20	>20	>20	>20	
68-34	>20	>20	>20	>20	
68-35	>20	>20	>20	>20	
68-36	>20	>20	>20	>20	
68-37	>20	>20	>20	>20	
PXL[2] (nM)	4.8 ± 0.6	5.9 ± 1.9	5.8 ± 0.2	2405.4 ± 44.8	

[1] Values are means ± standard deviation; [2] Paclitaxel (PXL; nM) was used as an experimental control.

Among the analogs of **68**, four C-11 mono-substituted alkaloids (**68-15**, **68-20**, **68-24**, and **68-32**) and two C-11,15 di-esterified alkaloids (**68-5** and **68-19**) exhibited average IC$_{50}$ values of less than 10 μM. Certain C-11 (**68-7**, **68-10**, and **68-22**), C-6,11 (**68-4** and **68-12**) and C-6,15 (**68-13**) esterified alkaloids were generally less potent, while all C-6 (**68-3**, **68-6**, **68-14**, and **68-23**) and C-15 (**68-1**, **68-11**, **68-16**, **68-25**, **68-28**, and **68-30**) mono-substituted alkaloids, as well as the tri-substituted analog (**68-18**), were inactive. Thus, all more active (IC$_{50}$ < 10 μM) C_{20}-diterpenoid alkaloids in this classification had an ester or ether group on the C-11 hydroxy and were 11-monoester/11,15-diester analogs of **68** (OH at C-6).

The data in Table 6 led to noticeable observations about the degree and comparative ratio of KB/KB-VIN potency. Six alkaloids (**68-5**, **68-15**, **68-19**, **68-20**, **68-24**, and **68-32**) were quite potent (IC$_{50}$ < 10 μM) against KB-VIN. Indeed, alkaloid **68-32** exhibited a low IC$_{50}$ value of 5.2 μM. The ratios of KB to KB-VIN (IC$_{50}$ KB/IC$_{50}$ KB-VIN) were greater than 0.70 for all active alkaloids, with many alkaloids displaying comparable potency against the two cell lines, in contrast with paclitaxel (ratio of 0.0067).

Alkaloids **68-12**, **68-13**, and **68-20** showed over 1.3-fold selectivity with their greatest cytotoxic activity against KB-VIN (IC$_{50}$ KB/IC$_{50}$ KB-VIN: 1.34, 1.48, and 1.44, respectively).

In mechanism of action studies on selected diterpenoid alkaloids, the hetisine-type C$_{20}$-diterpenoid alkaloid derivatives **68-7** and **68-22** showed important suppressive effects against Raji cells. Further study indicated that **68-22** inhibited extracellular signal-regulated kinase phosphorylation but induced enhanced phosphoinositide 3 kinase phosphorylation, leading to accumulation of Raji cells in the G1 or sub G1 phase [20]. More investigation is certainly warranted.

4. Discussion

We have synthesized acylated derivatives of various C$_{19}$- and C$_{20}$-diterpenoid alkaloids. Totally, 199 natural alkaloids and their derivatives were evaluated against four to five human tumor cell lines. Among all alkaloids, 128 alkaloids were non-toxic (IC$_{50}$ > 20 or 40 µM) and 51 alkaloids showed moderate antiproliferative effects (average IC$_{50}$ = 10–40 µM). General summaries are described briefly below, and the most active compounds are shown in Figure 8.

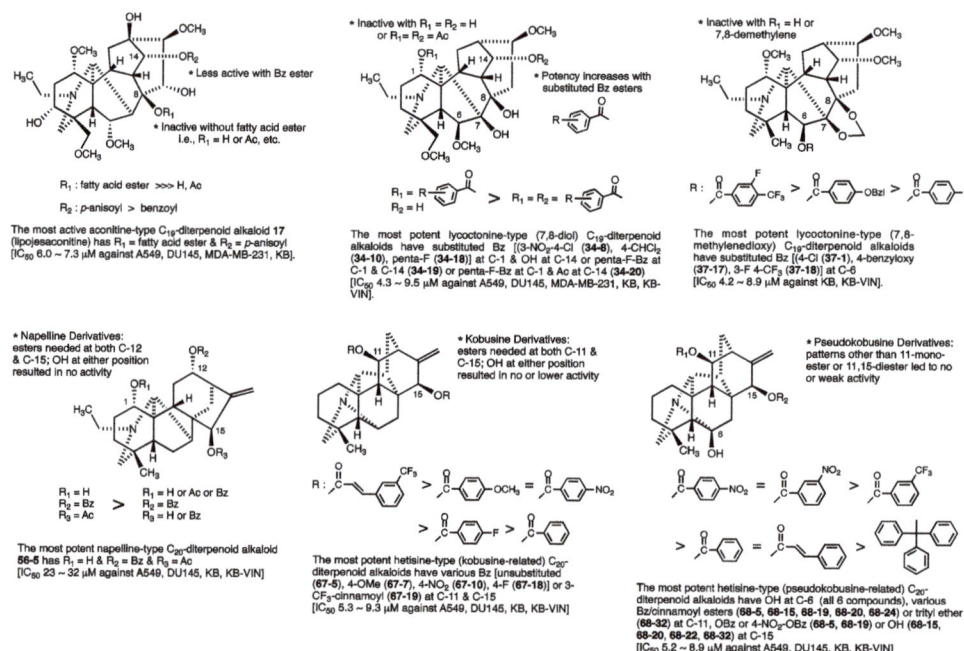

Figure 8. Most potent tested diterpenoid alkaloids & structure-activity correlations.

Among the aconitine-type C$_{19}$-diterpenoid alkaloids, the fatty acid ester at C-8 and the anisoyl group at C-14 found in **17** may be important to the cytotoxic activity. Compounds without the fatty acid ester at C-8 were inactive, and compounds with an unsubstituted benzoyl group at C-14 were less potent.

Among the C$_{19}$-diterpenoid alkaloids, the most active alkaloids were lycoctonine-type C$_{19}$-diterpenoid alkaloids with two different substitution patterns, C-1 (delcosine derivatives) and C-6 (delpheline derivatives). Delcosine derivatives **34-6**, **34-8**, **34-10**, and **34-18**, which are acylated at the C-1 hydroxy, as well as delpheline derivatives **37-1**, **37-17**, and **37-18**, which are acylated at the C-6 hydroxy, exhibited the greatest potency over all tested cell lines, including MDR KB-VIN.

Among the lycoctonine-type (7,8-diol) C$_{19}$-diterpenoid alkaloids, a C-1 acyloxy group and C-14 hydroxy group were important for improved antiproliferative activity. The C-1,14 diacylated delcosine derivatives were generally less potent than corresponding C-1 monoacylated delcosine derivatives. The 1-monoacylated alkaloids with the highest potency (IC$_{50}$ 4–6 µM) against five tested cell lines contained 3-nitro-4-chloro- (**34-8**) and pentafluoro- (**34-18**) as well as 4-dichloromethyl- (**34-10**) benzoyl esters. Two or one pentafluorinated benzoyl esters were also found in the two most consistently potent alkaloids (**34-19** and **34-20**) among the 1,14-diacyl and 1-acyl-14-acetyl derivatives.

Among the lycoctonine-type (7,8-methylenedioxy) C$_{19}$-diterpenoid alkaloids, none of the tested compound reached the potency levels of the most active 7,8-diol compounds. However, three 6-acylated delpheline derivatives **37-17~37-19** did show significant potency against the KB-VIN cell line (IC$_{50}$ 4.22, 4.40, and 4.71 µM, respectively). Interestingly, the two latter compounds contained fluorinated benzoyl esters. In addition, among 19 tested delpheline derivatives, four compounds (**37-12**, **37-16**, **37-13**, and **37-19**) showed over two-fold selectivity between the MDR and parental cell lines (ratio of IC$_{50}$ KB/IC$_{50}$ KB-VIN: 2.15, 2.28, 2.31, and 2.57, respectively).

None of the 15 tested actaline- and napelline-type C$_{20}$-diterpenoid alkaloids showed significant antiproliferative potency. Only 12-benzoyllucidsuculine (**56-5**) with C-1 hydroxy, C-12 acyloxy, and C-15 acetoxy groups showed even weak potency.

Among C$_{20}$-diterpenoid alkaloids, the most active alkaloids were hetisine-type C$_{20}$-diterpenoid alkaloids with two different substitution patterns, C-11,15 (kobusine) and C-6,11,15 (pseudo-kobusine). Hetisine-type C$_{20}$-diterpenoid alkaloids **67-5**, **67-7**, **67-10**, **67-18**, **67-19**, **68-5**, **68-15**, **68-19**, **68-20**, **68-25**, and **68-32**, which are acylated or tritylated at the C-11 hydroxyl, exhibited the greatest potency over all tested cell lines, including MDR KB-VIN. All five most active kobusine derivatives (**67-5**, **67-7**, **67-10**, **67-18**, and **67-19**) are acylated at both C-11 and C-15. All tested derivatives with a hydroxy group at either C-11 or C-15 were inactive or much less active. All six most active pseudo-kobusine derivatives (**68-5**, **68-15**, **68-19**, **68-20**, **68-25**, and **68-32**) contain a free hydroxy group at C-6. The substituent at C-11 is either a benzoyl/cinnamoyl ester (**68-5**, **68-15**, **68-19**, **68-20**, and **68-25**) or a trityl ether (**68-32**). Finally, the moiety at C-15 is a hydroxy group (**68-15**, **68-20**, **68-25**, and **68-32**) or benzoyl ester (**68-5**, **68-19**).

Furthermore, previously our study, Antitumor properties and radiation-sensitizing effects of various types of novel derivatives prepared from C$_{19}$- and C$_{20}$-diterpenoid alkaloids were also investigated [19]. Two novel hetisine-type C$_{20}$-diterpenoid derivatives (**68-7** and **68-20**) showed significant suppressive effects against the Raji non-Hodgkin's lymphoma cell line [20].

5. Conclusions

We have synthesized acylated derivatives of various C$_{19}$- and C$_{20}$-diterpenoid alkaloids. All alkaloids and their derivatives were screened against four to five human tumor cell lines. Alkaloids **37-2**, **37-9**, **37-17**, **37-18**, **56-5**, **67-7**, **67-14**, **67-19**, **68-4**, **68-12**, **68-20**, **68-22**, **68-24**, and **68-32** showed comparable potency against KB and KB-VIN cancer cell lines, and some alkaloids showed tumor-selective activity. Alkaloids **37-12**, **37-13**, **37-16**, and **37-19** exhibited greater inhibitory activity against drug-resistant KB-VIN cells (2.15~2.57-fold) than the parental KB cells. These results demonstrate that modified lycoctonine-type C$_{19}$-diterpenoid alkaloids and hetisine-type C$_{20}$-diterpenoid alkaloids are not substrates of P-gp and could be effective against P-gp overexpressing MDR tumors. These promising new lead alkaloids merit continued studies to evaluate their potential as antitumor agents, particularly with enhanced resistant tumor selectivity. In addition, our results from modification-based antitumor activity studies can be used for further development of anticancer drugs overcoming an MDR phenotype.

Funding: This study was supported in part by NIH grant CA177584 from the National Cancer Institute awarded to K.H.L. as well as the Eshelman Institute for Innovation, Chapel Hill, North Carolina, awarded to M.G.

Acknowledgments: The author gratefully acknowledges Lee, K.H., Goto, M., Morris-Natschke, S.L., Ohkoshi, E., Zhao, Yu., Li, K.P., Bastow, K.F., Natural Products Research Laboratories, UNC Eshelman School of Pharmacy, University of North Carolina at Chapel Hill; and Mizukami, M., Kaneda, K., Suzuki, Y., Shimizu, T., Kusanagi, N., Takeda, K., Haraguchi, M., Abe, Y., Kuwahara, N., Suzuki, S., Terui, A., Masaka, T., Munakata, N., Uchida, M., Nunokawa, M., Chiba, R., Kanazawa, R., Matsuoka, K., Suzuki, M., Ikuta, N., Asakawa, E., Tosho, Y., Nakata, A., Hasegawa, Y., Katoh, M., Kokubun, A., Uchimura, A., Mikami, S., Takeuchi, A., Department of Medicinal

Chemistry, Faculty of Pharmaceutical Sciences, Hokkaido University of Science, for their helpful advice and support throughout this work.

Conflicts of Interest: The authors declare no conflict of interest.

References

1. Dzubak, P.; Hajduch, M.; Vydra, D.; Hustova, A.; Kvasnica, M.; Biedermann, D.; Markova, L.; Urban, J.; Sarek, J. Pharmacological activities of natural triterpenoids and their therapeutic implications. *Nat. Prod. Rep.* **2006**, *23*, 394–411. [CrossRef]
2. Cragg, G.M.; Newman, D.J. Nature: A vital source of leads for anticancer drug development. *Phytochem. Rev.* **2009**, *8*, 313–331. [CrossRef]
3. Kingston, D.G. Tubulin-interactive natural products as anticancer agents. *J. Nat. Prod.* **2009**, *72*, 507–515. [CrossRef]
4. Lee, K.H. Discovery and development of natural products-derived chemotherapeutic agents based on a medicinal chemistry approach. *J. Nat. Prod.* **2010**, *73*, 500–516. [CrossRef]
5. Grothaus, P.G.; Cragg, G.M.; Newman, D.J. Plant natural products in anticancer drug discovery. *Curr. Org. Chem.* **2010**, *14*, 1781–1791. [CrossRef]
6. Kinghorn, A.D.; Pan, L.; Fletcher, J.N.; Chai, H. The relevance of higher plants in lead compound discovery programs. *J. Nat. Prod.* **2011**, *74*, 1539–1555. [CrossRef]
7. Dall'Acqua, S. Natural products as antimitotic agents. *Curr. Top. Med. Chem.* **2014**, *14*, 2272–2285. [CrossRef]
8. Hussain, M.; Khera, R.A.; Iqbal, J.; Khalid, M.; Hanif, M.A. Phytochemicals: Key to effective anticancer drugs. *Mini-Rev. Org. Chem.* **2019**, *16*, 141–158. [CrossRef]
9. Agarwal, G.; Carcache, P.J.B.; Addo, E.M.; Kinghorn, A.D. Current status and contemporary approaches to the discovery of antitumor agents from higher plants. *Biotechnol. Adv.* **2019**. [CrossRef]
10. Wang, F.P.; Chen, Q.H. The diterpenoid alkaloids. The Alkaloids: Chemistry and Biology; Cordell, G.A., Ed.; Academic Press: San Diego, CA, USA, 2010; Volume 69, pp. 1–577.
11. Wang, F.P.; Chen, Q.H.; Liu, X.Y. Diterpenoid alkaloids. *Nat. Prod. Rep.* **2010**, *27*, 529–570. [CrossRef]
12. Benn, M.H.; Jacyno, J.M. The toxicology and pharmacology of diterpenoid alkaloids. In *Alkaloids: Chemical and Biological Perspectives*; Pelletier, S.W., Ed.; Wiley-Interscience: New York, NY, USA, 1983; Volume 1, pp. 153–210.
13. Bock, J.H.; Norris, D.O. Introduction to forensic plant science. In *Forensic Plant Science*; Elsevier Academic Press: Boston, MA, USA, 2016; pp. 1–22.
14. Amiya, T.; Bando, H. Aconitum alkaloids. In *The Alkaloids*; Brossi, A., Ed.; Academic Press: San Diego, CA, USA, 1988.
15. Chan, T.Y.K. Aconite poisoning. *Clin. Toxicol.* **2009**, *47*, 279–285. [CrossRef]
16. Chan, T.Y.K. Aconite poisoning following the percutaneous absorption of *Aconitum* alkaloids. *Forensic Sci. Int.* **2012**, *223*, 25–27. [CrossRef]
17. Povšnar, M.; Koželj, G.; Kreft, S.; Lumpert, M. Rare tradition of the folk medicinal use of *Aconitum* spp. is kept alive in Solčavsko, Slovenia. *J. Ethnobiol. Ethnomed.* **2017**, *13*, 45. [CrossRef]
18. Wada, K.; Hazawa, M.; Takahashi, K.; Mori, T.; Kawahara, N.; Kashiwakura, I. Inhibitory effects of diterpenoid alkaloids on the growth of A172 human malignant cells. *J. Nat. Prod.* **2007**, *70*, 1854–1858. [CrossRef]
19. Hazawa, M.; Wada, K.; Takahashi, K.; Mori, T.; Kawahara, N.; Kashiwakura, I. Suppressive effects of novel derivatives prepared from *Aconitum* alkaloids on tumor growth. *Invest. New Drugs* **2009**, *27*, 111–119. [CrossRef]
20. Hazawa, M.; Wada, K.; Takahashi, K.; Mori, T.; Kawahara, N.; Kashiwakura, I. Structure-activity relationships between the *Aconitum* C_{20}-diterpenoid alkaloid derivatives and the growth suppressive activities of non-Hodgkin's lymphoma Raji cells and human hematopoietic stem/progenitor cells. *Invest. New Drugs* **2011**, *29*, 1–8. [CrossRef]
21. Wada, K.; Hazawa, M.; Takahashi, K.; Mori, T.; Kawahara, N.; Kashiwakura, I. Structure-activity relationships and the cytotoxic effects of novel diterpenoid alkaloid derivatives against A549 human lung carcinoma cells. *J. Nat. Med.* **2011**, *65*, 43–49. [CrossRef]
22. Bando, H.; Kanaiwa, Y.; Wada, K.; Mori, T.; Amiya, T. Structure of deoxyjesaconitine. A new diterpene alkaloid from *Aconitum subcuneatum* Nakai. *Heterocycles* **1981**, *16*, 1723–1725.

23. Mori, T.; Bando, H.; Kanaiwa, Y.; Wada, K.; Amiya, T. Studies on the constituents of *Aconitum* Species. II. Structure of deoxyjesaconitine. *Chem. Pharm. Bull.* **1983**, *31*, 2884–2886. [CrossRef]
24. Wada, K.; Bando, H.; Mori, T.; Wada, R.; Kanaiwa, Y.; Amiya, T. Studies on the constituents of *Aconitum* Species. III. On the components of *Aconitum subcuneatum* NAKAI. *Chem. Pharm. Bull.* **1985**, *33*, 3658–3661. [CrossRef]
25. Bando, H.; Wada, K.; Watanabe, M.; Mori, T.; Amiya, T. Studies on the constituents of *Aconitum* Species. IV. On the components of *Aconitum japonicum* THUNB. *Chem. Pharm. Bull.* **1985**, *33*, 4717–4722. [CrossRef]
26. Bando, H.; Wada, K.; Amiya, T.; Fujimoto, Y.; Kobayashi, K. Structures of secojesaconitine and subdesculine, two new diterpenoid alkaloids from *Aconitum japonicum* THUNB. *Chem. Pharm. Bull.* **1988**, *36*, 1604–1606. [CrossRef]
27. Yamashita, H.; Takeda, K.; Haraguchi, M.; Abe, Y.; Kuwahara, N.; Suzuki, S.; Terui, A.; Masaka, T.; Munakata, N.; Uchida, M.; et al. Four new diterpenoid alkaloids from *Aconitum japonicum* subsp. *subcuneatum*. *J. Nat. Med.* **2018**, *72*, 230–237. [CrossRef]
28. Yamashita, H.; Miyao, M.; Hiramori, K.; Kobayashi, D.; Suzuki, Y.; Mizukami, M.; Goto, M.; Lee, K.H.; Wada, K. Cytotoxic diterpenoid alkaloid from *Aconitum japonicum* subsp. *subcuneatum*. *J. Nat. Med.* **2019**, submitted.
29. Wada, K.; Bando, H.; Kawahara, N.; Mori, T.; Murayama, M. Determination and quantitative analysis of *Aconitum japonicum* by liquid chromatography atmospheric pressure chemical ionization mass spectrometry. *Biol. Mass Spectrom.* **1994**, *23*, 97–102. [CrossRef]
30. Wada, K.; Ohkoshi, E.; Zhao, Y.; Goto, M.; Morris-Natschke, S.L.; Lee, K.H. Evaluation of *Aconitum* diterpenoid alkaloids as antiproliferative agents. *Bioorg. Med. Chem. Lett.* **2015**, *25*, 1525–1531. [CrossRef]
31. Wada, K.; Bando, H.; Amiya, T. Two new C_{20}-diterpenoid alkaloids from *Aconitum yesoense* var. *macroyesoense* (NAKAI) TAMURA. Structures of dehydrolucidusculine and N-deethyldehydrolucidusculine. *Heterocycles* **1985**, *23*, 2473–2477.
32. Bando, H.; Wada, K.; Amiya, T.; Fujimoto, Y.; Kobayashi, K.; Sakurai, T. Studies on *Aconitum* Species. V. Constituents of *Aconitum yesoense* var. *macroyesoense* (NAKAI) TAMURA. *Heterocycles* **1987**, *26*, 2623–2637.
33. Wada, K.; Bando, H.; Kawahara, N. Studies on *Aconitum* species. XI. Two new diterpenoid alkaloids from *Aconitum yesoense* var. *macroyesoense* (NAKAI) TAMURA V. *Heterocycles* **1989**, *29*, 2141–2148.
34. Wada, K.; Kawahara, N. Diterpenoid and norditerpenoid alkaloids from the roots of *Aconitum yesoense* var. *macroyesoense*. *Helvetica Chimica Acta* **2009**, *92*, 629–637. [CrossRef]
35. Wada, K.; Yamamoto, T.; Bando, H.; Kawahara, N. Four diterpenoid alkaloids from *Delphinium elatum*. *Phytochemistry* **1992**, *31*, 2135–2138. [CrossRef]
36. Wada, K.; Ishizuki, S.; Mori, T.; Bando, H.; Murayama, M.; Kawahara, N. Effects of alkaloids from *Aconitum yesoense* var. *macroyesoense* on cutaneous blood flow in mice. *Biol. Pharm. Bull.* **1997**, *20*, 978–982.
37. Wada, K.; Mori, T.; Kawahara, N. Application of liquid chromatography–atmospheric pressure chemical ionization mass spectrometry to the differentiation of stereoisomeric C_{19}-norditerpenoid alkaloids. *Chem. Pharm. Bull.* **2000**, *48*, 660–668. [CrossRef]
38. Wada, K.; Goto, M.; Shimizu, T.; Kusanagi, N.; Lee, K.-H.; Yamashita, H. Structure-activity relationships and evaluation of esterified diterpenoid alkaloid derivatives as antiproliferative agents. *J. Nat. Med.* **2019**. [CrossRef]
39. Bando, H.; Wada, K.; Tanaka, J.; Kimura, S.; Hasegawa, E.; Amiya, T. Two new alkaloids from *Delphinium pacific giant* and revised ^{13}C-NMR assignment of delpheline. *Heterocycles* **1989**, *29*, 1293–1300. [CrossRef]
40. Wada, K.; Chiba, R.; Kanazawa, R.; Matsuoka, K.; Suzuki, M.; Ikuta, M.; Goto, M.; Yamashita, H.; Lee, K.H. Six new norditerpenoid alkaloids from *Delphinium elatum*. *Phytochem. Lett.* **2015**, *12*, 79–83. [CrossRef]
41. Wada, K.; Asakawa, E.; Tosho, Y.; Nakata, A.; Hasegawa, Y.; Kaneda, K.; Goto, M.; Yamashita, H.; Lee, K.H. Four new norditerpenoid alkaloids from *Delphinium elatum*. *Phytochem. Lett.* **2016**, *17*, 190–193. [CrossRef]
42. Yamashita, H.; Katoh, M.; Kokubun, A.; Uchimura, A.; Mikami, S.; Takeuchi, A.; Kaneda, K.; Suzuki, Y.; Mizukami, M.; Goto, M.; et al. Four new C_{19}-diterpenoid alkaloids from *Delphinium elatum*. *Phytochem. Lett.* **2018**, *24*, 6–9. [CrossRef]
43. Wada, K.; Ohkoshi, E.; Morris-Natschke, S.L.; Bastow, K.F.; Lee, K.H. Cytotoxic esterified diterpenoid alkaloid derivatives with increased selectivity against a drug-resistant cancer cell line. *Bioorg. Med. Chem. Lett.* **2012**, *22*, 249–252. [CrossRef]

44. Wang, F.P.; Liang, X.T. C$_{20}$-Diterpenoid alkaloids. In *The Alkaloids: Chemistry and Biology*; Cordell, G.A., Ed.; Academic Press: San Diego, CA, USA, 2002; Volume 59, pp. 1–280.
45. Wada, K.; Mori, T.; Kawahara, N. Application of liquid chromatography-atmospheric pressure chemical ionization mass spectrometry to the differentiation of stereoisomeric diterpenoid alkaloids. *Chem. Pharm. Bull.* **2000**, *48*, 1065–1074. [CrossRef]
46. Wada, K.; Ishizuki, S.; Mori, T.; Fujihira, E.; Kawahara, N. Effects of *Aconitum* alkaloid kobusine and pseudokobusine derivatives on cutaneous blood flow in mice. *Biol. Pharm. Bull.* **1998**, *21*, 140–146. [CrossRef] [PubMed]
47. Wada, K.; Ishizuki, S.; Mori, T.; Fujihira, E.; Kawahara, N. Effects of *Aconitum* alkaloid kobusine and pseudokobusine derivatives on cutaneous blood flow in mice; II. *Biol. Pharm. Bull.* **2000**, *23*, 607–615. [CrossRef] [PubMed]
48. Wada, K.; Bando, H.; Kawahara, N. Studies on *Aconitum* Species. XIII. Two new diterpenoid alkaloids from *Aconitum yesoense* var. *macroyesoense* (NAKAI) TAMURA VI. *Heterocycles* **1990**, *31*, 1081–1088. [CrossRef]
49. Wada, K.; Bando, H.; Wada, R.; Amiya, T. Analgesic activity of main components from *Aconitum yesoense* var. *macroyesoense* (NAKAI) TAMURA and pseudokobusine derivatives. *Shouyakugaku Zasshi* **1989**, *43*, 50–54.

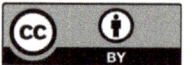

© 2019 by the authors. Licensee MDPI, Basel, Switzerland. This article is an open access article distributed under the terms and conditions of the Creative Commons Attribution (CC BY) license (http://creativecommons.org/licenses/by/4.0/).

MDPI
St. Alban-Anlage 66
4052 Basel
Switzerland
Tel. +41 61 683 77 34
Fax +41 61 302 89 18
www.mdpi.com

Molecules Editorial Office
E-mail: molecules@mdpi.com
www.mdpi.com/journal/molecules

www.ingramcontent.com/pod-product-compliance
Lightning Source LLC
LaVergne TN
LVHW070219100526
838202LV00015B/2063